Atlas of

Orthopedic
Pathology

with Clinical and Radiologic Correlations

2nd edition

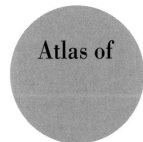

Atlas of Orthopedic Pathology

with Clinical and Radiologic Correlations

2nd edition

Peter G. Bullough, M.B., Ch.B.

Director of Laboratory Medicine
Hospital for Special Surgery

Professor of Pathology
Cornell University Medical College
New York

Forewords by

Lauren V. Ackerman, M.D.

Professor of Surgical Pathology and Pathology
State University of New York at Stony Brook
New York

Philip D. Wilson Jr., M.D.

Professor of Surgery (Orthopedics)
Cornell University Medical College

Surgeon-in-Chief Emeritus
Hospital for Special Surgery
New York

Gower Medical Publishing
New York · London

Distributed in the USA and Canada by:

J B Lippincott Company
East Washington Square
Philadelphia, PA 19105
USA

Distributed in the UK and Continental Europe by:

Gower Medical Publishing
Middlesex House
34-42 Cleveland Street
London W1P 5FB

Distributed in Australia and New Zealand by:

HarperEducational (Australia) Pty Ltd.
P.O. Box 226
Artarmon
NSW 2064
Australia

Distributed in Southeast Asia, Hong Kong, India and Pakistan by:

APAC Publishers Services
30 Jalan Bahasa
Singapore 1129

Distributed in Japan by:

Nankodo Co. Ltd.
42-6 Hongo 3-chome
Bunkyo-ku
Tokyo 113
Japan

Distributed in South America by:

Harper Collins Publishers Latin America
701 Brickell Avenue - Suite 1750
Miami, FL 33131
USA

Editors: Jane Hunter, Sharon Rule
Art Director: Jill Feltham
Designer: Surachara Wirojratana
Illustrators: Sue Ann Fung Ho, Margaret Marino, Patricia Gast

Library of Congress Cataloging-in-Publication Data

Bullough, Peter G., 1932–
    Atlas of orthopedic pathology : with clinical and radiologic correlations / Peter G. Bullough ; forewords by Lauren V. Ackerman, Philip D. Wilson, Jr. — 2nd ed.
        p.   cm.
    Includes bibliographical references and index.
    ISBN 0-397-44621-7
    1. Bones—Diseases—Atlases.   2. Joints—Diseases—Atlases
I. Title. II. Title: Orthopedic pathology.
    [DNLM: 1. Bone and Bones—radiography—atlases.   2. Bone Diseases––pathology—atlases.   3. Joint Diseases—pathology—atlases.
4. Joints—radiography—atlases.   5. Muscles—radiography—atlases.
6. Muscular Diseases—pathology—atlases.   WE 17 B938a]
RC930.4.B84   1991
616.7'1—dc20
DNLM/DLC

British Library Cataloguing in Publication Data

Bullough, Peter G.
    Atlas of orthopedic pathology with clinical and radiologic correlations. – 2nd ed.
    I. Title
    616.7

    ISBN 1-397-44621-7

Printed in Singapore by ImagoProductions (PE) Pte Ltd.

10   9   8   7   6   5   4   3   2   1

D E D I C A T I O N

**To the memory of my
Mother and Father,**

*And many more, whose names on
Earth are dark,
But whose transmitted effluence can
not die,
So long as fire outlives the
parent spark.*

—Percy Bysshe Shelley

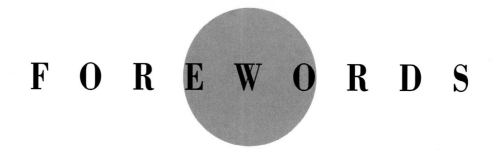

F O R E W O R D S

This book was first published in 1984, and it is now time for a new edition. The present volume has been completely revised, its contents rearranged, and the text expanded by a third, with five new chapters. There are 350 additional illustrations.

This is an elegant book. Textbooks are often marked by complicated prose, poor grammar, and faulty syntax. The present volume is a wonderful exception, a pleasure to read, for each sentence has been constructed with care and each sentence adds information that is directly relevant to the subject. The text is not cluttered with references and numbers but at the end of the book there is a carefully selected current set of references corresponding to each section. This appendix will serve readers interested in expanding their knowledge without being obliged to decide among 300 references on a given subject.

Although the title indicates an atlas, this book goes far beyond that category, including an extensive discourse on arthritis, and other areas such as metabolic bone disease and rare entities. To substitute adequately for Bullough's work one would have to buy a book on metabolic bone disease, another on arthritis, and a third on neoplasms. The thorough presentation of arthritis is alone worth the price of the book.

Another unique feature of the text is the presence of line drawings accompanying illustrations such as gross photographs, photomicrographs, x-rays, and electron microscopy. Each of these illustrations was chosen to provide a visual representation of a particular bit of information.

Although the book has been discovered by orthopedic surgeons, pathologists have not as yet realized its value, since many pathologists are afraid to look at a piece of bone. This book will soothe their fears and open up an area of knowledge in which many are deficient. It has been a rewarding pleasure for me to read the new edition and I recommend it to you with the greatest confidence.

Lauren V. Ackerman, M.D.
Professor of Pathology
State University of New York at Stony Brook
Stony Brook, New York

This new edition of Peter Bullough's *Atlas of Orthopedic Pathology* has been entirely reorganized, updated, and enlarged into 19 chapters. Along with new information, most of the previous text has been rewritten. As with the first edition, a correlated slide atlas is available and extends the suitability of the material's use for study, lectures, and seminars.

The illustrations are superb, the supporting text and legends comprehensive, clear, and concise. Specific points in the photographs are highlighted and clarified by accompanying line drawings. The resulting presentation is not only informative but beautiful to behold. To review the book's pages is a pleasing experience.

In the seven years since the first edition, there have been many advances in orthopedic and rheumatologic knowledge and understanding, and new data and practices have been worked into the second edition. The material is sensibly organized into six major sections: *Normal*, which includes structure and examination methods; *Response to Exogenous Injury*, including infections; *Metabolic Disturbances*, which includes congenital and developmental chondro-osseous dystrophies, "aging" conditions of bone, mineral metabolic and endocrine changes, marrow storage diseases, and hematologic disorders; *Arthritis*, with special chapters on spondyloarthropathies and tissue responses to implanted material; *Tumors*, with four separate chapters; and *Common but Unexciting Orthopedic Conditions* in two chapters.

The clinical significance and applications of the pathologic information are highlighted, making this an essential text for all orthopedists, rheumatologists, and radiologists as well as pathologists, whether generalist or specialist oriented. Also, all those who want to acquire or maintain a broad knowledge base in musculoskeletal pathology and its clinical correlations will find this book to be an important resource. It is useful, therefore, to student and teacher alike. At this point in time when maintenance of competence through continuing education is being emphasized, and even demanded, I cannot think of a better method for doing so than by a thorough study of this atlas.

Dr. Bullough is to be complimented for his exhaustive labor in revising and expanding this edition, which reaffirms the atlas's position as a masterpiece in the field of orthopedic literature. Gower is to be thanked for making the resulting volume available to us in such a beautiful form.

Philip D. Wilson Jr., M.D.
Professor of Surgery (Orthopedics)
Cornell University Medical College
and
Surgeon-in-Chief Emeritus
The Hospital for Special Surgery

PREFACE

Musculoskeletal conditions are the third most frequent cause of acute disease resulting in a visit to a doctor, the fifth most frequent cause of hospitalization, and the third most frequent cause of surgery. They impact principally on the quality of life, with the elderly suffering the most, usually from arthritis and osteoporosis. Unfortunately, medical school curricula and most pathology training programs assign disproportionately little time for the study of bones and joints. At autopsy, attention is given to the study of parenchymal organs, rather than to the study of bones and joints. A great deal of pathology is being overlooked as a result.

From Virchow's time to the present, there have been students for whom musculoskeletal diseases have held a particular interest, and a few excellent texts have been written on the pathology of bones and joints. When this book was first published in 1984, the intention was to provide a concise, yet lavishly illustrated and comprehensive, account of the pathology of musculoskeletal diseases. In the process, we hoped to stimulate interest and enthusiasm for this important branch of pathology.

In this new edition, the text has been completely revised and is now 50% longer. Five new chapters have been added as well as 363 new figures. However, the object remains the same, to provide an up-to-date and concise account of bone and joint disease.

This book has been written for the use of busy practicing surgical pathologists as well as for orthopedic surgeons who would like to better understand their subject. Radiologists having a special interest in skeletal radiology will also find this book helpful. For orthopedic surgeons and radiologists, chapters on normal bone and on histologic preparation of bone have been included, as has a chapter describing the histologic processes involved in injury and repair in general, and of the connective tissues in particular. These chapters provide background information for the pathologic descriptions that follow.

The clinician visualizes the morbid anatomic changes associated with disease by various imaging techniques, which figure extensively throughout the book. Line drawings are used liberally to indicate specific features in a photograph. Where the three-dimensional and/or temporal aspects of structure must be communicated, color schematic and anatomic drawings are provided.

The bibliography is arranged by chapter, and then further divided by condition. The references per condition have been chosen to best amplify the presentations in this book and to provide further access to the literature.

Most of the gross photographs and photomicrographs used were taken over the many years of my professional life: first, as a fellow at the Hospital for Joint Diseases in New York; next, as a lecturer in orthopedics at the Nuffield Orthopaedic Center in Oxford, England; and finally, over the past 22 years, as a pathologist at The Hospital for Special Surgery in New York. Most of the clinical radiographs are from the radiology department at The Hospital for Special Surgery and are used with the kind permission of Dr. Robert Freiberger and Dr. Jeremy Kaye. Additional illustrations have been generously contributed by numerous colleagues throughout the world, to whom I am extremely grateful.

Our interest and understanding depends upon our teachers and upon our students, but perhaps even more importantly upon our colleagues, and I feel myself extremely fortunate in having had so many stimulating and helpful colleagues. I am most particularly grateful to the members of the New York Bone Club, who have met together once a month for the past 12 years and have shared their experience and their knowledge. From this exceptional group I have learned more of my profession than from any other source.

In the preparation of the first edition of this book, I was fortunate to have the assistance of Dr. Vincent Vigorita who had just completed his fellowship at Memorial Hospital before joining our staff as assistant pathologist. For this edition, I have had the invaluable help of Dr. Rafael Castro, who has been with the pathology department for the last two years. Through his organizational skills he managed the logistics of cataloging illustrations, checking the references, tracking down radiographs, and many, many other tasks which are entailed in such a project as this. I am extremely grateful to him for all his help and support.

I am also indebted to the staff of the pathology department at The Hospital for Special Surgery—both past and present—for their excellent work in this and other projects over the years. Finally, I thank the staff of Gower Medical Publishing for the care that went into the preparation of this book: to Sharon Rule and Jane Hunter for their editing, to Surachara Wirojratana for her satisfying design, and to Abe Krieger for his keen interest and unflagging support throughout.

Peter G. Bullough

CONTENTS

SECTION VI   COMMON BUT UNEXCITING
ORTHOPEDIC CONDITIONS

S E C T I O N I

NORMAL

The explanation of disease, *pathology*, from the Greek Παθος (suffering, disease) and λογος (reason, discourse), has always been central to the practice of medicine. In Western medicine throughout the nineteenth and twentieth centuries, the explanation of disease has been based on the scientific observation of departure from normal anatomy to morbid anatomy (Morgagni 1761), from normal tissue (histology) to disturbed tissue (Bichat 1800), from normal cell structure to abnormal cell structure (Virchow 1858), and at each of these levels from normal function (physiology) to abnormal function (pathophysiology).

Acute disease, a subjective state, is the result of acute malfunction, malfunction being in general the consequence of mechanical trauma, infection or metabolic injury. In any tissue, acute disease may become chronic either as the result of continuing injury, or as the consequence of ineffective or imperfect repair.

In the connective tissues, acute injury may lead to profound and immediate malfunction. Fracture of bone and rupture of a ligament are examples. In the connective tissues in particular, the processes of repair will restore normal function only if they first restore the normal anatomy.

The recognition of normal anatomy, normal histology, and normal cytology, together with an understanding of function at each of these levels, is thus essential to the recognition and understanding of disease processes.

CHAPTER 1

Normal bone structure and development

The microscopic examination of bone dates back to the earliest days of microscopy. In 1674, Anton van Leeuwenhoek read a letter to the Royal Society on the topic; soon afterwards, in 1691, Clopton Havers published his *Osteologia Nova*, in which he described the pores in the cortical bone to which we now refer as haversian canals. Since then, major contributions to the study of bone anatomy and histology have been made by many of the most famous names in pathology and medicine. To name but a few, Cheselden, in 1733, wrote the *Osteographia*, which contained full and accurate descriptions of all human bones gained with the use of the camera obscura; the beautiful and accurate work of Albinus on bone and muscle, in 1754, established a new standard in anatomical illustrations; the experiments of Haller in 1763 contributed greatly to the understanding of bone formation; Hunter, in 1772, did much to elucidate the mechanism of bone growth, particularly the appositional mechanism rather than that of interstitial growth such as occurs in other organ systems; Winslow's *Anatomical Exposition*, in 1776, systematized the approach to bone anatomy; Bichat, in the early 1800s, stressed the importance of the tissue elements shared among the different organ systems (hence histology) and, in particular, described the synovial membrane; and Virchow, in the latter half of the nineteenth century, wrote classic descriptions of several bone tumors and metabolic disturbances.

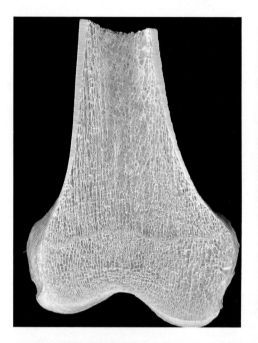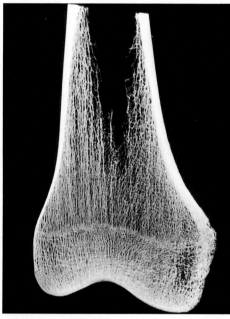

FIGURE 1.1 Cleaned and macerated specimen of lower femur demonstrates the distribution of cancellous bone and the thickening of the cortex approaching the diaphysis *(left)*. Radiograph of the same specimen *(right)*. Note the horizontal plate of bone which marks the site of the previous cartilage growth plate (the "epiphyseal scar").

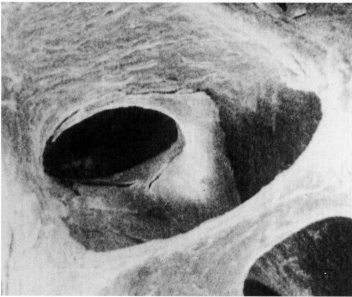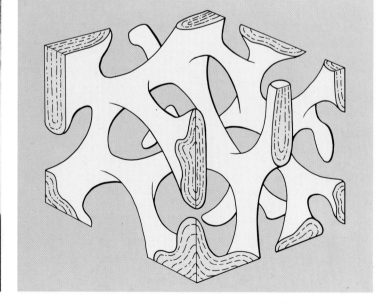

FIGURE 1.2 *(left)* Scanning electron micrograph (x 400), and *(right)* schematic representation, of the plates and rods of bone in the cancellous bone.

Bone, cartilage, ligaments, and tendons have a primarily mechanical function: they provide movement, support, and protection. Unlike the parenchymal organs, eg, the liver or kidneys, which are composed mainly of cellular elements with a metabolic function, the connective tissues are formed mostly of an extracellular material (or matrix) made up of substances (both fibrous materials and packing materials) well-suited for the mechanical functions of those tissues.

THE BONES

GROSS STRUCTURE AND FUNCTION

Each bone has a limiting surface shell known as the cortex. Enclosed by the cortical shell are plates and rods of bone tissue known as the spongy, cancellous, or trabecular bone (Figs. 1.1 and 1.2).

Cortex thickness varies considerably, both within a single bone and among different bones. For example, in normal vertebral bodies the cortex is very thin, whereas in long bones, such as the femur and the tibia, the cortex in the mid-diaphysis may reach more than a quarter inch in thickness. Even in the long bones, however, there is great variation in thickness between the ends of the bone (in which the cortex is thin) and the midshaft of the bone (in which the cortex is thick).

A moment's reflection will make the reason for these differences obvious. The thick cortical bone is well constructed to resist bending, and it is in the middle of the long bones that this force occurs. In contrast, the cancellous or trabecular bone is concentrated where compressive forces predominate, ie, in the vertebral bodies and in the expanded ends of long bones. Thus, the architecture of the bone reflects its function. This concept of an organized distribution of structural elements is summarized in Wolff's law, which can be simply stated as: "Every change in the function of a bone is followed by certain definite changes in internal architecture and external conformation in accordance with mathematical laws" (Fig. 1.3).

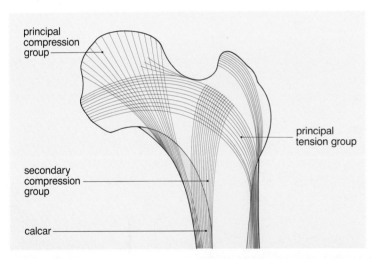

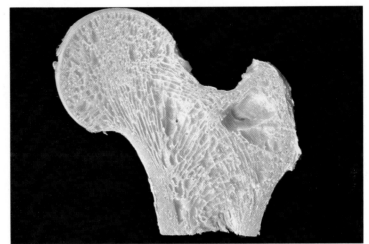

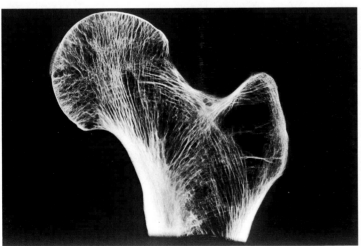

FIGURE 1.3 *(upper left)* Wolff's law is well demonstrated in the head and neck of the femur, in which the bone trabeculae radiate from the articular surface down onto the medial cortex of the femoral neck (the calcar), which is much thicker than the cortex on the lateral side of the femoral neck. *(upper right)* In this slice through the upper end of the femur, the marrow fat has been washed out of the specimen to better demonstrate the distribution of the cancellous bone. *(lower left)* The best way to demonstrate the arrangement of the bone trabeculae is by radiographs of the specimen.

As we shall see shortly, the arrangement of the elements of the extracellular matrix, both in the bone itself and in all other connective tissues—eg, cartilage, tendon, meniscus, intervertebral disc—is also no less precisely organized for its mechanical function.

The bones are often compartmentalized by the morphologist into three indistinct zones: the bone end or epiphysis—the region above the growth plate (or, in adults, the zone above the closed growth plate); the metaphysis—the region immediately below the growth plate (in the growing animal, the area of growth and most active modeling); and the diaphysis—the region between the metaphyses (ie, the shaft of the long bones). The terms epiphysis, metaphysis, and diaphysis are useful in the description of disease, because many diseases have predilections for one or another of these compartments (Fig. 1.4).

Periosteum

Except at the musculotendinous insertions and at their articular ends, the bones are covered by a thin but tough fibrous membrane, the periosteum. At the articular margins and tendinous insertions the periosteum blends imperceptibly with the surface fibers of those tissues.

The periosteum is attached to the surface of the bone cortex by collagen fibers (the fibers of Sharpey) which are direct continuations of periosteal fibers. Where these fibers enter the bone they are encrusted with hydroxyapatite, which cements them into the bone (Fig. 1.5). Therefore, any attempt at separation of the periosteum from the bone requires physical tearing of these fibers.

On microscopic examination, the periosteum is seen to have two layers: an outer fibrous layer and an inner cambium layer, which forms bone. In children the cambium layer provides for the increasing diameter of the bone with growth (Fig. 1.6). In adults, the bone-forming potential of the periosteum is reactivated by trauma and infection, and in association with some tumors. In children, the periosteum is only loosely attached to the underlying bone, whereas in adults it is firmly attached. Thus the clinical extent of periosteal reaction, which in similar conditions is much greater in children than in adults (Fig. 1.7).

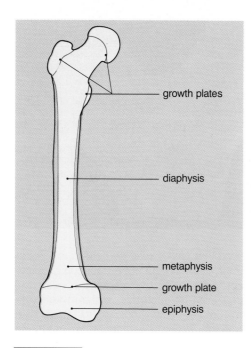

growth plates

diaphysis

metaphysis

growth plate

epiphysis

FIGURE 1.4 Bone compartments in the femur.

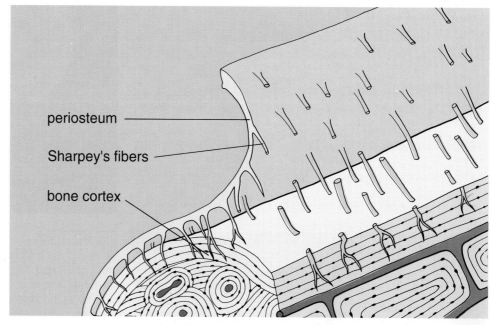

periosteum

Sharpey's fibers

bone cortex

FIGURE 1.5 The fibers of Sharpey are direct continuations of periosteal fibers extending into the bone cortex.

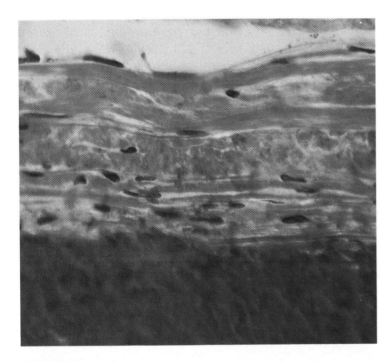
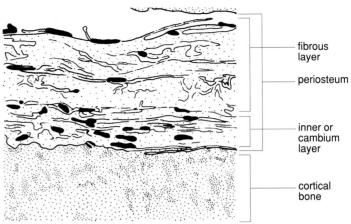

fibrous layer

periosteum

inner or cambium layer

cortical bone

FIGURE 1.6 Photomicrograph of the periosteum and underlying cortical bone. Note the double layer, of which the inner or cambium layer is more active in producing bone (H & E, x 25 obj.).

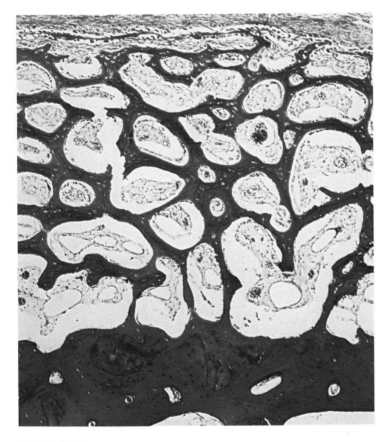
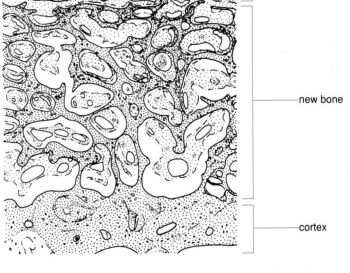

periosteum

new bone

cortex

FIGURE 1.7 Photomicrograph of periosteal new bone layer produced by the cambium of the periosteum after trauma in a child (H & E, x 4 obj.).

Blood Supply

Many capillaries enter the bone through the periosteum. This periosteal blood supply augments the principal nutrient arteries, which enter the medullary cavity by penetrating the cortex (usually at about the middle of the diaphysis), and the epiphyseal and metaphyseal vessels at the ends of the bone (Figs. 1.8 and 1.9).

THE MATRIX

A knowledge of the matrix components is essential to the understanding of connective tissue diseases. Collagen fibers, the principal extracellular components of connective tissues, are made up of bundles of fibrils which, in turn, are composed of stacked molecules formed from polypeptide chains arranged in a helical pattern (Fig. 1.10). Collagen is well suited to resist pulling and is the principal component of the tendon matrix: however, it does not resist bending or compression, and because the matrices of both bone and cartilage are subjected to these latter types of forces, they contain stiffening substances in addition to collagen.

In bone, the stiffening substance takes the form of crystals of calcium phosphate (hydroxyapatite: $Ca_{10}(PO_4)_6(OH)_2$) (Fig. 1.11). The crystals are too small to be seen by light microscopy but can be visualized by electron microscopy in mineralized tissue. They are approximately 2 x 9 x 25 nm in size. The hydroxyapatite provides strength in compression, although, as would be expected, it is weak in tension.

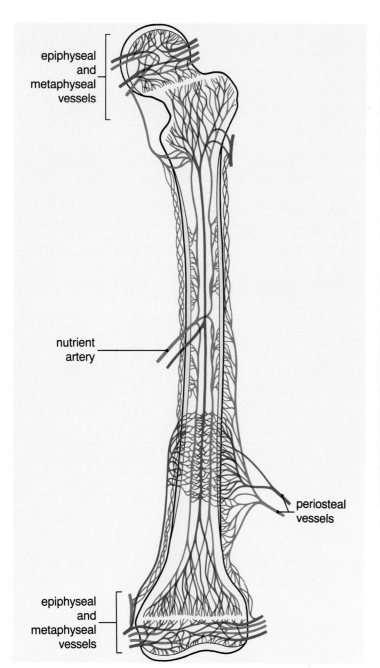

epiphyseal
and
metaphyseal
vessels

nutrient
artery

periosteal
vessels

epiphyseal
and
metaphyseal
vessels

FIGURE 1.8 Diagram of blood supply to the bone.

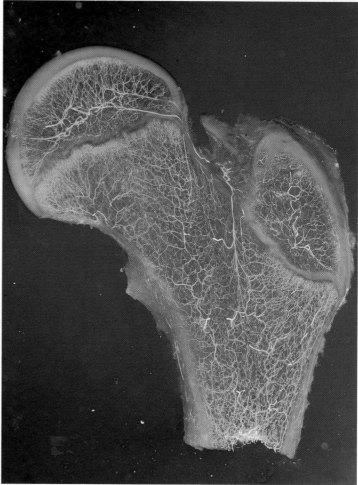

FIGURE 1.9 Coronal section of femur showing blood supply. Note separate vascular supply to diaphysis, femoral epiphysis and trochanteric apophysis. (Courtesy of H.V. Crock)

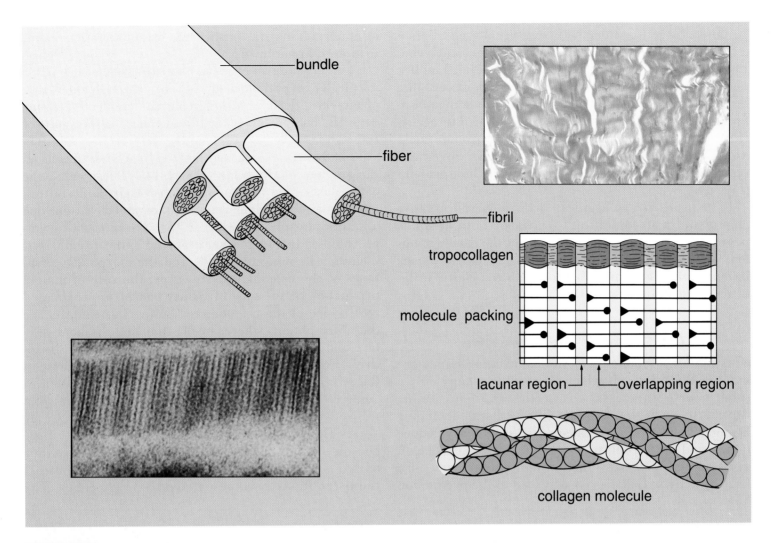

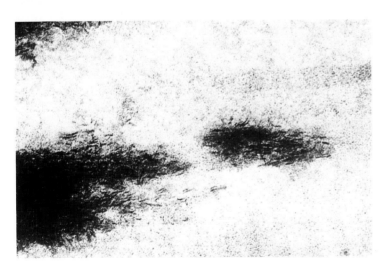

FIGURE 1.10 In histologic section stained with H & E, the wavy homogeneous strands of pink material represent bundles of collagen fibers. The collagen molecule is a triple helix formed of polypeptide chains, which in turn are formed of repeating tripeptide sequences of glycine-x-y-glycine-x-y, etc., in which x and y are frequently proline and hydroxyproline. Visualized by transmission electron microscopy the individual collagen fibrils are seen to have two orders of banding. As can be seen from the drawing, the larger bands result from the gaps between the individual molecules of collagen, which then overlap the adjacent molecules.

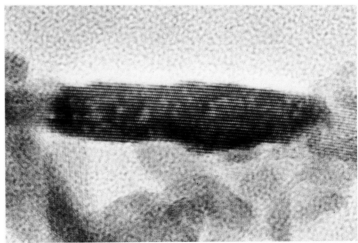

FIGURE 1.11 Electron micrographs of bone mineral crystals: at a magnification factor of x 101,500 *(left)* the crystal structure can be clearly seen. At higher magnification, x 2,110,000 *(right)*, the lattice formation of the crystals can be appreciated. (The various stains for demonstrating calcium salts in undecalcified sections are described in Chapter 2.)

In cartilage, the filler between the collagen fibers is a large negatively charged molecule of proteoglycan. Proteoglycan has a molecular weight of several million and a spatial configuration somewhat reminiscent of a test tube brush. The proteoglycan macromolecule is formed from long chains of repeating sulfated disaccharides, which are covalently linked to a protein backbone. Large numbers of these protein cores are attached to a hyaluronic acid molecule by link proteins (Fig. 1.12).

The proteoglycan aggregate has an overall negative charge and a strong affinity for water, both of which provide for a swelling pressure within the cartilaginous matrices, which maintains the collagenous framework in tension and is responsible for the visco-elastic properties of the tissue (Fig. 1.13).

Cell Synthesis and Breakdown

The matrix components of the connective tissues are manufactured by cells which themselves occupy only a small volume of the tissues. Nevertheless, these cells, ie, fibroblasts (cells that produce fibrous tissue, including ligaments and tendons), osteoblasts (cells that produce bone), and chondroblasts (cells that produce cartilage), are essential to the production and maintenance of a healthy matrix. Cell disease may lead to the production of abnormal matrix constituents or, on the other hand, to altered breakdown.

The breakdown of matrix constituents, either physiologically or pathologically, occurs through the action of enzymes derived either from the connective tissue cells themselves or from blood-borne inflammatory cells.

The bone matrix is synthesized by a layer of cells on the surface of the bone (Fig. 1.14). These cells, the osteoblasts, are mesenchymal in origin and contain abundant endoplasmic reticulum, as well as the enzyme alkaline phosphatase (Fig. 1.15). There is an incomplete correlation between actual bone formation, including its mineralization, and the morphologic features of the osteoblasts. However, the rate of matrix production at the time of biopsy can be approximated by the size of the osteoblasts. "Active" osteoblasts are therefore plump, whereas cells that line the bone surface and are flat can be considered quiescent or "inactive" (Fig. 1.16). Because there is a gradual increase in the size of bone-forming cells, the point at which an "inactive" cell becomes an "active" cell is necessarily a subjective determination.

As the osteoblasts produce bone matrix, they become surrounded by the matrix formed and are thus buried within the surface of the bone. By this process the osteoblasts become osteocytes (Fig. 1.17). The

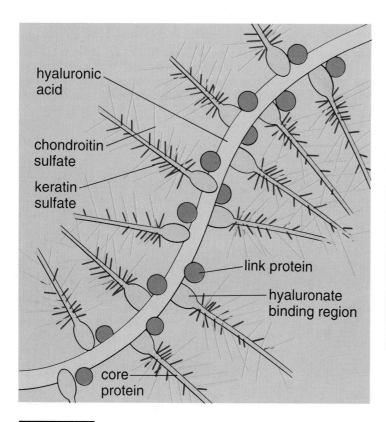

FIGURE 1.12 Schematic drawing of the proteoglycan macromolecule. The proteoglycan in histologic sections can be stained by various techniques, including safranin O, alcian blue, and toluidine blue.

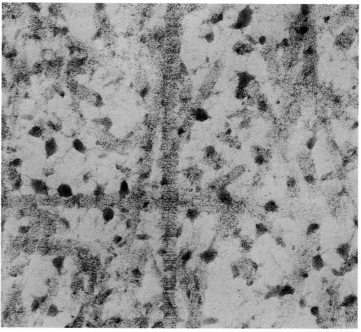

FIGURE 1.13 Electron microscopic examination of cartilage demonstrates amorphous electron-dense deposits of proteoglycan between collagen fibers (x 102,900).

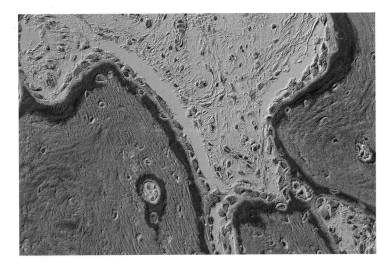

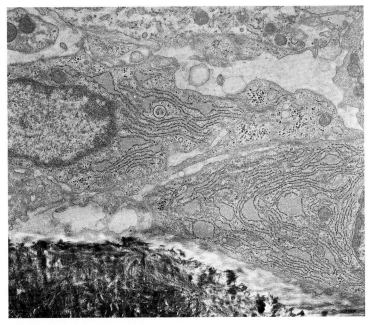

FIGURE 1.14 Photomicrograph showing a layer of active, plump osteoblasts at the bone surface. The layer of red-stained tissue beneath the osteoblastic layer represents unmineralized matrix or osteoid, (Goldner Stain, x 10 obj.).

osteoblasts

rough endoplas-
mic reticulum

unmineralized
bone matrix

mineralized
bone matrix

FIGURE 1.15 Electron photomicrograph shows a portion of two osteoblasts. The cytoplasm is rich in rough endoplasmic reticulum. Underlying the cell is a layer of nonmineralized collagenous matrix (osteoid), which in light microscope sections is seen as a smooth pink layer on the bone surface. Directly under the osteoid seam is a thin layer of mineralized bone (x 10,000).

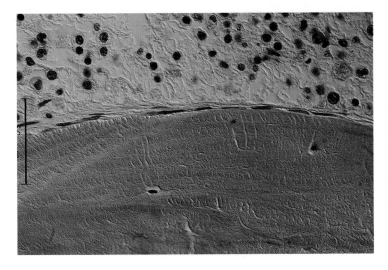

FIGURE 1.16 Photomicrograph shows a layer of inactive flat osteoblasts at the bone surface (H & E, x 10 obj.).

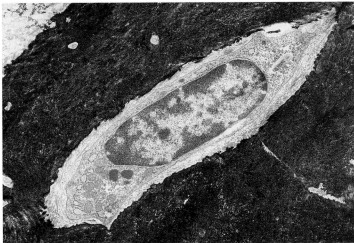

FIGURE 1.17 Electron micrograph of an osteocyte. In the upper left-hand corner is a portion of the bone surface. Within the mineralized matrix, cross-sections of several osteocytic canaliculi and osteocytic processes can be seen (x 10,000).

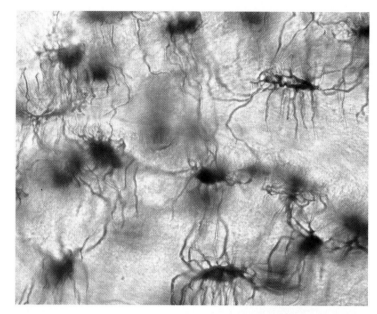

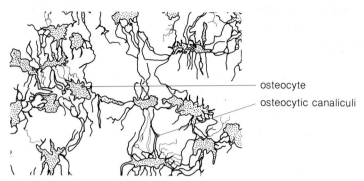

FIGURE 1.18 Photomicrograph of osteocytes and osteocytic canaliculi seen by transmitted light in ground bone section (x 10 obj.).

— osteocyte
— osteocytic canaliculi

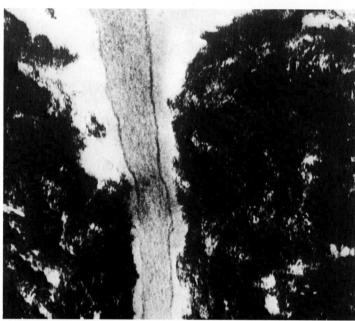

FIGURE 1.19 Electron photomicrograph of a portion of an osteocytic process in an osteocytic canaliculus in mineralized bone (x 50,000).

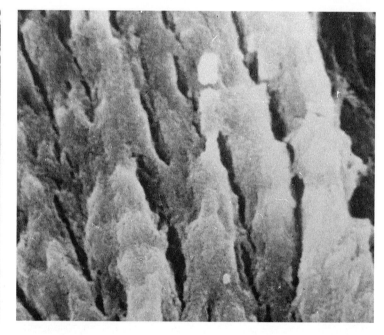

FIGURE 1.20 Scanning electron micrograph of the bone surface shows the opening of the canaliculi only onto the surface (x 8000).

FIGURE 1.21 Photomicrograph of a section of undecalcified bone shows a prominent layer of active osteoblasts lying on an osteoid seam, with underlying mineralized bone. The calcification front is seen as a deeply staining basophilic line (H & E, x 25 obj.).

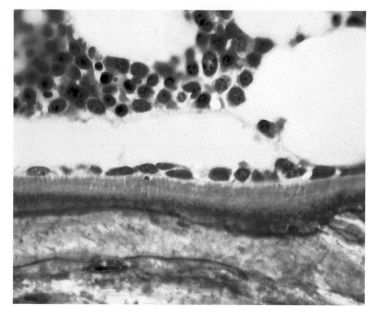

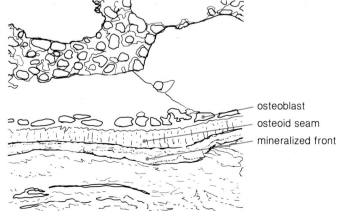

— osteoblast
— osteoid seam
— mineralized front

osteocytes communicate with each other and with the osteoblasts on the surface of the bone by a series of connecting cell processes which run through canals permeating the bone tissue (Figs. 1.18–1.20). These canals are called the osteocytic canaliculi. The syncytium of osteocytes that permeate the bone probably plays an important role in physiologic calcium homeostasis, and may also act as a sensing device to regulate skeletal homeostasis in accordance with Wolff's law. Note that the osteocytic canaliculi do not cross the cement lines (see Fig. 1.29 for description of cement lines).

Associated with the cells that are actively forming bone matrix, a thin layer of nonmineralized bone matrix (osteoid), normally approximately 10 μm thick, can be seen underlying the cellular layer (Fig. 1.21). The time between the deposition and subsequent mineralization of the matrix, called the "mineralization lag time," is about 10 days. The recognition of osteoid in histologic sections usually depends on the preparation of undecalcified sections. The ability to identify this nonmineralized bone is a key factor in the diagnosis of certain metabolic disturbances of bone.

On histologic examination it can be seen that actively forming bone surfaces, as well as inactive already formed surfaces, are smooth. However, some bone surfaces have an irregular or "gnawed out" appearance, and these surfaces either have been resorbed or are actively resorbing (Fig. 1.22). The cells concerned with resorption are the osteoclasts, large, often multinucleated cells with abundant cytoplasm. Osteoclasts frequently lie in cavities in the bone surface known as Howship's lacunae (Fig. 1.23). The osteoclast is usually a multinucleate cell, but mononuclear forms of resorbing cells can also be seen.

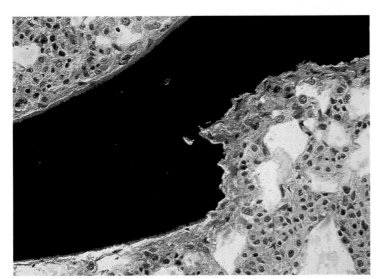

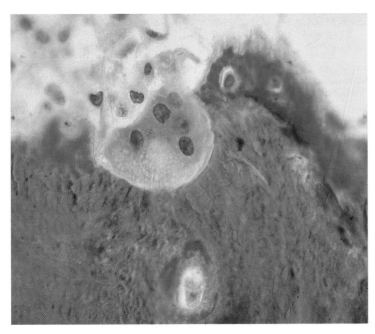

FIGURE 1.22 Photomicrograph shows contrast of bone-forming surface with osteoid seam *(upper left)* with a resorbing surface *(lower right)* (H & E, x 10 obj.).

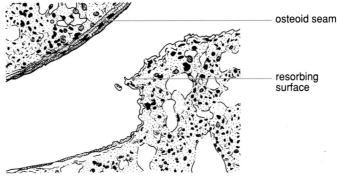

osteoid seam

resorbing surface

FIGURE 1.23 Photomicrograph shows an osteoclast in a Howship's lacuna. Osteoclasts are identified by their abundant cytoplasm and multiple nuclei (Goldner stain, x 25 obj.).

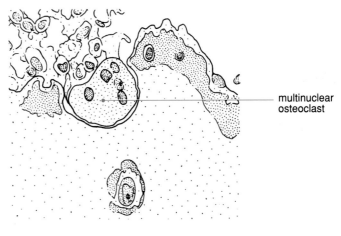

multinuclear osteoclast

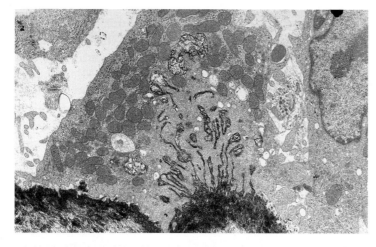

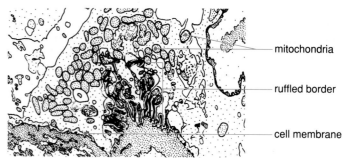

mitochondria

ruffled border

cell membrane

FIGURE 1.24 Electron photomicrograph of an osteoclast. Note the interdigitating ruffles of the osteoclast and the underlying mineralized bone. Apatite crystals are seen deep within the sub-stance of the osteoclast. Note the abundant mitochondria and lysosomal inclusion bodies (x 15,000).

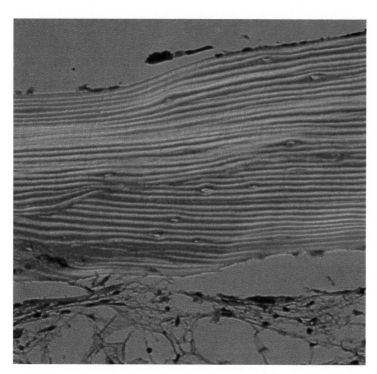

FIGURE 1.25 Segment of trabecular bone microscopically examined with polarized light (x 10 obj.).

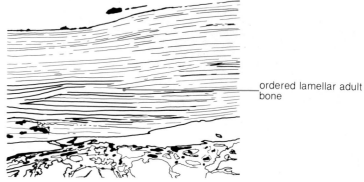

ordered lamellar adult bone

FIGURE 1.26 Diagrammatic representation of the layered (lamellar) appearance of bone shows how the alternating dark and light layers are explained by the change in direction of the collagen fibers in each layer.

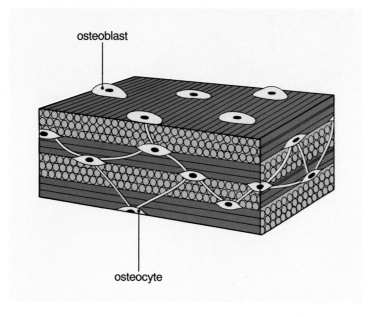

osteoblast

osteocyte

By electron microscopy the osteoclast is seen to have a ruffled border adjacent to the bone and to contain many lysosomal bodies, mitochondria, and vesicular inclusions (Fig. 1.24). Although complete agreement with regard to the origin of the osteoclast has not yet been reached, this cell probably derives from blood-borne monocytes.

HISTOLOGY

Mature Bone

In mature bone tissue the collagen fibers of the matrix are arranged in layers or lamellae (hence "lamellar

bone"), and in each of these layers the collagen bundles lie parallel to each other (Figs. 1.25 and 1.26). However, the orientation of the collagen bundles changes significantly from one layer to another, in a way similar to the structure of plywood. Therefore, bone tissue gains much of its strength from its internal construction.

In cortical bone the lamellae are arranged concentrically around a vascular core (haversian canal) to form an osteon (Figs. 1.27 and 1.28). On histologic examination it becomes apparent that surrounding each osteon, and also irregularly distributed throughout the trabecular bone, there are distinct lines that appear deep blue after hematoxylin and eosin staining.

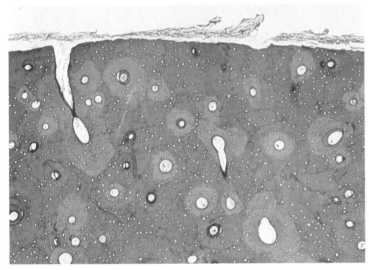

FIGURE 1.27 Photomicrograph of cortical bone shows lamellae surrounding haversian canals to form osteons (H & E, x 4 obj.).

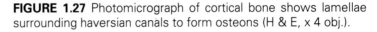

periosteum

perforating periosteal vessel

haversian canal

osteon

interstitial lamellae

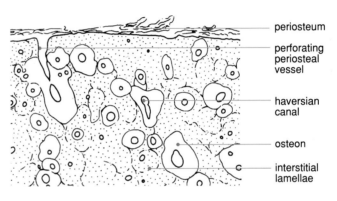

circumferential lamellae

osteon

lacuna   osteocyte

Volkmann's canal

haversian canal

vessel

FIGURE 1.28 Schematic diagram of some of the main features of the microstructure of mature bone. Note the general construction of the osteons, the distribution of the osteocytic lacunae, the haversian canals and their contents.

These lines are the cement lines (Fig. 1.29). When histologic sections are examined by polarized light, a discontinuity of the collagen can be seen on either side of the cement line. From this observation it can be inferred that the bone is constructed of separate pieces like a three-dimensional jigsaw puzzle. (It has been experimentally demonstrated that fractures occur along the cement lines.)

Primary osteons are formed in the infant by the ingrowth of periosteal blood vessels following a "cutting cone" of osteoclasts, which tunnels through the existing cortex deposited by the periosteum. The tunnel formed by the osteoclasts and containing the vessel then becomes partially filled in by osteoblasts, which deposit

concentric layers of bone matrix. Secondary and subsequent osteons are formed during the process of remodeling by the outgrowth from existing haversian systems of vessels, which are also preceded by a cluster of osteoclasts (Fig. 1.30).

Immature Bone

In addition to lamellar bone, another form of bone tissue exists in which the collagen matrix is irregularly arranged in a woven pattern resembling the warp and woof threads in a fabric (Figs. 1.31 and 1.32). The cells within this matrix are larger, more rounded, and closer together than those in normal bone. This type of bone,

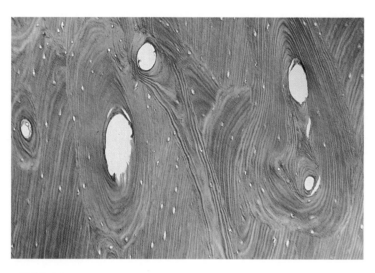

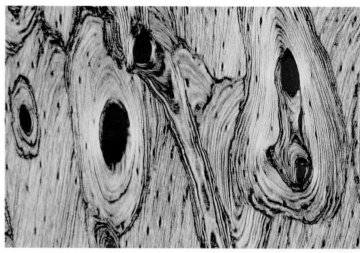

FIGURE 1.29 *(left)* Photomicrograph of a portion of the cortical bone in cross-section (H & E, Nomarski optics, x 10 obj.). *(right)* The same histologic field photographed using polarized light. The

structural discontinuity between the various osteons is seen as dark lines which correspond to cement lines. Cement lines may stain blue on H & E sections but are often difficult to see.

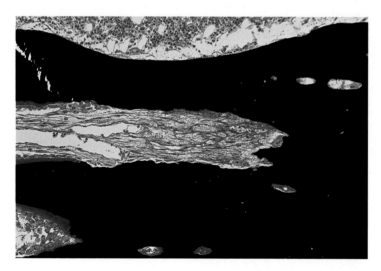

FIGURE 1.30 Photomicrograph of a portion of the cortical bone shows a cutting cone. Note the osteoclasts at the advancing nose of the cone and the active osteoblastic activity behind. The osteoblasts are associated with a thin layer of osteoid (von Kossa, x 10 obj.).

which has been variously called woven bone, primitive bone, fiber bone, and immature bone, is seen during development, in fracture callus, in bone-forming tumors, and in conditions characterized by a highly accelerated rate of bone formation (eg, Paget's disease and other hypermetabolic states). The recognition of this kind of bone by the pathologist is important, because it usually indicates the presence of a disease process.

Marrow

The tissue space between the osseous elements is occupied by fat, hematopoietic tissue, and neurovascular tissue. Although hematopoietic tissue is found in all the bones at birth, with maturation this tissue becomes largely confined to the axial skeleton, ie, the skull, ribs, vertebral column, sternum, and pelvic girdle. The appearance of cellular marrow at other sites during adult life is abnormal and warrants investigation. In areas where hematopoietic tissue is normally present the ratio of fat to hematopoietic tissue is normally 50:50. An increase or decrease in this ratio may indicate hematologic disease and should be further investigated. (Interestingly, although in certain disease states hyperplastic marrow may again be seen in adult long bones, it is often arrested at the site of the closed epiphyseal plate.)

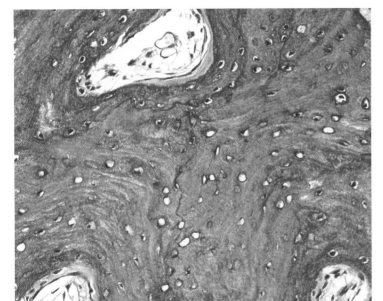

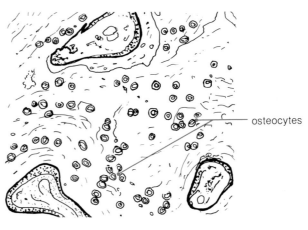

FIGURE 1.31 Photomicrograph of immature bone from a patient with osteogenesis imperfecta. Note the crowded oval to round osteocytes (H & E, x 10 obj.).

osteocytes

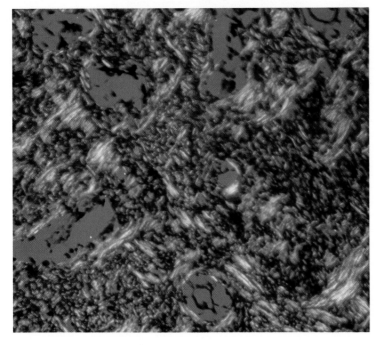

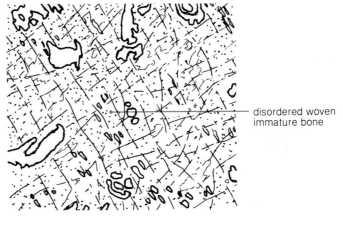

FIGURE 1.32 Photomicrograph of immature bone taken with polarized light demonstrates the irregular woven appearance of the collagenous matrix (H & E, x 10 obj.).

disordered woven immature bone

THE JOINTS

GROSS STRUCTURE

The ends of contiguous bones, together with their soft tissue components, cartilage, ligaments, and synovium, constitute a functioning unit: the joint. Of the three types of joints, the most common is the diarthrodial joint, which has a cavity and forms a movable connecting unit between two bones (Fig. 1.33). Hyaline cartilage (articular cartilage) covers the articulating surfaces of the diarthrodial joints, with the exception of the sternoclavicular and temporomandibular joints, which are covered by fibrocartilage.

The normal function of a diarthrodial joint depends principally on three factors. These factors are: the freedom of the articulating surfaces to move over each other, the ability of the joint to maintain stability during use, and a proper distribution of stress through the tissues which comprise the joint so that these tissues are not damaged. These aspects of joint function are governed by the interdependent actions of the shape of the articulating surfaces of the joint (Fig. 1.34); by the integrity of the ligaments, muscles, and tendons that support the limb; and by the biologic cellular control of the mechanical properties of the matrices of the bone, cartilage, and the other tissues that together comprise the joint.

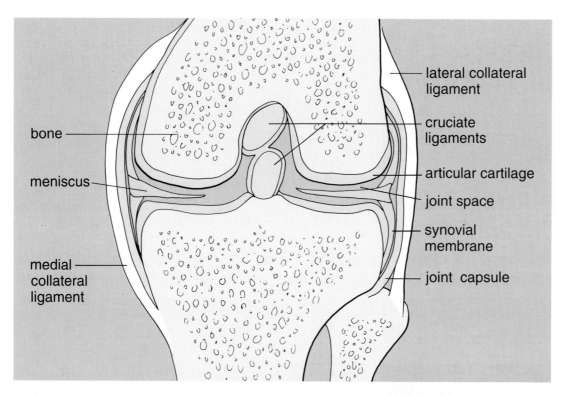

bone

meniscus

medial collateral ligament

lateral collateral ligament

cruciate ligaments

articular cartilage

joint space

synovial membrane

joint capsule

FIGURE 1.33 Diagram of the knee joint. The radiologic joint space consists of the radiolucent articular cartilage plus the joint cavity.

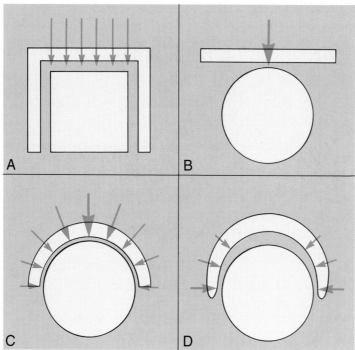

A

B

C

D

FIGURE 1.34 The shape of the joint determines the freedom of the joint surfaces to articulate, the stability of the joint, and the distribution of stress on the tissues. *A* does not allow acceptable freedom of movement. *B* permits total freedom of movement, but is unstable. *C* allows freedom of movement and is stable; however, the shape is not optimal because it does not provide space between the articulating surfaces for lubrication or nutrition (ie, it is completely congruent). Furthermore, when the joint is loaded, the stress is not equally distributed over the joint surfaces. *D* is the optimal shape for a joint because it is stable, it articulates easily, and there is some space between the joint surfaces so that the synovial fluid can move into the joint space to provide for the nutrition of the cartilage and the lubrication of the surfaces. This shape also distributes an increasing load equally, because the deformability of cartilage and bone enables the tissues to respond and conform to stresses imposed on them.

The second type of joint is the amphiarthrodial joint, which is characterized by limited mobility, eg, the intervertebral disc (Fig. 1.35). The disc is a fibrocartilaginous complex which forms the articulation between the vertebral bodies. It contributes to the mobility and stability of the spine as well as to the transmission of load through it. It should be noted that disc height, in general, is not the same in all segments of the spine, the cervical and thoracic discs being flatter than those of the lumbar region. Disc height also varies from front to back, relative to the curvature of the spine.

The intervertebral disc can be divided into two components: the outermost fibrous ring (anulus fibrosus) and the innermost gelatinous core (nucleus pulposus). The anulus, when viewed from above, is seen to contain fibrous tissue layers arranged in concentric circles. Each layer extends obliquely from vertebral body to vertebral body, with the fibers of one layer running in a direction opposite to that of the adjacent layer. These alternating layers provide for motion that is universal in direction but restricted in degree (Figs. 1.36 and 1.37). The fibers of the anulus are attached by

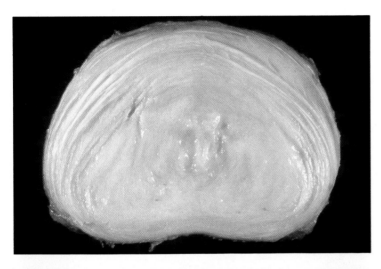

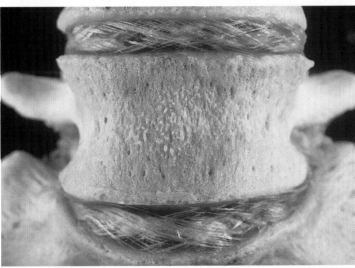

FIGURE 1.36 Photograph showing frontal view of L5 with the adjacent intervertebral disc. Note the oblique disposition of the collagen fibers of the anulus fibrosus in this macerated specimen.

FIGURE 1.35 Intervertebral disc seen from above. Note the circumferential fibers in the anulus fibrosus. The nucleus pulposus *(center)* is rich in proteoglycan and water, and acts to resist compression. The circumferential fibers of the anulus prevent lateral spread of the nucleus.

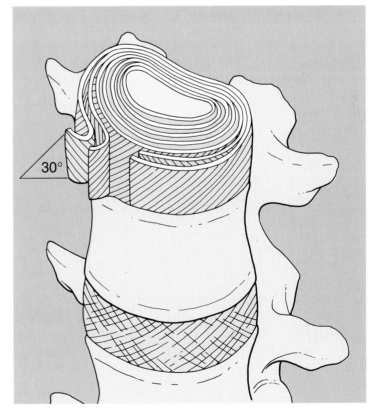

FIGURE 1.37 Schematic drawing of the intervertebral disc demonstrates the layered arrangement of collagen fibers in the anulus. The fibers of each layer run at an approximately 30° angle to the surface of the vertebral body and in a direction opposite to that of the adjacent layer.

Sharpey's fibers to the bony endplates of the adjacent vertebral bodies (Fig. 1.38). The fibrous lamellae are stronger and more numerous in the anterior and lateral aspects of the disc than in the posterior aspect, where they are sparser and thinner. The anterior anulus is therefore almost twice the thickness of the posterior anulus. The nucleus pulposus typically occupies an eccentric position within the disc space, usually being closer to the posterior margin. The tissue of the nucleus is separated from that of the bone by a clearly defined layer of hyaline cartilage which extends to the inner margins of the insertion of the anulus (Fig. 1.39).

On microscopic examination of the nucleus pulposus a large number of cells can be observed suspended in a loose fibrous matrix. Many of these cells are fusiform and resemble typical fibrocytes (Fig. 1.40).

Because no blood vessels are present in adult disc tissue, nutrients must travel by diffusion from capillary beds at the disc margins. The restricted flow of nutrients to the nucleus and inner annulus may contribute to or even underlie disc degeneration in the adult.

The third and final type of joint is the synarthrosis. Synarthoses, such as the skull sutures, are nonmovable joints.

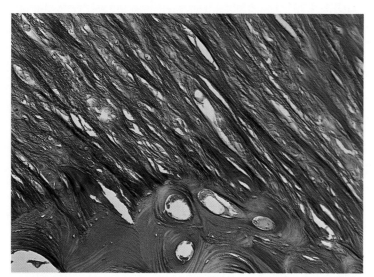

FIGURE 1.38 Photomicrograph showing the insertion of the fibers of the anulus fibrosus into the bone of the margins of the articular surface of the vertebral body. Where the collagen fibers of the anulus enter the bone (Sharpey's fibers) they are calcified (H & E stain, partially polarized light, x 4 obj.).

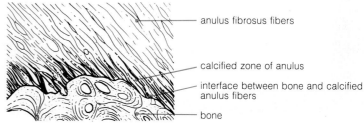

anulus fibrosus fibers

calcified zone of anulus

interface between bone and calcified anulus fibers

bone

FIGURE 1.39 Invertebral disc. Hyaline cartilage separates the tissue of the nucleus pulposus from that of the bone.

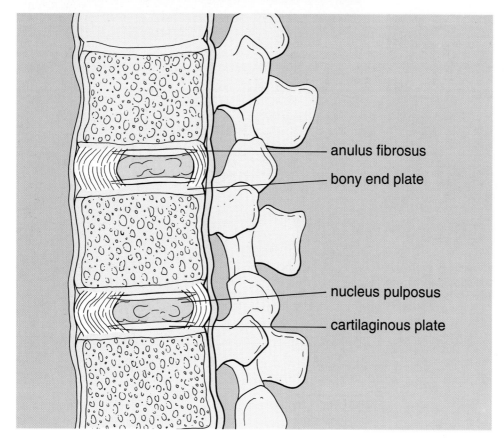

anulus fibrosus

bony end plate

nucleus pulposus

cartilaginous plate

ARTICULAR CARTILAGE

The articular ends of the bones are covered with hyaline cartilage, which is a nerveless, bloodless, firm and yet pliable tissue. In young people hyaline cartilage is translucent and bluish-white, and in older individuals it is opaque and slightly yellowish (Fig. 1.41). This change with age in the appearance of the articular cartilage is also seen in other connective tissues and is probably related to a number of factors, including dehydration of the tissues with age, increased numbers of cross-linkages in the collagen, and accumulation of lipofuscin pigment in the tissues of older individuals (Fig. 1.42).

Hyaline cartilage deforms under pressure but recovers its original shape on removal of the pressure. In growing children it is the precursor of the bony skeleton and is also the means by which the bones increase in length. Articular cartilage is characterized on microscopic examination by its abundant glassy extracellular matrix, with isolated, sparse cells located in well-defined spaces (lacunae). It is often described as having four layers or zones: the superficial, intermediate, deep, and calcified layers.

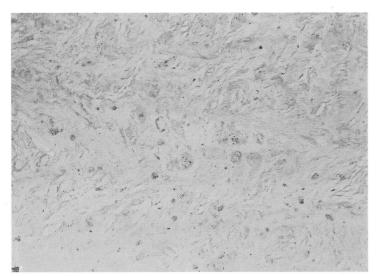

FIGURE 1.40 Photomicrograph of normal nucleus pulposus. The matrix is loose and fibrous, with scattered small stellate cells and occasional chondrocytes in clumps (H & E stain, x 4 obj.).

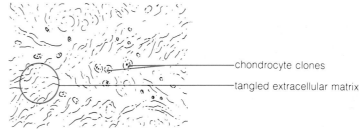

chondrocyte clones

tangled extracellular matrix

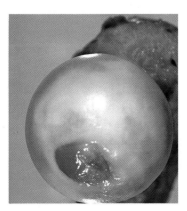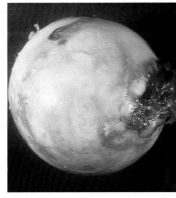

FIGURE 1.41 Femoral head from an 18-year-old shows a translucent bluish-white cartilage *(left)*, and from a 65-year-old shows an opaque slightly yellowish cartilage *(right)*.

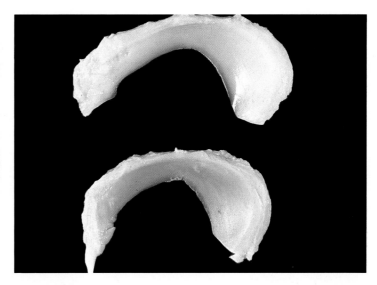

FIGURE 1.42 Gross photographs of menisci obtained from a young *(upper)* and an old *(lower)* patient. In contrast to the meniscus from the young patient, which has a bluish-white color and is supple, the meniscus from the old patient has a characteristically yellowish color and feels stiffer on palpation.

In the superficial layers the cells are flat. In the intermediate zone the cells have a tendency to form radial groups which apparently follow the pattern of collagen disposition. In the calcified zone, ie, the zone adjacent to the bone, the cells are apparently nonviable and the matrix is heavily calcified (Fig. 1.43).

That some fibrous system exists within normal articular cartilage is readily demonstrable by the sim-ple expedient of pricking its surface with a pin. A split results, and if the pricking is repeated all over the sur-face a constant pattern of split lines is revealed (Fig. 1.44). If we accept for the moment that the fissures reflect the internal fiber arrangement of the cartilage, then we can infer that on the surface the fibers run par-allel to the surface and in the general direction of the split line. If the superficial layer of the cartilage is

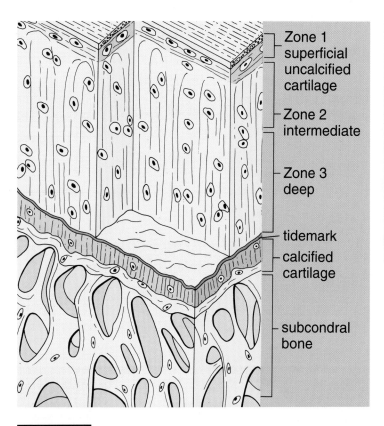

FIGURE 1.43 The zones of adult articular cartilage.

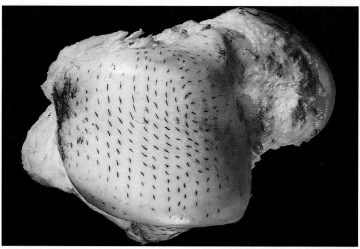

FIGURE 1.44 Photograph of the superior articular surface of the talus after the entire surface has been pricked with a pin whose tip had been dipped in India ink. Note the resulting pattern of split lines

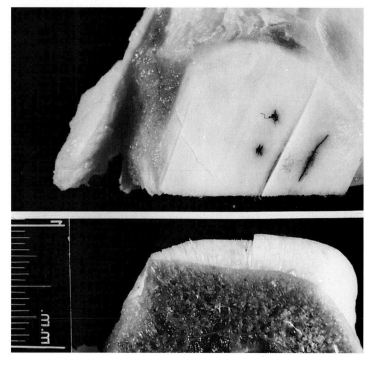

FIGURE 1.45 Photograph demonstrating that when the outer layer of cartilage is removed before the pin is inserted, only a round hole appears, rather than a split.

pared away and the exposed surface pricked, instead of fissures only small round holes appear (Fig. 1.45). If the cut edge of the cartilage is pricked a vertical split line is produced, and this occurs in all planes of section (Fig. 1.46). These experiments indicate that in the deeper layers of the cartilage the fibers are predominantly vertical (Fig. 1.47).

A combination of polarizing microscopy, transmission electron microscopy, and scanning electron microscopy confirms that the principal orientation of collagen in articular cartilage is vertical through most of its thickness and horizontal at the surface (Fig. 1.48).

The precise organization of collagen, as described for the cartilage, bone, and anulus of the intervertebral disc, serves a mechanical function. The mechanical requirements of all other connective tissues are similarly provided for by the architectural arrangement of the collagen matrix. For example, the menisci of the knee are composed mainly of collagen, although some proteoglycan is also present. Microscopic examination of carefully oriented sections has shown that the principal orientation of the collagen fibers in the menisci is circumferential. The few small, radially disposed fibers appear designed to withstand the circumferential ten-

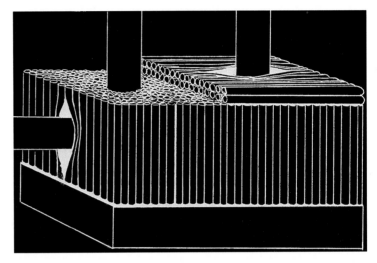

FIGURE 1.46 A photograph of a portion of the articular cartilage which has been sectioned vertically to show the cut edge and the underlying bone. The direction of pin pricks made on the surface can be seen and additional pin pricks have been made on the cut edge all of which result in vertical splits.

FIGURE 1.47 Model illustrating the experiments shown in Figures 1.44 -1.46.

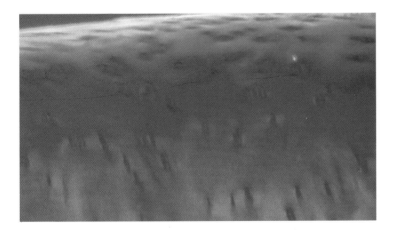

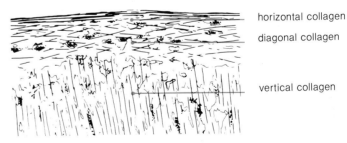

horizontal collagen

diagonal collagen

vertical collagen

FIGURE 1.48 Photomicrograph of the articular cartilage using polarized light and a first-order red compensating filter. The fibers at the surface of the cartilage are seen as blue, the fibers in the lower part of the cartilage as red, and between the two layers

there is less polarization. These observations can be interpreted as demonstrating that at the surface the fibers are horizontally disposed, in the deep part of the cartilage they are vertical, and in between there is a crossover of fibers (x 10 obj.).

sion within the meniscus during normal loading. The radially disposed fibers probably act as ties to resist any longitudinal splitting of the menisci that might result from undue compression (Fig. 1.49).

The distribution of proteoglycans in the cartilage matrix is also related to the mechanical requirements. It varies markedly from joint to joint, geographically within a single articular cartilage, and also as a function of age (in general, proteoglycan distribution is more diffuse in children than in adults). The surface layers of the cartilage contain much less proteoglycan than the deeper layers. In the deeper layers there is a higher concentration of staining with safranin O and toluidine blue around the cells (the pericellular matrix) than between the cells (the intercellular matrix) (Fig. 1.50).

In histologic sections stained with hematoxylin and eosin, the junction between the calcified cartilage and the noncalcified cartilage is marked by a basophilic line known as the tidemark. This basophilic line is not seen in the developing skeleton but is clearly visible in the adult (Figs. 1.51 and 1.52).

Mechanical failure in the cartilage rarely, if ever, gives rise to the separation of bone and cartilage. However, when such failure occurs it is seen as a horizontal cleft at the junction of the calcified and noncalcified cartilage (at the tidemark) (Fig. 1.53). Presumably, failure occurs at the tidemark because of the considerable change in the rigidity of the cartilage at this junction.

At its base, adult articular cartilage is bordered by the subchondral bone plate. The cartilage tissue is keyed into the irregular surface of the underlying bone, again somewhat like a jigsaw puzzle. Because the cartilage adjacent to the bone is calcified and has a rigidity similar to that of bone, the keying is rigid (Fig. 1.54).

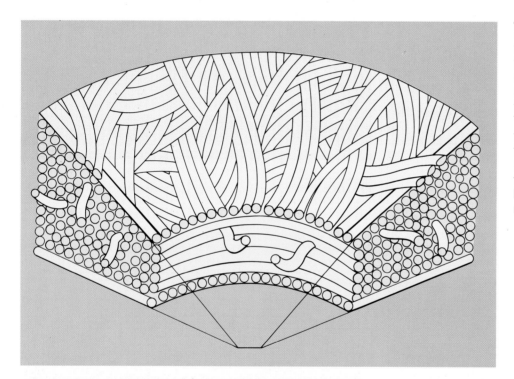

FIGURE 1.49 Diagrammatic representation of the distribution of collagen fibers in the meniscus of a knee. Collagen is oriented throughout the connective tissues in such a way as to maximally resist the forces brought to bear on these tissues. The majority of the fibers are circumferentially arranged; a few radially arranged fibers, particularly on the tibial surface, resist lateral spread of the meniscus. In the meniscus, tension is generated between the anterior and posterior attachments.

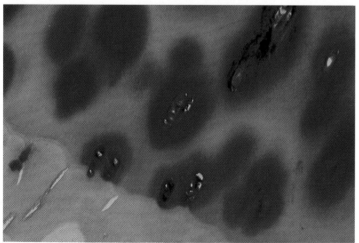

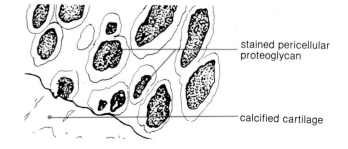

stained pericellular proteoglycan

calcified cartilage

FIGURE 1.50 Portion of cartilage stained by toluidine blue shows intense metachromasia around the chondrocytes in the deep part of the noncalcified cartilage. This represents staining of the proteoglycan, and there is much less staining in the interterritorial matrix than around the cell. Even less staining is seen in the calcified cartilage (x 10 obj.).

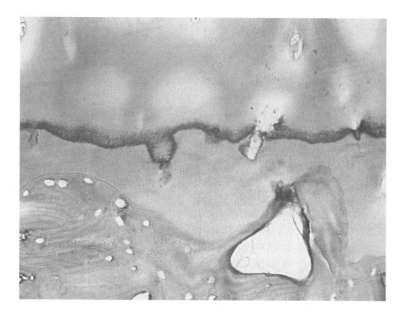

FIGURE 1.51 Photomicrograph of the junction of articular cartilage with bone shows the basophilic line (tidemark) that separates the noncalcified from the calcified cartilage. This line represents the mineralization front of the calcified cartilage. In normal adult cartilage it is clearly defined and relatively even, but in arthritic conditions the line may become widened and diffuse, with duplication of the line a common finding (H & E, x 10 obj.).

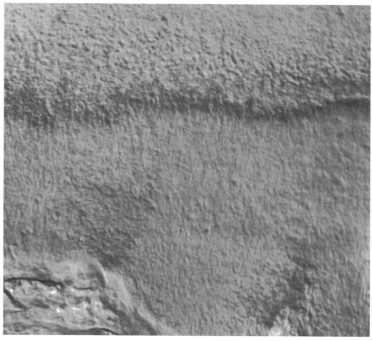

FIGURE 1.52 Photomicrograph demonstrates the tidemark at a somewhat higher power than in Figure 1.51. By the use of this technique a granular appearance of the tidemark can be appreciated (H & E, x 25 obj., Nomarski optics).

FIGURE 1.53 Photomicrograph demonstrates a traumatic separation of the cartilage in the region of the tidemark. This defect has become filled by reparative fibrous tissue (H & E, x obj.).

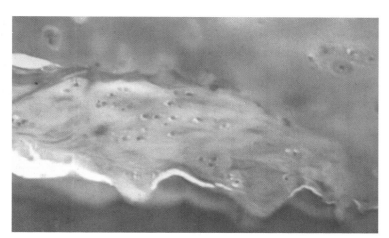

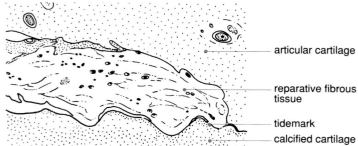

articular cartilage

reparative fibrous tissue

tidemark

calcified cartilage

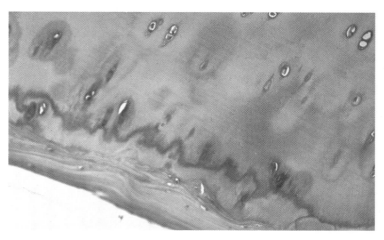

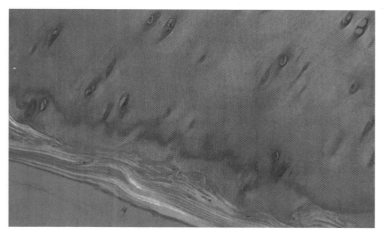

FIGURE 1.54 Photomicrographs of the bone–cartilage interface. In the section on the left the tidemark, which indicates the upper edge of the calcified cartilage, can be seen as a wavy blue line, but bone–cartilage interface is poorly visualized. When the same histologic field is examine by polarized light using a first-order red compensator filter *(right)* the bone, which is seen as red, and the cartilage (blue) are easily differentiated and the tidemark can still be seen (H & E, x 10 obj.).

The insertions of ligaments and tendons into the bone are effected by a similar keying, and at their insertions ligaments and tendons are also calcified (Fig. 1.55).

In addition to the hyaline cartilage of which articular cartilage is composed, two other forms of cartilage can be histologically identified. Fibrocartilage is a tissue in which the matrix contains a high proportion of collagen, the fibers of which are usually visible by transmitted light microscopy. Fibrocartilage is found in the menisci of the knee, the anulus fibrosus, at the insertions of ligaments and tendons into the bone (Fig. 1.56), and on the inner side of tendons as they angle around pulleys, eg, at the malleoli. The second type of nonhyaline cartilage is elastic cartilage, in which the matrix contains a high proportion of elastic tissue. Elastic fibers are found in the ligamentum flavum, external ear, and epiglottis (Fig. 1.57).

Both the fibrocartilage and the elastic cartilage incorporate the term "cartilage" because the cells are rounded and lie in lacunae, which gives them a superficial resemblance to the cells of hyaline cartilage. However, the mechanical functions of these tissues are very different from those of hyaline cartilage. Both fibrocartilage and elastic cartilage function principally as resisters of tension, with, however, some element of compression. On the other hand, hyaline cartilage is mainly subject to and resists compressive forces.

SYNOVIAL MEMBRANE

The synovial membrane lines the inner surface of the joint capsule and all other intra-articular structures, with the exception of articular cartilage and the meniscus. Synovial membrane consists of two components. The first of these is the synovial lining (or intimal layer) bounding the joint space. This layer is predominantly cellular. The second component is a subintimal, supportive, or backing layer formed of fibrous and adipose tissues in variable proportions. The surface of the synovial lining is smooth, moist, and glistening, with a few small villi and fringe-like folds (Fig. 1.58).

The cellular elements of the joint lining consist of intimal cells (or synoviocytes) and other connective tissue cells, including fat cells, fibroblasts, histiocytes,

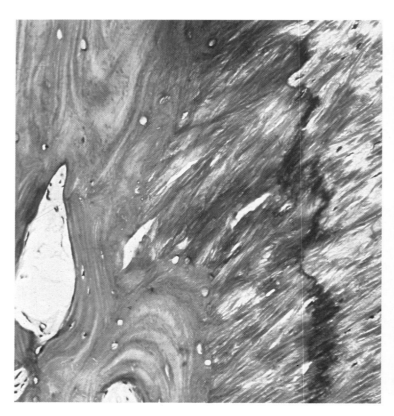
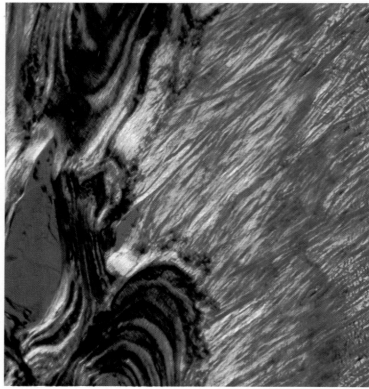

FIGURE 1.55 Photomicrographs of the insertion of a ligament into bone. In the section on the left the wavy blue line, which represents the edge of the calcified portion of the ligament, is clearly seen, but the interface of ligament and bone is not well visualized. When the same histologic field is examined by polarized light *(right)*, the interface of calcified ligament and bone is clearly demonstrated (H & E, x 10 obj.).

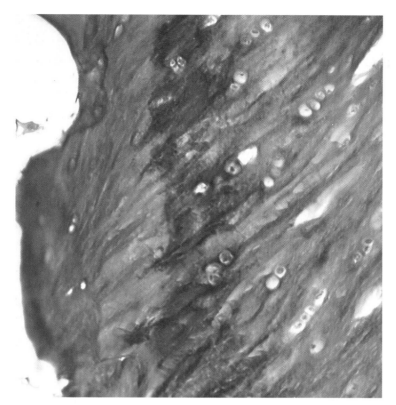

FIGURE 1.56 Photomicrograph of tendon insertion. Note that the cells of the tendon are rounded and lie in lacunae. This appearance is described as fibrocartilage (H & E, x 10 obj.).

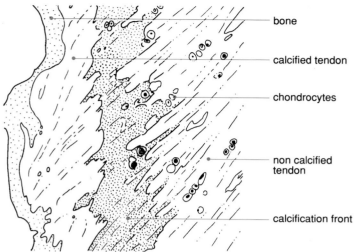

bone

calcified tendon

chondrocytes

non calcified tendon

calcification front

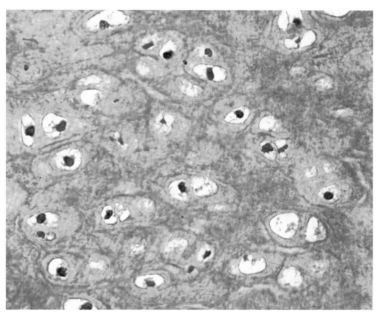

FIGURE 1.57 Photomicrograph of ear cartilage. Although the cells resemble those seen in hyaline cartilage, the matrix contains many elastic fibers which appear bright red in this section stained with phloxine and tartrazine (x 25 obj.).

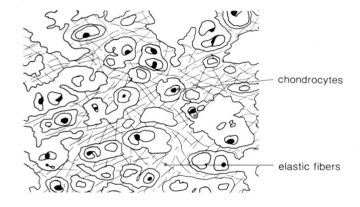

chondrocytes

elastic fibers

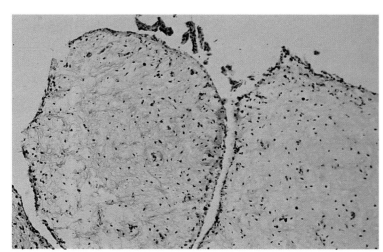

FIGURE 1.58 Photomicrograph of synovium showing the simple lining and the fibro-adipose subsynovial tissue (H & E, x 4 obj.).

and mast cells (mast cells are omnipresent in connective tissue). Sections of synovial membrane reveal, along the edge facing the synovial cavity, a single row or sometimes multiple rows of closely packed cells with large elliptical nuclei (Fig. 1.59).

Electron microscopic studies have revealed two principal types of synovial cells, which have been designated by Barland as Types A and B. (Many cells have features of both types and have been called intermediate.) The predominant cell (Type A) has many of the features of a macrophage, and there is good evidence that it is structurally adapted for phagocytic functions (Fig. 1.60). The less common Type B cells are richly endowed with rough endoplasmic reticulum, contain Golgi systems, and often exhibit pinocytotic vesicles (Fig. 1.61). Normal synovial intima contains far more Type A than Type B cells.

The synovial membrane has three principal functions: secretion of synovial fluid hyaluronate (B cells); phagocytosis of waste material derived from the various components of the joint (A cells); and regulation of the movement of solutes, electrolytes, and proteins from the capillaries into the synovial fluid, thus providing for the metabolic requirement of the joint chondrocytes and possibly also providing a regulatory mechanism for maintenance of the matrix through the role of various mediators such as interleukin 1.

In addition to lining the joints, synovial membrane lines the subcutaneous and subtendinous sacs known as bursae, which permit freedom of movement over a limited range for the structures adjacent to the bursae. Synovial membrane also lines the sheaths that form around tendons wherever they pass under ligamentous bands or through osseofibrous tunnels.

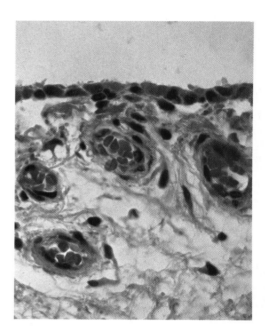

FIGURE 1.59 Photomicrograph of synovium shows a delicate synovial lining resting on a fibroadipose subintimal layer which is rich in capillaries, lymphatics, and nerve endings (H & E, x 25 obj.).

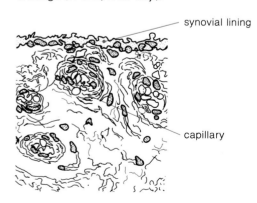

synovial lining

capillary

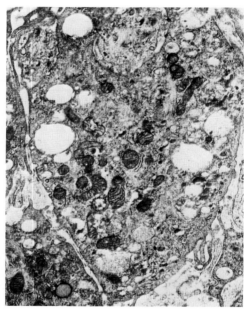

FIGURE 1.60 Electron micrograph of an A cell shows abundant mitochondria and dense inclusion bodies (x 10,000).

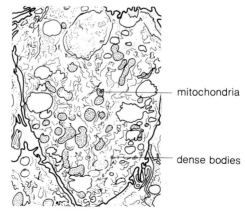

mitochondria

dense bodies

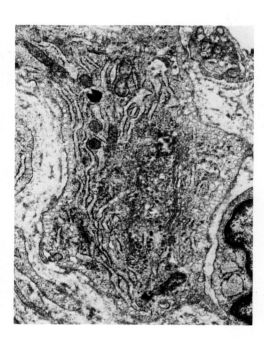

FIGURE 1.61 Electron micrograph of a B cell shows abundant rough endoplasmic reticulum and many pinocytotic vesicles (x 10,000).

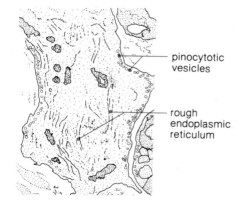

pinocytotic vesicles

rough endoplasmic reticulum

BONE GROWTH AND DEVELOPMENT

Unlike most tissues, bone can grow only by apposition on the surface of an already existing substrate such as bone and/or calcified cartilage. As Hunter put it, "Bones do not grow by fresh matter being put into all parts, so as to push the old matter to a greater distance but by new matter laid upon the external surface." In contrast, cartilage grows by interstitial cell proliferation and matrix formation. It is perhaps because of the capacity of cartilage for interstitial growth that most of the embryonic skeleton is first formed in the cartilage, and that cartilage proliferation plays such an important role in skeletal growth and development. With the exception of the cranial vault, the skeleton appears in the embryo as a cartilaginous structure.

Even before any bone tissue formation has occurred, it can be seen in an embryonic cartilage skeleton that the cartilage cells towards the middle of the bone model are larger and more separated by interstitial matrix than those towards the end of the bone model, which are fairly small and closely packed together (Fig. 1.62). As the cells in the center of the bone shaft continue to enlarge, the cartilage matrix lying between the cells becomes calcified, and the cells die (Fig. 1.63). The mechanisms responsible for calcification of the matrix are not completely understood, but it is generally believed that the initiators of calcification are small membrane-bound vesicles known as matrix vesicles, which are found in the interstitial matrix between the cells. After calcification of the cartilage matrix, the periosteum surrounding this portion of the

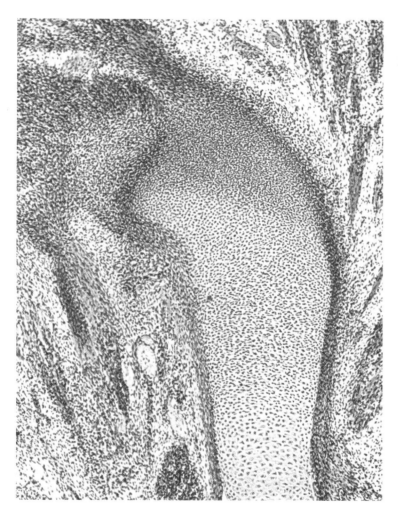

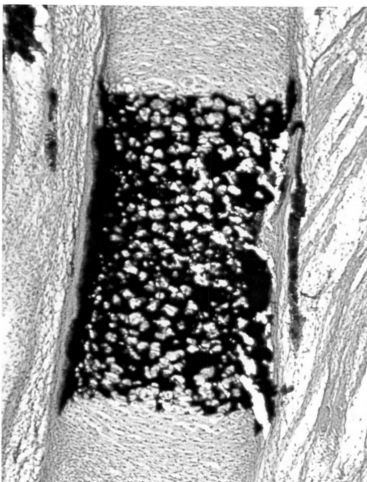

FIGURE 1.62 Photomicrograph of the upper end of the femur and hip joint in a 5-week fetus. The bone is already modeled in cartilage and is covered by a condensation of mesenchymal cells, which will eventually become the periosteum. Note that the cells in the diaphysis of the cartilage model of the bone are larger and paler than those at the end of the bone (H & E, x 4 obj.).

FIGURE 1.63 Photomicrograph of the shaft of the long bone in a 7-week fetus (cut, undecalcified, and stained with von Kossa stain). Note the calcification of the cartilage matrix (black) in the diaphysis of the bone (x 4 obj.).

bone begins to produce a primitive bone matrix which is quickly formed into a cuff of bone (Fig. 1.64). After formation of this cuff of bone, small capillaries can be seen penetrating through the periosteum and the periosteal bone cuff into the calcified cartilage matrix, destroying the now empty cartilage lacunae and establishing a vascular network through the calcified cartilage (Fig. 1.65). Cells, perhaps derived from the vessel walls, are seen lining up on the surface of the remaining calcified cartilage and depositing a bony matrix.

This process of cartilage calcification followed by vascular invasion and deposition of bony matrix on the remaining calcified cartilage is known as endochondral ossification, and is the normal means by which cartilage is transformed into bone. The bone that is first laid down, ie, with a core of calcified cartilage and primitive bone on the surface, is commonly known as the primary spongiosa (Fig. 1.66; see also Fig. 1.77). As the primary spongiosa is remodeled and the calcified cartilage removed, the bone trabeculae come to be formed

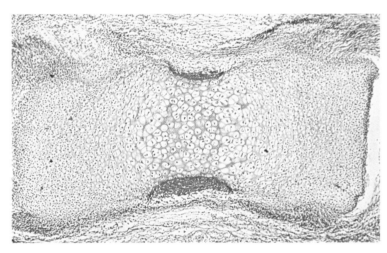

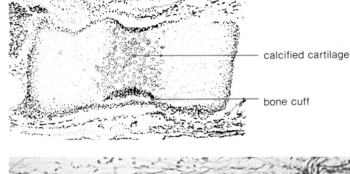

FIGURE 1.64 Photomicrograph of a section through a metacarpal bone from a 7-week fetus. In the diaphysis the cartilage matrix stains with a deeper blue, indicating that it is calcified. Around the calcified cartilage matrix is a narrow cuff of immature bone (trichrome stain, x 4 obj.).

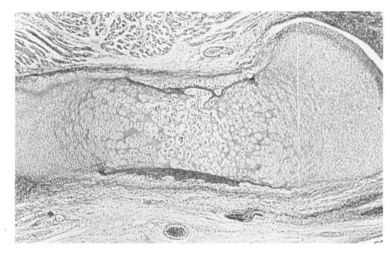

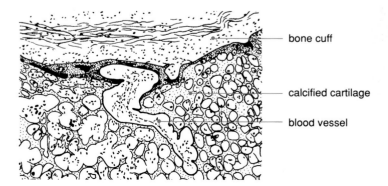

FIGURE 1.65 *(left)* Photomicrograph of a long bone removed from a 10-week fetus (trichrome, x 4 obj.). *(right)* Close-up shows the calcified cartilage below and the diaphyseal bone cuff above, covered by the condensed mesenchymal tissue that forms the periosteum. Penetrating through the bone cuff into the calcified cartilage is a blood vessel. This blood vessel will eventually erode through the calcified cartilage entirely, bringing in osteoblasts to form the earliest primary spongiosa (trichrome, x 16 obj.).

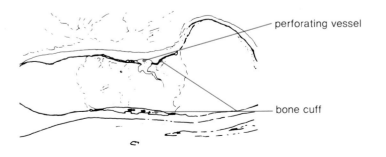

entirely of bone tissue, and at this stage they are usually referred to as the secondary spongiosa.

In the fetus, the process of endochondral ossification continues until such a stage is reached that a considerable portion of the shaft of the bone has been converted into an osseous tissue and only the ends of the bone are still formed of cartilage (Fig. 1.67). The carti-

lage at the bone ends continuously proliferates and lengthens by a process of interstitial growth. The cartilage cells, as they approach the midshaft of the bone, enlarge and degenerate; the cartilage matrix calcifies, and eventually vascular invasion and formation of primary spongiosa occur. Thus it is that the bone grows in length (Fig. 1.68).

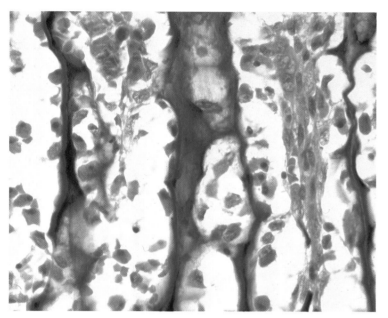

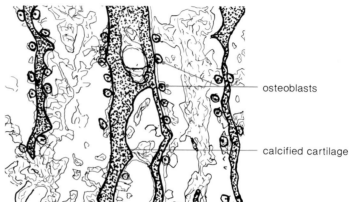

FIGURE 1.66 A portion of the primary spongiosa from the diaphysis of a long bone in a 10-week fetus. Notice the delicate cores of calcified cartilage covered by plump cells (osteoblasts), which are forming the seams of immature bone matrix (H & E, x 25 obj.).

osteoblasts

calcified cartilage

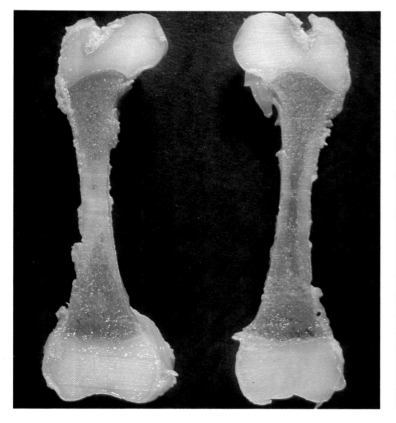

FIGURE 1.67 Gross photograph of a femur from a 6-month stillborn baby. At this stage the epiphyseal ends of the bone are still entirely cartilaginous.

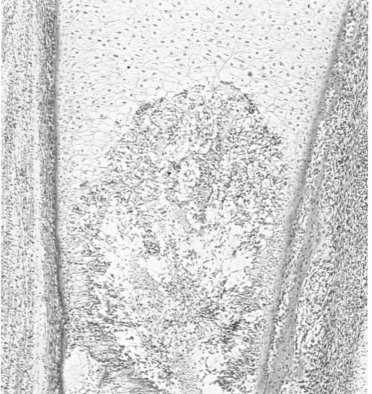

FIGURE 1.68 Photomicrograph of the upper end of the femur shows the junction between the newly formed bone and the epiphyseal cartilage. The bone grows in length by the process of endochondral ossification, in which the calcified cartilage is invaded by blood vessels and replaced by bone (H & E, x 10 obj.).

During the early stages of skeletal development, the locations of joints are marked by a condensation of mesenchymal cells. Only after the fifth to eighth week of intrauterine life do these cells undergo solution to form a joint cleft (Figs. 1.69, 1.70, and 1.71).

At some point during development a secondary center of ossification is formed within the cartilaginous end of the bone (Figs. 1.72, 1.73, and 1.74). Calcification occurs initially at the middle of the secondary center. This area is then invaded by blood vessels and the process of endochondral ossification ensues. The vessels leading to the degenerated and calcified cartilage in the center of the epiphysis are carried in canals that develop from invagination of the surface covering of the

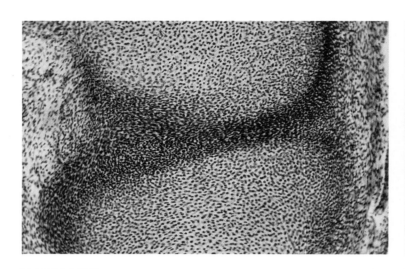

FIGURE 1.69 Photomicrograph of a sagittal section through the fetal knee joint at the sixth week of gestation, showing the condensation of the mesenchyme marking the future joint space (H & E, x 10 obj.).

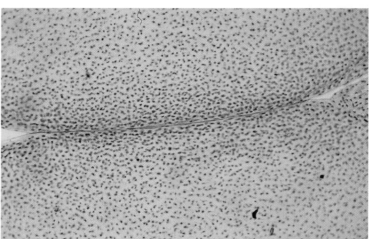

FIGURE 1.70 Photomicrograph of a sagittal section through the knee joint at the ninth week of gestation, showing the development of the joint space from the periphery towards the center of the joint (H & E, x 10 obj.).

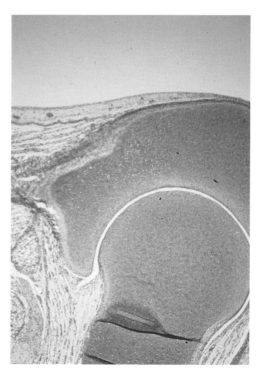

FIGURE 1.71 Photomicrograph of a section through the hip joint at the tenth week of gestation, showing a fully developed joint space (H & E, x 4 obj.).

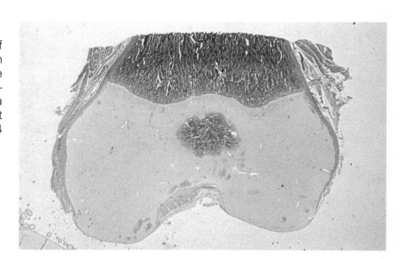

FIGURE 1.72 The secondary center of ossification is demonstrated in the lower end of the femur. This area increases in size by the process of maturation and calcification of the cartilage around the secondary center, with subsequent endochondral ossification (H & E, x 1 obj.).

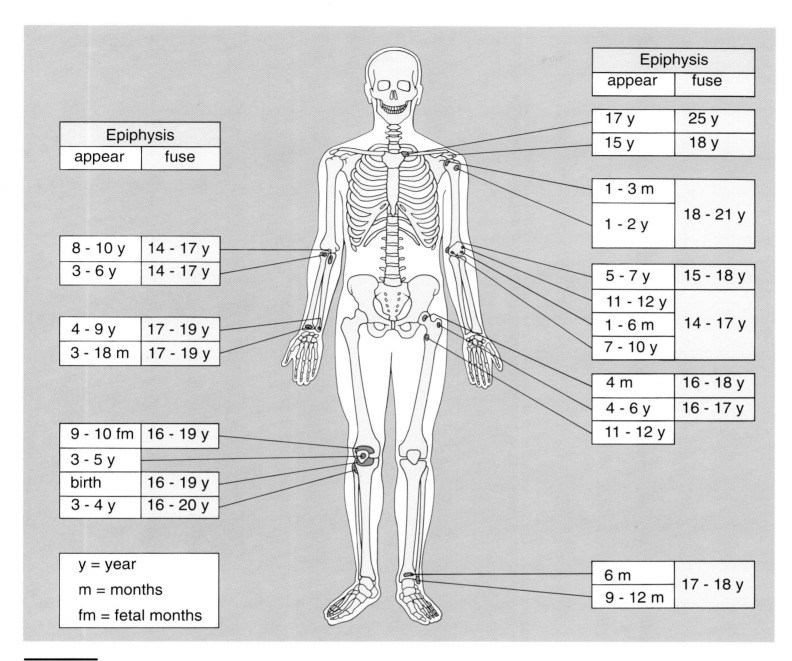

Epiphysis

appear	fuse
17 y	25 y
15 y	18 y

appear	fuse
1 - 3 m	
1 - 2 y	18 - 21 y

appear	fuse
5 - 7 y	15 - 18 y
11 - 12 y	
1 - 6 m	14 - 17 y
7 - 10 y	

appear	fuse
4 m	16 - 18 y
4 - 6 y	16 - 17 y
11 - 12 y	

appear	fuse
6 m	17 - 18 y
9 - 12 m	

Epiphysis

appear	fuse
8 - 10 y	14 - 17 y
3 - 6 y	14 - 17 y

appear	fuse
4 - 9 y	17 - 19 y
3 - 18 m	17 - 19 y

appear	fuse
9 - 10 fm	16 - 19 y
3 - 5 y	
birth	16 - 19 y
3 - 4 y	16 - 20 y

y = year

m = months

fm = fetal months

FIGURE 1.73 Schematic diagram showing of the times of ossification of the skeleton.

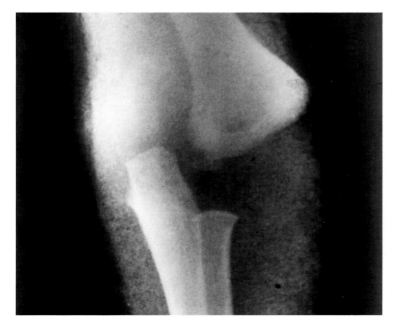

growth plate

secondary ossification center

cartilaginous epiphysis

FIGURE 1.74 The post-traumatic radiograph of a 2-year-old child illustrates the importance of full awareness of the secondary centers of ossification. It might initially appear that there has been a dislocation of the elbow. However, since the ossification center of the capitulum is still in place, it can be inferred that the joint is intact and the displacement of the humerus results from a fracture through the region of the growth plate.

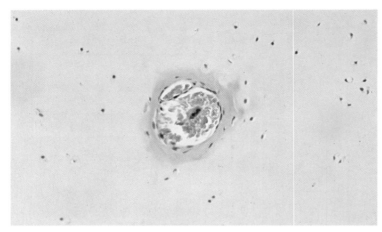

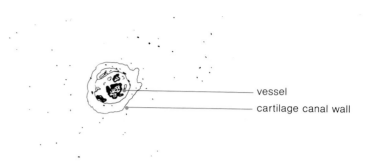

FIGURE 1.75 The vessels that feed the ossification center are carried in canals through the epiphyseal cartilage; one of these canals is demonstrated here (H & E, x 25 obj.).

vessel
cartilage canal wall

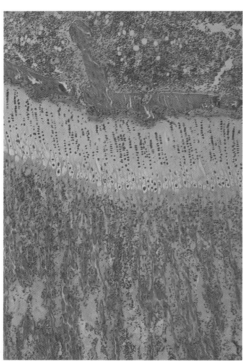

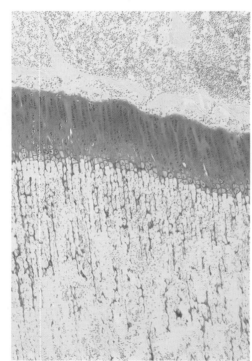

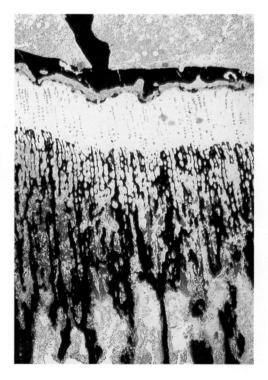

FIGURE 1.76 Photomicrograph demonstrating the appearance of the growth plate during active bone growth. At the top of the field is a portion of the epiphysis, and the cartilage cells in this region are proliferating cells. Further down the cells begin to pal-isade into vertical columns, and as they approach the metaphysis the cells hypertrophy and the matrix calcifies. The calcified matrix is then invaded by blood vessels. (*left,* H & E; *center,* safranin O; *right,* von Kossa; all x 4 obj.)

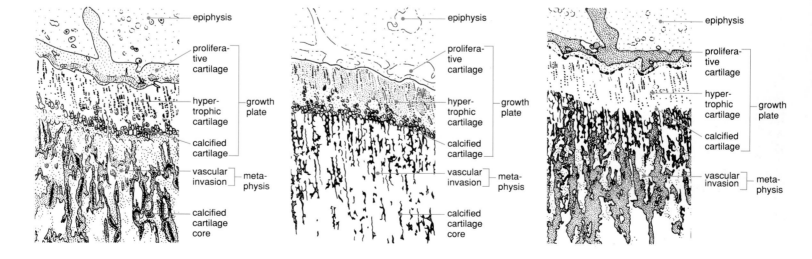

embryonal cartilage (Fig. 1.75). As the secondary center of ossification grows, the only remaining cartilage is that which covers the articular end of the bone and a thin layer or plate of cartilage lying between the secondary center of ossification and the main part of the bone shaft. This plate is known as the growth plate or physis (Figs. 1.76 to 1.78).

The epiphysis therefore comprises the portion of the bone that lies between the growth plate or physis and the articular surface. The metaphysis is that portion just below the growth plate (the area occupied by the primary spongiosa) and, in general, corresponds to the flared zone in the shaft below the growth plate. The diaphysis is the portion that lies between the two metaphyses. The cartilage of the growth plates continues to proliferate and to undergo endochondral ossification until apparent growth ceases at adolescence. At adolescence the growth plate is perforated by blood vessels

and becomes obliterated (Fig. 1.79). However, a trace of the growth plate scar continues in the form of an epiphyseal bone plate, which is recognizable on radiologic examination and in anatomic specimens throughout life (Fig. 1.80). Acute illness may lead to a temporary cessation of growth, and the stigma of this cessation may remain for many years in the shaft of the bone as a linear density, known as a Harris line or growth arrest line, paralleling the epiphyseal scar (Fig. 1.81).

The bones of the skull, as well as some of the facial bones and most of the clavicle form in the same manner as the initial periosteal bone cuff, ie, without a preexisting cartilage model, from undifferentiated connective tissue cells (mesenchyme). These bones are termed membranous bones, and they grow only by the apposition of new bone on the surface. Membranous bones have no cartilaginous growth plates (Figs. 1.82, 1.83, and 1.84).

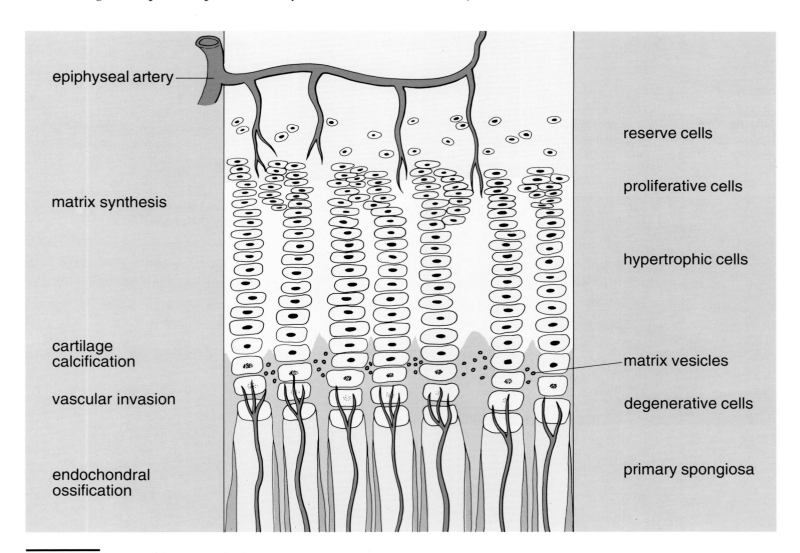

FIGURE 1.77 Diagram of the growth plate.

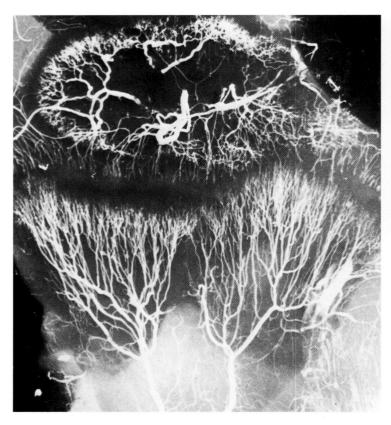

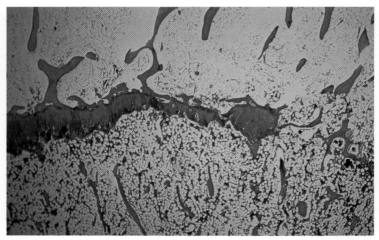

FIGURE 1.79 Photomicrograph of the epiphyseal growth plate from the upper end of the tibia in a 17-year-old boy. Although the growth plate is still open on the left side of the field, it can be seen at the right side that a bony continuity has been established between the metaphysis and the epiphysis. At this point growth can be said to have ceased. In general, the plate first closes in its central portion, and the peripheral portion of the plate is the last part to close (H & E, x 4 obj.).

FIGURE 1.78 Specimen of the upper end of the tibia in an immature pig. The vessels have been injected with barium sulfate and the bone decalcified. The ramifying vessels in the metaphysis which provide for endochondral ossification are clearly seen.

FIGURE 1.80 Radiograph of the ankle in an adult shows the epiphyseal scar in the lower end of the tibia.

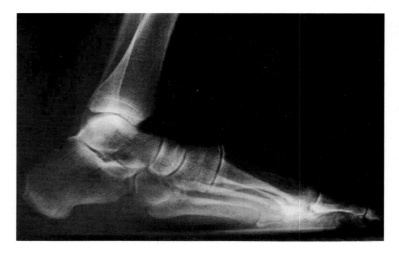

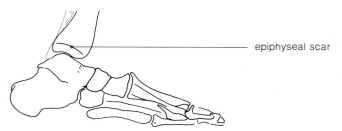

epiphyseal scar

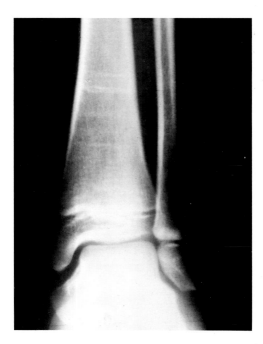

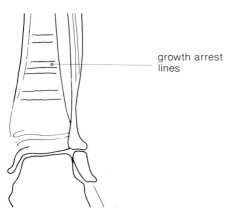

FIGURE 1.81 Radiograph of the tibia in a child with an open epiphyseal plate. In the shaft of the tibia a number of radiopaque lines are clearly visible, representing episodes of growth arrest.

growth arrest lines

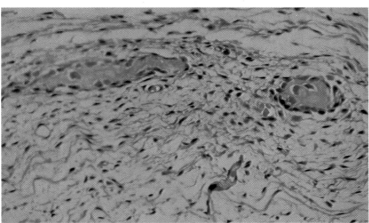

FIGURE 1.82 Photomicrograph of a section taken through the skull area of an 11-week fetus. The bone presents first as cell condensations which secrete an extracellular matrix of immature bone (H & E, x 16 obj.). Two islands of bone matrix are clearly seen in the upper third of the section.

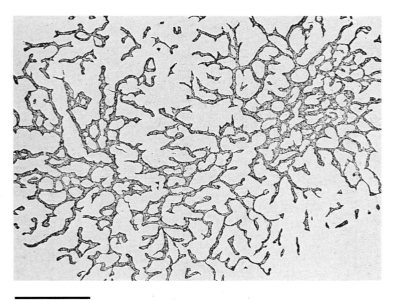

FIGURE 1.83 Drawing of a macerated specimen of the parietal bone demonstrates how individual foci of secreted bone matrix fuse together to form first a network of bone and later a plate.

FIGURE 1.84 Photomicrograph of a calvarial bone from a 19-week fetus shows a section through the bone plate. The dural surface is on the lower border of the field, and the epidermal surface is on the upper border. Note the resorptive activity along the dural surface and the blastic activity along the epidermal surface, which allows for expansion of the cranium (H & E, x 4 obj.).

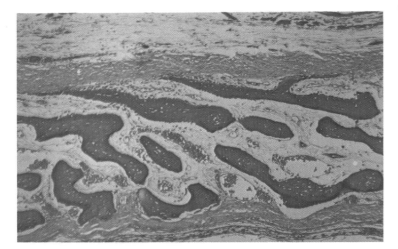

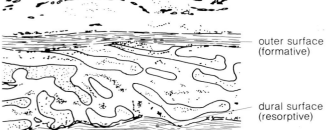

outer surface (formative)

dural surface (resorptive)

Methods of examination

The techniques used by the pathologist to examine diseased tissue are dealt with exhaustively in a number of texts and will not be discussed in detail here. However, for the general reader to fully comprehend the topic under discussion some aspects of tissue examination need to be understood, and these aspects are dealt with in this chapter.

GROSS EXAMINATION

Bone specimens received by the surgical pathologist often consist only of fragments, and the anatomic site cannot be recognized. When it is important for the fragments to be differentiated, it is the surgeon's responsibility to ensure that the individual pieces are separately submitted and correctly labeled. On the other hand, when a larger piece of bone is submitted, anatomic landmarks should be carefully sought. If a photographic record is warranted, careful dissection of the soft tissue adherent to the bone surface will prepare the specimen for photography at this stage. Photographs without this step are likely to be morphologically less informative and visually disappointing (Fig. 2.1).

Cutting the specimen into thin slices (3 to 5 mm) will enable one to get an impression of the appearance of the interior of the bone and will also ensure proper fix-

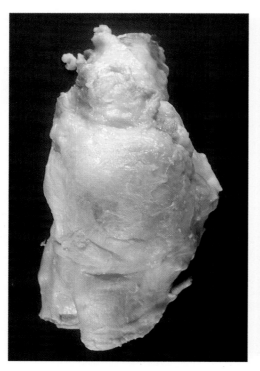
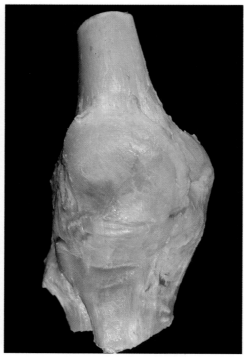

FIGURE 2.1 *(left)* Photograph of partially dissected knee joint. The residual soft tissues obscure the anatomy. *(right)* Once the remnants of muscle and fat are dissected away the gross anatomy of the knee is more obvious.

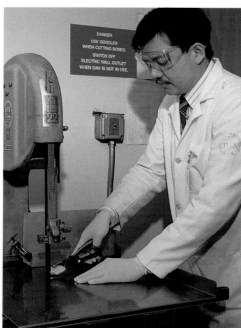
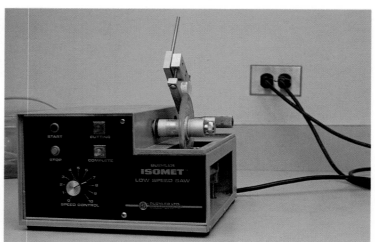

FIGURE 2.2 *(left)* A band saw is used to cut large specimens. Note that soft tissue left attached to the bone is liable to catch in the saw blade and be torn. *(right)* Small pieces of bone can be cut on a circular saw such as shown here, using a diamond blade and a micrometer screw to advance the specimen.

ation. Large specimens can be cut on a band saw, and smaller specimens on a small circular saw (Fig. 2.2). After sawing the bone, it is important to wash the cut surface of the tissue carefully under running water, brushing gently with a soft nailbrush. This procedure ensures that any fragments of bone dust and other tissue debris generated by the sawing are washed out of the interstices of the marrow space. Unless this is done, microscopic artifacts will appear on the histological sections (see below).

Visual examination of the cut surface is particularly helpful with tumors in which the character of the tissue may enable one to assess the viability of the tumor and, in some cases, to make a preliminary diagnosis, eg, car-

tilage tumors or aneurysmal bone cysts (Fig. 2.3). It may also be useful for assessment of an infiltrative condition, such as lymphoma, or a metabolic disturbance, such as Gaucher's disease, in both of which the normal red or yellow marrow is replaced by a somewhat firmer tissue with a pink, fleshy appearance. Bone necrosis is easily recognized because of its opaque yellow appearance, in contrast to the translucent appearance of living bone tissue (Fig. 2.4). We have found that a dissecting microscope mounted directly over the grossing area in the surgical pathology laboratory is particularly useful for recognition of morbid anatomy and for correlating the gross appearance of a tissue with the microscopic histology (Fig. 2.5).

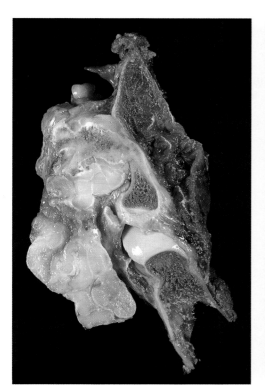

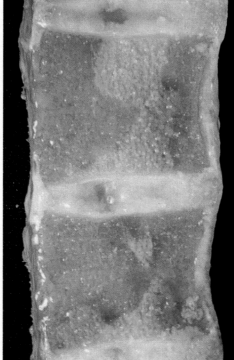

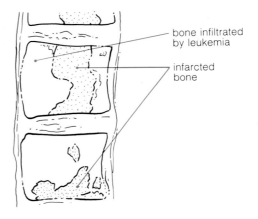

FIGURE 2.4 Segment of the spine from a child who died of leukemia. Within the vertebral bodies are geographic areas of necrosis which appear as yellow opacification of the bone and marrow. These are surrounded by a thin rim of hyperemic tissue. Note that the viable bone marrow has a fleshy tan color, reflecting the leukemia infiltrate.

bone infiltrated by leukemia

infarcted bone

FIGURE 2.3 This patient had a large tumor projecting from the scapula surface. The glassy blue-white appearance is most consistent with a tumor of cartilaginous origin.

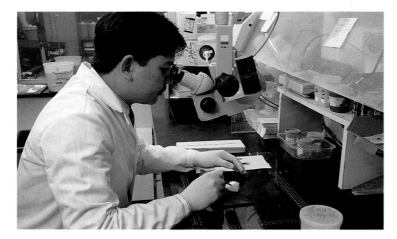

FIGURE 2.5 Photograph of the dissecting microscope used in the grossing area of the surgical pathology laboratory at the Hospital for Special Surgery.

The pathologist should also assess the texture and the porosity of the bone, whether increased or decreased from normal. Although this is often done by a prosector who presses on the tissue with his thumb, this practice should be avoided because it distorts the microscopic histology. Porosity and texture are much better assessed radiographically.

RADIOGRAPHIC EXAMINATION OF BONE SPECIMENS

A useful adjunct to gross visual examination of bone specimens is the preparation of radiographs using low-voltage x-rays (Faxitron; *Field Emission Corporation*, McMinnville, OR) and industrial film (Kodalith Orthofilm type 3) (Fig. 2.6). The detail revealed by such films depends on the thickness of the specimen: the thinner the slice, the more detail will be revealed (Fig. 2.7). The radiograph is particularly useful for assessing alterations in bone texture and organization (Fig. 2.8). It can be helpful in finding a lesion that may not be apparent on gross examination, such as the nidus of an osteoid osteoma (Fig. 2.9). The radiograph is also a useful guide in deciding which portions of the tissue should be submitted for microscopic examination (Fig. 2.10).

SPECIMEN PHOTOGRAPHY

Thirty-five millimeter color photographs are useful both for research and for teaching purposes. In either case, as mentioned earlier, before taking the photograph the specimen must be adequately cleaned so that the bone and the lesion area are readily recognizable. It should be carefully washed and dried so that there are no abnormal highlights from reflections of the floodlamps, and also so that the lesion areas are clearly demarcated from normal tissue. The specimen for photography should be aligned according to anatomic principles. A scale should also be included in the photograph (Fig. 2.11).

For publication purposes, it is sometimes necessary to prepare black-and-white photographs, a generally

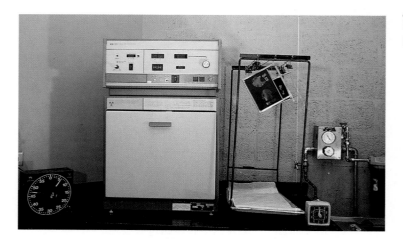

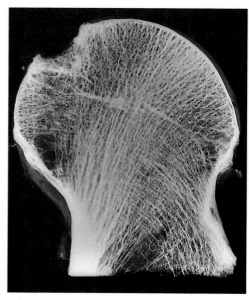

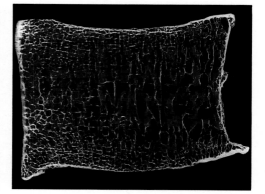

FIGURE 2.6 In a small darkroom adjacent to the surgical pathology laboratory is a low-voltage x-ray machine, shown here.

FIGURE 2.7 (*left*) Radiograph of a slice of the femoral head, 5 mm thick. (*right*) Radiograph of a slice of a vertebral body <1 mm thick. Less overlay of structure results in improved discrimination.

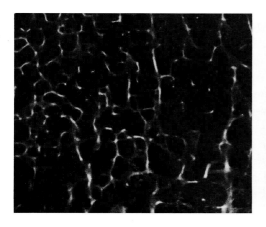
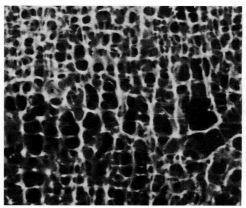
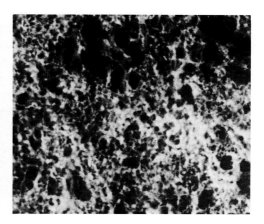

FIGURE 2.8 Radiographs of osteopenic *(left)*, normal *(center)*, and osteosclerotic *(right)*, vertebrae demonstrate the relative radiolucency *(left)* and density *(right)* of bone in two pathologic conditions. The normal vertebra has readily identifiable vertical and horizontal bone trabeculae.

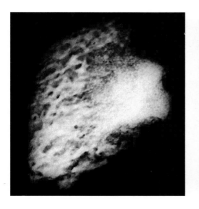
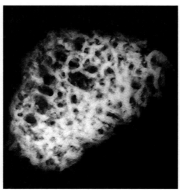

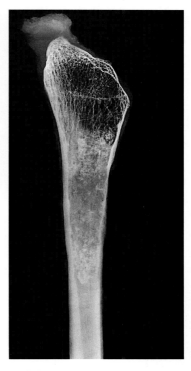

FIGURE 2.10 Radiograph of the upper end of a fibula resected because of an intra-osseous tumor. The margins of the tumor are clearly seen on the radiograph, which is therefore an excellent guide to mapping of the section.

FIGURE 2.9 Thirteen fragments of bone were submitted from a patient with an osteoid osteoma. *(left)* Fragment 6 showed a portion of the nidus, recognizable by the dense, finely packed area of bone. *(right)* Compare with fragment 13, which is entirely cancellous bone.

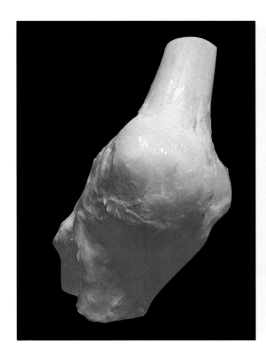
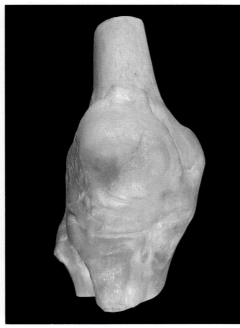

FIGURE 2.11 *(left)* This photograph shows a number of photographic errors, including dirty background, slight lack of focus on the front of the patella, highlights caused by an improperly dried specimen, poor positioning, poor lighting, and no scale or identification. *(right)* A more correctly taken photograph of the same specimen for comparison.

difficult procedure owing to the uniformity of color normally present and especially because of the natural translucency of the tissue. The usual photographic methods using white light, which has a broad wavelength range, result in variable penetration of light into the translucent object, thereby precluding a sharp focus. These problems can be largely overcome by the use of short-wave monochromatic light. For this purpose, we have found a black (UV) light source to be inexpensive and to provide very satisfactory photographs (Figs. 2.12 and 2.13).

PREPARATION OF TISSUE FOR MICROSCOPIC EXAMINATION

Preparation of tissue sections containing the maximum information depends on choice of the right piece of tissue and on proper processing of the tissue blocks.

To ensure adequate penetration of the processing fluids, the submitted tissues should not exceed 3 to 4 mm in thickness. It is important to use an adequate amount of fresh solution for fixation, because the fixative is being used up in the process. Far too frequently, specimens from the operating room are received barely covered by fixative, and irreversible tissue breakdown may have taken place as a result of inadequate fixation.

In general, the volume of fixative should be at least ten times the volume of the tissue. For most purposes, formalin provides adequate fixation. However, the formalin should be buffered to prevent the formation of formalin pigment, which can interfere with the proper interpretation of other pigments that may be present, such as iron or gold. Buffering the formalin also prevents the formation of formic acid, which might otherwise result in undesirable decalcification.

If decalcification is desired after adequate fixation of the tissue, 5% nitric acid will produce decalcification in a reasonable time with good preservation of the tis-

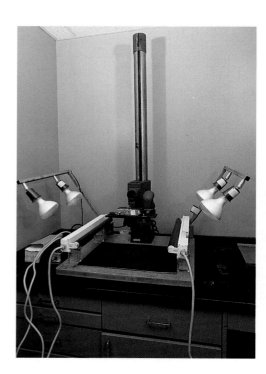

FIGURE 2.12 Illustration of the set-up used in our laboratory for UV photography. When in use, a developed x-ray film is used for the background to the specimen. Apart from the UV lights the other lights in the room are switched off.

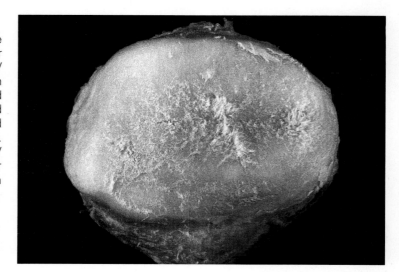

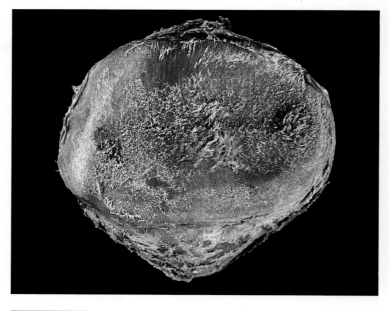

FIGURE 2.13 The articular surface of a patella with early degenerative joint disease. *(top)* Photograph with white floods as illumination. *(bottom)* The same illuminated only with black (UV) light.

sue. However, an adequate volume of acid should be used, approximately ten to twenty times that of the tissue. Because the acid is neutralized as the calcium is removed from the bone, it should be changed frequently; in our laboratory we change the acid twice a day. To ensure access of the acid to the tissue, gentle agitation using a shaker is a helpful procedure (Fig. 2.14). The adequacy of decalcification can be assessed by preparing radiographs of the specimens, and this can be done with the tissues in their cassettes (Fig. 2.15).

After decalcification has been achieved, it is essential to wash the tissue adequately in running water for at least 12 hours, to ensure good differentiation of the hematoxylin and eosin stain. If the bone tissue is overdecalcified or if the acid is inadequately removed, poor staining will result.

For paraffin embedding of the tissue, the use of a vacuum, which is available in most modern processing machines, is strongly recommended to achieve better infiltration, thus making sectioning easier and ensuring better sections.

The preparation of histologic sections of bones for routine microscopic examination has, in general, required the removal of the inorganic mineral component by acidic solutions, as just described. For this reason, the quantity and quality of mineralization have been impossible to assess. The technique of embedding bone in methyl methacrylate, although very time consuming, not only allows thin histologic sections of bone to be cut without prior decalcification but also has the considerable advantage of achieving a better preservation of tissue relationships. Because of the tough col-

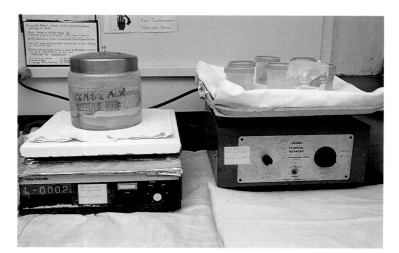

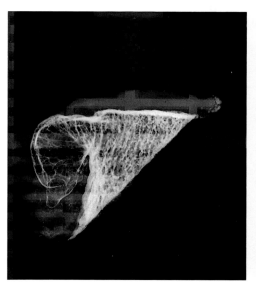

FIGURE 2.14 A shaker ensures adequate mixing of the acid and that it gets to the surface of the bone. Shown here are a shaker and a magnetic stirrer used for the same purpose.

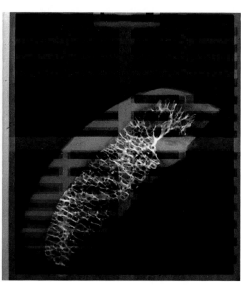 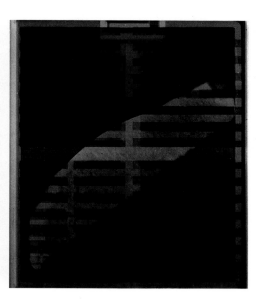

FIGURE 2.15 Radiograph of three bone specimens in their cassettes, showing the stages of decalcification.

lagenous nature of the organic matrix, such preservation is often difficult to obtain when routine paraffin embedding is used (Fig. 2.16).

Bone can also be prepared for electron microscopy by fixing diced tissue in paraformaldehyde or in glutaraldehyde. The tissue can be decalcified using EDTA, or the calcified tissue can be sectioned with a diamond knife.

Stains

A variety of staining techniques are used to demonstrate the different components of the matrix. Collagen can be demonstrated by a trichrome stain or the van Gieson stain (Fig. 2.17). (As we shall see later under the discussion of microscopic examination, perhaps the most useful technique for examining collagen is polarized light microscopy.) The proteoglycans can be demonstrated by the safranin O stain, the alcian blue stain, and less specifically by toluidine blue and periodic acid–Schiff (PAS) (Fig. 2.18). Mineral components, can be demonstrated only in undemineralized tissue, and the mineral can be stained by two techniques: alizarin red, which stains the calcium components of hydroxyapatite red, and the von Kossa method, which stains the phosphate component as well as other calcium salts (eg, carbonate and oxalate), black (Fig. 2.19). The distribution of mineral in the tissue can also be studied by microradiography, using low-kilovoltage x-rays from an x-ray tube with a fine focal spot. These radiographs are prepared using thin slices of bone cut with a diamond saw at approximately 100 μm (Fig. 2.20). A fine-grained film (as is generally used with light photography) should be used to facilitate low-power microscopic examination. This will naturally require a correspondingly longer exposure than is needed with a coarse-grained x-ray film.

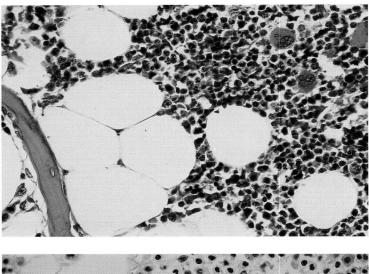

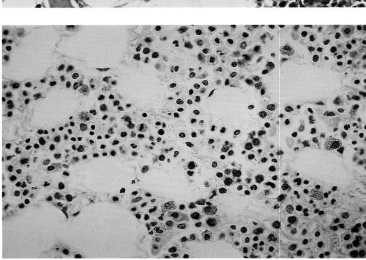

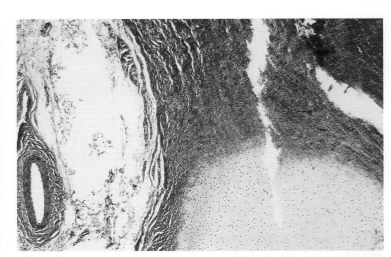

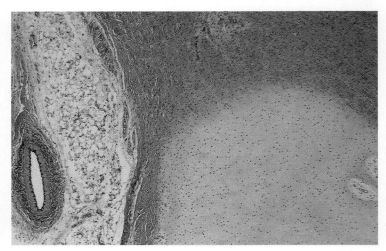

FIGURE 2.16 *(top)* Photomicrograph of a section of bone marrow decalcified and embedded in paraffin. *(bottom)* Photomicrograph of a section of bone marrow undecalcified and embedded in methyl methacrylate. Note that this is a thinner section than that demonstrated above and therefore has more cytologic detail without obscuring overlay (both views H & E, x 10 obj.).

FIGURE 2.17 *(top)* Photomicrograph of a portion of developing cartilage, tendon, and vascularized adipose tissue stained by Masson's trichrome stain. Muscle stains red, as seen in the media of the artery in the lower left, and collagen stains blue. *(bottom)* The same tissue stained with Verhoeff's elastic stain (van Gieson as counterstain), where the collagen stains red and the elastic tissue black. The muscle fibers stain yellow-green (x 4 obj.).

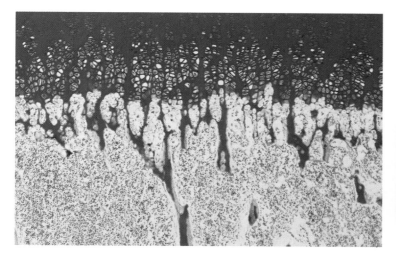

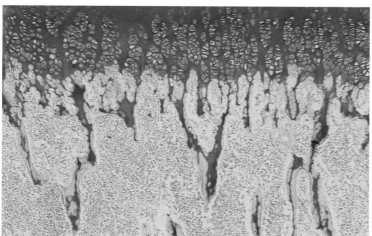

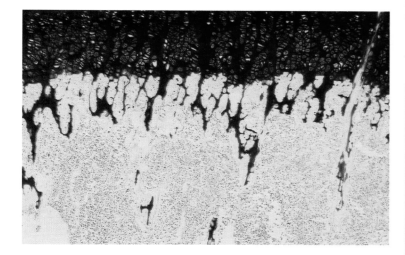

FIGURE 2.18 Photomicrograph of a portion of growth plate and underlying metaphysis stained with safranin O *(top)*, alcian blue *(center)*, and toluidine blue *(bottom)*. With toluidine blue the cartilage is stained purple, ie, it exhibits metachromasia (x 4 obj.).

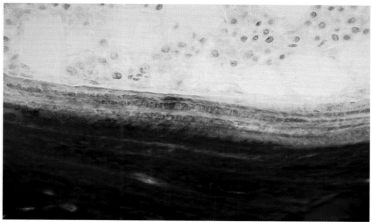

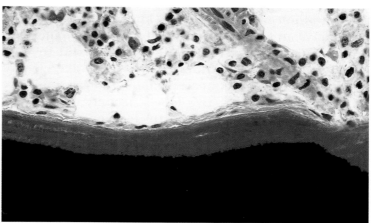

FIGURE 2.19 *(top)* Section of undecalcified bone stained with alizarin red, which stains the calcium salts red. The osteoid is counterstained with azure blue (alizarin red, x 10 obj.). *(bottom)* Section of undecalcified bone stained by the von Kossa method, in which the calcium salts are stained black. The osteoid is counterstained with acid fuchsin (von Kossa, x 10 obj.).

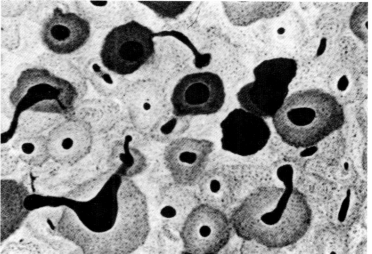

FIGURE 2.20 Microradiograph of a portion of cortical bone, to show the variation in the calcium content of various osteons and the generally increased calcium content of the interstitial osteons (x 10 obj.).

Osteoblasts and osteoclasts can be stained using alkaline phosphatase and acid phosphatase stains, respectively. These stains can be done on unfixed frozen sections or on glycol methacrylate sections prepared after brief fixation.

Antibodies prepared against various collagen types and against constituents of proteoglycan aggregates have been used as investigative tools to study the distribution of the matrix constituents. Immunoperoxide staining has been proven useful for the identification of various mesenchymal tumors.

Fluorescence Labeling

The autofluorescing antibiotics known as the tetracyclines have an affinity for mineral at actively mineralizing surfaces. They serve well as supravital in vivo markers of mineralization because they are clearly visualized when a section is examined microscopically using ultraviolet light. Two labels, usually of different tetracyclines, must be used to determine both the extent and the rate of mineralization. The protocol for tetracycline labeling used in our laboratory is as follows: 250 mg of oral oxytetracycline are given four times a day for three days. After an interval of 12 days, demeclocycline, 300 mg four times a day, is given for a further three days. The bone biopsy is then performed four to seven days after the last dose of demeclocycline. The specimen is fixed in 70% alcohol, which helps to protect against leaching of both the label and the mineral from the tissue. Unstained sections should always be stored in the dark. At the time of fluorescence microscopy they should be covered with an optically inactive oil for optimal visualization of the label. In our experience, 5 µm thick sections are adequate for the visualization of properly applied labels. In a normal biopsy, both single and double labels may be observed, and these labels are usually sharp and distinct (Fig. 2.21). In case of certain metabolic disturbances the labels have specific morphologic features that reflect the condition of the mineralizing bone–osteoid interface (see Chapter 7).

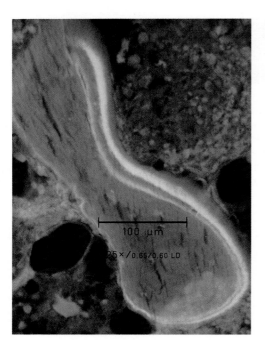

FIGURE 2.21 Photomicrograph showing two distinct tetracycline labels. The yellow label is demeclocyline, the green oxytetracycline. The scale is superimposed at the time of photography (ultraviolet, x 25 obj.).

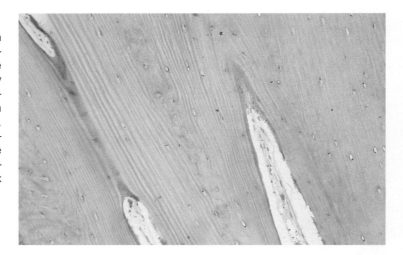

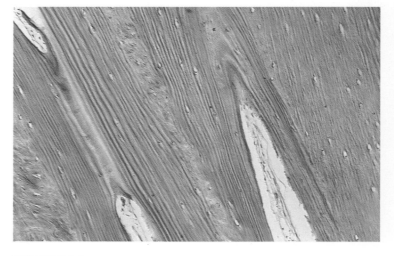

FIGURE 2.22 (top) Photomicrograph of a longitudinal section of cortical bone (H & E, x 10 obj.). (bottom) The same field as illustrated above photographed using Nomarski optics (H & E, x 10 obj.).

MICROSCOPIC EXAMINATION

In addition to the commonly used transmitted light optical microscopy, a number of other techniques are particularly useful for examination of connective tissues. Differential interference contrast (DIC, or Nomarski optics) is especially valuable because it provides a pseudo-three-dimensional appearance to the tissue, which can be helpful in understanding the structure. In addition, this system gives some improvement of resolution, so that the resulting photographic images are somewhat clearer than those obtained with transmitted light microscopy (Fig. 2.22).

Perhaps the most useful microscopic technique utilizes polarized light, especially for the examination of connective tissues, not only because it clearly reveals the collagen fibers but also because it enables one to determine the orientation of the collagen and to study the microarchitecture of the tissue (Fig. 2.23). This information can be very helpful in the interpretation of disease states, eg, Paget's disease, or in delineating reparative scars.

An important diagnostic procedure in the clinical diagnosis of crystal synovitis is the examination of synovial fluid for crystals, which also requires the use of polarized light microscopy. Performance of this examination requires a polarizing microscope with a compensating first-order red filter. (See Chapter 11 for a complete discussion of this procedure.)

Sodium urate crystals are usually needle-shaped and show strong negative birefringence; that is, they appear bright yellow when aligned parallel with the line on the compensating filter. Calcium pyrophosphate dihydrate crystals are usually rhomboidal crystals which show a weak positive birefringence, ie, when their long axis is aligned with the line on the compensating filter they appear blue and much less bright than urate crystals. There are two important caveats to note. First, when a crystal is oriented at 90° to the line on the compensating filter it appears the opposite color to its color in the parallel orientation. Second, the shape of the crystal may be misleading, because pyrophosphate crystals are occasionally needle-shaped, and urate crystals may be broken up into short, squared-off fragments.

The most common and one of the most troublesome artifacts encountered in sections of bone is the presence in the marrow space of irregular fragments of basophilic material, that may be mistaken for tumor or some other morbid condition (Fig. 2.24). These frag-

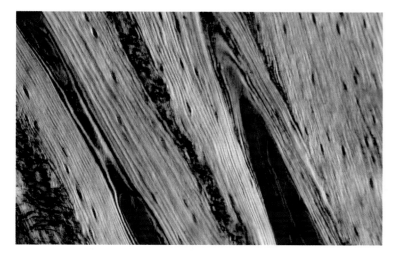

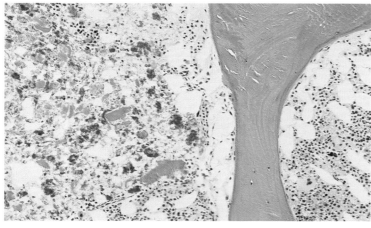

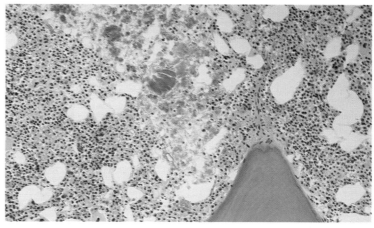

FIGURE 2.23 Photomicrograph of the same field as illustrated in Figure 2.22, photographed with polarized light (H & E, x 10 obj.).

FIGURE 2.24 Two examples of bone dust artifact. This artifact is common and can be avoided by washing the tissue after it has been cut on the saw and by cutting deeply into the block (H & E, x 4 obj.).

ments represent bone dust and other debris which is driven into the interstices of the bone during the slicing process. This artifact can be avoided by washing the surface after sawing and by cutting into the block before taking sections for microscopic examination.

HISTOMORPHOMETRY

Histomorphometry is the measurement of tissue and cell features on thin sections. Because of its rigid nature, bone is more suitable for histomorphometry than most other tissues, as the tissue and cell relationships are not significantly altered during proper processing and thin sectioning.

There are essentially two reasons to perform histomorphometry on bone: first, to quantify the features of bone tissue as they reflect cell activity in health and disease; and second, to study the structure of bone as a

mechanical system under normal and abnormal conditions (see Chapter 7).

Two methods are predominantly used for the routine generation of histomorphometric values: the manual and semiautomated methods. The manual method requires the use of integrating grids, usually set in the eyepiece of the microscope, which are optically overlaid onto the histologic section. In this method, the results of point and intercept counts provide the primary data from which the final figures are generated (Fig. 2.25). The semiautomated method employs a number of different computer-controlled procedures and devices, such as video monitors and digitizing tablets, for gathering and manipulating the primary data. In this method, an operator identifies the features of interest and the computer program automatically calculates the area and linear measurements and keeps track of the counts. Final results are then generated from these data (Fig. 2.26).

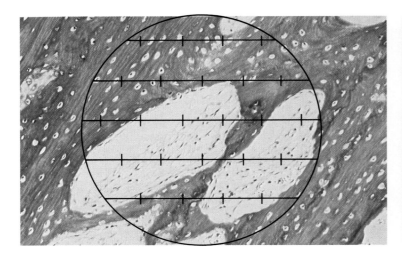

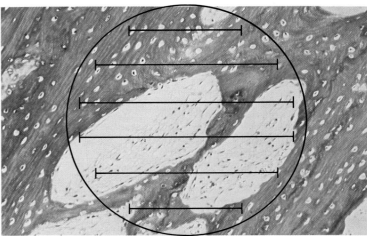

FIGURE 2.25 The types of integrating eye pieces employed to estimate various bone parameters. *(left)* The type I eyepiece is employed to estimate bone mass (volume). The eyepiece contains a series of lines on which are 25 points. Trabecular bone area is measured by recording the number of points that lie on bone. *(right)* The type II eyepiece contains a series of lines and is used to measure the extent of different bone surfaces. Total surface is recorded as the number of intersections of lines with bone surfaces, and each specific type of bone is estimated in a similar manner and expressed as a percentage of the total number of intersections.

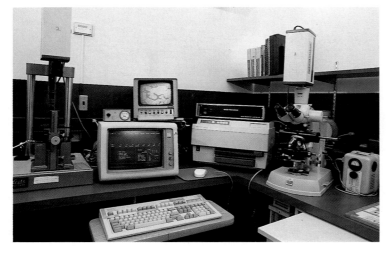

FIGURE 2.26 The semiautomated histomorphometry system used at the Hospital for Special Surgery.

SECTION II

RESPONSE TO EXOGENOUS INJURY

This section is concerned with the physiologic response to exogenous injuries. For most of human history the two greatest threats to survival have been trauma and infection; in the West, we sometimes tend to forget that this is still true for most people in other parts of the world.

Two important questions must be addressed when the effects of injury are considered. First, what happens to the cell, to the extracellular matrix, to the tissue, and to the organ when they are injured? Second, how does the body deal with injury and bring about repair?

These questions have formed the basis of pathology research for more than a hundred years, and the results of these investigations are reviewed in depth in a number of texts devoted to general pathology. For the sake of readers who are not pathologists, Chapter 3 briefly reviews the processes associated with injury and repair, especially mechanical trauma to and repair of connective tissue. It then considers some specific connective tissue injuries, including fracture repair, cartilage repair, and repair of a torn meniscus. Chapter 4 is concerned with the response of skeletal tissue to infection and its associated morbidity.

CHAPTER 3

Injury and repair

he publication in 1858 of Virchow's book, *Die Cellularpathologie in ihrer Begründung auf physiologische und pathologische Gewebelehre* (The Cellular Basis of Disease and Its Foundations in Physiology and Tissue Pathology), brought to the medical profession a completely new understanding of the fundamental nature of disease. For the first time, the cell was seen as the basic unit of the living organism, and alterations in cellular function were seen as being ultimately responsible for disease states. Thus pathology, the study of disease, was no longer to be limited to gross anatomic description. It is this correlation of molecular biology, physics, and chemistry with anatomy that is the key to our present and future understanding.

Some of the most fundamental questions for the pathologist are as follows: what happens to a cell, and to the tissue of which the cell is a unit, after injury? How much injury can the cell sustain before it dies? How does the body deal with the injured cells and effect repair?

EFFECTS OF INJURY

In pathology reports, as well as in other medical reports, a commonly used term is "degeneration" or "degenerative change." This terminology is more emotive than substantive. We would be better informed if a pathology report detailed the etiology of and the response to the injury. For example, instead of "fragment of degenerated intervertebral disc," a better descriptive diagnosis would be "fragment of lacerated anulus fibrosus with granulation tissue and early scarring."

Degeneration is defined in the Oxford Dictionary as "A morbid change in the structure of parts consisting in a disintegration of tissue or in a substitution of a lower for a higher form of structure." Such a disintegration may simply be the normal result of getting older. It may also be the result of disuse atrophy or of abuse (injury). Although degeneration caused by injury is the subject of this chapter, it is important to bear in mind that injury is not the only cause of degeneration.

FIGURE 3.1 Diagram of a cell showing the basic cytoplasmic organelles and their function.

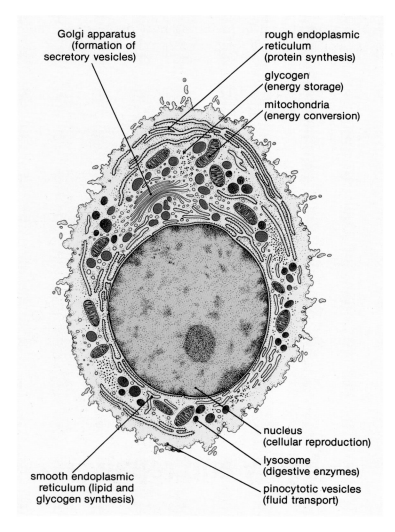

Golgi apparatus
(formation of
secretory vesicles)

rough endoplasmic
reticulum
(protein synthesis)

glycogen
(energy storage)

mitochondria
(energy conversion)

nucleus
(cellular reproduction)

lysosome
(digestive enzymes)

smooth endoplasmic
reticulum (lipid and
glycogen synthesis)

pinocytotic vesicles
(fluid transport)

Injury may be caused by physical agents (mechanical trauma, extremes in temperature, or ionizing radiation), chemicals, or biologic agents (bacteria, viruses, fungi, or other organisms). Regardless of the etiology, two effects can be expected: a local effect at the site of injury, and a general effect on the body as a whole. (Shock following severe hemorrhage in association with an open fracture is an example of the generalized effect of injury.)

The cell is a complex structure in which the basic processes of energy conversion, protein synthesis, and other vital activities are constantly taking place (Fig. 3.1). Each cell exists in an ever-changing environment, and its ability to adapt to new conditions determines its continued functional activity. Injury to the cell occurs when conditions in the local environment are such that the cell is unable to maintain its physiologic equilibrium.

The physiologic results of injury are altered synthesis (anabolism) and/or altered breakdown (catabolism). The nature of the injurious agent and the duration of its application determine which process predominates. If only transient alterations occur in the intracellular or extracellular regulatory mechanisms, the cell may revert to its normal basal state when the adverse conditions cease. A more severe yet sublethal injury may result in adaptive changes, recognizable microscopically by the presence of hypertrophy, atrophy, or hyperplasia. When the insult is lethal, the necrosis (death) of the cell can be recognized microscopically by loss of staining, disintegration of the nucleus, and breakdown of the cell membranes.

Because of the variability in types of injury and the widely differing susceptibility of various body tissues, it is difficult to generalize about the morphologic effects of injury. However, mechanical injury usually causes cell disruption; freezing depresses cell metabolism and

ultimately leads to the formation of destructive intracytoplasmic ice crystals; heat increases rates of metabolism, enzyme inactivation, and protein coagulation and, at extreme temperature, may even cause tissue charring. The effects of ionizing radiation are focused mostly on the nucleus, where it causes chromosome breakage and gene mutation. Chemicals act either locally or systemically by interfering with metabolic processes in the cell, especially by inactivation of enzymes and also by denaturation of cellular protein. Finally, many biologic agents manufacture toxins that cause disturbances of cell metabolism.

In addition to the types of injurious agents (physical, chemical, or biologic), other considerations affect the degree of injury. Among these is the intensity of application of an injurious agent, which may eventually result in irreversible cell damage. Another consideration is the site of injury. For example, anoxia rapidly produces irreversible damage to brain cells and cardiac muscle, whereas connective tissue can usually withstand anoxia for considerable periods of time. Furthermore, the effects of injury are influenced by the individual's general health, including nutritional state, the presence or absence of drugs in the body, and so on.

HISTOLOGIC OBSERVATIONS

The most commonly observed microscopic change associated with altered cell homeostasis is a change in cell volume. This results from the cell's loss of ability to regulate electrolyte and fluid metabolism, owing to altered function of the mitochondria and the cell membrane. Hypoxia, which affects lipoproteins as well as protein synthesis and secretion, may lead to accumulation of lipid droplets in cells and of amorphous eosinophilic material in both the cell and the extracellular space (Fig. 3.2).

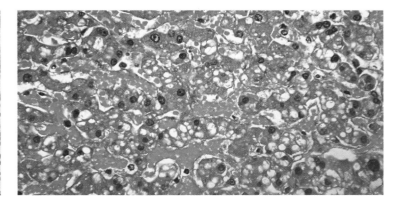

FIGURE 3.2 Cell changes due to hypoxia are well demonstrated in these photomicrographs of the centrilobular part of the liver. (*left*) On the left can be seen normal liver tissue, while on the right some vacuolization is apparent within the cytoplasm and there is swelling of the cell outline. (*right*) In tissue adjacent to the central veins, congestion of the liver sinuses is readily apparent, with marked vacuolization and some shrinkage and darkening of nuclei also in evidence. This appearance is characteristic and indicative of chronic anoxic conditions (H & E, x 25 obj.).

A fundamental characteristic of living cells is their ability to sense and to adapt to changes in the environment. This ability to adjust enables cells to survive under conditions that might otherwise prove lethal. Such adaptations, which include atrophy, hypertrophy, and hyperplasia, are commonly observed in the course of many disease processes (Fig. 3.3).

Atrophy

Atrophy refers to a decrease in the size and activity of a cell, and is particularly striking clinically when it occurs in the musculoskeletal or the central nervous system. It may occur as an adaptation to diminished use, or as a result of reduction in blood supply, poor nutrition, or a decrease in normal hormonal stimulation. Cell atrophy is usually accompanied by shrinkage of the affected organ. In parenchymal organs, atrophy may result solely from a decrease in cell size. However, in the later stages of disease the decrease in cell size may also be accompanied by actual loss of cells. In con-

nective tissue, atrophy may be more difficult to recognize. It is caused by a loss of the extracellular matrix, which in turn reflects an alteration in cell activity.

Hypertrophy

Hypertrophy refers to an increase in cell size caused by augmentation of the intracellular organelles, especially the endoplasmic reticulum; as a result, protein synthesis is generally enhanced. Hypertrophy is frequently a compensatory reaction, as in the heart muscles of patients with increased cardiac workload who develop an increased number of myofibrils.

Hyperplasia

Hyperplasia, an increase in the number of cells, is commonly seen in the synovium of patients with arthritis. The accelerated breakdown of the joint constituents (cartilage and bone) that occurs in all forms of arthritis leads to enhanced phagocytosis by the synovium. This

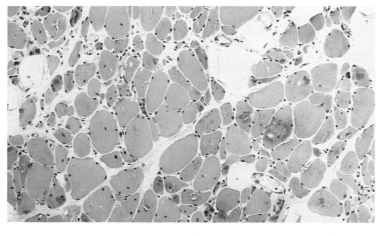

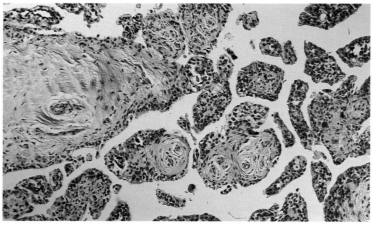

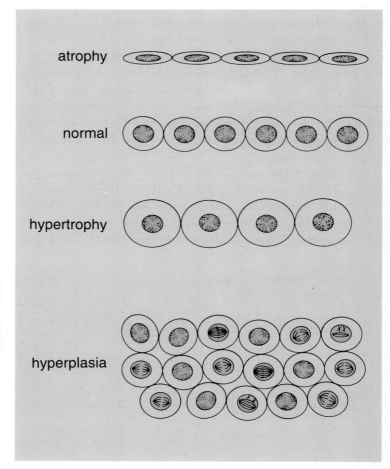

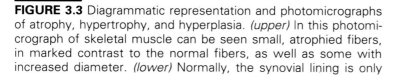

FIGURE 3.3 Diagrammatic representation and photomicrographs of atrophy, hypertrophy, and hyperplasia. *(upper)* In this photomicrograph of skeletal muscle can be seen small, atrophied fibers, in marked contrast to the normal fibers, as well as some with increased diameter. *(lower)* Normally, the synovial lining is only one cell thick; however, in this photomicrograph of the synovial lining from a patient with chronic osteoarthritis, one can readily see a marked proliferation of synoviocytes, characteristic of hyperplastic condition (H & E, x 4 obj.).

increased activity is associated with augmentation of the synovial lining cells, thus increasing not only the thickness of the synovial lining but also the absolute area of the synovium, which is frequently thrown up into papillary projections that extend into the joint cavity.

Necrosis

Cell necrosis (death) is usually recognized microscopically by changes in the nucleus. These changes include swelling of the nucleus, which is followed by condensation of the nuclear chromatin (pyknosis) and finally by dissolution of the nucleus (karyolysis) (Fig. 3.4).

The gross and microscopic appearance of necrotic tissue depends on the organ involved and on the type and extent of injury. In tissue necrosis associated with sudden and complete cessation of the blood supply (an infarct), the affected tissue usually has an opaque appearance and a firm consistency, like boiled egg white. Microscopic examination of infarcted tissue usually reveals maintenance of structural anatomy, with preservation of the ghost-like outlines of the cells (Fig. 3.5). Conversely, in most bacterial injuries the cells are totally broken down, resulting in a soft area of necrotic

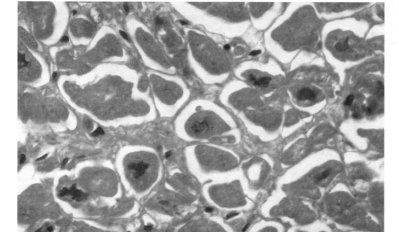

FIGURE 3.4 High-power photomicrograph of necrotizing myocardium shows a number of dense, shrunken and fragmented nuclei, characteristic of cell necrosis (H & E, x 40 obj.).

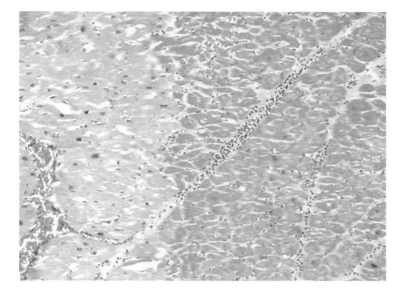

FIGURE 3.5 The right side of this photomicrograph of myocardial tissue exhibits fibers with granular, eosinophilic cytoplasm devoid of nuclei. In addition, acute inflammatory infiltration between the muscle fibers and along the course of the myocar-dial capillaries can be seen. All of these features are characteristic of necrotic tissue. By contrast, note the pale cytoplasm and intact nuclei in the normal, viable tissue on the left (H & E, x 4 obj.).

material in which no structural elements of the cell are recognizable microscopically (Fig. 3.6).

Necrosis may be easily overlooked in connective tissue, because the extracellular matrix which gives form to the tissue is often unchanged. In bone, the most obvious evidence of necrosis can be seen in the marrow, either as fat necrosis and dystrophic calcification or as ghosting of the hematopoietic tissue (Fig. 3.7). Changes in the osteocytes may be difficult to recognize (Fig. 3.8). In cartilage, ghosting or calcification of the chondrocytes is a frequent finding in osteoarthritis (Fig. 3.9). Inflammatory arthritis is often characterized by enlarge-

ment of the chondrocyte lacunae, which contain either pyknotic nuclei or no obvious cellular elements; these are referred to as Weichselbaum's lacunae (Fig. 3.10).

Calcification

Dead tissue that does not undergo rapid absorption frequently becomes calcified. This type of calcification, which is not related to a disturbance in calcium homeostasis as in the case of metabolic dysfunction, is called dystrophic calcification. It is common in areas of infarction, fat necrosis, and also in caseous necrosis,

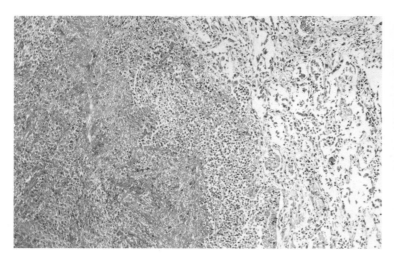

FIGURE 3.6 Photomicrograph shows the cell degradation within an abscess. Note that at the periphery of the abscess (at right) there is infiltration of acute inflammatory cells as well as fibrin. However, towards the center of the abscess there is complete loss of tissue architecture, with an accumulation of cell debris and acute inflammatory cells (H & E, x 4 obj.).

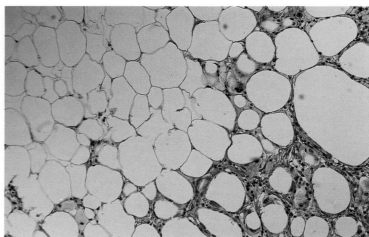

FIGURE 3.7 Photomicrograph showing stages of necrosis in the fatty marrow. In the upper left there is complete necrosis; on the right, ischemia has resulted in breakdown of the fat cells, with reactive chronic inflammation and foamy histiocytes (H & E, x 10 obj.).

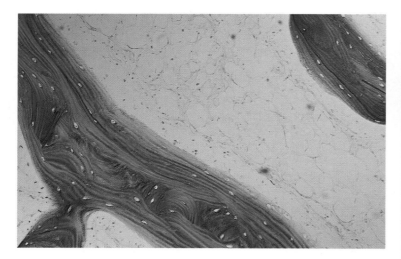

FIGURE 3.8 Necrotic cancellous bone. There is no hematoxylin staining of the fat cells in the marrow or of the osteocytes in the bone, although the ghosts of the cells remain. Recognition may be difficult in such cases without areas of viable bone for comparison (H & E, x 10 obj.).

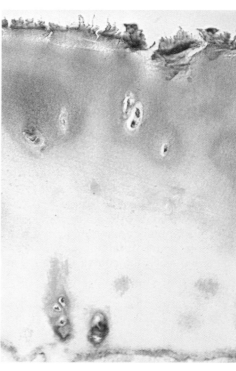

FIGURE 3.9 Photomicrograph revealing chondrocyte necrosis in the articular cartilage. Isolated chondrocytes are still staining with hematoxylin (H & E, x 4 obj.).

which occurs in patients with tuberculosis. Of particular interest to orthopedic surgeons is the calcification commonly found in areas of injured tendons or ligaments (Fig. 3.11).

Injury to the Extracellular Matrix

The extracellular matrix, which is composed of collagen, proteoglycan, various noncollagenous proteins, and inorganic constituents, is a nonviable material. Nevertheless, it shows the effects of both mechanical and chemical injury. Fibrillation of the cartilage is an example of mechanical injury with disruption of the collagen framework (Fig. 3.12). The so-called "hyalin-

ization" of collagen is caused by chemical (enzyme) denaturation of the fibrillar structure, especially of the intermolecular and possibly the intramolecular cross-linkage of the collagen molecules (Fig. 3.13). Such injured matrices invariably have altered mechanical properties. The fibrillated cartilage does not function as well as normal cartilage, either in the transmission of load or in providing a low-friction articulating surface. The "hyalinized" collagen, with its weakened cross-links, has lost much of its tensile strength. On the other hand, a piece of "dead bone" (ie, one in which both marrow cells and bone cells are dead), is exactly as strong as a similar piece of viable bone unless structural changes of the bone matrix have occurred.

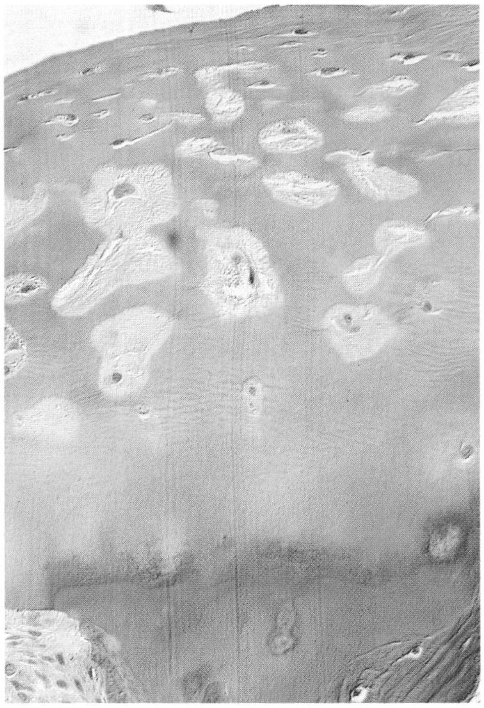

FIGURE 3.10 Photomicrograph illustrating the dissolution of the matrix that occurs around dying chondrocytes in cases of inflammatory arthritis (typically rheumatoid arthritis). Chondrocyte lacunae with this alteration in appearance are known as Weichselbaum's lacunae (H & E, x 10 obj.).

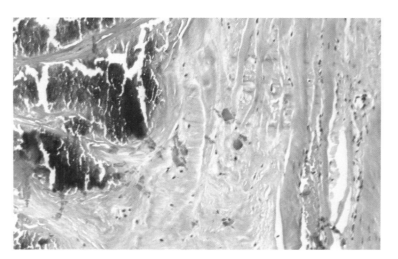

FIGURE 3.11 Photomicrograph shows extensive calcification in the capsule of the shoulder joint. Such dystrophic calcification is a common complication of tissue necrosis following injury (H & E, x 10 obj.).

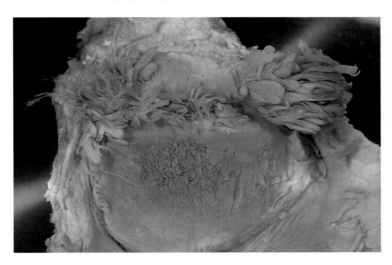

FIGURE 3.12 Photograph of the articular surface of a patella, illustrating loss of integrity due to collagen disruption or fibrillation.

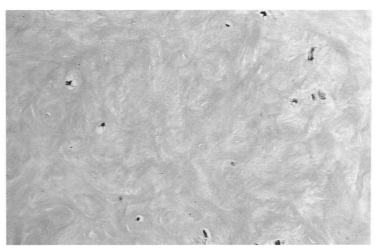

FIGURE 3.13 Photomicrograph of fibrous tissue to show some loss of nuclei and smudging, or hyalinization, of the collagen (H & E, x 50 obj.).

THE RESPONSE TO INJURY

The inflammatory reaction comprises the collective response of the body to both local and systemic injury. These responses, which are directed towards the restoration of homeostasis include: removal and/or sequestration of the necrotic tissue and the injurious agents; defense against further injury; and replacement of injured cells with restoration of tissue architecture by reparative tissue. The inflammatory reaction is not confined to an acute, local cellular response; it involves the entire body's defense mechanisms, and it is not completed until a homeostatic state has been restored.

After local injury the damaged area experiences vascular dilatation and increased blood flow. The blood vessel wall becomes more permeable. White blood cells attach themselves to the vascular endothelium and pass through the wall of the vessel to the extravascular space (Fig. 3.14). These observations, first made in the nineteenth century by Julius Cohnheim, explain Celsus' four cardinal signs of inflammation:
1. Redness, caused by vasodilatation.
2. Heat, the result of increased blood flow.
3. Swelling, caused by exudation of fluids and cells into the extravascular spaces.
4. Pain, the result of swelling of the nerve endings.

Swelling is caused by the accumulation of fluid in the injured tissue; it is always present to a greater or lesser degree during the acute stage of inflammation. This excessive accumulation of fluid occurs because the vessels of the inflamed tissue become more permeable and allow plasma proteins to leak out into the extravascular space. This protein-rich fluid is called an exudate.

There are two basic reasons for leakage of fluids from the vessels in injured tissue. The first is direct injury to the wall of the vessel; the second is increased permeability of the vessels brought about by substances released from or produced by the damaged tissue. These substances are referred to as the mediators of inflammation. They are derived from both the blood (the blood-clotting system itself, platelets, and the components of the complement system) and the tissues (histamine, prostaglandins—particularly PGE and PGE_2—and various lysosomal enzymes).

The migration (diapedesis) of leukocytes across the

endotheiium

capillary

leukocyte

bacilli

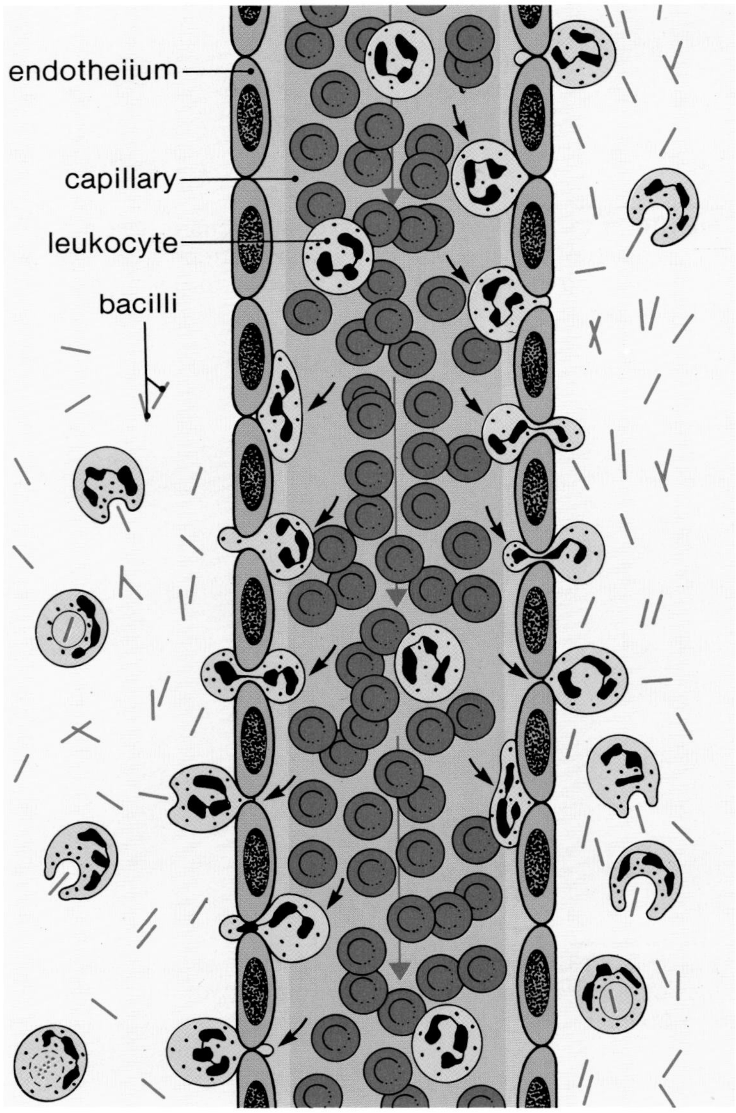

FIGURE 3.14 Schematic diagram illustrates the migration of leukocytes across the vascular endothelium into the adjacent tissue. Once in the tissue, the leukocytes may encounter and engulf any existing microbes by means of phagocytosis.

wall of the venule is an active rather than a passive phenomenon. Even after fluid exudation has passed its peak, leukocyte migration continues, presumably as a result of a persistent chemotactic effect of the injurious agent and the injured tissue.

Although Cohnheim described the migration of white blood cells through the vessel walls, it was Elie Metchnikoff who, a few years later, determined the function of these cells. He observed that they were capable of engulfing foreign matter, including bacteria, and he called this process phagocytosis (see Fig. 3.14).

Because both large and small cells are involved in phagocytic activity, he called the large cells macrophages and the small cells microphages (Fig. 3.15). (The microphages are now referred to as polymorphonuclear leukocytes (PMNs) or neutrophils; the macrophages are sometimes called histiocytes.)

The type of cell seen microscopically in the cell infiltrate depends on the nature of the injury (eg, bacterial injury results in a marked neutrophilic infiltrate, whereas a mechanical injury does not) and the time that has elapsed since the injury. Within the first few

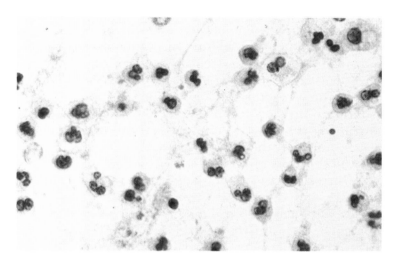
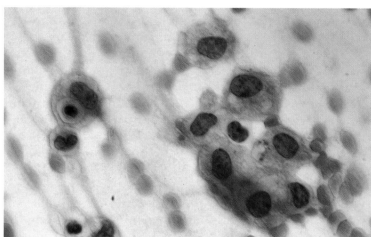

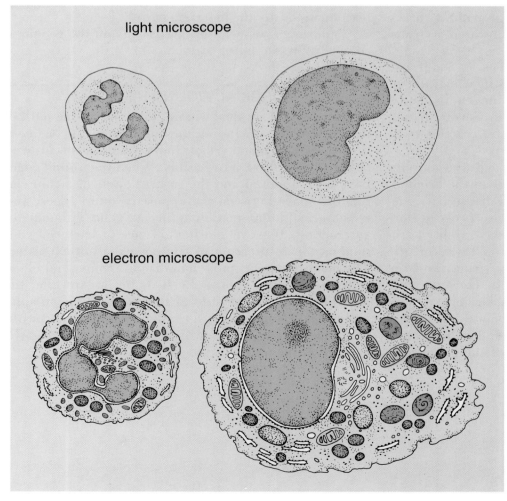

FIGURE 3.15 Photomicrograph of polymorphonuclear (PMN) leukocytes *(upper left)* and histocytes *(upper right)* (H & E, x 100 obj.). Diagrammatic representations of the light microscopic and electron microscopic characteristics of a PMN leukocyte *(lower left)* and a histiocyte *(lower right)*.

light microscope

electron microscope

hours, and up to a day or so, the predominant cells in the tissue exudate are polymorphonuclear leukocytes. However, after a period of 24 to 48 hours, more and more of the cells in the exudate are seen to be mononuclear—lymphocytes and macrophages. This biphasic response may be the result of a sequential action by specific chemical mediators.

Polymorphonuclear and mononuclear phagocytes migrate into the damaged tissues, where they engulf and digest bacteria and necrotic cells (Fig. 3.16). Phagocytes are equipped for this task by their possession of large numbers of cytoplasmic granules, including large dense granules (lysosomes), which contain various enzymes such as acid phosphatase, an antibacterial substance called lysozyme, and peroxidase.

The acute inflammatory reaction may either subside, as is usually the case or, in the presence of continuing cell injury, it may persist and become chronic. On histologic examination, chronic inflammation is distinguished from acute inflammation by a marked increase in the number of mononuclear cells in the inflamed area. These mononuclear cells include macrophages, lymphocytes, and plasma cells (Figs. 3.17 and 3.18).

Chronic inflammation occurs as a result of many types of infection, including tuberculosis, syphilis, and fungal infection, as well as in certain autoimmune diseases (eg, rheumatoid arthritis and systemic lupus erythematosus). Inflammation is also seen in response to the introduction of foreign bodies, eg, around suture material or in particulate debris generated by total joint replacement procedures.

The inflammatory reaction serves as a defense against further tissue damage, a means by which the injurious agent is removed or rendered innocuous, and a means for removal or sequestration of necrotic tissue. The final component of the inflammatory reaction to be considered is the healing phase (repair).

Eventual restoration of the damaged area may involve cell regeneration of tissue similar to the original, or replacement by fibrous connective tissue (scar tissue); usually a combination of these two processes occurs. The tissues of the body differ in their ability to regenerate. In general, the epithelium of the skin, the gastrointestinal tract, the respiratory tract, and the connective tissues all regenerate well. However, the more specialized and differentiated tissues have a more limited regenerative capacity. Furthermore, it is important to note that regeneration of tissue does not imply restoration of anatomy. In the case of the connective

tissues, failure to restore anatomy may lead to failure of function.

Perhaps the most characteristic histologic finding in the reparative stage, is the proliferation of capillaries and fibroblasts that comprise granulation tissue (Fig. 3.19). In granulation tissue, the fibroblasts produce the structural extracellular matrix, composed of collagen, proteoglycan, and other noncollagenous proteins which give body and strength to the new scar tissue.

In the medical and surgical management of injured tissues, the prevention of both delayed healing and excessive scarring is important. The clinician should take every opportunity to promote regulated healing. Therapeutic measures include wound debridement, adequate administration of antibiotics, use of nonreactive suture material, and good surgical technique. The avoidance or at least the limitation of drugs that suppress the inflammatory reaction (eg, cortisone) is important, and adequate intake of substances necessary for wound healing (protein and vitamin C) is essential. In some cases, however, the use of corticosteroids may be necessary to suppress excessive scar formation.

During most of the inflammatory response, the exudative and reparative events take place simultaneously, although the exudative features predominate in the early stages of the process, and the reparative aspects become more prominent after the removal or neutralization of injurious agents and the removal of necrotic tissue by the macrophages.

Following is a series of discussions on the repair of connective tissues after trauma.

SURGICAL WOUND HEALING

In the case of a surgical wound, all tissue in the path of the knife blade (including the epithelium, fibrous connective tissues, blood vessels, nerves, and fat) is injured either reversibly or irreversibly. When the wound edges have been apposed and the sutures applied, a thin clot fills the space between the apposed wound edges, and mediators of inflammation induce an acute inflammatory reaction. However, in the absence of bacterial contamination, infiltration of leukocytes is not extensive. The macrophages rapidly mobilize to remove red blood cells, fibrin, and damaged cell tissue. Meanwhile, the fibroblasts on either side of the wound hypertrophy and migrate, together with capillary sprouts, and within a few days circulation is reestablished across the margins of the wound.

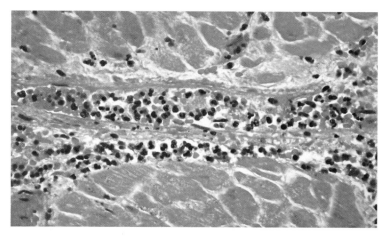

FIGURE 3.16 This photomicrograph illustrates the events during an acute inflammatory reaction brought on by tissue necrosis (in this case, specifically, by myocardial infarction). A small capillary is congested with blood and with many more PMNs than would normally be expected. These PMNs have infiltrated through the vessel wall by diapedesis and are now seen in the perivascular tissue (H & E, x 32 obj.).

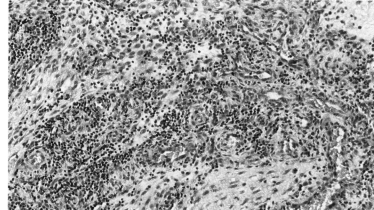

FIGURE 3.17 In this photomicrograph, a chronic inflammatory reaction can be identified by the extensive infiltration of mononuclear cells (H & E, x 10 obj.).

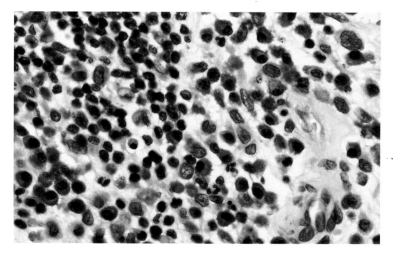

FIGURE 3.18 This high-power photomicrograph reveals a chronic inflammatory infiltrate within the perivascular tissue, which exhibits the characteristics of lymphocytes and plasma cells (H & E, x 100 obj.).

FIGURE 3.19 Photomicrograph of granulation tissue in an early stage of repair. Note the fibrin clot on the left, and the proliferating fibroblasts and capillaries interspersed with chronic inflammatory cells towards the right (H & E, x 4 obj.).

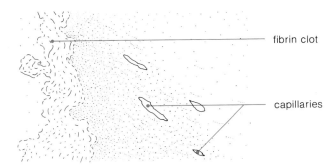

fibrin clot

capillaries

As the fibroblasts begin to lay down collagen, the cellular inflammatory infiltrate diminishes. The epithelial cells at the surface begin to undergo mitosis and to migrate over the vascularized granulation tissue. In the case of a nonlinear wound, as the epithelial cells migrate over the granulation tissue they extend beneath the fibrin clot (scab) that closes off the surface of the wound. When the epithelium is firmly reestablished underneath the scab, the scab usually sloughs off (Fig. 3.20).

The suture material used to appose the wound edges frequently causes a foreign body giant-cell reaction (Fig. 3.21), and may also act as a track along which bacteria may travel. If infection is thus induced, healing is delayed until the infection has been overcome. Healing may also be delayed if there is poor circulation in the area, or if the patient is severely debilitated.

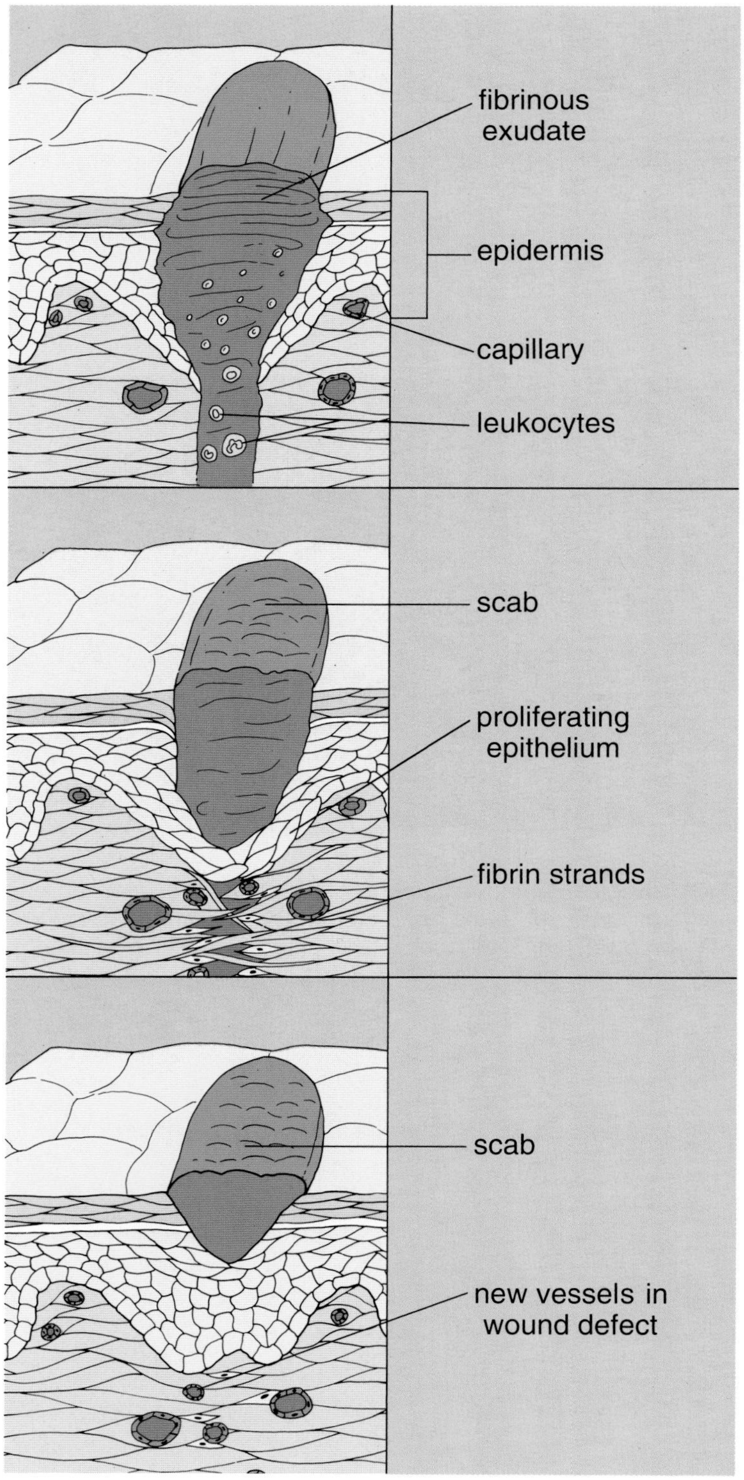

FIGURE 3.20 Schematic diagram illustrates the healing process in epithelial tissue after ulceration. The wound is first filled with a fibrinous exudate composed of acute inflammatory cells. This is gradually replaced by granulation tissue, with proliferating epithelium extending from the margins of the wound, over the granulation tissue, and beneath the residual fibrin of the surface. As the epithelium completely re-covers the wound, the dried-up layer of fibrin forms a scab, which eventually falls off.

MUSCLES

Contrary to widespread belief, muscle tissue regenerates well, but the restoration of normal structure and function is strongly dependent on the type of injury sustained. In severe infections the muscle fibers may be extensively destroyed. However, the sarcolemmal sheaths usually remain intact and rapid regeneration of muscle cells within the sheaths occurs, so that the function of the muscle may be completely restored (Fig. 3.22).

After the transection of a muscle, muscle fibers may regenerate either by growth from undamaged stumps or by growth of new, independent fibers. The nuclei for both of these processes are derived from the satellite or reserve cells found in the endomysium. It should be noted that as the muscle fibers regenerate and grow, there is also an ingrowth into the damaged muscle of capillaries and fibroblasts, with accompanying produc-

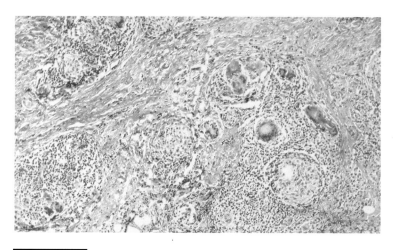

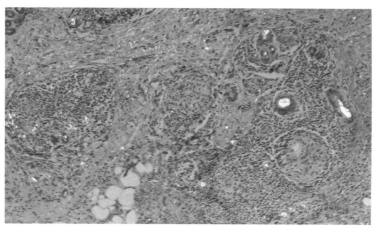

FIGURE 3.21 The introduction of foreign matter into tissue frequently leads to a chronic inflammatory reaction, with proliferating macrophages digesting the foreign material. Photomicrograph (*left*) shows giant cells and chronic inflammatory cells, giving the appearance of a granulomatous inflammation. However, under polarized light (*right*), one can clearly see the fragments of suture material that gave rise to this reaction (H & E, x 4 obj.).

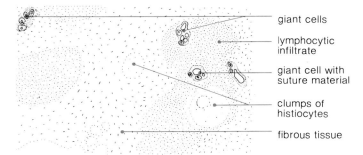

- giant cells
- lymphocytic infiltrate
- giant cell with suture material
- clumps of histiocytes
- fibrous tissue

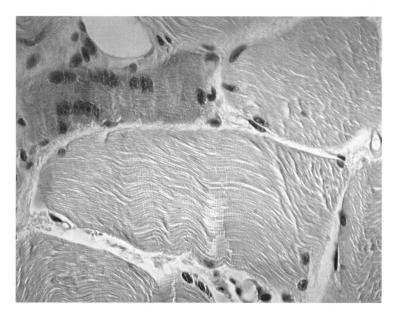

FIGURE 3.22 Photomicrograph shows a regenerating muscle fiber. Note the basophilic cytoplasm and the centrally located nuclei (H & E, x 40 obj.).

tion of collagen; this scarring usually overrides and prevents muscle fiber regeneration (Fig. 3.23). In muscle regeneration and healing, much depends on the correct alignment of the supportive structures by meticulous surgical restoration.

TENDONS

Tendons may heal either as a result of proliferation of the tenoblasts from the cut ends of the tendon, or, more likely, as a result of vascular ingrowth and proliferation of fibroblasts derived from the surrounding tissues that were injured at the same time as the tendon. Because the surrounding tissues contribute so much to the healing of a tendon, adhesions are very common. To avoid this complication, the repair of tendons requires meticulous atraumatic technique. With rupture of the achilles tendon or of the cruciate ligament, functional restoration frequently requires apposition and suturing of the cut ends.

PERIPHERAL NERVES

When a nerve fiber is divided, the peripheral portion rapidly undergoes myelin degeneration and axonal fragmentation. The lipid debris is removed by macrophages mobilized from the surrounding tissues. In the central stump, the nerve fibers retract and the axons adjacent to the cut degenerate. However, within 24 hours of section, new axonal sprouts from the central stump can usually be demonstrated, together with proliferation of Schwann cells from both the central and peripheral stumps (Fig. 3.24). With careful microsurgical approximation of the nerve, function may be achieved. The most important feature of nerve regeneration is the maintenance of the neurotubules along which the new axonal sprouts can pass.

BONE

Bone Injury

Fracture of the bone results from mechanical injury. However, the force required to produce a fracture in bone depends on the strength of the bone itself. Many fractures seen in hospital practice are in elderly people; in these patients, fractures of the vertebral bodies, the femoral neck, and the wrist are common, usually as the result of osteoporosis and weakening of bones. Fractures may also result from weakening of the bone caused by local disease, such as tumor or infection.

Because bone is a composite material and is also anisotropic (see Chapter 1), the gross appearance of a fracture depends on the microstructure of the bone tissue. Bone's most important features, in terms of fracture propagation are its many weak interfaces (cement lines) and the osteocyte lacunae and canaliculi dispersed throughout its structure. The osteocyte lacunae can act as sites of crack initiation, and the cement lines provide the major planes of fracture propagation (Fig. 3.25) The alignment of the cement lines in the cortical bone in a predominantly longitudinal direction is partially responsible for the obliquity of most fractures in the shafts of long bones. In diseases in which the microstructure of bone is markedly disturbed [eg, osteopetrosis or Paget's disease (see Chapter 6)], the patterns of fracture (usually transverse in a long bone) reflect the disturbance in microarchitecture.

The direction in which a load is applied also determines the direction of the fracture. In general, tensile load causes flat fractures, whereas compressive load results in oblique fractures, usually, with greater damage to the bone. Bending forces cause fractures that combine the features of tensile and compressive fracture, and torsional loads usually lead to helical fractures

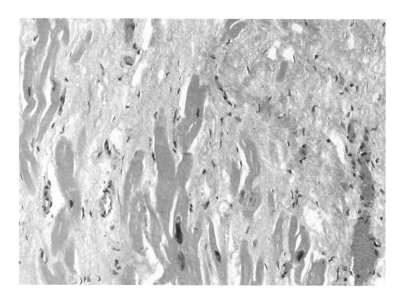

FIGURE 3.23 Photomicrograph of damaged myocardial tissue shows extensive fibrous scarring, with only a few muscle fibers enmeshed in the dense scar tissue. This scarring blocks any potential for regeneration and restoration of the muscle tissue (H & E, x 25 obj.).

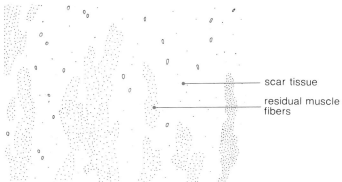

scar tissue

residual muscle fibers

FIGURE 3.24 After nerve damage, the proximal stump of the damaged nerve demonstrates proliferation of Schwann cells and eventually of axons. Unless the nerve fascicles are meticulously approximated, adequate restoration of the nerve fibers will not occur. This photomicrograph shows the proximal stump at right, and a tangled mass of proliferating (regenerative) Schwann cells and axons at left (H& E, x 4 obj.).

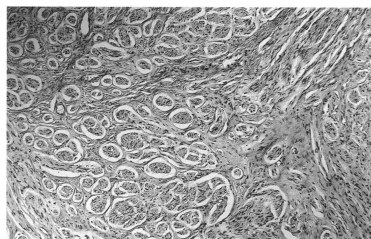

FIGURE 3.25 As a bone fracture develops, the propagation of cracks is likely to follow the cement lines. In this photomicrograph, the cement lines are indicated by cracks which have developed during tissue sectioning (H & E, x 40 obj.).

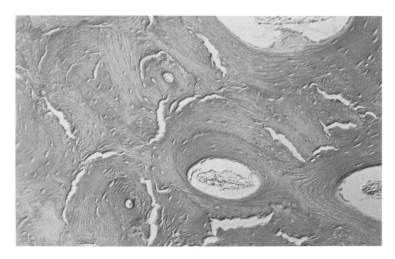

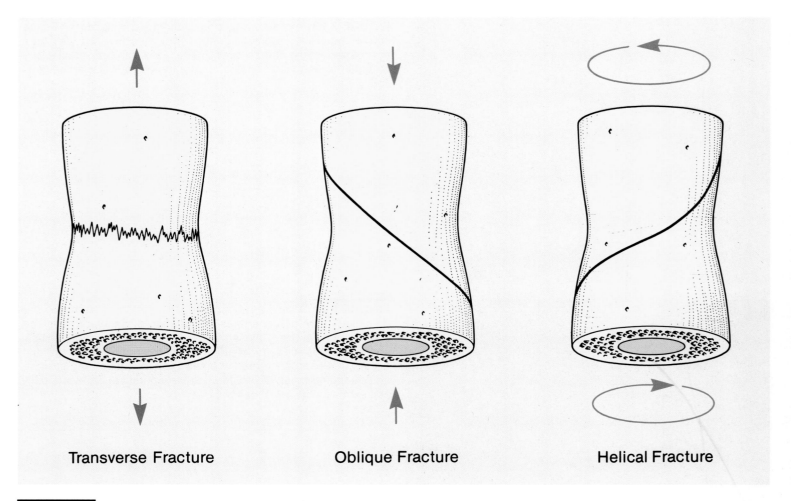

Transverse Fracture   Oblique Fracture   Helical Fracture

FIGURE 3.26 The following diagrams illustrate three different kinds of fractures, and how they are caused. *(left)* Transverse fracture, caused by traction (pulling force). *(center)* Oblique fracture, caused by compression. *(right)* Helical fracture, caused by torsion.

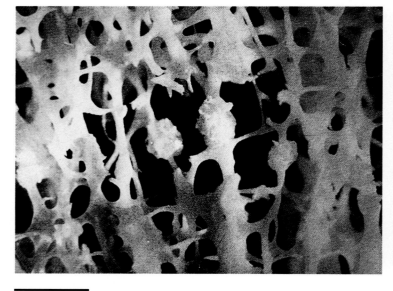
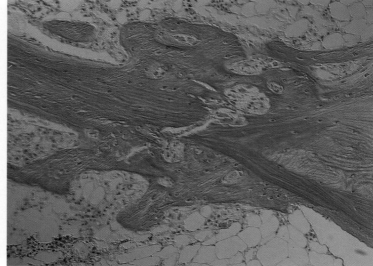

FIGURE 3.27 *(left)* Enlarged photograph of an area of subarticular cancellous bone, showing 3 microfractures which are recognized by the presence of cocoon-like microcallus attached to the trabeculae. *(right)* Photomicrograph of a microfracture through a single trabeculum. Note the fracture line, the resorption at the fracture line, and the surrounding reactive immature bone of the microcallus (H & E, Nomarski optics, x 4 obj.).

(Fig. 3.26). Daily injuries of everyday life are the probable cause of individual trabecular fractures in cancellous bone, called microfractures (Fig. 3.27).

Repeated stress to the bone, as occurs in long-distance running and walking, may result in the development of stress (or fatigue) fractures usually in the feet or in the tibia, in which an accumulation of microfractures eventually leads to a complete fracture through the bone cortex (Fig. 3.28). Such a lesion occurs without a history of significant mechanical trauma, and therefore the lesion may be misinterpreted by the clinician, radiologist, or pathologist as a neoplasm. Repeated trauma at ligamentous and tendinous insertions

that results in an avulsion fracture may exhibit a pseudosarcomatous appearance, both radiographically and histologically. In young adolescents, such injuries are most likely to occur in and around the pelvis, particularly at the origins of the adductor muscles along the inferior pubic ramus adjacent to the symphysis pubis; the lower head of the rectus femoris just above the acetabulum; and the origins of the hamstring muscles at the ischial tuberosity, as well as the insertions of the gluteus at the greater trochanter and the psoas at the lesser trochanter (Fig. 3.29). Repeated trauma at the insertion of the adductor muscles of the thigh may lead to the formation of a bony spur on the lower medial aspect

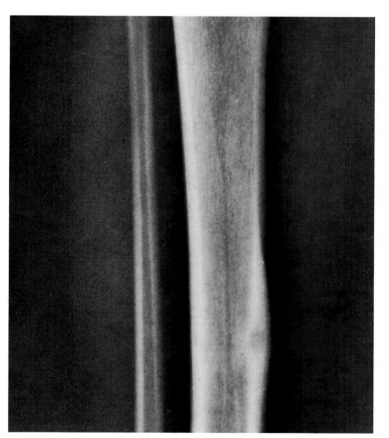

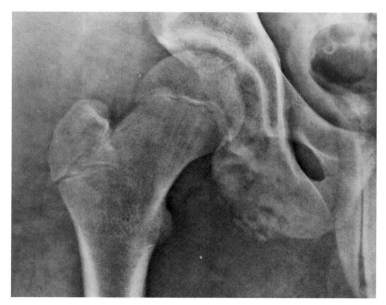

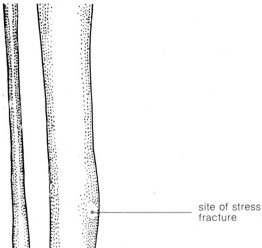

FIGURE 3.28 Clinical radiograph of a stress fracture of the leg. A patient with this type of fracture usually does not have a history of trauma, and presents clinically with pain and swelling in the affected parts after strenuous physical activity. The periosteal elevation, combined with a lack of displacement or obvious fracture line through the bone, may lead to this fracture being misdiagnosed radiographically as a tumor. Even if a biopsy is obtained, the hypercellular appearance of the callus may lead the pathologist to believe that this is a cellular bone-forming neoplasm or, as in this case, an osteoid osteoma.

site of stress fracture

FIGURE 3.29 Clinical radiograph shows an avulsion fracture in the pelvis. Note the fragmentation due to avulsion injury of the ischial tuberosity. This fracture, like the stress fracture in Figure 3.28, may easily be misdiagnosed as a tumor.

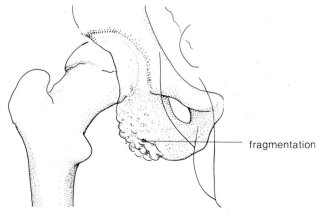

fragmentation

of the femur, often referred to as a rider's spur because it is commonly seen in those who ride horseback.

In children around the ages of 10 and 11 years, avulsion fractures are also seen at the tibial tubercle, where the effects of the injury and eventual repair result in a lesion known as Osgood–Schlatter disease (Fig. 3.30).

Bone Repair

Fortunately, the healing of bone is one of the great successes of nature. Under favorable conditions, bone can be regenerated and remodeled to function optimally, provided the fractured ends are properly aligned.

The single most important factor in the primary healing of a fracture is complete immobilization of the fractured ends. In nature, this immobilization is achieved through the production of immature bone and cartilage matrix by the cambial layer of cells in the periosteum and from undifferentiated mesenchymal cells in the soft tissues around the broken ends of the bone. This reparative tissue is referred to as the fracture callus (Fig. 3.31).

The amount of callus produced depends on a number of factors, including the degree of instability and the vascularity of the injured bone. The amount of callus is usually increased in unstable fractures and the callus often contains much cartilage tissue (Fig. 3.32). In poorly vascularized areas of the skeleton (eg, the midshaft of the tibia), callus formation may be scant; consequently, healing may be delayed, sometimes indefinitely. This delay gives rise to chronic nonunion of the fracture site (Fig. 3.33).

When a fracture occurs, the amount of injury sustained by the bone itself and by the soft tissues surrounding it depends on the direction and magnitude of the force applied. The bone fragments may be displaced. The fracture line may be single (a simple fracture) or the bone may be broken into many fragments (a comminuted fracture). If the skin over the fractured bone is also broken, the injury is considered a compound fracture, and infection is a common complication. In some cases, soft tissue may become interposed between the fractured ends of the bone, causing healing to be significantly delayed. For all these reasons, the histologic appearance of the reparative tissue surrounding a fracture may vary greatly.

Tissue obtained within a few days of injury usually shows areas of hemorrhage and acute tissue damage (Fig. 3.34). The bone and bone marrow on either side

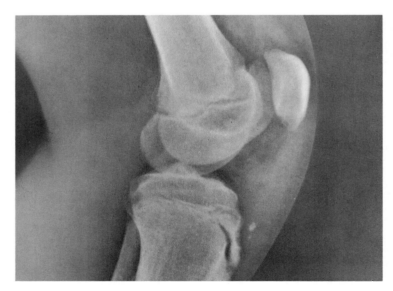

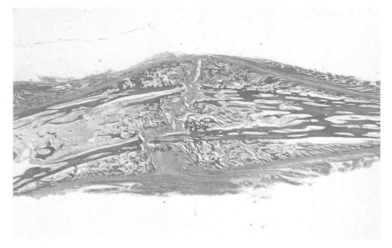

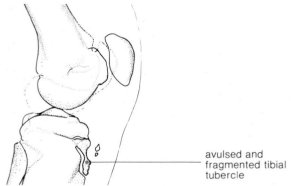

FIGURE 3.30 Clinical radiograph of the knee in a 12-year-old child shows fragmentation and avulsion of the tibial tubercle. This condition, known as Osgood–Schlatter disease, is almost certainly post-traumatic.

avulsed and
fragmented tibial
tubercle

FIGURE 3.31 Low-power photomicrograph shows reparative new bone that has formed in the soft tissue and periosteum surrounding a fractured rib. Restoration of bone cortex and medulla depends on complete immobilization of the fracture site, which is naturally accomplished through the formation of external callus. However, when a fracture is treated by rigid internal fixation external callus may not be evident (H & E, x 1.5 obj.).

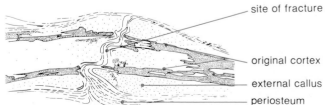

site of fracture

original cortex

external callus

periosteum

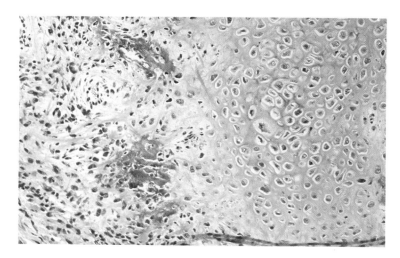

FIGURE 3.32 A normal fracture callus contains variable amounts of bone, cartilage, and fibrous tissue. However, when a fracture is unstable or when the fracture site is poorly vascularized, an abundance of cartilage will be found, as seen in this photomicrograph (H & E, x 25 obj.).

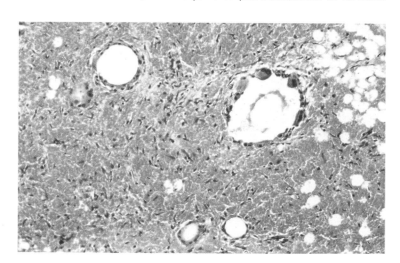

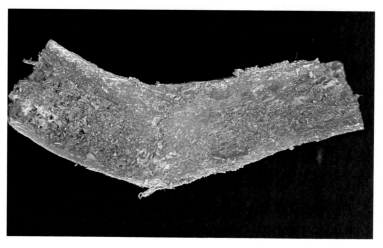

FIGURE 3.33 Healing may be delayed in a poorly vascularized or extremely unstable fracture, and sometimes may not even occur at all. In such a case, a false joint or pseudarthrosis is formed.

(left) Gross specimen of a false joint. *(right)* Histologic appearance of a false joint (H & E, x 1.5 obj.).

FIGURE 3.34 Photomicrograph of tissue obtained from the area around a fracture site shows extensive hemorrhage and a large fat cyst surrounded by giant cells, characteristic of fat necrosis (H & E, x 10 obj.).

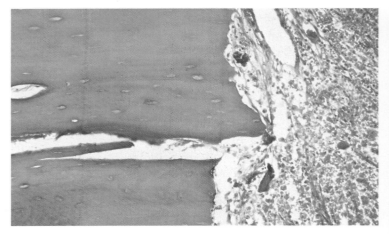

FIGURE 3.35 Photomicrograph of the broken end of a bone taken 1 week after the fracture demonstrates both hemorrhage and bone necrosis. Note that the osteocyte lacunae in the bone are completely empty (H & E, x 1 obj.).

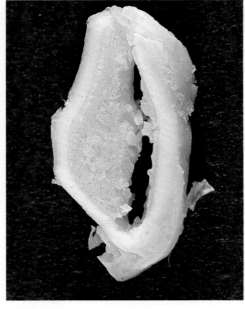

FIGURE 3.36
After injury, the blood supply may be so compromised as to cause complete necrosis of the affected tissue. In this gross specimen, complete osteonecrosis of the carpal lunate bone has occurred. The necrotic bone is recognized by its opaque yellow appearance.

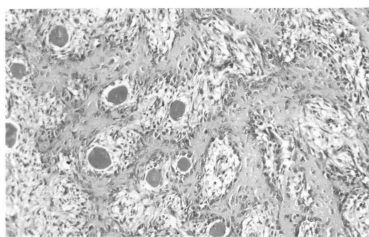

FIGURE 3.37 Photomicrograph of a fracture callus obtained from the soft tissue around a 2-week-old fracture demonstrates proliferating trabeculae of immature cellular bone growing around and between muscle fibers. This histologic finding could be misdiagnosed as an infiltrating bone-forming tumor (phloxine and tartrazine, x 10 obj.).

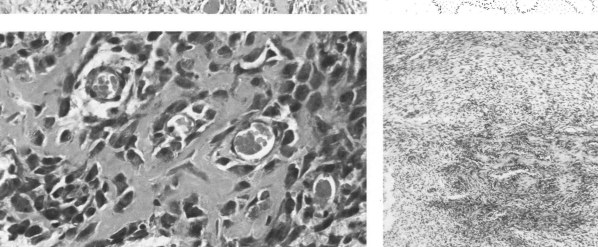

proliferating immature bone

muscle fibers

FIGURE 3.38 Higher-power photomicrograph demonstrates the immature and cellular appearance of a fracture callus (H & E, x 32 obj.).

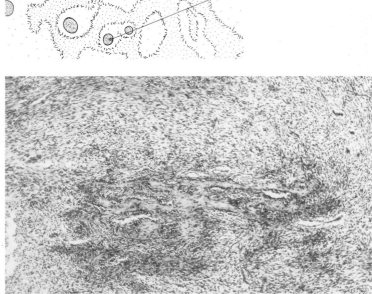

FIGURE 3.39 Lower-power photomicrograph demonstrates the hypercellular, proliferative appearance of callus, which in this case shows only minimal bone matrix formation. The pseudosarcomatous appearance of this tissue may lead to misdiagnosis (H & E, x 10 obj.).

of the fracture undergo necrosis, the extent of which depends on the local anatomy (Fig. 3.35). Fractures of the femoral neck, of some of the carpal and tarsal bones, and of the patella frequently demonstrate widespread bone necrosis because the local vascular supply is so severely compromised (Fig. 3.36). In a comminuted fracture the separate bone fragments are likely to undergo necrosis, and if the necrosis is extensive healing will be delayed.

Microscopic examination of tissue from a two-week-old fracture callus shows markedly cellular tissue, usually hypervascular, which produces irregular islands and trabeculae of immature bone (Figs. 3.37 and 3.38). The hypercellularity and the disordered organization may produce a pseudosarcomatous appearance in the tissue (Figs. 3.39 and 3.40). Because a biopsy is not likely to be performed unless the clinician has failed to recognize the traumatic origin of the patient's complaints, the pseudosarcomatous appearance of the callus can easily lead to errors in interpretation by the pathologist. It cannot be too strongly emphasized that because stress fractures without an obvious history of injury are common in young people (the same age group as osteosarcomas), recognition of the true nature of the problem is important and, on occasion, is among the most difficult problems in differential diagnosis for the pathologist (Fig. 3.41).

Once the callus is sufficient to immobilize the fracture site, repair occurs between the fractured cortical and medullary bones. When union has been achieved,

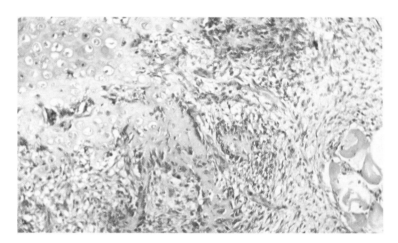

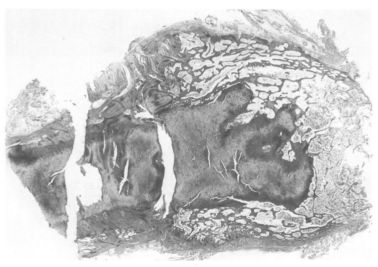

FIGURE 3.40 Photomicrograph of a fracture callus taken from the area around a 10-day-old fracture. Note the proliferating cartilage and immature bone to the left, and the degenerate muscle fibers to the right (H & E, x 10 obj.).

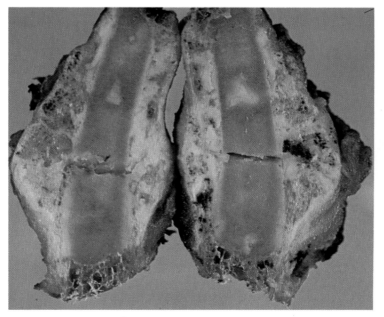

FIGURE 3.41 A segment of the costochondral junction was resected from a patient who presented with a swelling in the region *(left)*. Radiographic examination revealed extreme density, which was interpreted by both the clinician and the radiologist as a form of neoplasm. However, the histologic preparation of the resected specimen *(right)* shows a fracture through the calcified costal cartilage, surrounded by a mass of firm tissue. This is the histologic picture expected of a fracture callus (H & E, x 1.5 obj.).

the callus is remodeled and eventually disappears. Very little callus is produced when a fracture is treated with rigid internal or external surgical fixation, where primary healing of the bone proceeds without the abundant external callus seen in association with unstable fractures.

Many factors influence the repair of a fracture. These include the particular bone involved (the tibia being especially difficult), the portion of the bone involved (the diaphysis is worse than the metaphysis), the type of fracture (comminuted vs. simple), the degree of soft tissue injury and interposition, and the stability of the site after fixation. Evaluation of fracture repair in any clinical study must consider the effects of these fac-

tors. When there is nonunion of a previous fracture or when large bone defects are present, grafting with autografts (from another anatomic site in the same patient), allografts (from other human subjects), or xenografts (from animals) is an accepted practice (Fig. 3.42).

Histologic evidence from experimental studies of fracture repair and ectopic ossification point out the necessity for a rigid framework so that lamellar bone can be deposited. The composition of this framework may be calcified cartilage, calcified woven bone, or even foci of dystrophic calcification. When such a framework exists and lamellar bone is produced, it is said to be osteoconductive, playing the role of a filler to assist in the bridging of a gap (usually a fracture line).

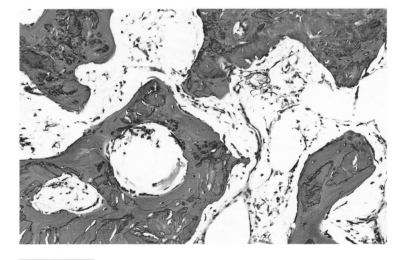
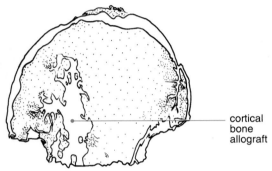

cortical
bone
allograft

FIGURE 3.42 This patient with a history of segmental avascular necrosis of the femoral head had been treated with a cortical bone allograft 18 months before the resection of the femoral head. This cut section through the femoral head clearly shows the incorporated graft.

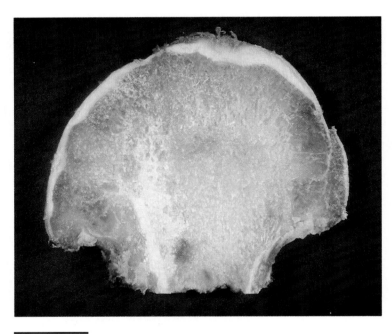
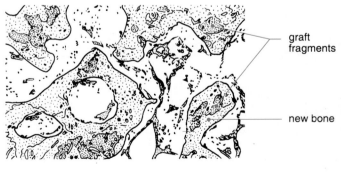

graft
fragments

new bone

FIGURE 3.43 Photomicrograph of tissue obtained from an area previously grafted with bone tissue broken into very small pieces. New bone has formed and surrounds the fragments of grafted bone (H & E, x 4 obj.).

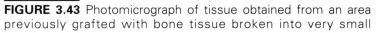

Most bone grafts act in this way (Fig. 3.43). However, it has been shown that certain proteins derived from bone and bone marrow are osteoinductive, ie, they stimulate the formation of bone matrix by the cell. A mixture of xenograft material (osteoconductive) and admixed bone marrow (osteoinductive) will work better as a graft than a xenograft alone.

Fractures can also lead to systemic complications, eg, shock syndrome and myoglobinuria, the latter occurring when there is significant muscle injury. Associated with all fractures is a disruption of the bone marrow, with the potential for embolization of the fatty marrow through the locally damaged venous system. Fat embolization becomes a clinical problem in severe multiple fractures and extensive orthopedic surgery,

eg, bilateral joint replacements resulting in petechial hemorrhages, cerebral ischemia, and/or pulmonary insufficiency (Fig. 3.44). The effects of fat emboli on the tissues are, first, mechanical obstruction of the capillary bed and, second, an inflammatory response resulting from breakdown of the fat into free fatty acids.

CARTILAGE

Healing of cartilage is adversely affected by two factors: its avascularity and its low cell-to-matrix ratio. Nevertheless, it is essential to recognize that cartilage cells can indeed proliferate, and that in arthritis, in which the cartilage is damaged, cartilage regeneration with both cartilage cell proliferation (Fig. 3.45) and

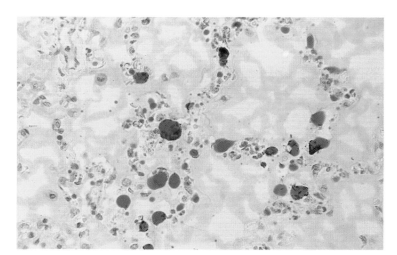

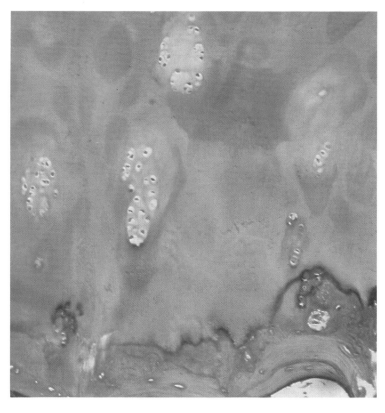

FIGURE 3.44 Photomicrograph of a piece of lung showing globules of fat in the alveolar walls (frozen section; oil red O stain, x 4 obj.).

FIGURE 3.45 After injury to cartilage tissue resulting in cell death, proliferation of groups or clones of reparative chondrocytes may appear, as seen in this photomicrograph (H & E, x 25 obj.).

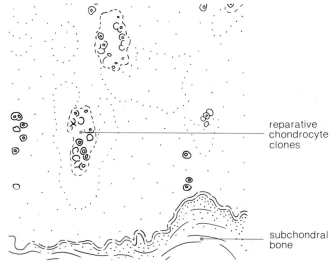

reparative chondrocyte clones

subchondral bone

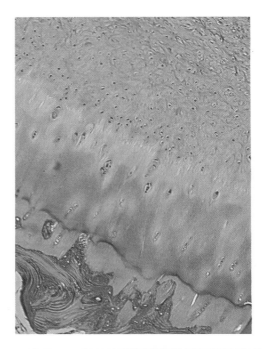

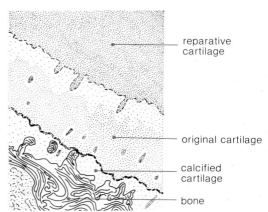

FIGURE 3.46 After cartilage damage there may be regeneration of both cartilage cells and matrix. The photomicrograph shows normal cartilage covered by a thick layer of reparative cartilage. When viewed under polarized light, as here, one can appreciate the alteration in the collagen structure of the matrix. The concept of articular cartilage repair is an important consideration in the management of patients with arthritis (H & E, x 10 obj.).

reparative cartilage

original cartilage

calcified cartilage

bone

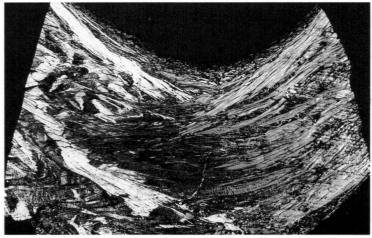

FIGURE 3.47 *(left)* Photomicrograph of a section cut along the length of the meniscus in its mid-zone demonstrates that the collagen fibers run circumferentially (polarized light, x 1 obj.). *(right)* Cross-section of the meniscus about halfway along its length demonstrates that most of the collagen fibers are cut across.

However, especially on the tibial surface of the meniscus the collagen fibers are cut lengthwise, indicating their radial disposition (polarized light, x 1 obj.). These figures should be compared with Figure 1.49.

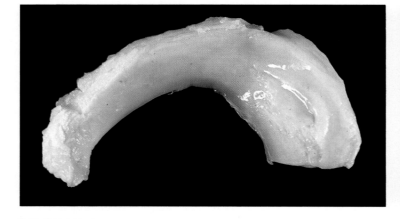

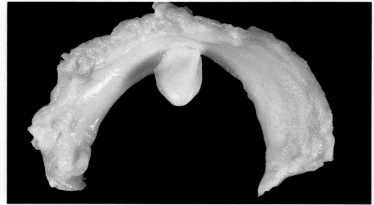

FIGURE 3.48 Gross photograph of a medial meniscus with an early tear in the posterior horn. These tears characteristically occur as clefts in the substance of the meniscus and run in the direction of the collagen fibers.

FIGURE 3.49 Occasionally, a tear such as that shown in Figure 3.48 will extend onto the medial margin and form a tag that extends into the joint space. Such a tag may become smoothed off at its margins, as seen in this specimen.

cartilage matrix production (Fig. 3.46) is a regular feature.

The ability of cartilage cells to produce an adequate matrix and to restore functional tissue probably depends on their mechanical environment. After an injury to the articular surface, as might occur in an athletic injury, continued irritation will probably result in worsening of the condition. The features of cartilage repair will be discussed at greater length in Chapter 9.

THE MENISCI OF THE KNEE

The menisci are composed mainly of collagen, although some proteoglycan is also present. Examination of carefully oriented sections has revealed that the principal orientation of the collagen fibers in the menisci is circumferential (Fig. 3.47). The few small, radially disposed fibers that do occur exist primarily on the tibial surface. The circumferential orientation of most of the collagen fibers appears designed to withstand the circumferential tension within the meniscus during normal loading. The radially disposed fibers probably act as ties to resist longitudinal splitting of the menisci that might result from undue compression.

The menisci of young individuals are usually white, have a translucent quality, and are supple on palpation. The menisci in older individuals lose their translucency, become more opaque and yellow in color, and feel less supple (see Fig. 1.42).

Lacerations of the meniscus cause symptoms that require surgical treatment in two groups of patients: young active patients in whom injury is frequently related to athletic activity, and older individuals in whom degeneration leads to laceration. Most lacerations take place in the posterior horn of the meniscus and, more commonly, in the medial meniscus. They usually occur as clefts that run along the circumferentially directed collagen fibers (Fig. 3.48). Over time, such a cleft may extend to the medial margin of the meniscus and create a tag, which eventually may become quite smooth (Fig. 3.49). Extension of the tear may lead to the bucket-handle deformity (Fig. 3.50). Sometimes, the meniscus shows peripheral detachment, usually posteriorly. A horizontal cleavage in the posterior horn of the meniscus is found at autopsy in over 50 percent of older individuals.

The advent of arthrography and arthroscopy has assisted in the clinical diagnosis of tears in the menisci. These techniques help localize tears and, when the scope of the injury is limited, can facilitate partial meniscectomy.

In histologic sections of torn menisci, evidence of both injury and repair may be seen, with the findings likely to be time dependent (Fig. 3.51). It is difficult to determine whether histologic degenerative changes observed at meniscectomy result from or contribute to the tear (Fig. 3.52).

SYNOVIUM

Injury to any of the joint structures necessarily affects the synovium. Traumatic synovitis is usually characterized microscopically by evidence of hemorrhage (hemosiderin staining), hypertrophy and hyperplasia of the synovial lining cells, mild chronic inflammation, and occasionally by included fragments of detached bone and cartilage (Fig. 3.53). Sometimes the severity of the synovial response may mask the underlying traumatic etiology.

CONCLUSION

After injury, the effects are noted both locally, in the cells and the tissue, and systemically. The response to injury (the inflammatory response) is effected mainly through the vascular system; its purpose is to restore the body to its status quo. In the case of minor injuries that frequently befall all of us, the status quo is indeed restored. In the case of more severe injury, however, a new status quo that may result in some disability is likely to occur.

Trauma is a major cause of disease attributable to skeletal malfunction. Trauma also plays a contributory role in a number of other morbid conditions, including but not limited to osteoarthritis, slipped capital femoral epiphysis, congenital pseudarthrosis, myositis ossificans, and interdigital (Morton's) neuroma of the foot. It is probable that predisposing conditions exist in many of these disease states, all of which are not clearly understood at this time.

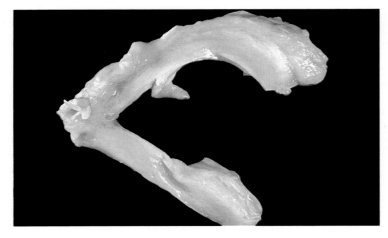

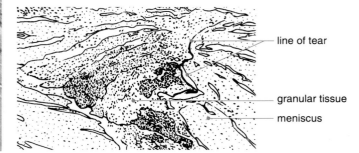

FIGURE 3.50 Extension of the meniscal tear along the length of the meniscus may result in a bucket-handle tear, as demonstrated here.

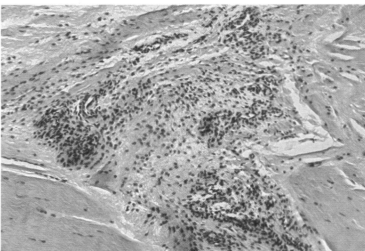

FIGURE 3.51 Photomicrograph of an area of laceration in a meniscus. On both the right and left side intact collagen fibers can be seen, while in the center a defect filled with granulation tissue is evident. Repair is much more likely to be seen in the peripheral third of the substance of the meniscus where the tissue is vascularized (H & E, x 10 obj.).

line of tear

granular tissue

meniscus

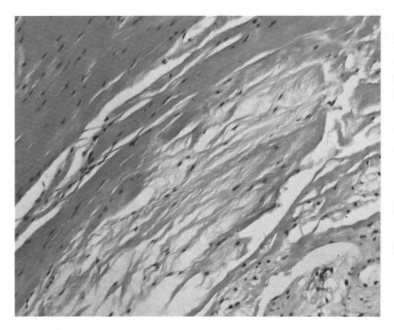

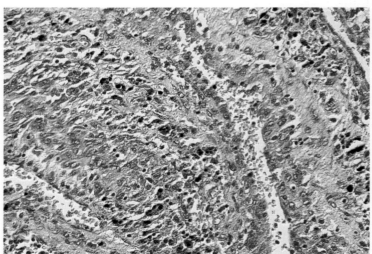

FIGURE 3.53 Photomicrograph of synovial tissue obtained from a knee joint about 1 to 2 months after injury to the joint. The synovial lining is both hypertrophied and hyperplastic. There is extensive hemosiderin deposition in the subsynovial tissue (H & E, Nomarski optics, x 10 obj.).

FIGURE 3.52 Photomicrograph of meniscal tissue shows foci of normal-appearing collagen at the upper left; splitting of the collagen fibers, which appear to be frayed and open, in the middle; and some myxomatous tissue, possibly the result of degenerative changes, at lower right (H & E, x 25 obj.).

Bone and joint infection

I nflammation is the most common of all pathologic processes, and clinically significant inflammation is most frequently the result of infection. However, inflammation also accompanies many other pathologic processes, including those caused by trauma, some metabolic diseases (eg, gout), and even neoplasia. Because it is so common, the physician may understandably think first of infection when signs of inflammation are present, and it is important to guard against neglect of the other possible etiologies.

During the late nineteenth century, it became recognized that bone marrow infection (osteomyelitis) is caused by microorganisms and tends to involve the ex-

tremities and the juxtaepiphyseal area of the bone. Before the era of antibiotics, bone and joint infections were common; they presented serious clinical problems that led to high rates of morbidity and mortality. In the present day, the incidence of osteomyelitis and its associated mortality have decreased dramatically; however, even with the use of antibiotics, morbidity connected with the disease remains high.

The proper diagnosis and management of osteomyelitis depends on careful correlation of clinical, radiologic, and histopathologic findings. Occasionally, there are problems in differential diagnosis, especially with regard to differentiating osteomyelitis from round-

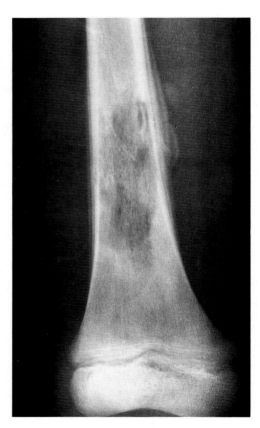

FIGURE 4.1
A 7-year-old boy had pain in his right leg for 3 weeks. AP radiograph demonstrates a lesion in the medullary portion of the distal femoral diaphysis with a moth-eaten type of bone destruction, associated with a lamellated periosteal reaction and a small soft tissue prominence. These radiographic features may suggest a diagnosis of Ewing's sarcoma, however the lack of a definite soft tissue mass and the short symptomatic period, point to the correct diagnosis of osteomyelitis, which was confirmed by biopsy.

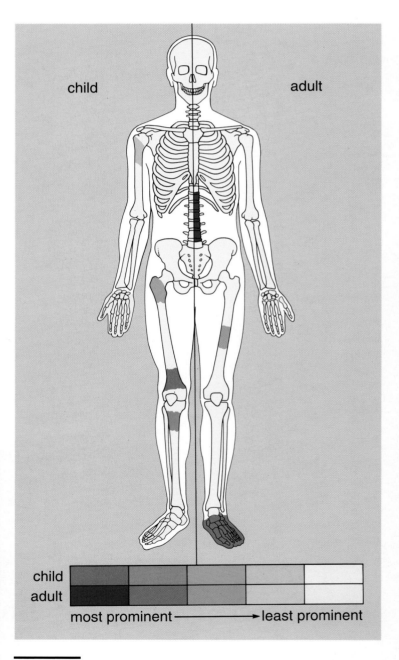

FIGURE 4.3 Distribution of osteomyelitis in children and adults.

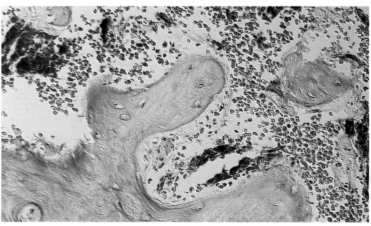

FIGURE 4.2 Photomicrograph of tissue obtained by bone biopsy shows nest of dark hyperchromatic cells crushed at the time of biopsy, rendering accurate microscopic diagnosis impossible (H & E, x 10 obj.).

cell tumors and eosinophilic granuloma. Diagnostic problems are encountered not only radiologically but also microscopically, especially with small crushed specimens (Figs. 4.1 and 4.2). In such cases, the diagnosis of osteomyelitis may depend on the results of intraoperative cultures and the subsequent postoperative course.

The majority of bone and joint infections are caused either by organisms that produce pus (pyogenic infections) or by organisms that produce multiple nodules or granules in the tissue (granulomatous infections). In general, pyogenic infections more commonly present as bone disease, whereas granulomatous infections present as joint disease.

PYOGENIC AND OTHER NONGRANULOMATOUS INFECTIONS

CLINICAL CONSIDERATIONS

Infection of the skeletal tissues results from microbial organisms that are either blood borne (hematogenous infection) or implanted directly into the bone. The latter most often occurs as a complication of a compound fracture or of surgery.

Hematogenous Osteomyelitis

The majority of patients with acute hematogenous osteomyelitis are children, who usually present with high fever and local pain. In most cases, the organism responsible for the infection in patients over the age of 3 years is *Staphylococcus aureus* (coagulase positive). The most frequent sites of infection in children are the distal femur, the proximal tibia, the proximal femur, the proximal humerus, and the distal radius, all of which are areas of rapid growth and increased risk of trauma (Fig. 4.3). It has been suggested that the large caliber of the metaphyseal veins in children leads to marked slowing of blood flow, and consequently predisposes to post-traumatic thrombosis and colonization by blood-borne bacteria (Fig. 4.4).

Hematogenous osteomyelitis is uncommon in otherwise healthy adults. However, cases of acute hematogenous osteomyelitis are sometimes seen in debilitated

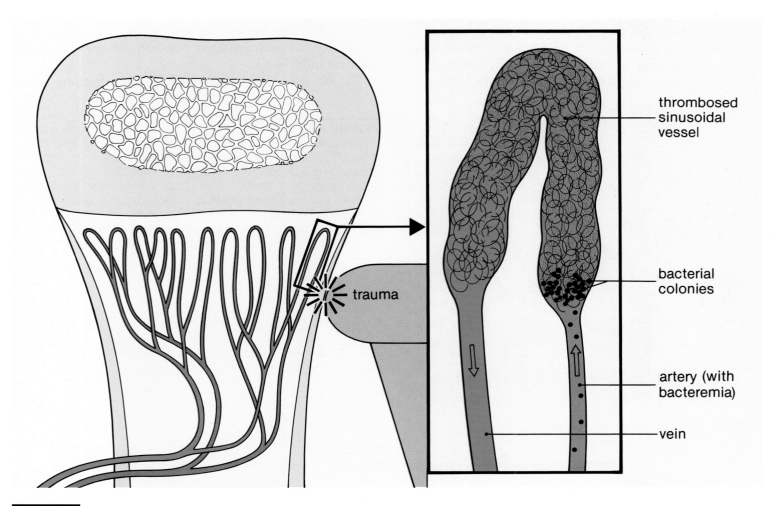

FIGURE 4.4 After mechanical trauma to the bone in children, the large venous channels in the metaphysis are liable to thrombose (see vein on right). In the presence of bacteria from infection elsewhere in the body, such a site of thrombosis can act as a nidus for bacterial growth and subsequent development of osteomyelitis.

adults (eg, those with chronic disease or drug addiction). In debilitated elderly adults with genitourinary infections, in whom spinal osteomyelitis is not uncommon, the responsible organisms (usually gram-negative rods) probably gain access to the spine via Batson's venous plexus (Fig. 4.5).

Another group of elderly patients in whom osteomyelitis may be a problem are those with peripheral vascular insufficiency, which in many cases is associated with diabetes. In these patients, the infection usually involves the small bones of the feet. The etiology is frequently polymicrobial, and may be due to anaerobic organisms.

Recent studies of osteomyelitis in drug addicts have shown Pseudomonas to be the responsible organism in the majority of those affected. In most of these patients, fever and chills were conspicuously absent, and local pain was often the sole clinical finding suggestive of osteomyelitis. In drug addicts, the focus of osteomyelitis is usually the spine (Fig. 4.6) or the pelvis, although the disease may occur anywhere in the skeletal system (sometimes in unusual sites, such as the clavicle). Organisms are carried from the skin and from unclean hypodermic needles. In addition, intravenous injection of drugs—often "cut" and thus contaminated with other particulate matter—may produce microvascular occlusion, thereby providing a site for bacterial colonization.

It is important to realize that adult patients with bone infections frequently present only with pain; therefore, the diagnosis of osteomyelitis is often not made immediately. As already mentioned, in these patients, radiographic changes in the bone may be misinterpreted by the radiologist as resulting from a malignant tumor (Fig. 4.7).

In recent years, probably because of the widespread and somewhat indiscriminate use of antibiotics, cases of osteomyelitis caused by organisms of low virulence have been reported. When long bones are involved, these cases pursue a course similar to that described above; however, the radiographic changes, which include lysis of the affected bone, as well as sclerosis and periosteal reaction (sometimes in the onion-skin pattern) often lead to problems of differential diagnosis.

Neonatal Osteomyelitis

Neonatal osteomyelitis, which also commonly involves the joint adjacent to the involved bone, is usually the result of hematogenous infection by one of three organisms: *Staphylococcus aureus*, group B streptococcus, or *Escherichia coli*. Group B streptococcus is commonly found in the vagina, and the unborn child presumably becomes infected during delivery. *E. coli*, a common contaminant at the time of delivery, is pathogenic in the neonatal period because of the infant's lack of immunity, a condition that persists for approximately the first month of life.

In the case of *S. aureus* and *E. coli* infections, about

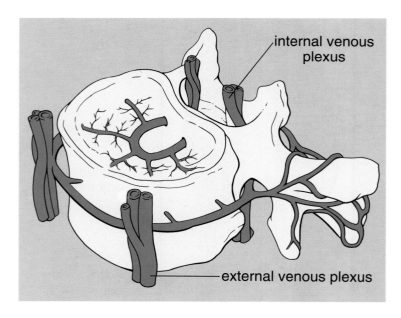

internal venous plexus

external venous plexus

FIGURE 4.5 The veins of the vertebral column form intricate plexuses around the column, along the spinal canal, and through the bone substance. These venous plexuses, also known as Batson's plexus, communicate freely with the segmental systemic veins and with the portal system. Because of these anastomoses and the lack of valves in these veins, retrograde flow frequently occurs and may result in metastatic infection, as well as metastatic tumors, to the vertebral bodies, spinal cord, brain, and skull.

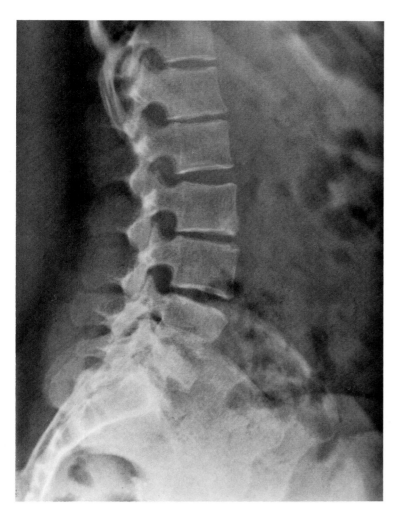

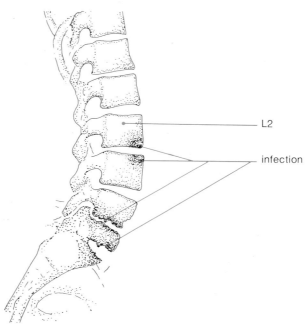

FIGURE 4.6 Radiograph of a lateral projection of the spine in a young drug addict shows bone destruction anteriorly on both sides of the disc between L2 and L3 and extensive destruction at L4–L5 and L5–S1, with collapse of L5. Bacteriologic culture showed that the offending organism in this case was *Staphylococcus aureus*.

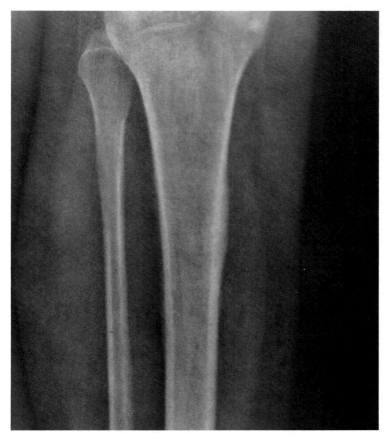

FIGURE 4.7 Radiograph of a young woman who complained of pain in the upper end of the tibia shows extensive periosteal reaction along the tibia. Clinical examination of the area revealed tenderness and swelling, although the patient's general health appeared good. The differential diagnosis was between a round-cell tumor (eg, non-Hodgkin's lymphoma) or infection. Biopsy proved the lesion to be infective in nature.

40 percent of the patients show polyostotic involvement. Polyostotic involvement with osteomyelitis is extremely rare except in neonate (Fig. 4.8). When streptococcus is the causative organism, usually only a single bone is involved. In some cases of neonatal osteomyelitis, the absence of systemic symptoms may delay the clinical diagnosis.

Osteomyelitis Resulting from Direct Inoculation of Bacteria

Acute hematogenous osteomyelitis of childhood, which used to be regularly encountered in orthopedic practice, is now much less common, at least in the developed Western countries. However, post-traumatic osteomyelitis has become much more of a clinical problem, usually resulting from puncture wounds, traffic accidents, and iatrogenic infections (Fig. 4.9).

Most traffic accidents involve high-impact collisions that result in compound and comminuted fractures. A significant amount of foreign material, including metallic debris, pieces of clothing, soil, etc., can usually be found in these wounds.

It is important to recognize the polymicrobial nature of the infection in accident cases. Both staphylococcus and streptococcus can be expected and, in addition, gram-negative organisms (including pseudomonas)

are often present. The most important procedure in the treatment of such infections is removal of all foreign and dead matter. If this step is omitted, elimination of the infection becomes difficult, if not impossible. Antibiotic therapy should not be continued for longer than is necessary to eliminate the signs of sepsis; otherwise, secondary contamination of the wound by resistant organisms can be expected.

In patients who have osteomyelitis as a complication of a fracture, it is important to achieve complete immobilization of the fracture fragments. Without immobilization, reestablishment of the vascular supply necessary to deal adequately with the inflamed and infected tissues becomes virtually impossible.

Iatrogenic infections may be a direct result of surgical intervention, associated with the internal fixation of a simple or compound fracture, or, more recently, with prosthetic joint replacement. (More than 500,000 prosthetic joint replacements are performed each year in the United States alone.) After a total joint replacement procedure, infection may occur as an acute complication of the operation or may present insidiously many months (or even years) later (Fig. 4.10). The causative organisms commonly identified in such cases are staphylococcus (both coagulase negative and coagulase positive), pseudomonas, and a variety of anaerobic organisms.

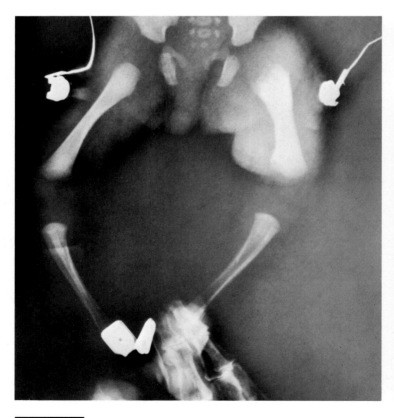
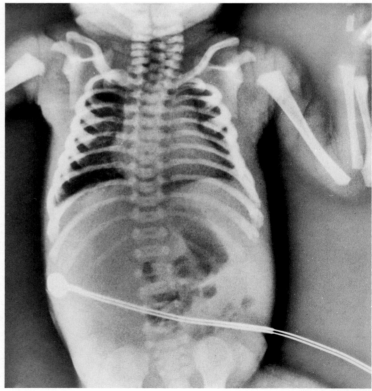

FIGURE 4.8 Polyostotic involvement in neonatal osteomyelitis. Radiograph of the lower limbs of a newborn child *(left)* shows marked periosteal reaction all along the left femur. Radiograph of the chest *(right)* shows involvement of some ribs as well as the right clavicle.

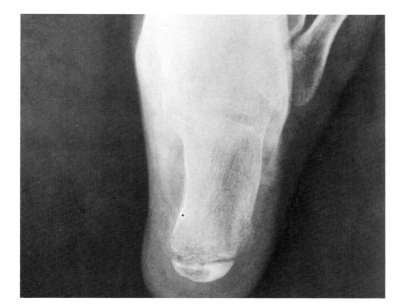

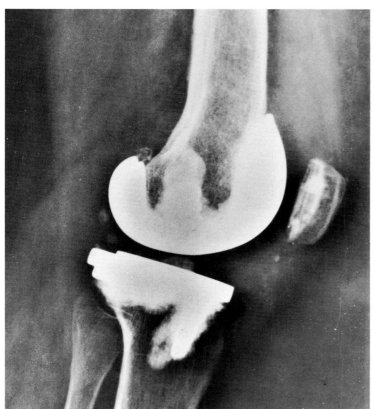

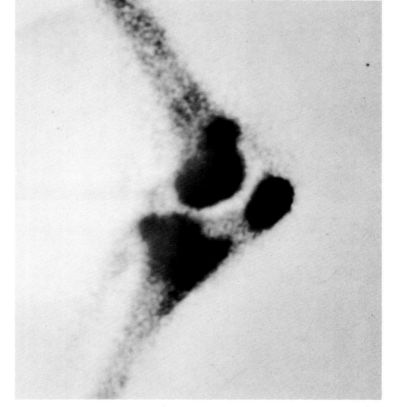

FIGURE 4.9 Radiograph of the heel in a 7-year-old child shows a lytic lesion in the apophysis of the os calcis, which proved on biopsy to be due to infection after a puncture wound.

FIGURE 4.10 Radiograph of a patient with a total knee prosthesis inserted 18 months previously *(left)*. The patient had recently experienced increasing pain in the knee; evidence of osteolysis can be seen around the prosthesis, particularly in the area of the tibial component. Such osteolysis can result either from infection or mechanical loosening. An isotope scan *(right)* shows intense uptake around all the components of the knee joint, typical of infection. In the case of prosthetic loosening, increased isotope uptake would also occur; however, one would expect it to be limited to the component that had been loosened (usually, in the case of the knee, the tibial component), and to be focal at the sites of maximal movement of the prosthesis.

Chronic Osteomyelitis

Although the mortality rate of acute hematogenous osteomyelitis has been reduced to almost zero, between 15 and 30 percent of patients with this disorder still develop chronic disease. Frequently, chronic osteomyelitis follows inadequate treatment with antibiotics, and inadequate surgical debridement of necrotic bone contributes to its development. The necrotic bone within the affected area (the sequestrum) provides a harbor for the bacteria in which they are inaccessible even to high levels of antibiotics. In patients with chronic relapsing osteomyelitis due to Staphylococcus, the organisms isolated in the microbiology laboratory, even after many years, are of the same phage type as the original infecting organisms.

Squamous cell carcinoma has been reported to be a late sequela of chronic osteomyelitis in about 1 percent of patients, occurring up to 30 to 40 years after the original infection (Figs. 4.11, 4.12, and 4.13). Systemic amyloidosis may also be a complication of chronic osteomyelitis.

In the tertiary stage of syphilis, a chronic necrotizing and destructive osteomyelitis characterized by heavy infiltration of plasma cells used to be a common occurrence. These lesions, referred to as gumma, were usually seen in the skull and the long tubular bones (Fig. 4.14). Nongummatous syphilitic periosteitis, a frequent complication of acquired syphilis, may be accompanied only by mild inflammation, comprising mainly fibrosis and perivascular chronic inflammation. Therefore, its infectious nature can easily be overlooked (Fig. 4.15).

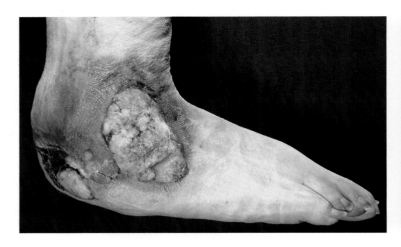

FIGURE 4.11 Gross photograph of the foot and ankle in a patient with long-standing osteomyelitis. Overgrowth of partially ulcerated hyperkeratotic skin is seen in the area of the ankle joint.

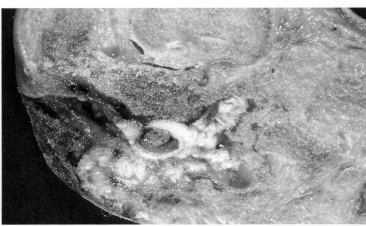

FIGURE 4.12 Sagittal section of the foot shown in Figure 4.11. A draining sinus from the infected bone opens onto the ulcerated skin. There is invasion of firm white tissue from the skin surface into the underlying soft tissue and bone.

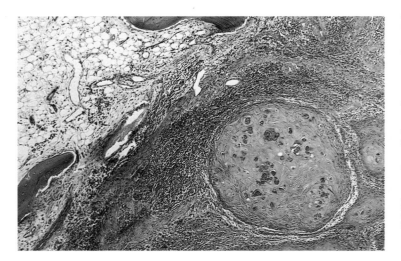

FIGURE 4.13 Photomicrograph of the bone from the patient in Figures 4.11 and 4.12 shows that the bone is being invaded by a well-differentiated epidermoid carcinoma (H & E, x 10 obj.).

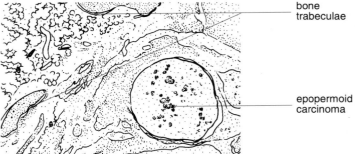

bone trabeculae

epopermoid carcinoma

Chronic Recurrent Multifocal Osteomyelitis

Chronic recurrent multifocal osteomyelitis (CRMO), a recently recognized variant of osteomyelitis in children and young adults, is characterized by the insidious onset of low-grade fever, local swelling, pain in affected bones, and radiologic findings suggesting osteomyelitis. Bone-seeking isotopes may reveal multiple asymptomatic sites of involvement. The lesions occur mainly in the metaphyses of tubular bones and clavicles and are sometimes symmetrically distributed. Prominent periosteal new bone formation in the region of the clavicle may lead to clinically identifiable swelling and thus raise the suspicion of a round-cell malignancy (Fig.

4.16). Cultures for bacterial, fungal, and viral organisms are negative. The clinical course is characterized by intermittent periods of exacerbation and improvement over a period of several years. In some patients, associated recurrent skin lesions (pustulosis palmoplantaris) closely parallel the exacerbations of the bone lesions.

The etiology of this disorder is completely unknown. There is evidence neither of a genetic component or of any abnormality common to all patients.

Acute inflammation, with polymorphonuclear leukocyte predominance, occurs in the early phases of the disease, and fibrosis of the marrow with chronic inflammation occurs in later phases. Microscopically, the

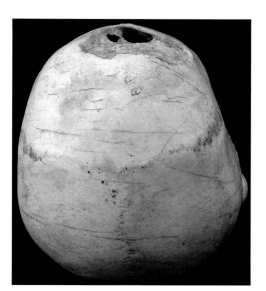

FIGURE 4.14 Photograph of the cranium showing thinning and fenestration of the frontal bone, in this case secondary to a gumma.

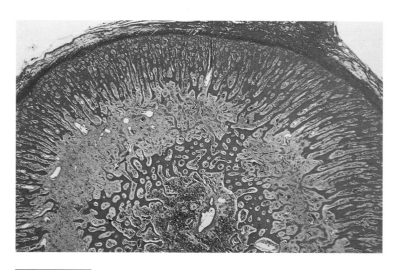

FIGURE 4.15 Photomicrograph showing severe periosteitis with fibrosis and chronic inflammation secondary to syphilitic infection (H & E, x 1 obj.).

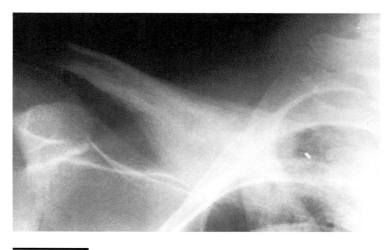

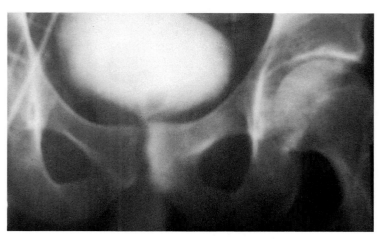

FIGURE 4.16 *(left)* Radiographs of a 23-year-old male who presented initially with pain and swelling in the clavicle. *(right)* Later he also developed lesions in the first and third ribs as well as in the pubis.

most common finding is subacute or chronic osteomyelitis with a predominance of plasma cells. Fragments of necrotic bone with associated multinucleated giant cell, are a common finding (Fig. 4.17).

Septic Arthritis

Joint infection may be caused by hematogenous infection of the synovium, by decompression of contiguous osteomyelitis (Fig. 4.18), or may be a consequence of direct inoculation of a joint following trauma. Septic arthritis is common in neonates and infants, affecting the hip, knee, or ankle. In patients with neonatal septic arthritis, severe residual growth disturbances often result from damage to the growth cartilage. For this reason, the importance of early diagnosis and treatment cannot be overemphasized (Fig. 4.19). Another group of patients particularly susceptible to developing septic arthritis are debilitated older adults with rheumatoid arthritis or other chronic inflammatory joint diseases.

The diagnosis is established by joint aspiration, preferably assisted by radiologic image intensification and performed under strict antiseptic conditions. The aspirate should be sent immediately to the laboratory for direct smear, aerobic and anaerobic cultures, and antibiotic sensitivity analysis. To increase the likelihood of bacterial growth, the aspirate should be inoculated into the medium as soon as possible. (The phenomenon of an apparently sterile infection may well result from difficulties in recovering and growing the bacteria.) The hip joint, situated deep in the body, is difficult to examine, and therefore the diagnosis of septic arthritis in

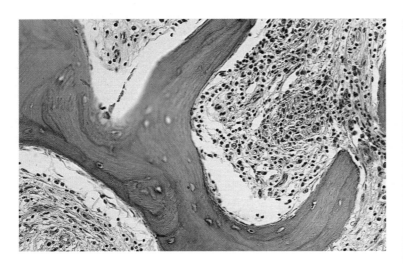

FIGURE 4.17 Photomicrograph of a bone biopsy obtained from the clavicle of the case illustrated in Figure 4.16. There is marrow fibrosis as well as an infiltration of chronic inflammatory cells. As is typical in such cases, no organisms could be isolated (H & E, x 10 obj.). (Case published with permission of Dr. Howard Dorfman)

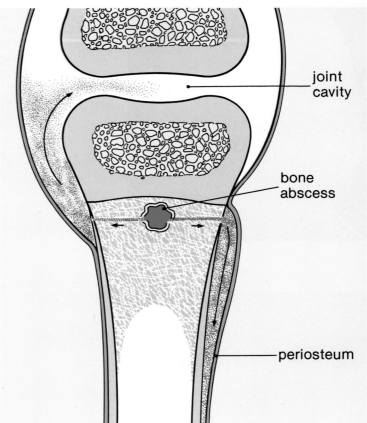

FIGURE 4.18 In patients with osteomyelitis, infected fluid material tracks through the bone to the bone surface, initially elevating the periosteum, and finally breaking through the periosteum into the soft tissues to drain onto the skin surface. In instances where the capsule of the joint is attached below the growth plate (as in the hip), the infection may extend directly into the joint cavity, giving rise to secondary septic arthritis.

this joint tends to be delayed, particularly in newborns and infants.

Cartilage is susceptible to the action of enzymes released by bacteria and disintegrating inflammatory cells, and consequently is rapidly destroyed in patients with septic arthritis (Fig. 4.20). For this reason, treatment of the disease consists of immediate surgical incision and drainage, followed by immobilization of the affected bone. Antibiotic therapy alone is usually insufficient.

Joint Infection Following Venereal Disease

Suppurative arthritis, which was once a frequent complication of gonorrhea, is now decidedly rare, presumably as a result of early and efficient chemotherapy. However, it is an important diagnostic alternative to bear in mind, because the true nature of the disease is likely to be missed unless a careful history is taken. As with other forms of bacterial arthritis, the knee joints are usually the first to be affected, but multiple joint involvement is much more common in patients with gonorrhea than in those with other types of infection. As *Gonococcus* is an extremely fastidious organism, its culture in these cases is extremely difficult.

Transient inflammatory arthritis may be a complication of the acute stage of gonorrhea. However, in these cases the arthritis usually is not caused by bacterial infection of the joint but rather is an immunologic response, often associated with a genetic predisposition. A similar type of arthritis may also complicate cases of nonspecific urethritis and AIDS (see Chapter 10).

Patients with syphilis may also develop arthritis, either as a result of the extension of gummatous osteitis into a joint or as a complication of congenital syphilis. (Charcot's joint, a rapidly destructive noninfectious arthritis which frequently complicates tabes dorsalis, is discussed in Chapter 11.)

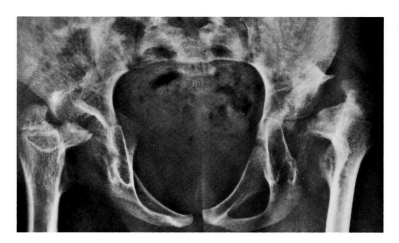

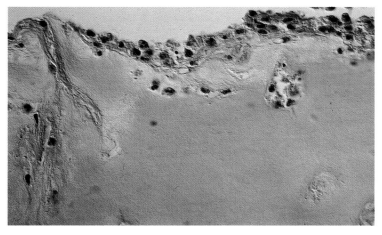

FIGURE 4.19 Radiograph of a 7-year-old boy with a history of multiple joint infections. Destruction of the articular cartilage and subchondral bone has led to total disappearance of both femoral heads and acetabulae with disintegration of the hip joints, characteristic of late septic arthritis.

FIGURE 4.20 Photomicrograph of a portion of articular cartilage obtained from an acutely inflamed joint to show polymorphonuclear leukocytes on the cartilage surface and underlying erosion of the cartilage (H & E, x 25 obj.).

Pyogenic Spondylitis

Pyogenic osteomyelitis of the vertebral column is rare in comparison with infections of the appendicular skeleton, and constitutes less than 1 percent of all cases of osteomyelitis. The disease can be seen at any age but is most common after the sixth decade. It should always be considered in the differential diagnosis of back pain in the elderly. As already mentioned, the predisposing factors include systemic urinary tract infection, diabetes, and IV drug addiction. The lumbar spine is involved twice as frequently as the thoracic spine; the cervical spine is only rarely affected.

This variation is probably associated with the source of the primary infection, as well as the route of infection via Batson's plexus.

Depending on the virulence of the infectious agent, pyogenic spondylitis may manifest as back pain, radiculopathy, and systemic signs of acute infection. Usually, however, the patient presents only with vague localizing symptoms and general malaise. Untreated infection may cause significant deformity of the spine and severe neurologic deficit.

An abscess in the vertebral body can spread posteriorly to involve the posterior arch or may violate the

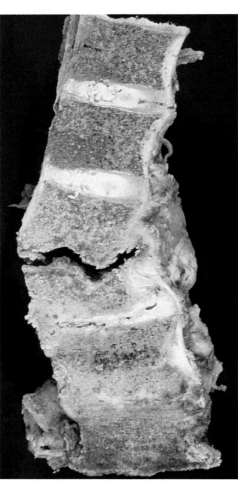

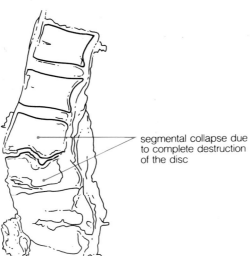

FIGURE 4.21
Photograph of sagittal section through the thoracolumbar spine of a patient with pyogenic spondylitis, showing involvement of few vertebral segments. Mild kyphotic deformity is apparent. Note the complete destruction of the disc by the disease process. (Courtesy of Dr. Krishnan K. Unni)

segmental collapse due to complete destruction of the disc

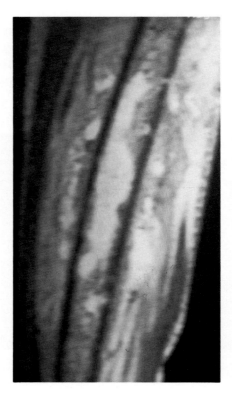

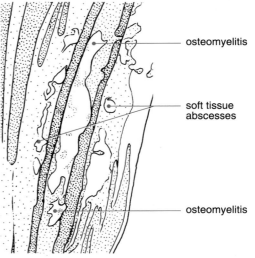

FIGURE 4.22
Magnetic resonance image showing a well-defined area of increased signal intensity in the medullary space of the midshaft of the femur representing osteomyelitis in this intravenous drug abuser. There are soft tissue inflammatory changes with multiple small abscesses adjacent to the femur.

osteomyelitis

soft tissue abscesses

osteomyelitis

anterior cortex and ligamentous structures to form paravertebral soft tissue abscesses. Retropharyngeal abscesses may arise from cervical infections, and abscess in the paraspinal muscle may follow thoracic infections. In the lumbar region, abscess in the psoas sheath may spread to the groin or even to the popliteal fossa. The central nervous system can become contaminated by spread of the infection into the neural canal, resulting in meningitis. The adjacent vertebra is often infected by spread along the vertebral ligaments; the intervertebral disc becomes sequestrated, and may eventually be destroyed (Fig. 4.21).

RADIOGRAPHIC CHANGES

No changes are visible on radiographs in the early stages of osteomyelitis and septic arthritis, although changes can sometimes be observed with MRI (Fig. 4.22). The morphologic changes in individuals with this disease cannot be demonstrated on radiographs until the disease is well established, significant bone destruction has occurred, and there is reactive new bone formation. These difficulties in radiologic diagnosis have

been partly solved by the considerable progress in radionuclide imaging, which permits earlier detection of osteomyelitic foci. Of the many radioactive substances used, technetium polyphosphates appear to produce the best results. In clinical studies, radionuclide uptake has been shown to occur in a sizable percentage of cases 10 to 14 days before changes are evident on radiographs (Fig. 4.23).

Despite its usefulness, radionuclide imaging has important limitations. First, in some patients multiple "hot spots" are detected in the bones at an early stage of Staphylococcus aureus septicemia, but these "spots" do not necessarily progress to clinical osteomyelitis. (It is not known whether these areas represent false-positive results or aborted bone infection.) Second, experimental and clinical studies have documented rare cases of osteomyelitis that have been confirmed by bacteriologic and histologic studies, even though bone scans were initially negative. (This phenomenon may be explained by impaired blood supply to or infarction of the infected area.) Third, technetium polyphosphate bone scanning performed after fracture or bone surgery does not differentiate bone repair from bone infection.

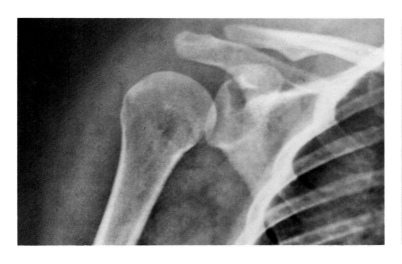 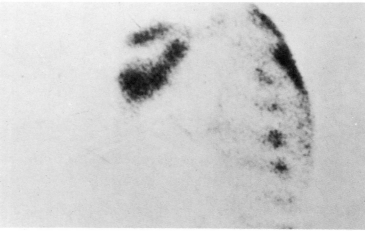

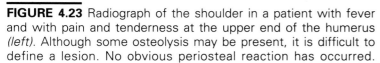

FIGURE 4.23 Radiograph of the shoulder in a patient with fever and with pain and tenderness at the upper end of the humerus *(left)*. Although some osteolysis may be present, it is difficult to define a lesion. No obvious periosteal reaction has occurred. However, in the isotope scan intense uptake of radioactive isotope is evident at the upper end of the humerus *(right)*. (A scan frequently demonstrates the presence of osteomyelitis before any changes are evident on radiographs.)

BACTERIOLOGIC DIAGNOSIS

The conclusive bacteriologic diagnosis of septic arthritis or osteomyelitis depends on the isolation of the pathogen from the lesion or from blood cultures (Fig. 4.24). However, the blood culture is positive only in about 50 percent of patients with acute, untreated hematogenous osteomyelitis. In patients for whom osteomyelitis is a likely diagnosis on the basis of clinical data, direct bone aspiration or surgical biopsy should be carried out when blood culture testing is negative. The importance of immediate inoculation into the medium of the material suspected of being infected cannot be overemphasized. Delay in getting the material from the operating room to the microbiology laboratory, and consequently in plating out and inoculating medium from swabs and tissue obtained from the diseased area, may lead to a reduced number of viable organisms, and therefore to a false-negative culture.

MORBID ANATOMY OF OSTEOMYELITIS

The presence of bacteria in a bone does not necessarily lead to osteomyelitis. It is generally believed that trauma is an important associated prerequisite, perhaps because it produces venostasis or thrombosis and thus provides a nidus for bacterial growth.

As with most infections, the clinical course of bone

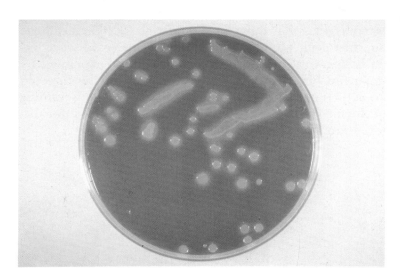

FIGURE 4.24 A blood-agar plate shows growth of beta-hemolytic staphylococci.

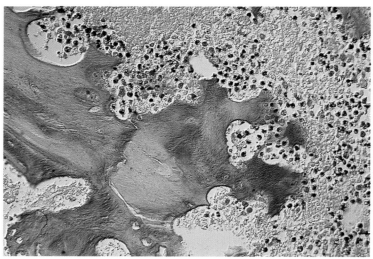

FIGURE 4.25 Photomicrograph of biopsy tissue from a case of osteomyelitis demonstrates a polymorphonuclear leukocyte infiltrate with focal areas of fibrinous exudate. The bone is necrotic and shows focal erosion secondary to enzymic digestion (H & E, x 10 obj.).

infection depends on the interaction between the injurious agent and the host tissue. In other words, the severity of the disease in a patient with osteomyelitis depends on the virulence of the invading organism, the site of infection, and the patient's age and general health.

The initial local response to infection with pyogenic bacteria is acute inflammation, which results in the production of an exudate containing polymorphonuclear leukocytes (neutrophils) and fibrin (Fig. 4.25). Continuing exudation raises the tissue pressure and, because bone is unable to expand, this pressure cannot be relieved by swelling, as is possible in most tissues.

Instead, the only potential space—the vascular space—is compromised, leading to widespread bone death (Fig. 4.26). Indeed, the major problem in treating patients with osteomyelitis is the extent of the resulting osteonecrosis, which interferes with the access of antibiotics.

Eventually, the exudate is forced through the medullary canal and the haversian systems of the cortical bone to the bone surface. In children, the cortex is thin and the periosteum is only loosely attached, so it is easily elevated (Fig. 4.27). New bone from the cambium layer of the periosteum produces a sleeve of reactive

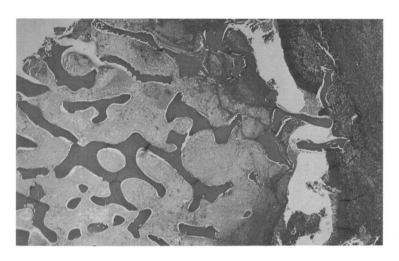

FIGURE 4.26 Photomicrograph demonstrates an area of necrotic bone surrounded by an acute inflammatory exudate (pus). A focus of necrotic bone such as this allows the sequestration of bacteria, and unless it is surgically removed, antibiotic therapy may not prevent the development of chronic relapsing osteomyelitis.

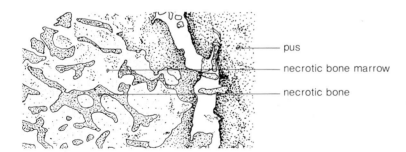

pus

necrotic bone marrow

necrotic bone

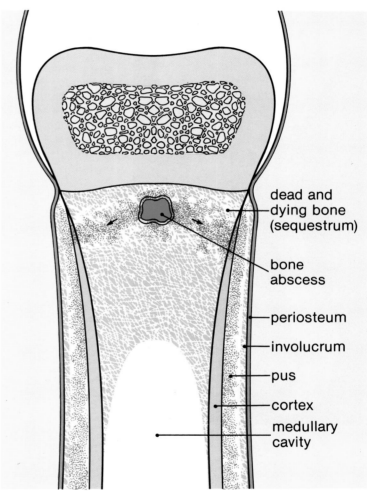

dead and dying bone (sequestrum)

bone abscess

periosteum

involucrum

pus

cortex

medullary cavity

FIGURE 4.27 As illustrated in this diagram, increased pressure in the medullary cavity eventually results in extension of the inflammatory exudate through the haversian systems of the cortex and beneath the periosteum. The elevated periosteum will lay down a sleeve of new bone (involucrum) around the infected segment. In children, this reaction is likely to be prominent: in adults, much less so.

bone (the involucrum) around the affected area. In very young children, the involucrum may be quite massive (Fig. 4.28). In adults (in whom the periosteum is firmly attached to the cortical bone), the periosteal elevation and new bone formation may be minimal. In children, the necrotic medullary bone becomes isolated within a large cavity and is referred to as the sequestrum (Fig. 4.29). The sequestrum may consist of a mere wafer of cortex, the devascularized cancellous bone having been absorbed, or it may be a large piece of bone or many small pieces. In adults, a large involucrum and the associated sequestrum formation are much less common. In untreated cases, the pus frequently extends beyond the confines of the periosteum into the soft tissue and ultimately through the skin, forming a draining sinus (Fig. 4.30).

The extent of the bone affected varies from case to case. When the entire diaphysis is surrounded by pus,

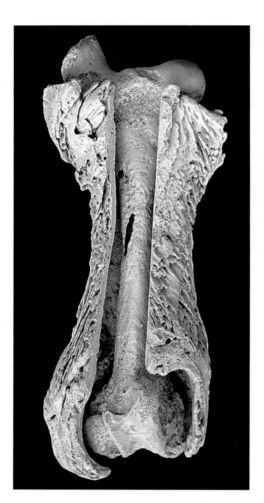

FIGURE 4.28
Gross photograph of a femur from a calf with osteomyelitis. The periosteal reaction has resulted in an extensive sleeve of new bone (the involucrum) which surrounds the necrotic, partially destroyed diaphysis of the femur (the sequestrum).

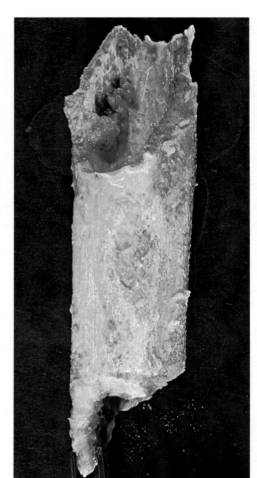

FIGURE 4.29
Gross photograph of a sequestrum removed from a patient with chronic osteomyelitis of the femur. It is important to remove such a focus of dead bone from an individual with osteomyelitis if persistent, chronic infection is to be avoided.

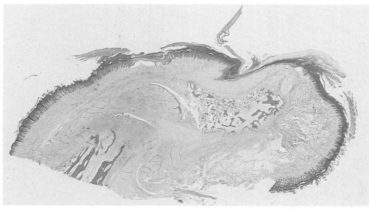

FIGURE 4.30 Photomicrograph of a toe removed from a diabetic patient who had developed osteomyelitis. The inflammatory response has led to destruction of the bone, the distal interphalangeal joint, and a sinus tract opening onto the skin dorsally (H & E, x 1 obj.).

it becomes completely necrotic. If only a small area of cortex is devascularized, the affected area may be gradually resorbed and will appear as a lytic zone on radiographic examination. Necrotic bone can undergo resorption only when there are viable cells in the marrow, because resorption depends not only on secretion of enzymes but also on active phagocytosis by osteoclasts.

If the infection is localized, an abscess (Brodie's abscess) will form (Fig. 4.31). The radiographic differential diagnosis of Brodie's abscess includes osteoid osteoma, eosinophilic granuloma, and malignant small-cell tumors (Fig. 4.32). In most cases, however, infection of the bone does not result in a localized abscess.

Osteomyelitis is often a complication of diseases that tend to result in vascular insufficiency. In the United States, perhaps the most common of these is sickle cell anemia (Fig. 4.33), in which patients often experience repeated attacks of bone infection.

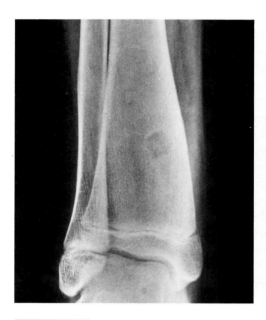

FIGURE 4.31 Radiograph of the ankle in a patient complaining of a dull aching pain in the lower leg reveals a lytic lesion with a well-defined sclerotic margin. Biopsy proved this lesion to have resulted from infection.

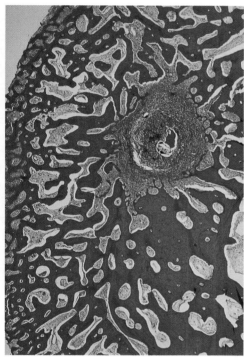

FIGURE 4.32 Photomicrograph of a cortical abscess, excised from the femoral neck of a 12-year-old boy, which was mistaken for an osteoid osteoma (H & E, x 1 obj.).

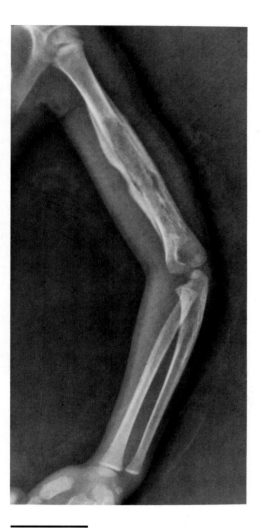

FIGURE 4.33 Radiograph of the arm in a patient with sickle cell disease shows permeative bone destruction of the humerus, with involucrum formation and extensive sequestration. At surgery, these complications were shown to be due to infection.

Among the organisms that may be isolated from these cases of osteomyelitis is Salmonella. It has been postulated that Salmonella organisms gain access to the blood through microinfarcts of the bowel. However, it should be pointed out that Salmonella is not the most common organism in patients with sickle cell disease; staphylococci are still the most common bacteria cultured from patients with osteomyelitis complicating sickle cell disease. Furthermore, not all cases of Salmonella osteomyelitis are seen in patients with sickle cell disease (Fig. 4.34).

Two other bone diseases that may be complicated by ischemia and infection are Gaucher's disease and osteopetrosis. In patients with Gaucher's disease, osteomyelitis sometimes follows a biopsy procedure. Therefore, if biopsy is performed for such patients the strictest asepsis is necessary (and even antibiotic coverage should be considered). In patients with osteopetrosis, it is the jaw that is often affected, probably via tooth infections.

GRANULOMATOUS INFLAMMATION OF BONES AND JOINTS

TUBERCULOSIS

Clinical Considerations

In 1779, Pott described the clinical presentation of paraplegia associated with the characteristic gibbus formation that bears his name. We now know that Pott's disease is usually associated with granulomatous inflammation. Approximately 1 percent of patients with tuberculosis develop musculoskeletal complications; and the most common site of skeletal involvement is the spine, owing to the primary tubercular foci in the lungs and the bowel.

Before the advent of modern chemotherapy for tuberculosis, and before the elimination of bovine tuberculosis in dairy cattle, bone and joint tuberculosis was one of the most common indications for admission to an orthopedic service. In less developed countries this is still the case. In developed countries, however, tuberculosis has become unusual enough that there is a real risk that it may remain clinically undetected. In many instances, the true nature of the disease becomes apparent only after the pathologist has examined the tissue. There is increased risk for tuberculous infection in individuals with chronic debilitating conditions (including narcotic addicts, patients receiving cortisone therapy, and other therapeutically immunosuppressed patients) and in AIDS patients.

In drug addicts, miliary tuberculosis may present as an acute febrile illness. However, in most patients the onset of symptoms is likely to be insidious and includes local pain as well as systemic signs of chronic debilitating illness.

Osseous tuberculosis is caused by metastatic spread of the disease from elsewhere in the body, usually from the lungs. In most patients, bony foci of infection coexist with arthritis, and multiple skeletal lesions are not uncommon. Skeletal manifestation of tuberculosis most often occurs in the spine (Figs. 4.35 and 4.36); the next

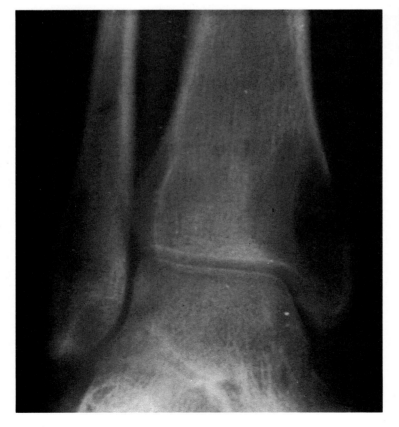

FIGURE 4.34 Radiograph of a middle-aged woman who was in good general health except for pain in the right ankle. The x-ray was interpreted as being most consistent with a giant cell tumor. Biopsy proved the lesion to be inflammatory, and *Salmonella typhosa* was isolated by culture.

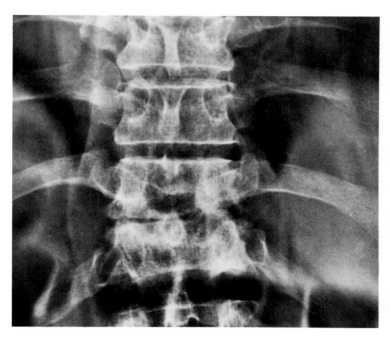 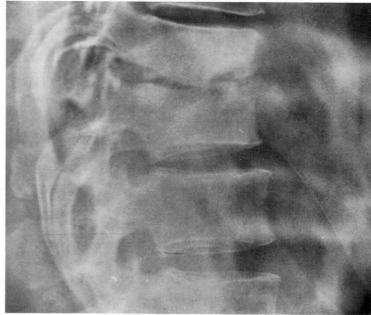

FIGURE 4.35 Anteroposterior radiograph of the spine *(left)* shows narrowing and destruction of the intervertebral disc at the level of T11–T12. Note also the paravertebral soft tissue swelling.

In the lateral radiograph *(right)*, destructive bone disease is seen anteriorly in the 11th and 12th thoracic vertebrae. This lesion was proved to be due to tuberculosis.

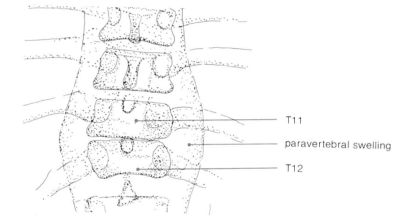

T11

paravertebral swelling

T12

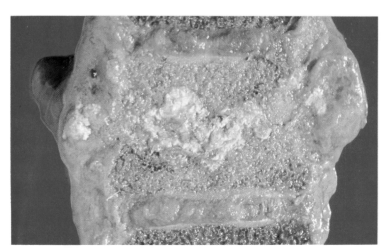

FIGURE 4.36 Gross photograph of a portion of the spine removed at necropsy from a patient with tuberculosis reveals destruction of the intervertebral disc space and contiguous bone, and the presence of a cheesy necrotic tissue (caseation necrosis). The caseating tissue extends into the soft tissue on either side of the spinal column.

most commonly affected area is the hip (Figs. 4.37 and 4.38), followed by the knee (Fig. 4.39). However, any joint may be involved, including those of the hand.

In general, osseous tuberculosis is a disease of young people, and both sexes are equally affected. Most patients are under the age of 25 years at diagnosis; however, the disease can occur at any age. Tuberculosis of the spine and hip is more common in children; tuberculosis of the knee is most common in adults.

The lower thoracic spine is the most frequent site of tuberculous spondylitis in both children and adults,

and involvement of several vertebral bodies occurs in 50 percent of cases. The disease often begins in one vertebral body and spreads underneath the spinal ligaments to affect other vertebrae.

At the time of presentation, the patient with tuberculous spondylitis may have radiculopathy caused by compression of the spinal cord or nerve roots. The disease may also spread to the meninges, with subsequent tuberculous meningitis.

In all age groups, paraplegia was the most serious complication before the advent of chemotherapy. Para-

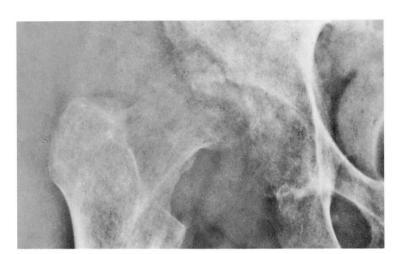

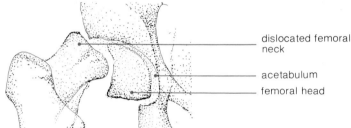

FIGURE 4.37 Radiograph of a patient with long-standing pain and limitation of motion in the right hip. Destructive joint disease with involvement of the bone is evident in both the femoral head and the acetabulum. In addition, a dislocation of the femoral neck has occurred. These are common manifestations of tuberculosis.

dislocated femoral neck

acetabulum

femoral head

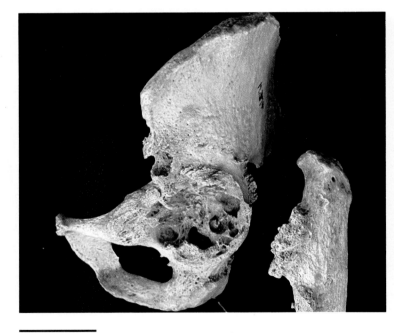

FIGURE 4.38 Macerated bone specimen obtained at necropsy demonstrates destructive disease of the hip joint in a patient with tuberculosis. Total destruction of the femoral head has occurred, with only a stump of the femoral neck remaining attached to the shaft of the femur.

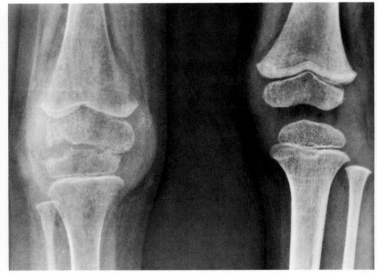

FIGURE 4.39 Radiograph of the knees in a child complaining of pain, swelling, and limitation of motion in the right knee. Note the narrowing of the joint, resulting from the destruction of cartilage and bone, that is evident in the right knee (the destruction is particularly obvious at the margins of the joint). In addition to the destructive changes, the radiograph also shows marked soft-tissue swelling. These changes were caused by tuberculosis.

plegia is caused by extension of the disease process into the peridural space with resultant pressure on the cord. This may be accentuated by the mechanical pressure associated with bone deformity. Dislocation of affected segments may lead to sudden paraplegia.

Because the initial lesion is most often seen in the lower thoracic spine, the psoas muscle sheath is frequently affected; patients may present with a fluctuant swelling, or cold abscess, in the groin or elsewhere as the result of tracking of the infected material from the paraspinal area. In untreated patients, this course eventually leads to vertebral collapse and angulation of the vertebral column (Pott's disease) (Fig. 4.40).

Radiographic Findings

Radiographic examination of an involved joint shows osteoporosis and soft-tissue swelling early in the disease. These changes are followed by marginal erosion of the bone and destruction of the subchondral bone, with narrowing of the joint space.

In non-weight-bearing joints such as the shoulder, but also occasionally in the knee joint, subchondral lysis may occur without obvious joint destruction. In such cases, which are sometimes referred to as "caries sicca," the lesion may mimic a tumor radiographically, and in children may be mistaken for a chondroblastoma (Fig. 4.41).

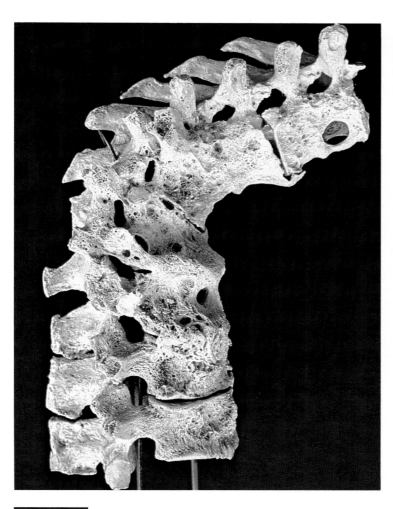

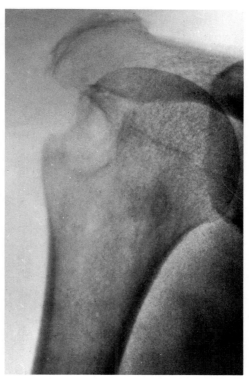

FIGURE 4.41 Radiograph showing a well-defined lytic lesion in the outer aspect of the humeral head which encroaches upon both the epiphysis and metaphysis. This lesion proved on biopsy to be due to tuberculosis.

FIGURE 4.40 Macerated specimen of spine removed at autopsy from a patient with chronic tuberculosis. In addition to extensive bone destruction, severe kyphosis and fusion of several vertebral bodies are seen.

In the spine, radiographic examination shows focal bony destruction with disc involvement and vertebral collapse. Unlike pyogenic osteomyelitis, reactive new bone around the infected focus and hypertrophied osteophytes is not common. The primary granulomatous abscess may be located in the vertebral body either anteriorly, paradiscally, or centrally, giving rise to three characteristic radiographic presentations (Fig. 4.42).

The anterior lesion, which accounts for approximately 20 percent of cases, usually leads to cortical bone destruction under the anterior longitudinal ligament. As the ligament lifts off the vertebral margin, infection spreads to the adjacent vertebral segment.

The paradiscal lesion, which accounts for over half the cases, begins in the vertebral metaphysis and erodes through the cartilaginous end plate, extending around and sequestrating the disc to extend into the adjacent vertebra. Disc space narrowing, bone destruction with subsequent kyphotic deformity, and eventual intervertebral body fusion occur, usually after 1 to 2 years.

The central lesion, which accounts for the remaining cases, begins in the mid-portion of the vertebral body. It then spreads to involve the entire vertebral body, leading to vertebral collapse and usually to pronounced gibbus deformity (Figs. 4.43 and 4.44).

Pathologic Findings

Gross examination of the areas affected by tuberculosis is likely to show thickened edematous tissue, frequently studded with grayish small nodules, sometimes with white opaque centers (granulomas). These granulomas often become confluent and produce larger areas of white necrotic material, so-called caseation (or cheesy) necrosis. In the joint, separation of the articular cartilage that is dissected from the underlying bone by granulomatous tissue is a characteristic feature. In the later stages of untreated disease, ankylosis is a frequent complication.

On microscopic examination, the typical tubercle (Figs. 4.45 and 4.46) consists of a central necrotic area surrounded by pale histiocytes, sometimes referred to as epithelioid cells. Among the epithelioid cells are some scattered giant cells, the nuclei of which are typically arranged at the margin of the cell (Langerhans giant cells). At the periphery of the tubercle is a rim of mixed chronic inflammatory cells. Often the tubercles are confluent, resulting in extensive central caseation. The acid-fast bacilli can be demonstrated with the Ziehl–Neelsen stain, and are characteristically seen in the giant cells and at the margin of the caseous area.

Occasional bone infections may result from atypical mycobacteria, such as *Mycobacterium avium* as is

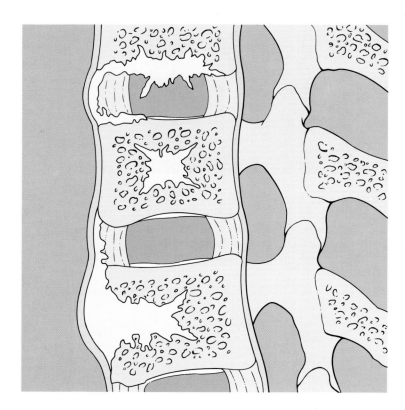

FIGURE 4.42 Schematic drawing showing three possible locations of the primary focus of tuberculous infection in the vertebral body. Each results in a characteristic radiographic presentation.

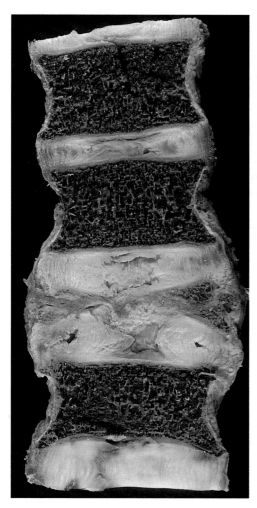

FIGURE 4.43
Frontal section through the thoracolumbar spine of a 67-year-old male. There is complete collapse of L3 secondary to tuberculosis which initially involved the mid-portion of the vertebral body.

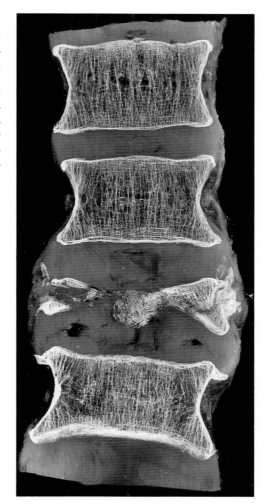

FIGURE 4.44
Radiograph of the specimen illustrated in Figure 4.43.

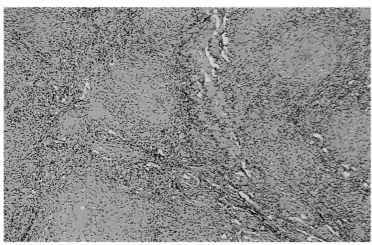

FIGURE 4.45 Photomicrograph of granulomatous tissue obtained from the synovium of a knee joint in a patient with tuberculosis. Many focal giant cells, nodular collections of histiocytes, and an infiltration of chronic inflammatory cells are present (H & E, x 4 obj.).

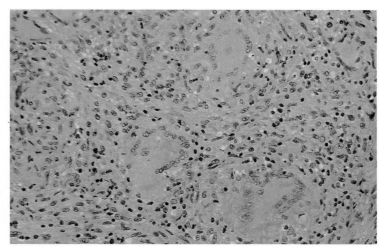

FIGURE 4.46 Photomicrograph showing the typical appearance of the giant cells in tuberculosis, with peripherally arranged nuclei—the so-called Langerhans giant cells (H & E, x 10 obj.).

the case in patients who are immunocompromised by AIDS. In this instance, typical granulomas may not form and only large numbers of histiocytes may be present. However, acid-fast staining will show large numbers of intracellular organisms, many more than are observed in a patient with the more typical presentation of tuberculosis (Fig. 4.47). Moreover, because atypical mycobacteria may be difficult to culture from synovial fluid, synovial biopsy may be necessary for diagnosis.

SARCOIDOSIS

About 10 percent of patients with sarcoidosis have joint involvement. In most cases this condition is a migratory polyarticular disease, often symmetrical and of only a few weeks' duration. In a small number of patients, a chronic granulomatous arthritis is present. Most often, this form of the disease is localized in the patient's fingers, where it clinically resembles rheumatoid disease (Fig. 4.48). Involvement of the synovium of large joints is rare, and therefore may lead to the mistaken diagnosis of tuberculosis (Figs. 4.49 and 4.50). However, certain histologic features help to distinguish sarcoidosis from tuberculosis, eg, the lack of caseation necrosis, the increased prominence of large, pale epithelioid cells with fewer chronic inflammatory cells, and the absence of acid-fast bacilli. (With regard to this last point, it should be noted that it is frequently difficult to demonstrate acid-fast bacilli in patients with bone and joint tuberculosis. In any individual suspected of having granulomatous tissue, smears should be taken for direct examination, and cultures for tuberculosis, brucellosis, fungus, and atypical mycobacteria should be prepared. In general, a firm diagnosis can be made only when positive cultures have been obtained.)

MYCOTIC INFECTIONS

The spine, as well as other bones and joints, can be affected by mycotic infections, with the lung being the usual portal of entry. The radiographic and pathologic features are similar to those of tuberculosis. For this reason, when granulomatous infection is found or suspected, it is important to make direct smears and to prepare cultures not only for acid-fast organisms but also for fungi. Common fungal conditions that have been found to be responsible for granulomatous infections include blastomycosis, coccidioidomycosis, cryptococcosis, and rarely actinomycosis.

Blastomycosis

Blastomycosis, endemic in the mid-Atlantic states, and in the Mississippi and Ohio Valleys, is acquired by inhalation of the spores of *Blastomyces dermatitidis*, a spherical, thick-walled yeast-like fungus found in the soil. The fungi induce a granulomatous infection of the lungs which, when established, may lead to dissemination of the fungi to other sites by way of the bloodstream. The most common skeletal sites are the vertebrae, ribs, tibia, and the tarsal and carpal bones. The

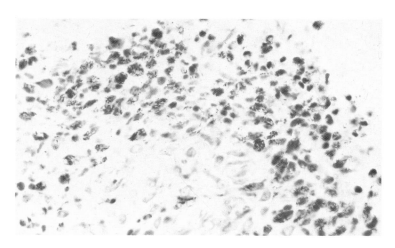

FIGURE 4.47 Photomicrograph of a specimen obtained from a patient with an atypical mycobacterial infection of the ankle joint. Innumerable acid-fast bacilli are present, and most of them are within histiocytes (Ziehl–Neelsen stain, x 100 obj.).

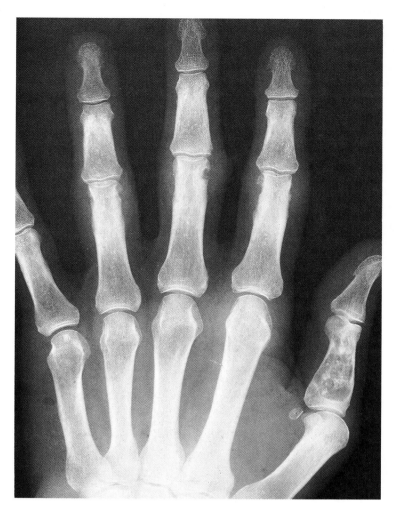

FIGURE 4.48 Radiograph of the hand in a patient with sarcoidosis demonstrates the two types of lesions that can be seen in this condition. Punched-out cortical erosions, some with obvious overlying soft-tissue lesions, are evident at the distal end of the proximal phalanx in the index, middle, and ring fingers. In the thumb is a central lytic lesion of the proximal phalanx, similar in appearance to the lesions of dactylitis tuberculosa seen in young adults.

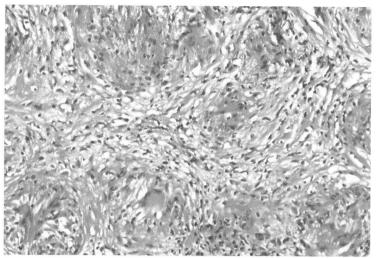

FIGURE 4.49 Photomicrograph of the synovium from a patient with sarcoidosis of the knee joint. Multiple nodules composed of pale histiocytes and giant cells are evident (H & E, x 10 obj.).

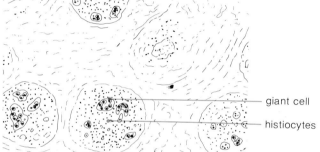

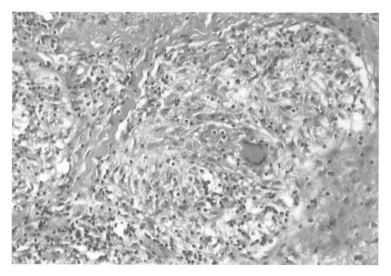

FIGURE 4.50 The noncaseating character of the granulomas can be seen in this higher power photomicrograph of the specimen shown in Figure 4.49. Note also the lack of lymphocytic cuffing of the granulomas. The rarity of sarcoidosis in large joints is likely to result in misinterpretation of the lesion as some other form of granulomatous inflammation, as was the case in this patient (H & E, x 40 obj.).

affected bones may exhibit necrosis and/or may be the site of an abscess. Therefore, if the vertebrae are involved, radiographic differentiation from tuberculous spondylitis can be difficult (Fig. 4.51). Microscopic examination of a stained smear of sputum, pleural fluid, or pus from the affected part will reveal the characteristic thick-walled, budding yeast cells.

Coccidioidomycosis

Coccidioidomycosis, also known as San Joaquin Valley fever, is caused by the fungus *Coccidioides immitis*. There is a high incidence of this disease in the arid southwestern United States. The lesions are usually lytic, with indiscriminate involvement and destruction of vertebral bodies, neural arches, and even contiguous ribs. Late changes of vertebral collapse may render differentiation from tuberculous spondylitis difficult.

Cryptococcosis

Skeletal cryptococcosis often occurs secondary to cases of chronic meningoencephalitis caused by *Cryptococcus neoformans*. The pelvis, femur, spine, and tibia are among the most common sites of involvement. Patients usually present with pain, swelling, and tenderness over the affected part. Radiographically, these lesions present as radiolucencies with or without local subperiosteal new bone formation. Histologically, the lesions reveal granulation tissue containing multinuclear giant cells, lymphocytes, and histiocytes. The presence of the yeastlike cryptococci may also be demonstrated (Figs. 4.52, 4.53, and 4.54).

Actinomycosis

Actinomycotic infections are usually insidious and chronic. The bone is rarely involved except as a result of a puncture wound (Figs. 4.55 and 4.56).

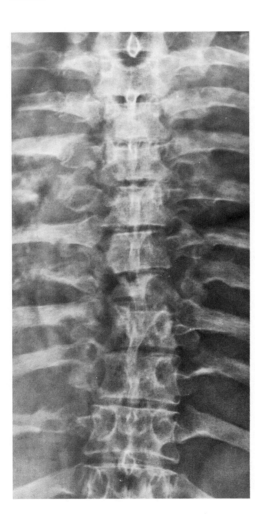
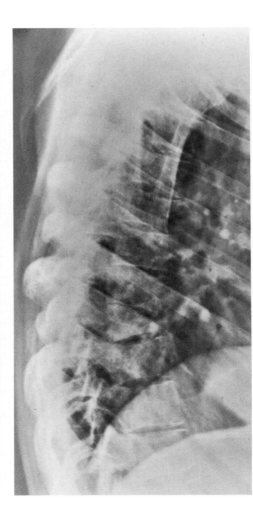
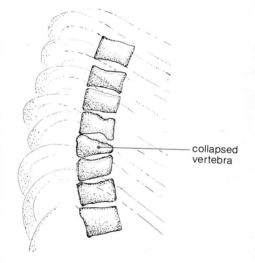

FIGURE 4.51 Anteroposterior *(left)* and lateral *(right)* radiographs of the thoracic spine demonstrate multiple destructive lesions involving several vertebral bodies, some of which are partially collapsed. Biopsy proved this to be due to blastomycosis.

collapsed vertebra

Other Fungal Infections

Sporotrichosis infection may result from the direct contamination of a joint by a puncture wound from the thorn of a contaminated plant (often a rose).

Patients with long-term indwelling intravenous catheters (eg, for parenteral nutrition) occasionally develop bone and joint infections due to Candida or Aspergillus.

Because blood cultures are likely to be negative with fungal infections, biopsy may be necessary for diagnosis.

PARASITIC INFECTIONS

Echinococcal Cysts

Echinococcal cysts (hydatid cysts) are not uncommonly seen in the bones of patients from sheep-raising countries in which the disease is endemic. The cyst is often seen initially at the epiphyseal end of the bone, usually affecting the spongiosa because localization is dependent on hematogenous dissemination. It should be noted that hydatid echinococcosis developing intraosseously does not resemble the classic unilocular hydatid of soft tissue. Rather, it is usually a multiloculated lesion, with an irregular outline that can be easily confused with a tumor on radiographs (Figs. 4.57 and 4.58). This is because the resistance offered by the osseous tissue causes the larva to develop by exogenous budding, resulting in the presence of many small cysts growing outside the original focus of implantation (Fig. 4.59). Scolices rarely develop in these cysts, and therefore, they are usually sterile (Fig. 4.60). Only when the cyst erupts to the surrounding soft tissue does the lesion assume the more conventional large unilocular appearance.

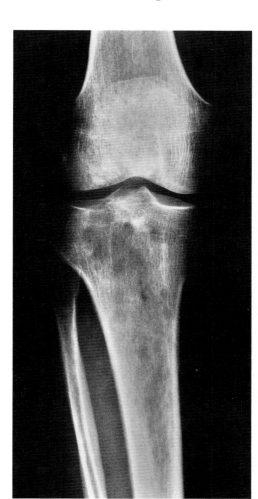

FIGURE 4.52
Radiograph of the right knee of a 60-year-old man complaining of mild pain for a few months. The film shows a poorly defined lytic lesion extending from the articular surface of the tibia into the diaphysis. The cortex appears intact. Biopsy proved this to be the result of infection with coccidioidomycosis. (Courtesy of Dr. A. Roessner)

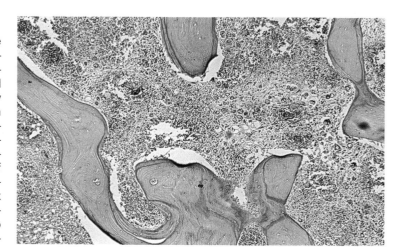

FIGURE 4.53 Low-power photomicrograph of tissue obtained from a patient with chronic spinal disease resulting from infection with *Coccidioides immitis*. The marrow space is infiltrated by chronic inflammatory tissue (H & E, x 4 obj.).

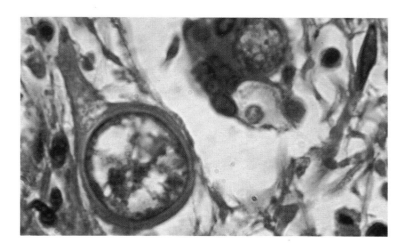

FIGURE 4.54 High-power view of the tissue shown in Figure 4.53 reveals two rounded, thick-walled fungal organisms containing endospores (H & E, x 100 obj.).

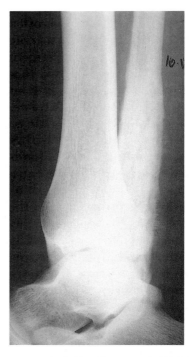

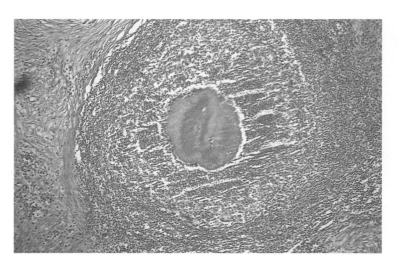

FIGURE 4.55 Radiograph of the ankle of a middle-aged shepherd with a sclerotic lesion of the lower fibula which on biopsy proved to be due to actinomycosis. (Courtesy of Dr. Juan Roig)

FIGURE 4.56 Photomicrograph of tissue obtained from the lesion shown in Figure 4.55 demonstrates an acute and chronic inflammatory reaction surrounding the typical eosinophilic "sulfur" granule seen in association with actinomycosis (H & E, x 10 obj.). (Courtesy of Dr. Miguel Calvo)

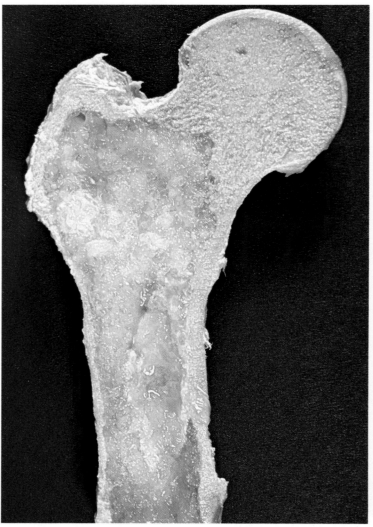

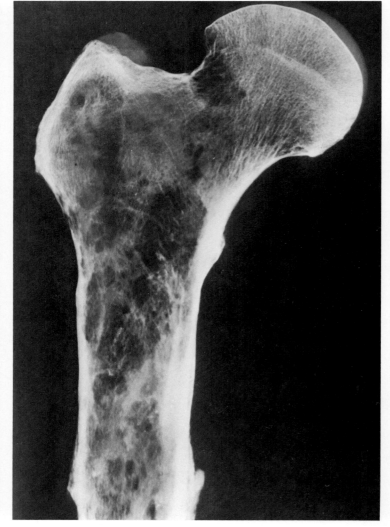

FIGURE 4.57 Gross photograph of the upper end of a femur removed at necropsy from a patient with hydatid disease. The medullary cavity is filled with glistening white nodular tissue, which on closer examination is found to be made up of fibrous-walled cysts.

FIGURE 4.58 Radiograph of the specimen shown in Figure 4.57. Note the multiloculated lytic appearance and the irregular thinning of the cortices. In those parts of the world where the occurrence of hydatid disease is rare, such radiographic findings will probably be interpreted by the radiologist as a tumor.

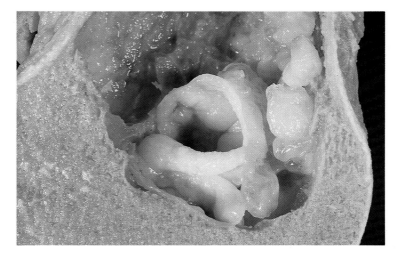

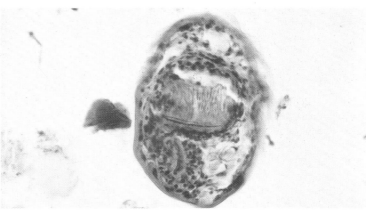

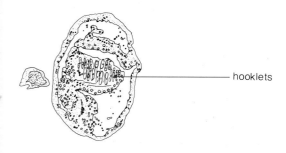

hooklets

FIGURE 4.59 Gross photograph of the many small cysts that are characteristic of echinococcal infestation of the bone.

FIGURE 4.60 Photomicrograph of material removed from a hydatid cyst reveals a scolex with hooklets (H & E, x 100 obj.).

SECTION III

METABOLIC DISTURBANCES

Metabolism, a term from the Greek μεταβωλη (metabolē: to change, convert, or transform), refers to the sum of all the physical and chemical processes by which a living organism is maintained (anabolism) and also to the transformation by which energy is made available for use by the organism (catabolism).

The maintenance of a functional skeleton depends on a continuing process of interactions between those cells that form and maintain the bone matrix (the osteoblasts and osteocytes) and those that remove bone matrix during the remodeling process (the osteoclasts). The term *metabolic bone disease* (MBD) is generally used to refer to those diseases that affect the skeleton as the result of cellular disturbances in the formation (anabolism) and breakdown (catabolism) of the extracellular matrices. Because the skeletal system has two major functions, mechanical and metabolic, there are two classes of MBDs: those caused by cellular disturbances that affect structural homeostasis, as in osteoporosis and Paget's disease, and those that affect mineral homeostasis, as in hyperparathyroidism and osteomalacia. It must be recognized that the two homeostatic systems are not independent: disturbances in structural homeostasis may influence calcium regulation, and disturbances in calcium regulation can and do alter structure, often resulting in mechanical failure.

In the nineteenth century and earlier, the MBDs were classified on the basis of the different skeletal deformities they produced. The introduction of radiography in the late 1800s enabled better anatomic and clinical characterization. Improvements in biochemical laboratory techniques permitted further diagnostic refinement and have shed much light on the mechanisms of physiologic control in the skeletal system. The development of procedures for plastic embedding of undecalcified bone specimens has made it possible to correlate the clinical, radiographic, and biochemical features with the microscopic histological features of this complex group of conditions.

No consensus presently exists concerning either the classification or the nomenclature of MBDs. For the purpose of discussion here, it is convenient to group these disorders according to their most significant pathologic feature. Chapter 5 deals with disturbances in the quality of the matrix caused by the synthesis of abnormal matrix constituents. These diseases, such as osteogenesis imperfecta, often result in severe deformities and can sometimes result in mechanical insufficiency. Chapter 6 discusses disturbances in cell linkage that give rise to quantitative differences in skeletal mass such as osteoporosis, the signs and symptoms of which are mainly confined to the bone. Chapter 7 deals with disturbances secondary to altered calcium homeostasis, in which both local disease in the bone and systemic disease caused by abnormal calcium levels in the blood and tissue are likely to be encountered. Finally, Chapter 8 discusses those diseases of the skeleton that result either from the deposition of extraneous metabolic products in skeletal tissue or from disease of the hematopoietic tissue.

**Diseases resulting from
abnormal synthesis of
matrix components**

s previously discussed in Chapter 1, the mechanical properties of the connective tissues are dependent upon the synthesis by the cells (eg, osteoblasts, chondroblasts, fibroblasts) of organic matrix constituents, both of the right type and in the right amount. These matrix constituents include collagen, proteoglycan, and other noncollagenous proteins. Disturbances in collagen synthesis may be congenital, as in osteogenesis imperfecta, or acquired, as in scurvy. The disturbance may be of intracellular origin, as in both osteogenesis imperfecta and scurvy, or extracellular origin, as in some cases of Ehlers–Danlos syndrome (Fig. 5.1). However, whether congenital or acquired, pretranslational or posttranslational, all of these conditions give rise to abnormalities in the connective tissue matrices that affect the mechanical properties of the skeleton. These mechanical properties are also very dependent on the calcification of the organic matrix. This, in turn, is dependent not only on adequate amounts of calcium and inorganic phosphates in the tissue fluid but also on the exercise of cellular control by means of the positive and negative influences of many substances, including alkaline phosphatase.

The final adult size (height, weight, build) of an individual is the result of many complex factors. Among the most important are the total number of connective tissue cells involved in production of the extracellular matrix, the quantity of extracellular matrix produced by each of the connective tissue cells, and the optimal functioning of the epiphyseal growth plate during the period of development.

Bone strength is determined by both genetic factors and nongenetic factors, such as diet and activity level.

OSTEOGENESIS IMPERFECTA

CLINICAL EVALUATION

Osteogenesis imperfecta (OI) is the most commonly recognized congenital disease affecting the production of collagen. It therefore involves the bone matrix as well as other connective tissues. The general category of OI includes a heterogenous group of conditions, for most of which the underlying biochemical defect is unknown.

The clinical disease state includes a number of distinct syndromes; some are transmitted as an autosomal dominant trait, others as a recessive trait, and still others occur as spontaneous ("point") mutations. On the basis of their pattern of inheritance, Silence has identified at least four types of OI. The largest group, Type 1, is inherited as an autosomal dominant trait and is characterized by osteoporosis and gray-blue sclerae.

Type 2 OI, with an autosomal recessive mode of inheritance, occurs in children who die before or soon after birth. The long bones are said to be characteristically broad and crumpled, and exhibit multiple fractures. Type 3, a severe form of the disease seen in children, results in progressive deformities and multiple fractures. The scleral color in these patients is almost normal, and both dominant and recessive autosomal inheritance patterns have been noted. The final group, Type 4, consists of osteoporosis with an autosomal dominant pattern of inheritance and is associated with normal scleral color.

These various syndromes have certain clinical features in common. The majority of patients are short in stature, and the most severely affected cases are dwarfed. There is an increased propensity to fracture due to osteopenia. However, the incidence of fracture varies considerably depending on the severity of the disease, and fractures are more common in children than in adults (Fig. 5.2). The standard treatment of fractures by immobilization results in disuse osteoporosis which, in turn, further increases the tendency to fracture, thereby setting up a vicious cycle (Fig. 5.3). Thus, once a fracture has occurred, these unfortunate patients have a tendency towards repeated fractures in the same area.

The presence in many patients of blue sclerae (Fig. 5.4), poorly formed dentin (Fig. 5.5), and ligamentous laxity indicates that the disease is not confined to the skeleton but rather involves a generalized disorder of the connective tissues. Collagen synthesis by the osteoblasts and other connective tissue cells is deficient quantitatively (Fig. 5.6) and has been shown to differ qualitatively, at least in some patients. The qualitative differences result from specific deletions in the genes that code for collagen production.

Two clinical forms of osteogenesis imperfecta are generally recognized. The more severe (congenita) type is manifest at birth and is associated with generalized osteoporosis, mutiple fractures with deformities, micromelia, and caput membranacea (Fig. 5.7). Patients afflicted by the less severe (tarda) type have far fewer fractures, usually two or less per year during the growing period, although the other stigmata of the disease (eg, ligamentous laxity, blue sclerae, deafness, dentinogenesis imperfecta) are usually present. These cases, which may or may not be manifest at birth, have been clinically separated into two groups according to the degree of functional disability (Fig. 5.8). Patients in the first group (tarda I) have deformities, usually confined to the lower limbs, that limit ambulation. Those in the second group (tarda II), although short, are without significant limb deformity and are therefore functionally much less disabled.

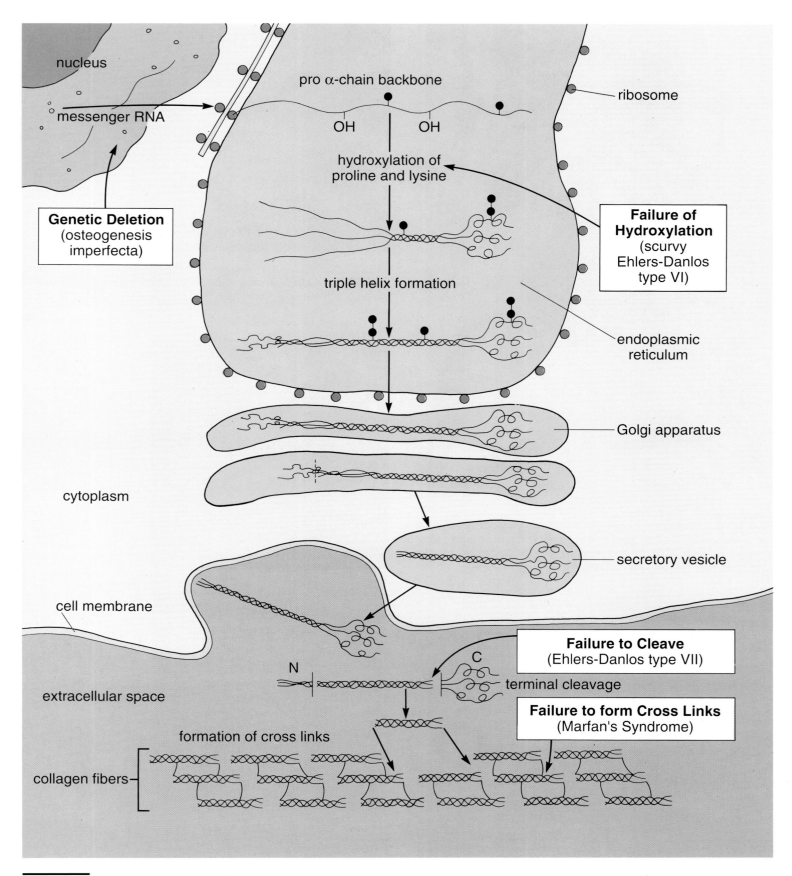

FIGURE 5.1 Schematic representation of sites of possible disturbances in collagen synthesis leading to various disorders.

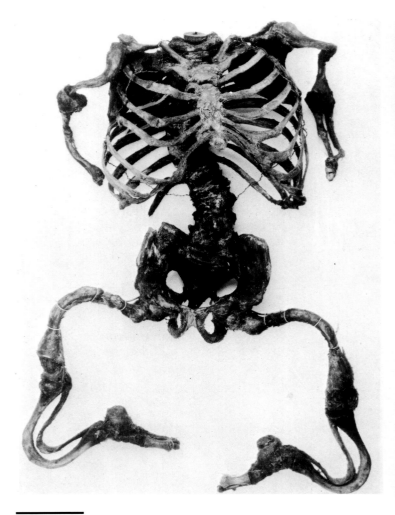

FIGURE 5.2 Skeleton of an older child with osteogenesis imperfecta congenita, who died after massive hemorrhage from a blow to the head. There are deformities in all four limbs, together with scoliosis, and chest and pelvic deformities.

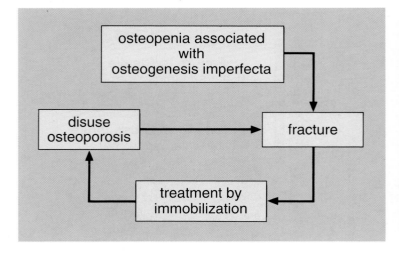

FIGURE 5.3 Fracture cycle in patients with osteogenesis imperfecta. These patients have a tendency towards fracture. The standard treatment of fractures by immobilization results in disuse osteoporosis, which in turn increases the tendency to fracture.

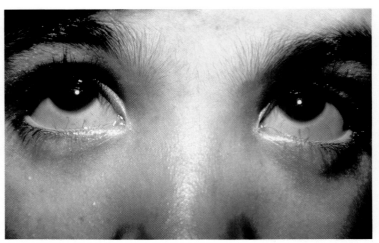

FIGURE 5.4 Osteogenesis imperfecta: clinical photograph showing blue sclerae. The color results in part from the thinness of the sclerae.

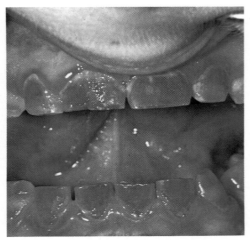

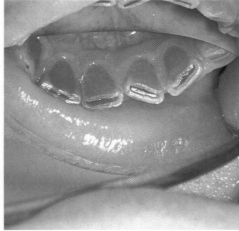

FIGURE 5.5 Two examples of the appearance of teeth in patients with osteogenesis imperfecta. Brown short teeth result from failure in the formation of dentin. The enamel appears to be normal.

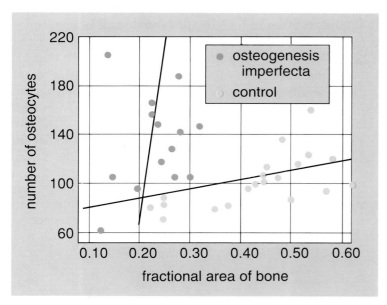

FIGURE 5.6 Graph showing that the number of osteocytes per area of bone is always greater in osteogenesis imperfecta patients than in age-matched controls. Stated another way, the volume of territorial matrix around each osteocyte is smaller in osteogenesis imperfecta than in age-matched controls.

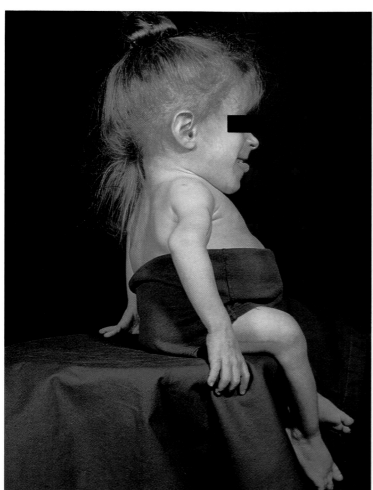

FIGURE 5.7 Patient with osteogenesis imperfecta congenita shows defect of all four limbs and increased anteroposterior diameter of the chest. Also note the spinal deformity.

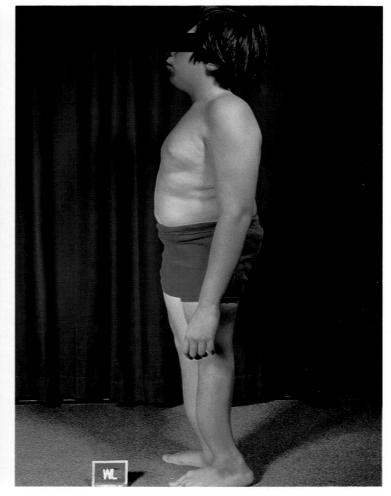

FIGURE 5.8 Patient with osteogenesis imperfecta tarda I shows anterior bowing of the tibia and short lower limbs. In comparison, the upper limbs appear relatively normal.

RADIOGRAPHIC FEATURES

The hallmark of OI is osteopenia associated with multiple fractures and, in the majority of cases, bone deformities. The entire skeleton is affected (Fig. 5.9).

In the spine, platyspondyly and biconcavity are evidence of compression fractures in the vertebral bodies, and in many cases these multiple fractures give rise to kyphoscoliosis (Fig. 5.10). In severely affected patients, the pelvis is often markedly deformed, and is sometimes referred to as being triradiate.

Skull films reveal a large cranial vault, with temporal bulging and typically with a small triangular face. Multiple centers of ossification may be observed in the skull, particularly in the occipital portion (wormian bones) (Fig. 5.11).

Fractures vary in number, depending on the severity of the disease, and are more common in the lower

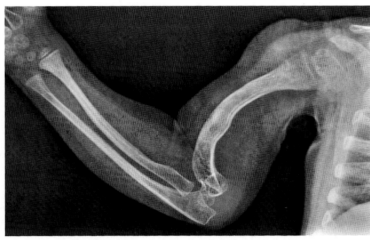

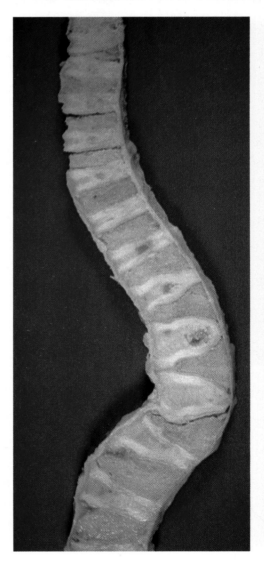
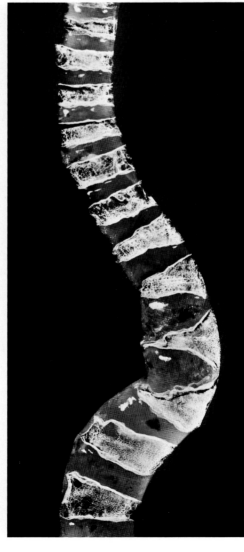

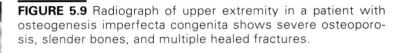

FIGURE 5.9 Radiograph of upper extremity in a patient with osteogenesis imperfecta congenita shows severe osteoporosis, slender bones, and multiple healed fractures.

FIGURE 5.10 *(left)* Dissected specimen of spine shows scoliosis subsequent to multiple compression fractures. *(right)* Specimen radiograph of spine demonstrates osteoporosis.

limbs. Usually they heal at the normal rate. The number of fractures sustained each year is maximal during the growing period because of rapid turnover and decreases after adolescence with growth stabilization. Fractures again become a problem with aging and the onset of senile osteoporosis. In a few fracture cases (usually in children), hyperplastic callus develops and causes excessive swelling, heat, throbbing pain, and tenderness. It may be difficult to differentiate this hyperplastic callus from an osteosarcoma or, on occasion, from osteomyelitis (Figs. 5.12 and 5.13).

Fairbank described three radiologic types of disease in the appendicular skeleton: the thick bone, slender bone, and cystic types. The thick bone type (which is rare) is usually seen in severely affected infants. It is believed to be due to multiple fractures, with telescoping of the bones. In most cases, however, the long bones are very slender (Fig. 5.14). The ribs may be so attenuated that one sees a "ribbon-like" configuration suggestive of neurofibromatosis.

Approximately 50% of the growing (epiphyseal) ends of the long bones in children with osteogenesis im-

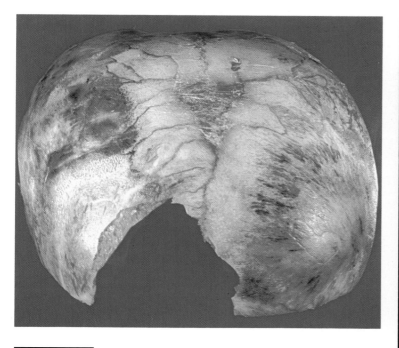

FIGURE 5.11 Skull from a 9-year-old child shows posterior fontanelle and multiple wormian bones.

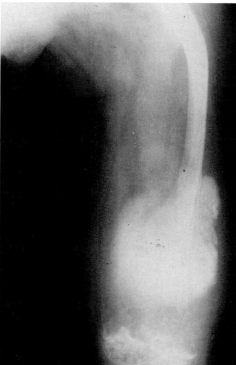

FIGURE 5.12 Radiograph of the femur of an adolescent patient with osteogenesis imperfecta tarda, who developed a rapidly growing, hyperemic tumor following injury. Radiographically, the tumor might suggest a neoplasm.

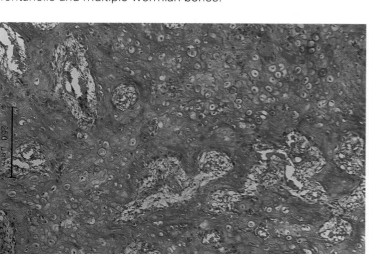

FIGURE 5.13 Photomicrograph of a biopsy obtained from the mass illustrated in Figure 5.12 demonstrates a cellular mass of immature bone and cartilage consistent with fracture callus (H & E, x 10 obj.).

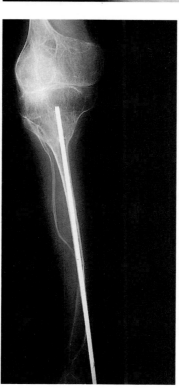

FIGURE 5.14 Radiograph of the leg of a patient with severe clinical osteogenesis imperfecta which has been treated by rodding of the tibia. The extreme attenuation and ribbonlike quality of the bones is apparent in the fibula.

perfecta congenita or tarda I (with equal incidence on the right and left sides of the body) exhibit a collection of rounded, scalloped radiolucencies with sclerotic margins. In some cases, this is accompanied by a ballooned-out epiphysis and metaphysis, giving a "popcorn bag" appearance similar to that described by Fairbank as cystic (Fig. 5.15). In all instances of such lesions, the cartilaginous growth plate is irregular, partially absent, or completely absent (Fig. 5.16). The lesions are most common in the lower limbs; in order of descending frequency, they occur in the distal femur, proximal tibia, distal tibia, and proximal femur. In the upper extremities, lesions are most frequently observed in the proximal and distal humerus. In some of our patients, films obtained during the neonatal period showed normal epiphyses and growth plates, indicating that these popcorn lesions are not congenital.

The radiographic differential diagnosis in cases of osteogenesis imperfecta in the neonate might include congenital hypophosphatasia. In a child, the differential diagnosis might include "battered child" syndrome or the early stages of leukemia. In the preadolescent, the self-limiting condition of juvenile osteoporosis may have to be considered. The diagnosis of osteogenesis imperfecta is made solely on clinical grounds, and there are no pathognomonic radiographic, pathologic, or biochemical findings.

A summary of the radiographic findings is shown in Fig. 5.17.

PATHOLOGIC FEATURES

Gross examination of the bones reveals a generalized loss of bone tissue, with thin, eggshell-like cortices and very little medullary cancellous bone. Many specimens demonstrate recent or healed fractures, with angulation and/or bowing (Fig. 5.18).

In general, the epiphyseal ends of the long bones, including the articular surfaces, retain a recognizable shape, although in proportion to the rest of the bone they appear larger and may show irregularity of the articular surface (Fig. 5.19). The secondary centers of ossification are often markedly distorted and may contain small cartilaginous nodules 1 to 4 mm in diameter (Fig. 5.20).

The appearance of the growth plate varies widely in appearance, ranging from normal, to exhibiting one or more indentations in the metaphysis, to total disruption of its regular outline (Figs. 5.21 and 5.22). These latter changes correspond to the scalloped or popcorn lesions seen on radiographic examination. It is probable that these epiphyseal changes are secondary to trauma and are not developmental in origin. The fragmentation of the growth plate might be reasonably expected to interfere with normal growth.

Microscopic examination of an intact growth plate may reveal disorganization of the proliferative and hypertrophic zones, increased permeation of the cartilage by metaphyseal blood vessels, and decreased thickness of the calcified zone of the growth plate cartilage. The primary spongiosa on the metaphyseal side is extremely scanty and is usually of the woven variety.

The large cartilage masses visible in the region of the metaphysis on both radiographic and gross examination result from fragmentation of the growth plate. On microscopic examination, the cartilage fragments show polarized maturation and columnization of the chondrocytes (Figs. 5.23 and 5.24).

Biopsy specimens from patients with the severe or congenita form of the disease are characterized by large

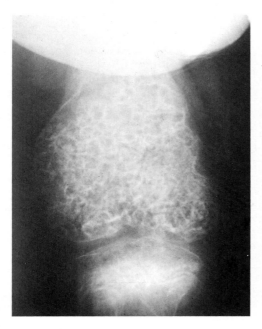

FIGURE 5.15
Radiograph of knee joint in an 8-year-old child with osteogenesis imperfecta congenita. The epiphysis and metaphysis of the femur contain nodular "popcorn" lesions with radiolucent centers and radiodense margins. No growth plate is seen in the femur. In the tibia the growth plate is visualized, but the central portion is disrupted. The buttock image obscures the femoral diaphysis.

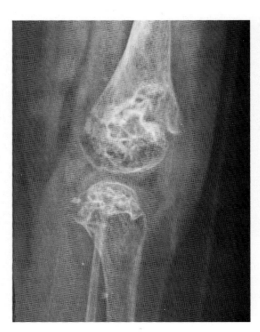

FIGURE 5.16
Radiograph of the knee in a patient with osteogenesis imperfecta congenita. There is irregularity and disruption of both the femoral and tibial growth plates, although less severe than that shown in Figure 5.15.

FIGURE 5.17

SUMMARY OF RADIOGRAPHIC FINDINGS IN OSTEOGENESIS IMPERFECTA

Bone Structure	Osteogenesis Imperfecta Tarda	Osteogenesis Imperfecta Congenita
Texture	Osteopenia with thin cortices and porous cancellous bone, proportional to the severity of the clinical disease	
Fractures	Generally seen during growth period; frequency 1–4 per year; most frequent in lower limbs; fractures may be present at birth, but not commonly; deformities usually confined to lower limbs, most often the tibia and fibula	Fractures present at birth; many fractures each year; occur in all four limbs, but always associated with severe deformities
Long Bones	Usually slender	May be widened during infancy due to telescoping; in older patients, usually very slender
Epiphyses	Usually normal in appearance, although irregularities may be present in the lower femoral and upper tibial epiphysis	Frequently irregular, with failure to recognize a normal growth plate, and replacement by bubbly calcified nodules; most frequently seen in lower femur, upper tibia, upper femur, and upper humerus
Spine	Osteopenia: platyspondyly; mild scoliosis	Severe osteopenia with biconcave vertebrae and frequently severe kyphoscoliosis
Ribs	Normal	Frequent deformities with thinning, malunited fractures
Pelvis	Normal	Triradiate
Skull	Wormian bones	

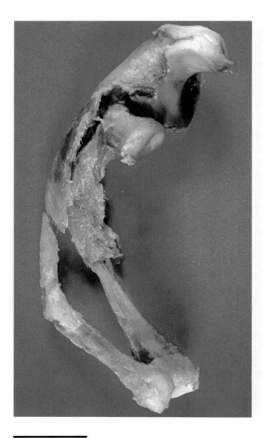

FIGURE 5.18 Dissected specimen of forearm bones shows multiple fractures, including fracture dislocation of the radial head.

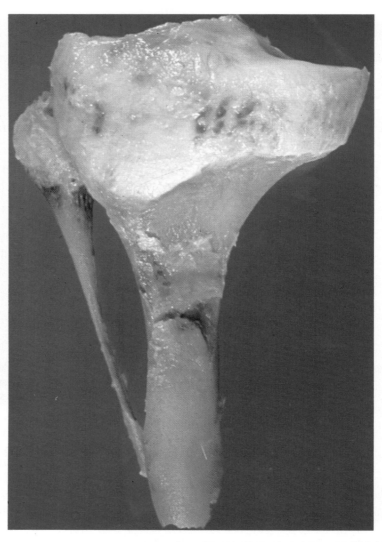

FIGURE 5.19
Upper end of tibia shows relative enlargement of the cartilaginous end of the bone and marked narrowing of the shaft of the fibula.

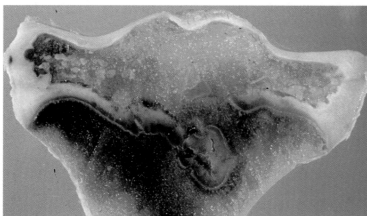

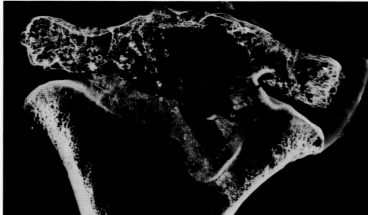

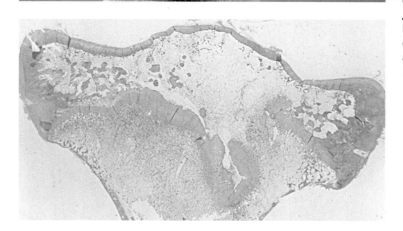

FIGURE 5.20 *(upper left)* Dissected specimen of the upper end of the tibia shows multiple cartilaginous nodules in the epiphysis and disruption of the growth plate. Radiograph of the specimen *(upper right)*. Histologic section *(lower left)*.

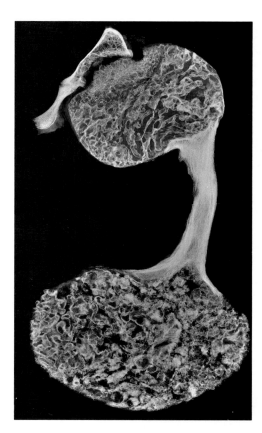

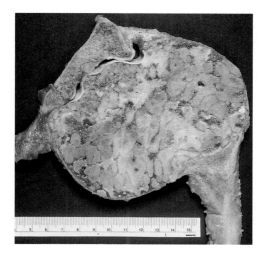

FIGURE 5.21 Specimen radiograph of the femur removed from a patient with osteogenesis imperfecta who was thought to have developed chondrosarcoma. However, these changes are compatible with fragmentation and continued growth of the epiphyseal cartilage plate (popcorn sign).

FIGURE 5.22 Photograph of a section through the upper end of the femur illustrated in Figure 5.21, showing the large cartilage fragments.

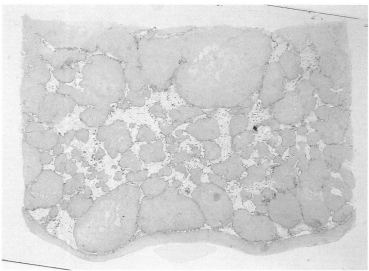

FIGURE 5.23 Photomicrograph of a portion of the epiphysis shown in Figure 5.22 (H & E, x 1 obj.).

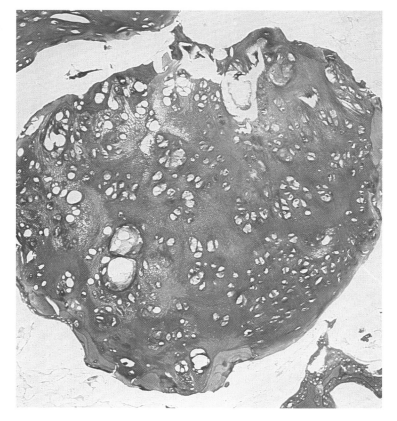

FIGURE 5.24 Histologic section of one of the cartilage nodules illustrated in Figure 5.23 shows hypercellularity and disorganization. A thin rim of bone is present around each of the nodules, giving rise to the rim of radiodensity seen in the radiograph (H & E, x 10 obj.).

areas of osseous tissue that is devoid of an organized trabecular pattern. Examination of the individual trabeculae reveals plump osteoblasts crowded along prominent osteoid seams, and large oval osteocytes surrounded by a small amount of matrix, which more often than not has a woven pattern (Fig. 5.25). Even in areas that display a lamellar pattern, the lamellae are thin. The osteoclasts appear to be morphologically normal, although both they and the resorptive surfaces are more numerous (Fig. 5.26).

Bone from less severely affected patients is characterized by a predominantly fine lamellar pattern, with only small areas of woven bone. Although osteoblasts are increased in number they appear smaller, more spherical, and less numerous than their counterparts in the congenita group. Osteoid seams are also prominent, probably due to an increased rate of bone formation. The osteocytes, although more mature in appearance than those in patients with osteogenesis imperfecta congenita, are more numerous, larger, and less homogeneously arranged throughout the trabeculae than the

osteocytes in normal patients (Fig. 5.27). Osteoclasts appear morphologically normal but are increased in number as compared with those in individuals not affected by osteogenesis imperfecta.

The histologic appearance of the bone suggests that at least one reason for the reduced bone mass and tendency to dwarfism is a decreased level of collagen production by the osteoblasts, evident morphologically as crowded osteocytes. Disruption of the growth plate secondary to fracture also interferes with growth and contributes to these patients' short stature.

EHLERS–DANLOS SYNDROME

Like osteogenesis imperfecta, Ehlers–Danlos syndrome, which gives rise to the "India rubber man" of the circus, comprises a heterogeneous group of connective tissue disorders which have only recently been classified into a number of different types. The underlying biochemical defect in the pathway of collagen synthesis is

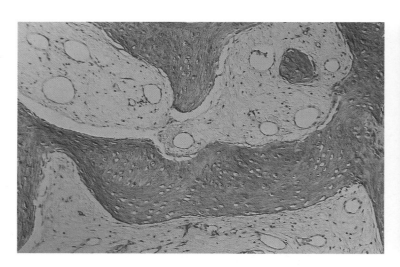

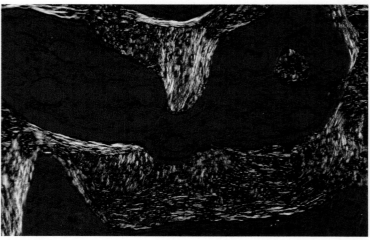

FIGURE 5.25 Photomicrograph of a biopsy of bone *(left)* obtained from a patient with osteogenesis imperfecta congenita showing irregular hypercellular bone which, on polarized light examination *(right)*, is seen to have a largely woven pattern (H & E x 4 obj.).

FIGURE 5.26 Osteogenesis imperfecta congenita: bone biopsy showing marked hypercellularity of the bone with a fine lamellar pattern and extensively eroded resorptive surfaces (H & E, x 10 obj.).

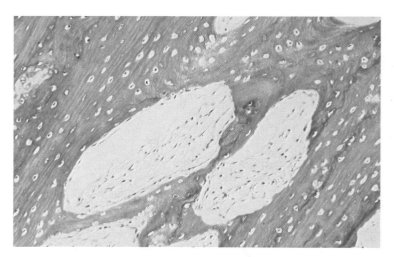

unknown in most cases. However, some cases of Ehlers–Danlos Syndrome type VI have demonstrated a hydroxylysine-deficient collagen, probably due to a lysyl hydroxylase deficiency which interferes with the formation of intramolecular cross-links in type I collagen. The type VII form of the disease is caused by a lack of procollagen peptidase. Thus, the conversion of procollagen to collagen is interfered with and the formation of collagen fibrils cannot proceed.

The characteristic features of Ehlers–Danlos syndrome are hyperextensibility of the skin, easy bruisibility, hypermobile joints which are prone to dislocation and, in type IV disease, dissecting aortic aneurysm. Blue sclerae are not uncommon in Ehlers–Danlos syndrome, and their presence should not be taken as evidence of an associated osteogenesis imperfecta.

In general, the bone is found on gross examination to be osteopenic. No characteristic histologic findings have been described (Fig. 5.28). Most patients exhibit a greater or lesser degree of kyphoscoliosis, which becomes worse during adolescence and may end in severe spinal curvature with pulmonary embarrassment (Fig. 5.29). Occasionally, severe spondylolisthesis is observed.

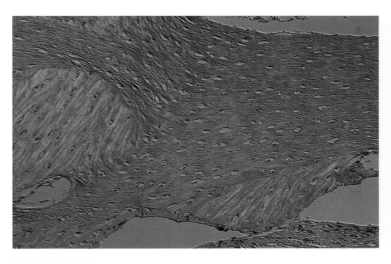
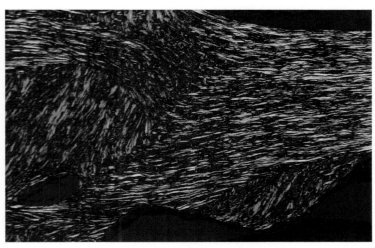

FIGURE 5.27 Photomicrograph of bone biopsy *(left)* from a patient with osteogenesis imperfecta tarda, showing fine, hyper-cellular lamellar bone. The lamellar pattern is more clearly seen in the polarized light picture *(right)* (H & E, x 10 obj.).

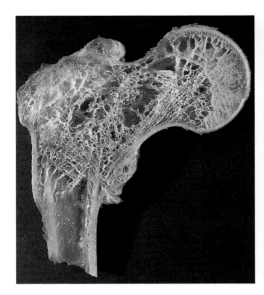

FIGURE 5.28 Photograph of an autopsy section through the femur of a young man with Ehlers-Danlos syndrome shows a healed pathologic fracture and severe osteoporosis.

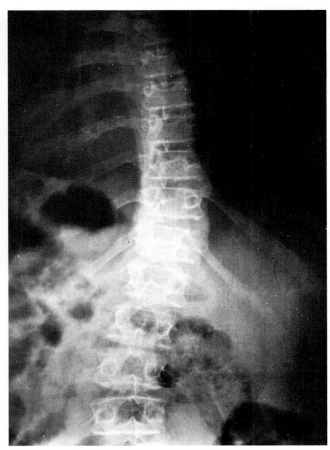

FIGURE 5.29 AP radiograph of a young adult with Ehlers-Danlos syndrome. The bone is markedly osteopenic, and there is a mild scoliosis with some rotational deformity.

SCURVY

Scurvy is now an extremely rare condition, although an occasional case may arise as the result either of deprivation or of food faddism. In the past, when infantile scurvy was common, the disorder was frequently associated with rickets.

The disease is characterized clinically by hemorrhage secondary to capillary fragility. The hemorrhages occur in the skin, gums, muscle attachments, serosal membranes and, especially in children, subperiosteally in the bones (Fig. 5.30). Affected individuals may also exhibit anemia, osteoporosis, intra-articular hemorrhages, and poor wound healing.

The recognition that scurvy is a deficiency state occurred in the late eighteenth century, when it became understood that the disease resulted from a deficiency of vegetables and fruit and that citrus fruit could prevent its onset. It is now known to be caused by a deficiency of ascorbic acid (vitamin C). Vitamin C is an essential cofactor for hydroxylation of the amino acids proline and lysine, an important step in the intracellular synthesis of collagen. In the absence of vitamin C, the conversion of proline and lysine to hydroxyproline and hydroxylysine cannot take place, with a resulting failure in the formation of intracellular bonds and thus failure in the formation of a stable triple-helical collagen molecule. In the vitamin C-deficient state, microscopic examination reveals that recently formed areas of connective tissue (eg, the metaphysis in a growing child) are markedly deficient in extracellular matrix formation. Indeed, the most prominent features in such areas are proliferating fibroblasts without collagen production and extravasated red blood cells (Fig. 5.31).

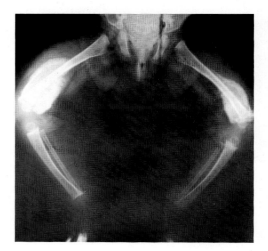

FIGURE 5.30 Radiograph of a young child shows extensive periosteal elevation in both femurs, with epiphyseal separation of the lower femoral epiphyses.

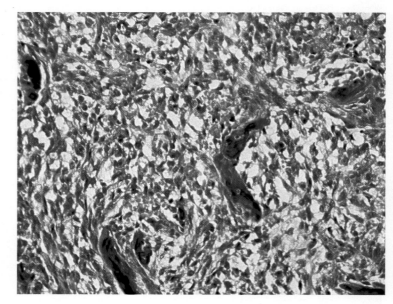

FIGURE 5.31 Photomicrograph shows extensive fibroblastic proliferation, with minimal bone and collagen production. Extravasation of red blood cells can be seen throughout the tissue (H & E, x 25 obj.).

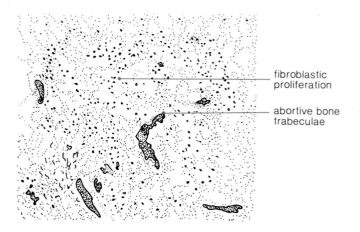

fibroblastic proliferation

abortive bone trabeculae

As mentioned earlier, in young children the bone lesions are characterized by subperiosteal hemorrhage that may be massive (Fig. 5.32). In addition, because the primary spongiosa fails to form adequately a fracture through the metaphysis frequently occurs, with a resulting separation of the epiphysis (Fig. 5.33), often clinically manifested by marked costochondral tenderness and swelling around major joints.

Because the periosteum is more securely attached to the bone in adults, subperiosteal hematomas are not a characteristic part of the clinical picture. However, adult patients may present with marked osteoporosis owing to the defect in collagen synthesis.

VITAMIN A INTOXICATION

Although uncommon, the effects of vitamin A (retinoic acid) intoxication are occasionally seen in food faddists. Irritability, loss of appetite, scaly skin, and hair loss

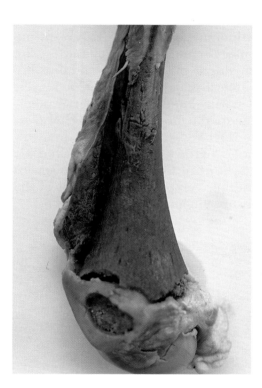

FIGURE 5.32 Photograph of a specimen showing periosteal elevation and subperiosteal hemorrhage. Separation of the lower femoral epiphysis has occurred.

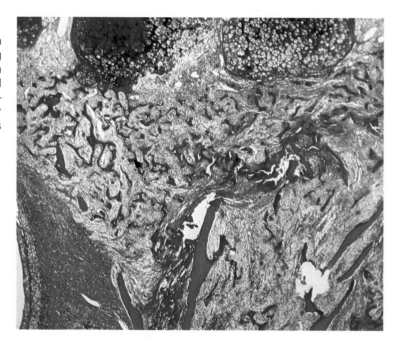

FIGURE 5.33 Photomicrograph of the region of the growth plate and metaphysis in a patient with scurvy. Subperiosteal hemorrhage and a fracture through the metaphysis are apparent.

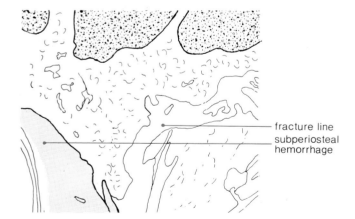

fracture line
subperiosteal hemorrhage

are the usual presenting symptoms. The mode of action on the bone cells is unclear. However, radiographic examination may reveal cortical hyperostosis, and infants and young children may exhibit accelerated maturation of the growth plates, resulting in a slow-down of bone growth activity (Fig. 5.34).

ies have shown that excessive amounts of hyaluronic acid are produced by the connective tissue cells of these patients. In addition, in some cases of Marfan's syndrome a defect in the formation of cross-linkages in the type I collagen fibrils has been found, contributing to the generalized connective tissue defect.

MARFAN'S SYNDROME

Marfan's syndrome consists of a heterogeneous group of connective tissue disorders characterized by an autosomal dominant pattern of inheritance. Affected individuals are usually tall and thin, with osteopenia, kyphoscoliosis, arachnodactyly, myopia, and often lens dislocation (Figs. 5.35 and 5.36). From a clinical standpoint, the most important aspects of the disease are cardiovascular abnormalities particularly affecting the heart valves and the aorta.

Microscopic examination of the heart valves and large arteries reveals a cystic necrosis of the media, with pools of mucoid material that stains metachromatically with toluidine blue (Fig. 5.37). Biochemical stud-

HOMOCYSTINURIA

Homocystinuria is an extremely rare autosomal recessive disease, characterized biochemically by a deficiency in the enzyme cystathionine-synthetase. The resulting elevated levels of homocysteine in the plasma affect the arterial walls, smooth muscle proliferation, and possibly collagen synthesis. Clinical signs include skeletal fragility, osteoporosis, tall stature, and arachnodactyly, similar to the changes seen in Marfan's syndrome. However, unlike the case with Marfan's syndrome, patients with homocystinuria are often mentally retarded. Disturbances in collagen fibril formation lead to severe osteoporosis, with multiple compression fractures of the vertebral bodies and subsequent kyphoscoliosis.

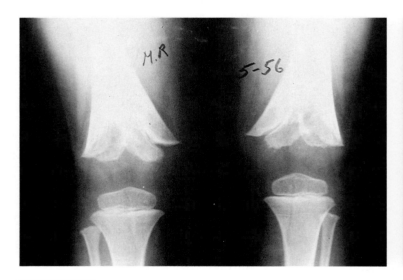

FIGURE 5.34 Radiograph of a patient suffering from vitamin A intoxication who developed fracture and displacement of the femoral epiphyses. An x-ray taken some years later after correction of the intoxication showed complete restoration of normal anatomy.

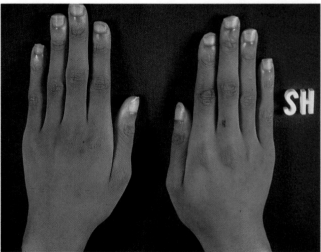

FIGURE 5.35 The hands of an adolescent female with Marfan's syndrome show the typical elongated fingers (arachnodactyly) associated with the syndrome. (Courtesy of Dr. David Levine)

MUCOPOLYSACCHARIDOSES

The extrafibrillar amorphous component of the extracellular tissue matrix is often referred to as the ground substance. It is particularly prominent in cartilage and plays an important role in the mechanical properties of cartilage and bone, as well as in the development of the shape of the bones.

The ground substance is a mixture of many components, and its composition differs among different tissues. The principal ground substance constituents of cartilage are the acid mucopolysaccharides which, combined with proteins, form the proteoglycan aggregates (see Chapter 1).

A number of heritable diseases, mostly autosomal recessive, are characterized by defects in the metabolism, storage, and excretion of these acid mucopolysaccharides (glycosaminoglycans). The majority of these diseases are associated with marked skeletal abnormalities, probably because the mucopolysaccharides are so important in the formation of the cartilage and its subsequent endochondral ossification.

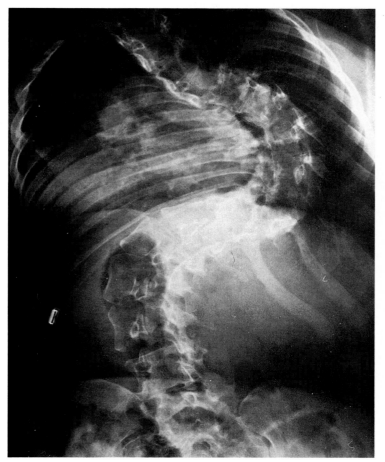

FIGURE 5.36 AP radiograph of the patient in Figure 5.35 demonstrates the severity of the spinal deformity.

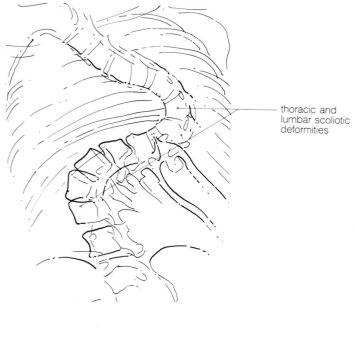

thoracic and lumbar scoliotic deformities

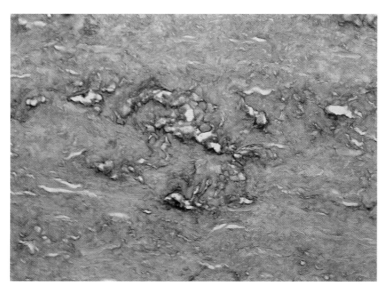

FIGURE 5.37 Photomicrograph of a portion of the wall of the aorta to demonstrating pools of mucoid material. The patient died of a dissecting aneurysm, a common complication in Marfan's syndrome (H & E, x 4 obj.).

More than six distinct syndromes have been described, many of which are characterized by the storage of dermatan sulfate and heparan sulfate in various tissues. Strikingly affected are the reticuloendothelial system, the heart (Fig. 5.38), and the central nervous system, the latter often resulting in severe mental retardation. Because of the important role played by the glycosaminoglycans in the formation of the vitreous humor and other components of the eye, blindness is a common complication.

The two most common mucopolysaccharidoses associated with severe skeletal abnormalities are Morquio's syndrome (MPS IV) and Hurler's syndrome (MPS I-H).

MORQUIO'S SYNDROME

Morquio's syndrome (mucopolysaccharidosis IV) is characterized biochemically by excessive amounts of keratin sulfate and chondroitin sulfate in the urine. This condition appears to be phenotypically, genetically, and chemically distinctive, probably involving a defect in metabolism of the proteoglycans of the cartilage. Affected patients are dwarfed, with characteristically flat vertebrae, epiphyseal dysplasia, and generalized osteoporosis. There is usually marked shortening of the trunk, with somewhat lesser shortening of the extremities (Figs. 5.39 and 5.40).

HURLER'S SYDROME

Hurler's syndrome (also known as gargoylism or MPS I-H) is caused by α-L-iduronidase deficiency. This condition may also involve some retardation of skeletal growth, although this is rarely severe. Although the vertebral bodies appear relatively normal, these patients frequently exhibit kyphotic deformity resulting from the malformation of at least one vertebral body

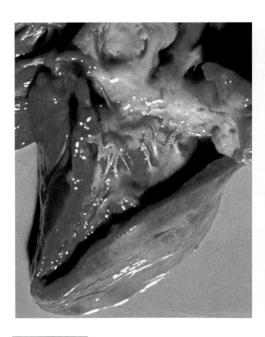

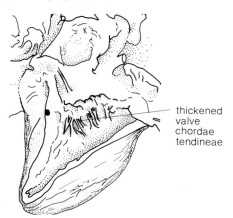

FIGURE 5.38 The heart from a child with Hurler's syndrome. Note thickening of the chordae tendineae cordis and opacity of the endothelial lining of the heart, both resulting from accumulation of macrophages filled with polysaccharides.

thickened valve chordae tendineae

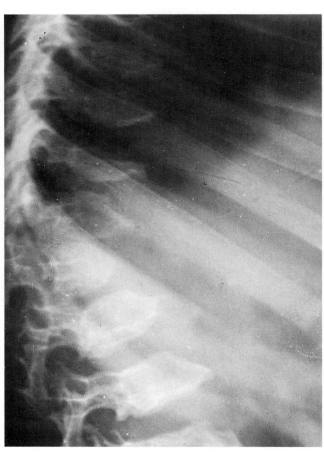

FIGURE 5.39 Lateral radiograph of the thoracolumbar spine in a 17-year-old girl with Morquio's disease, showing the typical tongue-like extensions of the anterior margins of the vertebral bodies. There also is a hemivertebra, which in this case has given rise to a thoracolumbar kyphosis, a typical occurrence in these patients.

usually the twelfth thoracic or the first lumbar (Fig. 5.41). For unknown reasons, a portion of the anterior half of the affected body or bodies fails to ossify, and the ensuing posterior displacement of one vertebral body on the other leads to kyphosis. However, in Hurler's syndrome the vertebral column does not show the general wedging of the vertebral bodies present in Morquio's syndrome. Unlike Morquio's syndrome, patients with Hurler's deteriorate rapidly and usually die within the first decade of life.

HYPOPHOSPHATASIA

Hypophosphatasia is a rare, genetically transmitted error of metabolism in which there is a disturbance in the synthesis of the enzyme alkaline phosphatase. Two forms of the disease have been described. The first,

inherited as an autosomal recessive trait, manifests in children who are severely affected; the second is an autosomal dominant form that becomes evident in adults, in whom the disease is less severe.

In infants, hypophospatasia is manifested clinically as a failure to thrive with growth retardation, and is accompanied by a wide range of symptoms including irritability, fever, and vomiting. In general, infants diagnosed before six months of age follow a rapidly progressive fatal course. In older children or adults, the disease is less severe and is usually asymptomatic. Hypophosphatasia is characterized by decreased levels of alkaline phosphatase in bone, intestines, liver, and kidney. Levels of serum phosphorus and calcium are usually high normal. Increased amounts of phosphoethanolamine, which is believed to be a substrate of alkaline phosphatase, are present in the urine and in the serum.

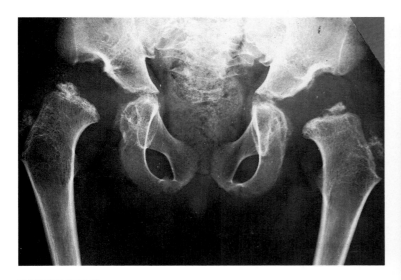

FIGURE 5.40 Radiograph of the hips of a boy suffering from Morquio's disease, demonstrating failure of development in the femoral heads as well as in the hip joints as a whole.

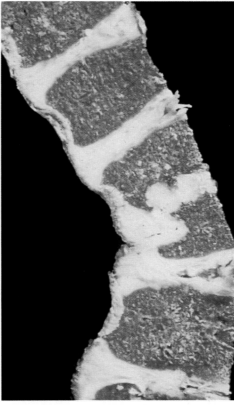

FIGURE 5.41
Photograph of a portion of the thoracolumbar spine in a patient with Hurler's syndrome showing a hemivertebra at the level of T-12. The vertebra above is also slightly deformed on its inferior surface, though the remaining vertebrae in this photograph appear to be within normal limits. (Courtesy of Dr James W. Milgram)

Radiographic manifestations of the disorder in children include poorly ossified and underdeveloped bones (Figs. 5.42 and 5.43). Gross and microscopic examination of the affected tissue reveals increased osteoid and irregular epiphyseal cartilage with lengthened chondrocyte columns (Figs. 5.44 to 5.46). The similarity to rickets is evident, and explains why this disease, for years, was called vitamin D-resistant rickets (see Chapter 7).

Hypophosphatasia may not present clinically until the fourth, fifth, or sixth decade of life, although there is often a childhood history of a rickets-like disorder. Edentia, short stature, and deformity of the extremities, including bowing, are not uncommon clinical findings. Radiographic features include pseudofractures and osteopenia. Histopathologic examination of bone from these patients reveals an osteomalacic picture, with increased amounts of nonmineralized bone. Unlike osteomalacia due to vitamin D or calcium deficiency, hypophosphatasia is characterized by a paucity of osteoblasts.

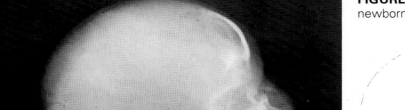

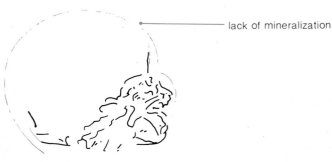

FIGURE 5.42 Hypophosphatasia: radiograph of the skull in a newborn baby shows poor mineralization of the vault of the skull.

— lack of mineralization

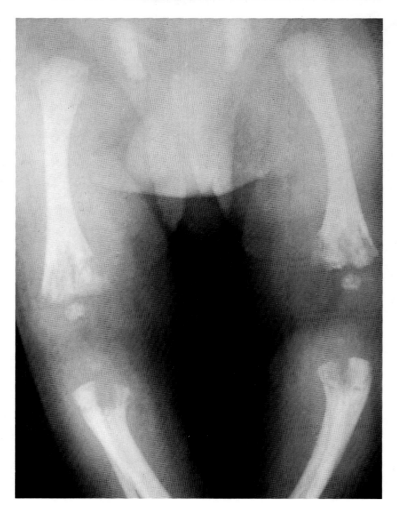

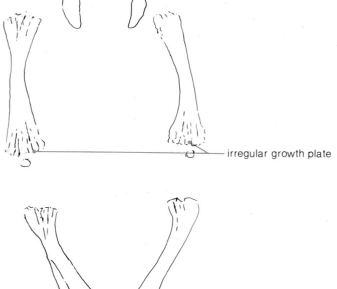

FIGURE 5.43 Hypophosphatasia: the lower limbs in a newborn child show marked irregularity of the growth plate, with streaks of radiodensity into the metaphysis. This appearance is indicative of poor endochondral ossification.

— irregular growth plate

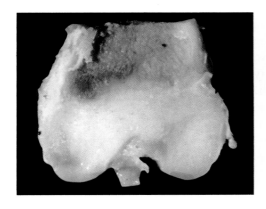

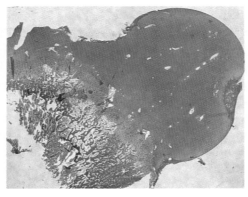

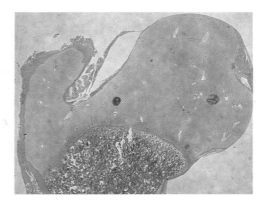

FIGURE 5.44 Hypophosphatasia: section through the lower femoral epiphysis and metaphysis show the irregularity of the growth plate.

FIGURE 5.45 Hypophosphatasia: low-power photomicrograph of the upper femoral growth plate *(left)*. The marked irregularity of the cartilage and the tongue of irregular cartilage extending to the

metaphyseal region are evident. For contrast, a normal upper femoral epiphysis in a patient of the same age is shown *(right)* (H & E, x 1 obj.).

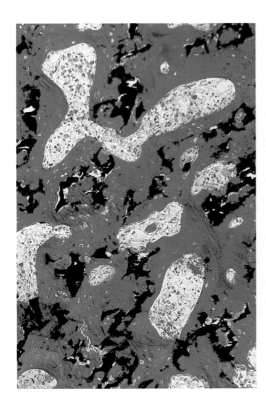

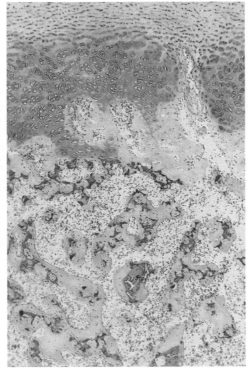

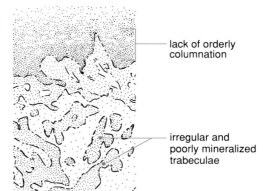

lack of orderly columnation

irregular and poorly mineralized trabeculae

FIGURE 5.46 Photomicrograph *(left)* shows the poor mineralization of the forming bone in hypophosphatasia. Only the areas stained black are mineralized (Von Kossa, x 25 obj.).

Photomicrograph *(right)* of a cross section of a vertebral body demonstrates disturbed endochondral ossification (H & E, x 10 obj.).

HYPERPHOSPHATASIA

Primary hyperphosphatasia, also known as juvenile Paget's disease, is a rare congenital autosomal recessive disorder characterized clinically by short stature, osteoporosis, and marked subperiosteal bone formation which may be confused with Caffey's disease (see Chapter 6). Patients with this condition have markedly elevated levels of serum alkaline phosphatase and acid phosphatase of bone origin, and an elevated level of urinary hydroxyproline.

On radiographic examination, a thickened skull with "cotton ball" radiodensities may be seen (Fig. 5.47). The long bones often exhibit an increase in width and loss of normal corticomedullary differentiation. these features are the result of the marked subperiosteal overgrowth (Fig. 5.48). Bowing due to fractures may be present, and in infants the disease must be distinguished from a "battered baby" syndrome.

Morphologic studies reveal that both the cortical and trabecular bone consists of immature fibrous (or woven) bone, with abundant osteoblasts and osteoclasts and prominent osteoid seams (Fig. 5.49). The marrow space is replaced by a well-vascularized fibrous connective tissue network. Using polarized light, one can observe a mosaic pattern of the bone matrix.

Hyperphosphatasia is distinguished clinically from Paget's disease by its early onset and the generalized symmetrical bone involvement.

FLUOROSIS

Fluoride substitutes for some of the hydroxyl ion in hydroxyapatite to form a more stable crystal fluorapatite, which is less soluble than hydroxyapatite.

Fluoride has been shown to stimulate bone production, although its degree of action is dependent on the length and magnitude of exposure. Fluoride intoxication may result from either industrial or endemic expo-

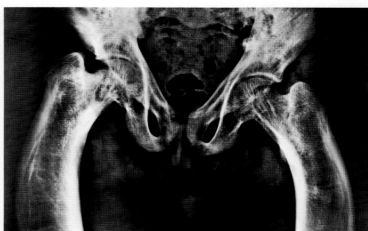

FIGURE 5.48 Radiograph of the pelvis and upper femurs in the patient seen in Figure 5.47 demonstrates marked thickening of the shafts of the femurs, with bowing of the femur and a dense irregular cortex.

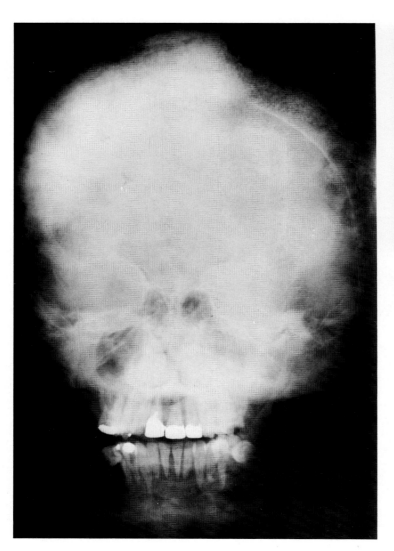

FIGURE 5.47 Radiograph of the skull in an 11-year-old patient with hyperphosphatasia. Note the marked thickening of the calvarium and the "cotton ball" radiodensities throughout.

sure to fluoride or, on the other hand, from therapeutic treatment of osteoporosis with fluoride. In populations exposed to a high fluoride content in water (in excess of 24 parts per 1,000,000), or in individuals exposed to high levels of industrial fluoride, the most dramatic radiographic change is marked coarsening and thickening of bone trabeculae, particularly involving the axial skeleton. Eventually, there is a significant increase in bone density, sometimes accompanied by periosteal new bone formation and marked spinal osteophytosis. The propensity for bone formation in this condition is by calcification of the muscles, ligaments, and tendons at the site of their attachment to the bone. Some patients in whom bone formation is particularly prominent in and around joints may develop debilitating arthrosis.

Affected individuals may also exhibit mottled tooth enamel and anemia.

In recent years, fluoride has been used to stimulate bone production in osteoporotic patients. Although the specific mechanism is not understood, fluoride in doses of approximately 1 mg per kg of body weight per day appears to produce increased bone density in some subjects (Fig. 5.50). However, its usefulness as a mode of treatment has been questioned and is presently a matter of controversy.

Microscopic examination of the sclerotic bone under polarized light reveals it to be predominantly lamellar. Increased osteocytes are seen, and there may be prominent cement lines. The osteocytes themselves do not appear normal, frequently displaying basophilic

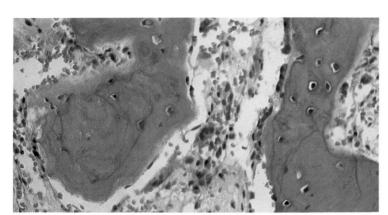

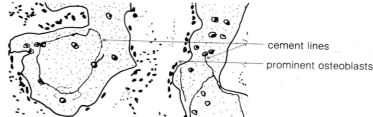

FIGURE 5.49 Hyperphosphatasia: photomicrograph of bone biopsy from the patient shown in Figures 5.47 and 5.48. The bone is somewhat immature, with large irregular cells. Note prominent cement lines and many osteoblasts on bone surface (H & E, x 25 obj.).

cement lines

prominent osteoblasts

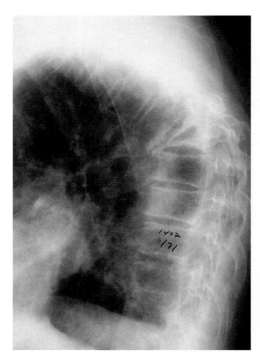

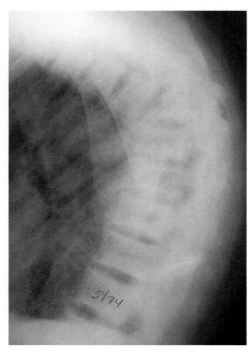

FIGURE 5.50 The effect of sodium fluoride on osteoporotic bone. Radiograph of an osteoporotic spine *(left)* shows collapse of thoracic vertebrae with marked osteopenia. After several years of treatment with sodium fluoride, calcium carbonate, and vitamin D *(right)*, spinal radiograph shows increased radiodensity.

mottling around the osteocytic lacunae or enlargement of the lacunae themselves. An increased amount of osteoid is also present (Figs. 5.51 to 5.53). A marked increase in the diameter of the cortical haversian systems gives a spongy appearance to the cortex.

DWARFISM
(CHONDRO-OSSEOUS DYSPLASIA)

Many of the diseases discussed in this chapter result in a stunting of growth which is sometimes dramatic, as in osteogenesis imperfecta and the various mucopolysaccharidoses, especially Morquio's syndrome. Dwarfism may also be caused by defects in the epiphysis or in the growth plate, either from a lack of an extrinsic factor necessary for cartilage growth, as occurs with deficiency of growth hormone (pituitary dwarfs), or from cellular deficiencies in the chondrocytes that might interfere

with endochondral ossification, such as appears to be the case with achondroplasia (Figs. 5.54 and 5.55). Although many different clinical syndromes have been described, mostly by radiologists, for the most part the molecular defects remain unknown.

The radiographic classifications is based either on the portion of the long bone (epiphysis, metaphysis, or diaphysis) involved and on the presence or absence of spinal involvement; or by the portion of the extremity involved.

Proximal shortening or disproportionate shortening of the humerus and femur is known as *rhizomelic dwarfism*; shortening of the bones of the leg or forearm is known as *mesomelic dwarfism*; and shortening of small distal parts is known as *acromelic dwarfism*.

The age of the patient at the time of presentation (eg, newborn, infant, child, or adult) is important in categorizing and analyzing the abnormalities which result in dwarfism.

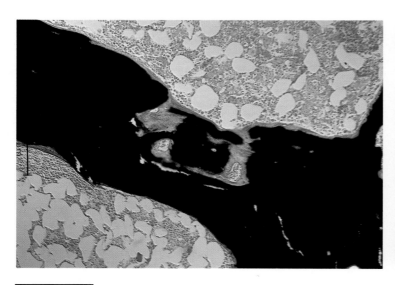

FIGURE 5.51 Photomicrograph of a section of undecalcified bone obtained from a patient treated with sodium fluoride showing increased amounts of osteoid, both extensively along the bone surfaces and patchily within the bone trabeculae (von Kossa, x 4 obj.).

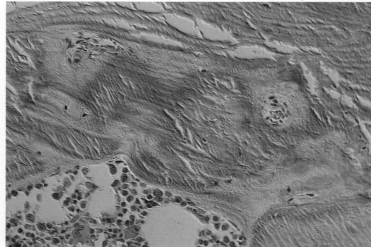

FIGURE 5.52 Photomicrograph of a section of undecalcified bone obtained from a patient treated with sodium fluoride to show the patchy basophilia which is seen in the affected bone (undecalcified specimen, H & E, x 10 obj.).

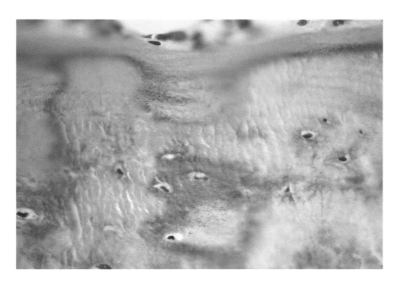

FIGURE 5.53 Photomicrograph of a section of undecalcified bone obtained from a patient treated with sodium fluoride showing the patchy basophilia seen in the previous illustration at a higher power (H & E, x 25 obj.).

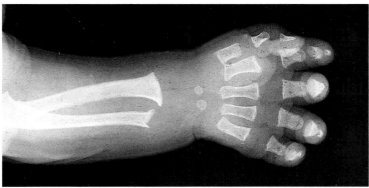

FIGURE 5.54 Radiograph of the arm of an achondroplastic infant to show the sharply defined sclerotic metaphysis indicating the absence of normal longitudinal growth and consequently, the shortened diaphyses and flared metaphyses.

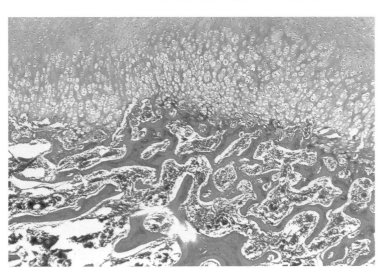

FIGURE 5.55 Photomicrograph of the growth plate and metaphyseal bone from an achondroplastic dwarf to show the lack of normal maturation and columnation in the growth plate and the presence of a bony end plate in the metaphysis (H & E, x 2.5 obj.).

**Diseases resulting from
disturbances in cell linkage**

A s discussed in Chapter 1, the skeletal tissues are in a continuous state of formation and breakdown, enabling them to constantly adapt to the mechanical demands made on them. Obviously, for the amount of tissue to remain the same there must be a balance between formation of the extracellular matrix by the osteoblasts and its breakdown by the osteoclasts. Any disturbance in the linkage between these two processes will result in either a decrease in bone density (osteopenia) or an increase in bone density (osteosclerosis) (Fig. 6.1). The first portion of this chapter deals with conditions in which there is increased bone tissue formation, either localized or generalized. The second portion discusses conditions characterized by osteopenia. In general, these diseases of disturbed cell linkage are not associated with disturbances of calcium homeostasis, and the blood calcium levels are essentially normal.

OSTEOSCLEROTIC CONDITIONS

Increased radiodensity is a common finding in the skeleton, usually associated with metastatic cancer (see Chapter 17). Bone sclerosis may also occur as a result of marrow disease, such as myelofibrosis (see Chapter 8), or disturbed calcification as occurs with fluorosis, as previously discussed in Chapter 5.

This section first discusses osteopetrosis and Paget's disease, in both of which the primary defect appears to be in the function of the osteoclasts. Discussion then follows of a group of conditions characterized by generalized osteosclerosis, which appears to result from overactivity of the osteoblasts.

OSTEOPETROSIS (MARBLE BONE DISEASE, ALBERS–SCHONBERG DISEASE)

Osteopetrosis is a rare congenital disorder characterized by a marked increase in the density of all the bones (Fig. 6.2). The bones are usually short, and frequently exhibit a modeling defect characterized by loss of the normal metaphyseal flare. The disease is often complicated by multiple fractures resulting from a disturbed microarchitecture (Fig. 6.3), and by anemia resulting from the marked reduction in the marrow space (Fig. 6.4). Two clinical presentations have been recognized: a severe (malignant) form that usually causes death in utero or in early childhood, and appears to be inherited as an autosomal recessive trait, and a less severe (benign) form in which the patients live into adult life, that appears to be inherited as an autosomal dominant. In the adult, the diagnosis may even be delayed until late middle age, and is usually made because of a pathologic fracture or as an incidental radiologic finding. In such cases, the condition must be differentiated from other causes of increased bone density, such as widespread osteoblastic metastases and myelosclerosis.

In severely affected patients, radiologic examination of the skeleton may reveal a uniform opacity of the skeletal tissue, with loss of the corticomedullary demarcation (Fig. 6.5). However, in less severely affected patients it is not unusual to find, particularly in the pelvis and the peripheral bones, alternating areas of affected and apparently normal bone, which results in a peculiar striped appearance of the tissue (Fig. 6.6). In the vertebral bodies, a central, horizontal lytic stripe is

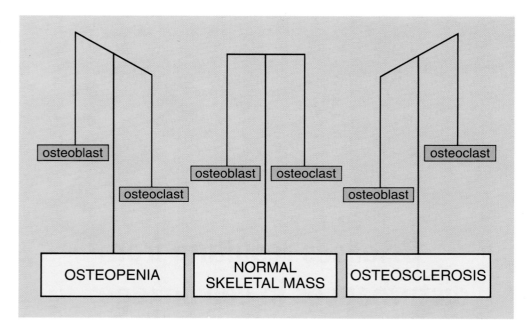

FIGURE 6.1 In each of these situations, it is the relative activity that matters, eg, in osteopenia there may be increased osteoblastic activity but osteoclastic activity is even greater.

often seen, which gives the vertebrae a sandwich-like appearance (Fig. 6.7). Occasionally, the spinal involvement may give rise to spondylolysis because of fractures through the pars interarticularis in the lumbar region.

Gross examination of the bones from fatal infantile cases usually shows widening in the region of the metaphysis and diaphysis, the characteristic Erlenmeyer flask deformity (Figs. 6.8 and 6.9). The affected bones have increased density and may weigh two to three times more than normal bone, despite the fact that they are usually somewhat smaller than normal. On sectioning, the bone tissue is very compact, with complete loss of the normal architecture.

Microscopic examination reveals extremely dense and irregular bone trabeculae, nearly all of which have a central core of cartilage (Fig. 6.10). (The primary spongiosa, which normally forms in the metaphysis during development, has a similar appearance but is rapidly remodeled to the adult form of bone. In pa-

tients with osteopetrosis, the mechanism by which this remodeling is effected appears to be deficient, and the primary spongiosa therefore persists.)

Although a paucity of osteoclasts has been reported in osteopetrosis, microscopic examination shows that osteoclasts are often abundant. However, electron microscopic studies have demonstrated that these osteoclasts lack ruffled borders and that although the cells are in proximity to the bone, they do not show the cytologic features normally present in an active osteoclast (Fig. 6.11). In other words, although osteoclasts are present they do not appear to be functioning. A possible explanation may lie in the observation that the enzyme collagenase is apparently absent in osteopetrotic bone.

In osteopetrotic mice, restoration of normal bone and cartilage resorption has followed the transplantation of normal bone marrow or spleen cells. This procedure has also been tried in humans with some promise of success.

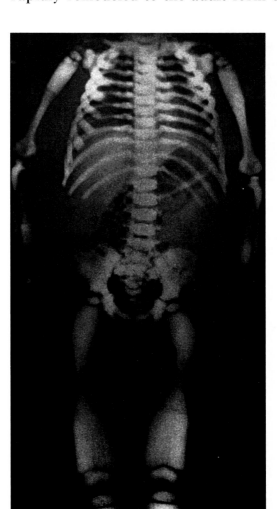

FIGURE 6.2
Whole body radiograph of a young child with osteopetrosis showing a marked increase in the density of the bones. In addition, there is the typical metaphyseal flaring, which is particularly prominent around the knees, hips, and upper humerus. The normal demarcation of cancellous bone and cortical bone is lost.

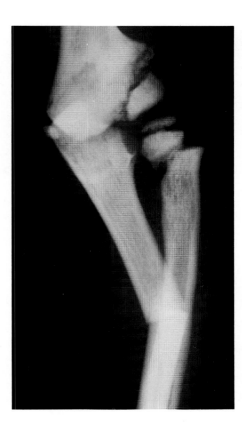

FIGURE 6.3
Multiple fractures of the forearm and elbow are demonstrated in this young patient with osteopetrosis.

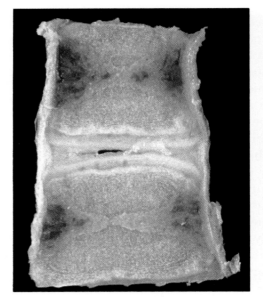

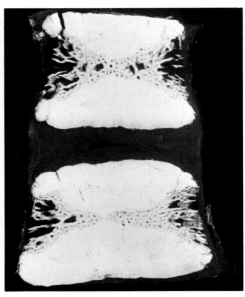

FIGURE 6.4 Osteopetrosis: gross appearance of two resected vertebral bodies in frontal section *(left)* and a radiograph of these vertebrae *(right)*. The obliteration of the marrow space results in extramedullary hematopoesis.

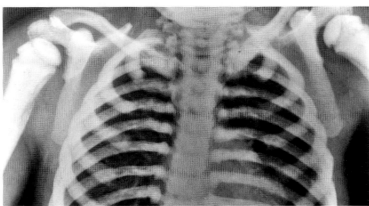

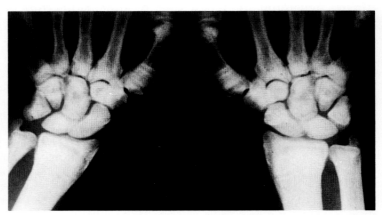

FIGURE 6.5 Radiograph of the upper body of a child with osteopetrosis. A marked increase in density of all the bones is apparent.

FIGURE 6.6 Clinical radiograph of the hands of an adult patient with osteopetrosis. The proximal end of the thumb clearly shows alternating stripes of dense involved bone, with less dense and apparently normal bone distally.

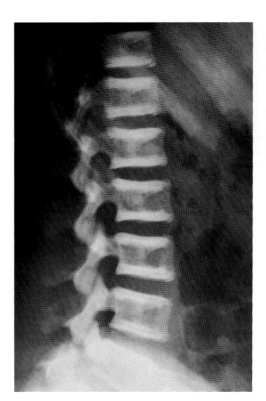

FIGURE 6.7
In this adult patient with osteopetrosis, a radiograph of the spine shows markedly increased density of the proximal and distal thirds of the vertebral bodies, giving a sandwich-like appearance.

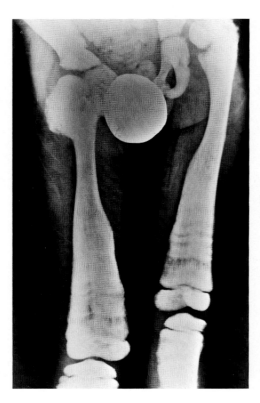

FIGURE 6.8
Radiograph of the legs in a child with osteopetrosis shows a lack of metaphyseal remodeling, which gives rise to an Erlenmeyer flask deformity. The normal cortical medullary differentiation is not seen, and the bones are strikingly dense.

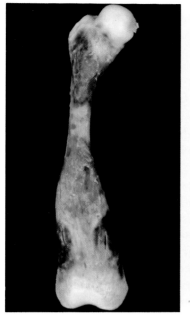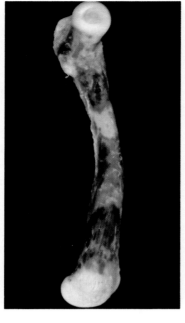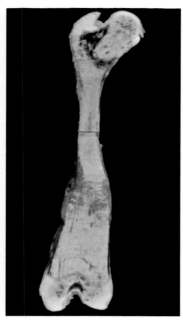

FIGURE 6.9 Gross appearances of a femur removed from a child with osteopetrosis seen in frontal *(left)*, lateral *(center)*, and cut section *(right)*. Note the characteristic Erlenmeyer flask deformity of the distal end of the femur, the exaggerated anterior bowing, subperiosteal hemorrhage, and uniform density of the bone on cut section.

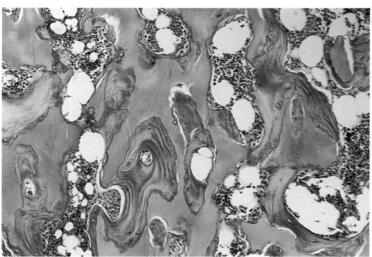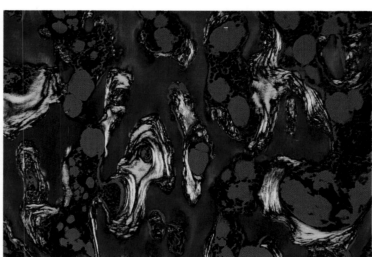

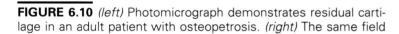

FIGURE 6.10 *(left)* Photomicrograph demonstrates residual cartilage in an adult patient with osteopetrosis. *(right)* The same field has been photographed using polarized light, which also clearly differentiates the bone and calcified cartilage (H & E, x 4 obj.).

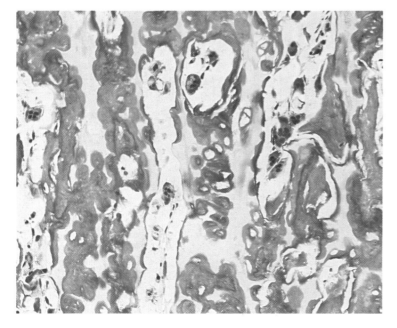

FIGURE 6.11 Histologic section taken from a young child with osteopetrosis shows numerous osteoclasts in the tissue, though these osteoclasts do not seem to be resorbing bone (H & E, x 10 obj.).

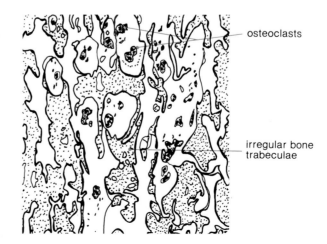

osteoclasts

irregular bone trabeculae

PAGET'S DISEASE
(OSTEITIS DEFORMANS)

Paget's disease, which is usually a localized condition, is characterized by disordered bone architecture which results from an increased rate of bone tissue breakdown by osteoclasts. In response to the increased osteoclastic resorption, there is a compensatory increase in the rate of bone tissue formation by osteoblasts, and the rate of bone turnover is thus increased (Fig. 6.12). Virtually any bone in the body may be involved, but the most common sites of disease are the lumbar spine, pelvis, skull, femur, and tibia. Less commonly, the disease is multifocal or even generalized.

The incidence of the condition varies with ethnicity; although common in northern Europeans, it is very rare in blacks and Asians. In two large autopsy series in northern Europe, the incidence of Pagets's disease was between 3 and 4 percent of all individuals over the age of 40. The disease was most often limited to a part of the vertebral column and/or the pelvis. Most of the individuals in whom the disease is discovered at autopsy had not been diagnosed during life. The clinical disease, characterized by widespread bone involvement, as described by Sir James Paget in 1877, actually represents only a small portion of the total number of affected individuals.

Radiologic and Gross Features

The radiologic appearance of the disease is variable. In the earliest stages, during which osteoclastic resorption predominates, there is a striking radiolucency without any thickening of the bone; in the skull this has been called osteoporosis circumscripta (Fig. 6.13). In the later stages of the disease, when resorption diminishes, the overall density of the bone increases (Fig. 6.14). The cancellous bone trabeculae can be seen to become thicker or coarser and more irregular. On the other hand, the cortical bone becomes radiographically less dense and there is loss of corticomedullary demarcation (Figs. 6.15 and 6.16). The periosteal and endosteal surfaces become irregular rather than smooth, often with an increase in the diameter of the bone.

Radiologic examination of the vertebral bodies may reveal either uniformly increased radiodensity or, more commonly, a "picture frame" appearance (Figs. 6.17 and 6.18). In the pelvis, it is common to find combina-

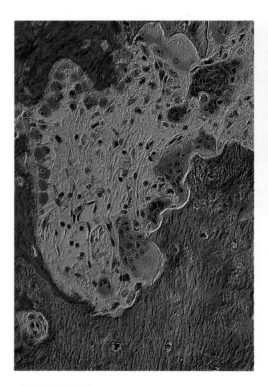

FIGURE 6.12 Photomicrograph of a histologic section obtained from a patient with Paget's disease demonstrates both bone resorption by large multinucleated giant cells and active bone deposition (undecalcified section, Goldner stain, x 10 obj.).

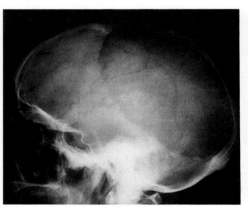

FIGURE 6.13 Clinical radiograph of a skull. Note large circular lytic defect involving the posterior half of the skull. One can also see some patchy osteoblastic reaction in the bone around the defect. This lesion, osteoporosis circumscripta, is a common radiologic presentation of Paget's disease.

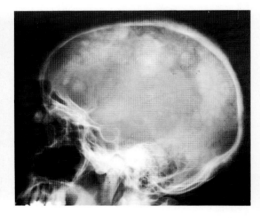

FIGURE 6.14 Clinical radiograph of the skull in the later stages of Paget's disease. Marked sclerosis appears in the bone, the diploetic architecture is lost, and the bone becomes extremely thick, on occasion becoming several times thicker than normal.

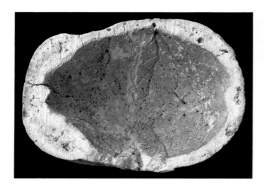

FIGURE 6.15 A striking example of late, severe Paget's disease in which the thickening of the skull, the loss of diploetic architecture, and the granular pumice-like appearance of the bone can be seen.

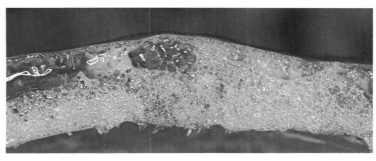

FIGURE 6.16 Paget's disease: close-up of the cut surface of a skull with large blood-filled lakes that may be present in pagetoid bone.

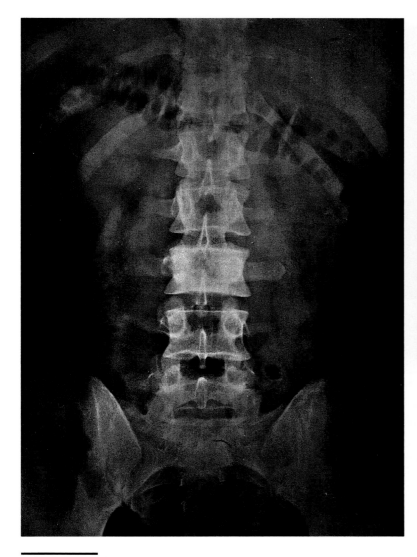

FIGURE 6.17 Clinical radiograph of a 38-year-old patient who presented with complaints of vague back pain. In this radiograph, a rather uniform sclerosis is seen in the body of L3; the initial radiographic diagnosis was lymphoma. Because of the sclerosis, a needle biopsy was obtained with difficulty which clearly demonstrated the mosaic-pattern, marrow fibrosis and increased osteoclastic resorption typical of Paget's disease.

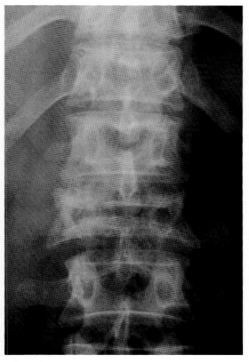

FIGURE 6.18 Clinical radiograph of the spine shows a solitary focus of pagetoid bone. There is a loss of height of the vertebra, some increases in the width of the vertebra, and a typical picture-frame appearance.

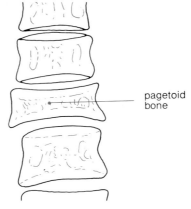

pagetoid bone

tions of increased density and lytic areas, as well as areas with a honeycombed or striated appearance.

In long bones, the process usually starts at one end, occasionally both, and spreads towards the center. The junction between the normal and diseased bone is demarcated as an advancing wedge of rarefaction frequently described as "flame-like" (Figs. 6.19 and 6.20).

In scintigraphic studies, isotope uptake is increased at all stages of the disease (Fig. 6.21).

Microscopic Appearance

Just as with the radiologic appearance, the microscopic appearance depends on the stage of the disease process, which can be divided into three phases. The osteolytic phase is characterized by active osteoclastic resorption and by an extremely vascular fibrous tissue that fills the marrow spaces. Inflammatory cells are absent (Fig. 6.22). In cancellous bone, the trabeculae are slender and sparse; in cortical bone, large resorption cavities

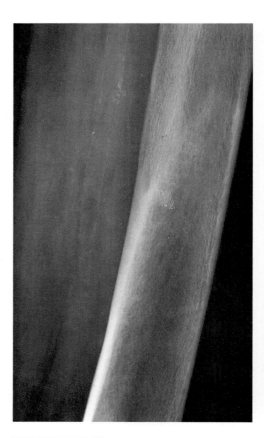

FIGURE 6.19 Radiograph of femur involved by Paget's disease. The cortex of the posterior femur in the proximal portion is irregularly thickened and more porotic than that in the distal part. At the junction between the involved upper bone and the normal lower bone, note a flame-shaped advancing edge.

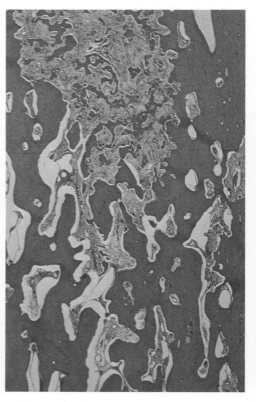

FIGURE 6.20 Histologic section of the advancing edge of involved bone shown in Figure 6.19. Note the involved fibrotic and pagetoid bone eroding the normal bone cortex (H & E, x 2.5 obj.).

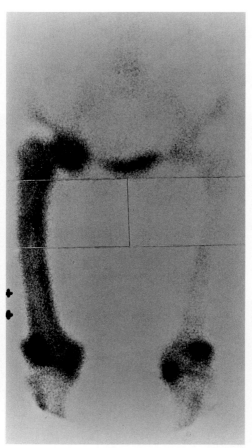

FIGURE 6.21 Scintigram shows increased ^{99}Tc uptake in a femur involved with Paget's disease. In this image, it is possible also to appreciate some bowing of the femur as well as varus deformity of the hip.

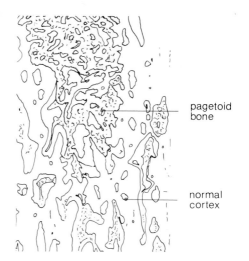

pagetoid bone

normal cortex

are seen. Concurrent with the osteoclastic activity, appositional new bone formation by prominent osteoblasts may be found. The bone tissue being formed is often of a woven type (Fig. 6.23). Both events are often observed on the same trabecula. The microscopic picture is one of frenetic cell activity, which may be confused with that of hyperparathyroidism.

This initial, mainly destructive phase is followed by an osteoblastic phase in which new bone formation predominates over resorption (Fig. 6.24). Massive trabecu-

lar plates are built up to a density that is neither cortical nor cancellous in its architecture.

The increased rate of bone formation and bone resorption results in an increased number of reversal fronts or cement lines, which give rise to the mosaic pattern (Fig. 6.25). The alteration in microarchitecture, together with the increased number of cement lines, facilitates the propagation of cracks and leads to structural weakness in the tissue. With the aid of polarized light microscopy, studies of the orientation of the

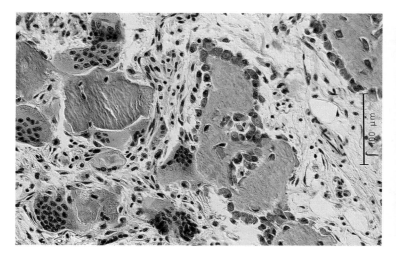

FIGURE 6.22 Photomicrograph demonstrates the acute phase of Paget's disease with very active osteoclastic resorption, marrow fibrosis, and the formation of new bone (H & E, x 10 obj.).

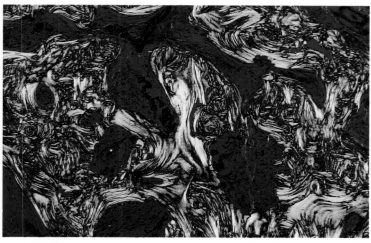

FIGURE 6.23 Photomicrograph taken using polarized light demonstrates woven bone formation in Paget's disease.

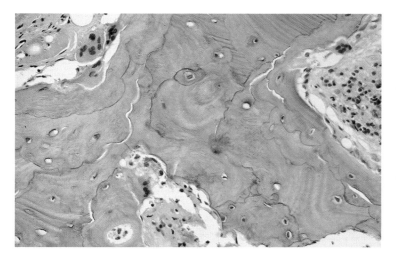

FIGURE 6.24 Photomicrograph demonstrates the thick, irregular plates of bone formed in Paget's disease. In this section, the basophilic cement lines are clearly seen. Note the microcracks which occur at the site of the cement lines and result in structural weakness in Pagetic bone (H & E, x 10 obj.).

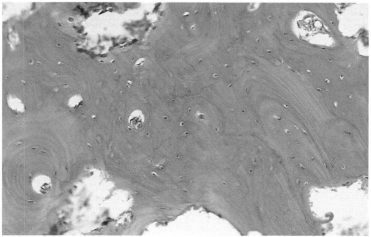

FIGURE 6.25 Histologic features of the late stages of Paget's disease. This section shows that the osteoblastic and osteoclastic reaction may be much less evident, and it can be difficult to appreciate the mosaic pattern, either because the tissue has been overdecalcified or because the staining is not adequate to show the basophilic lines clearly (H & E, x 10 obj.)

collagen in bone reveal the discordant nature of the new structure (Fig. 6.26).

A final "burnt-out" phase is generally described, during which cell activity is less intense and vascularity diminished. However, the turnover rate of the diseased bone may still be much greater than that of normal bone. The microscopic picture is that of heavily trabeculated bone showing a prominent mosaic pattern.

Clinical Laboratory Findings

An elevation of serum alkaline phosphatase activity (in association with the increased osteoblastic activity) to as much as 20 to 30 times the normal level has been recorded. The acid phosphatase level, too, tends to be at its upper limit or even slightly above normal. Regional blood flow studies have demonstrated increased vascularity, in some instances as much as 20 times the normal.

The serum calcium and phosphorus levels are ordinarily within normal limits in Paget's disease. However, hypercalcemia is an occasional complication following prolonged bed rest in a patient with extensive involvement. Elevated urinary hydroxyproline levels can also be expected as a consequence of increased bone tissue breakdown.

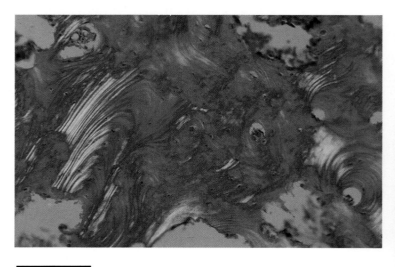

FIGURE 6.26 When the same histologic field as in Figure 6.25 is examined by polarized light with a first-order red filter, the disorganized pattern of the bone structure is clearly demonstrated.

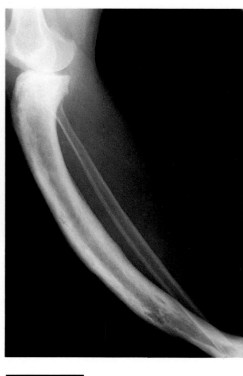

FIGURE 6.27 Radiograph of a patient with Paget's disease affecting the tibia but not the fibula shows an increase in length of the tibia, associated with bowing and irregularity of both periosteal and endosteal surfaces.

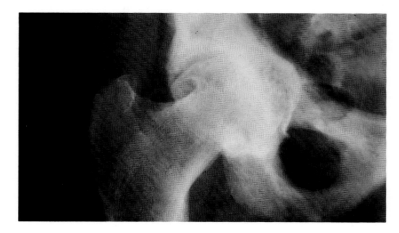

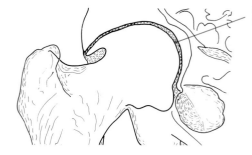

FIGURE 6.28 Clinical radiograph of a patient with Paget's disease. In the hip joint there is marked concentric narrowing, indicative of degenerative joint disease.

deformed narrowed joint

Clinical Presentation

The complaints that bring the patient to the physician are bone pain or symptoms of the complications of Paget's disease (fracture, arthritis, heart failure, or tumor). In patients with Paget's disease, small, incomplete cortical fractures may be numerous, particularly in weight-bearing bones. Progressive bowing of the femur and wedging of the vertebrae are the result of repeated microfractures (Fig. 6.27). Occasionally, these incomplete cortical fractures progress to complete transverse fractures.

Clinical evaluation of patients with Paget's disease reveals a high incidence of arthritis in the joints adjacent to involved bones (Figs. 6.28 and 6.29). Arthritis is most commonly seen in the hip joint, and is characterized on radiologic examination by concentric joint narrowing. This narrowing results from an accelerated rate of endochondral ossification in the calcified zone of the articular cartilage (Fig. 6.30) (consequent on the increased vascularity and turnover of the subchondral bone; see Chapter 9 for further discussion of this phenomenon). Bone deformity resulting from accelerated bone modeling also contributes to the arthritic process.

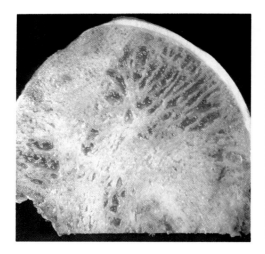
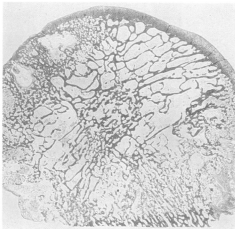
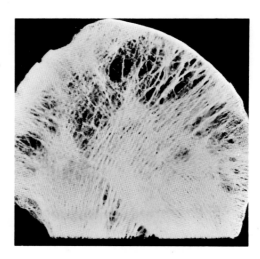

FIGURE 6.29 *(left)* A slice through a resected femoral head shows extensive involvement by Paget's disease and erosion of the cartilage on the medial side. Histologic section *(center)* of the femoral head and a radiograph *(right)* of a slice of the specimen. The pagetoid bone is seen to have a fine and disorganized trabecular pattern, which contrasts markedly with the normal cancellous bone that remains in some area.

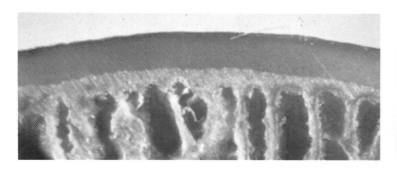
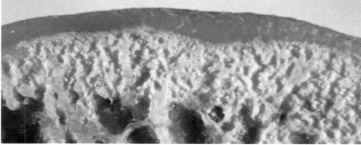
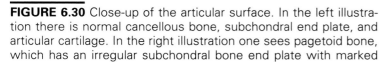

FIGURE 6.30 Close-up of the articular surface. In the left illustration there is normal cancellous bone, subchondral end plate, and articular cartilage. In the right illustration one sees pagetoid bone, which has an irregular subchondral bone end plate with marked thinning of the overlying cartilage. It may be that the accelerated remodeling of the affected subchondral bone has resulted in accelerated endochondral ossification of the overlying cartilage, which produces the evident thinning.

Sarcoma is reported to develop in 1 to 2 percent of patients with widespread Paget's involvement (Figs. 6.31 and 6.32). However, considering that most cases of Paget's disease are undiagnosed, the true incidence of sarcoma in Paget's disease must be very much lower. Sarcoma is a complication not only of widespread disease; it may rarely be engrafted on monostotic Paget's disease (Fig. 6.33). The sarcoma that develops usually shows a mixed pattern of osteosarcoma, fibrosarcoma, chondrosarcoma, and malignant fibrous histiocytoma, ie, a mixed mesenchymal pattern (Fig. 6.34). Occasionally a benign conventional giant cell tumor pattern may be seen, and in such cases the tumors may be multiple (Figs. 6.35 and 6.36). Myeloma, lymphoma and metastatic cancer have also been reported in association with Paget's disease. Pseudosarcomatous lesions, characterized by florid new bone and abundant periosteal bone formation, have also been described (Fig. 6.37), further

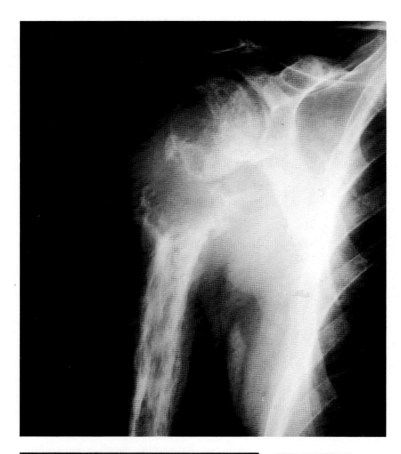

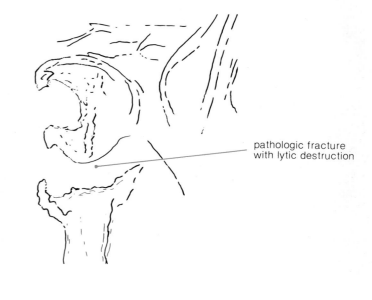

pathologic fracture
with lytic destruction

FIGURE 6.31 Clinical radiograph of a patient with widespread Paget's disease of the skeleton shows, in addition, at the proximal end of the humerus a destructive lytic lesion and a pathological fracture indicating sarcomatous degeneration.

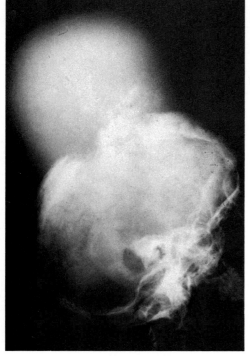

FIGURE 6.32 Radiograph of the skull of a patient with Paget's disease who had developed over the previous few months a large firm mass over the vault of the skull. Biopsy showed this to be a Paget's sarcoma.

emphasizing the need for biopsy in cases where tumor is suspected, so that treatment can be appropriate.

The cause of Paget's disease remains unknown. However, electron microscopic observations of the osteoclasts of patients with Paget's disease have demonstrated the presence of specific intranuclear inclusions composed of microcylinders (Fig. 6.38). These structures suggest an analogy with the myxovirus of the measles group. Studies with indirect immunofluorescence and immunoperoxidase techniques have lent further support to the hypotheses of a viral etiology in Paget's disease of bone.

GENERALIZED OSTEOSCLEROSIS ASSOCIATED WITH INCREASED OSTEOBLASTIC ACTIVITY

Increased osteoblastic activity not associated with any increase in osteoclastic activity leads to increased skeletal density. Physiologically, such an increase in density results from increased physical activity. Pathologically, osteosclerosis may result from a disturbance of normal cell linkage, but such cases are very rare. They are usually characterized by severe and unremitting bone pain, and their etiology is obscure.

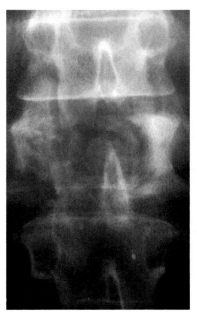

FIGURE 6.33 Spinal radiograph *(left)* of a 58-year-old female with a 2-month history of low back pain. Fourteen years earlier she had undergone hysterectomy for cervical carcinoma. A patchy sclerotic and lytic appearance was noted, which was interpreted to be consistent with metastatic disease. However, there is some widening of the body which is unusual in metastasis. Needle biopsy showed an anaplastic tumor with many giant cells, consistent with Paget's sarcoma; foci of bone obtained with this biopsy showed the typical mosaic pattern of Paget's. The patient died approximately 4 months later. Autopsy revealed local extension of the tumor, which involved T-12 and L-2, and compression and encasement of the vena cava. Extensive lung metastases had the pattern of a Paget's sarcoma. An H & E section *(lower left)* of a portion of bone adjacent to the tumor shows increased numbers of cement lines within the bone. In the polarized section *(lower right)* of the same field, the disorganized bony architecture is obvious (H & E, x 4 obj.). This case is significant because it demonstrates that even in monostotic Paget's disease, a sarcoma may rarely occur as a complication.

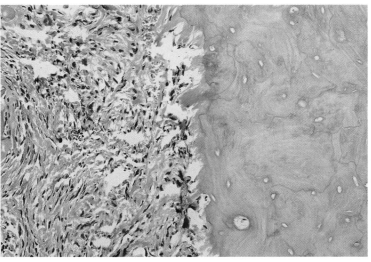

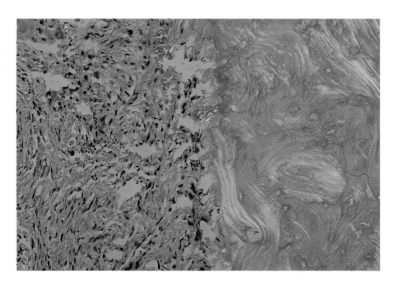

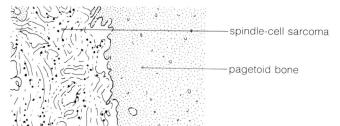

spindle-cell sarcoma

pagetoid bone

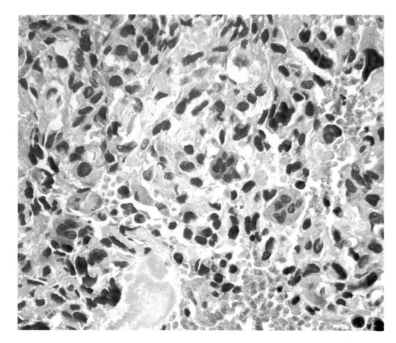

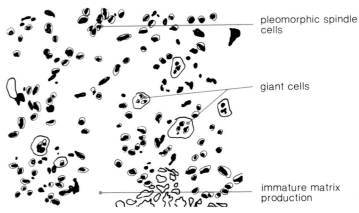

FIGURE 6.34 High-power view of a biopsy from the patient in Figure 6.31 shows a pleomorphic spindle cell tumor with many giant cells, which is typical of the histologic appearance of Paget's sarcoma (H & E, x 25 obj.).

pleomorphic spindle cells

giant cells

immature matrix production

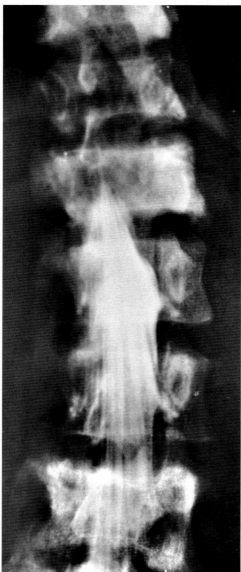

FIGURE 6.35 Radiograph of the spine of a patient with Paget's disease (note the irregular coarse density of several vertebral bodies). The myelogram shows an occlusion at the level of L1 with displacement of the dura by a soft tissue mass, which on biopsy proved to be a giant cell tumor.

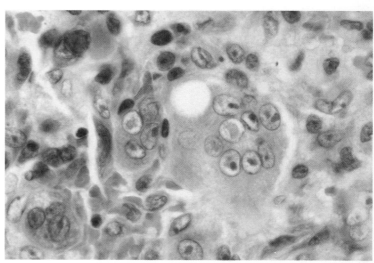

FIGURE 6.36 Photomicrograph of a giant cell tumor from a patient with Paget's disease. Note the intranuclear eosinophilic inclusions in addition to the more clearly defined basophilic nucleoli (H & E, x 50 obj.).

Camurati–Engelmann Disease

The clinical features of Camurati–Engelmann disease are painful legs, a waddling gait, and wasting muscles. The disease is usually hereditary, with an autosomal dominant mode of transmission. The symptoms usually become manifest early in life, commonly before the age of 10 years. However, occasional cases have been reported in which the patient's age at diagnosis has been as late as the fifth decade.

The disease is diagnosed primarily on the basis of radiologic examination. Symmetric sclerosis is observed, and often a fusiform enlargement of the diaphysis of the long bones, especially the femur and tibia. There may also be changes in the skull, and rarely in the pelvis, mandible, clavicle, ribs, spine, metacarpals, and phalanges (Fig. 6.39).

The disorder is characterized histologically by a thickened cortex, which results mainly from increased

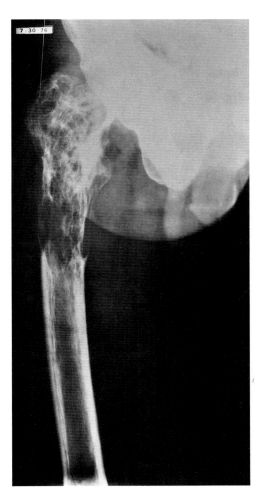

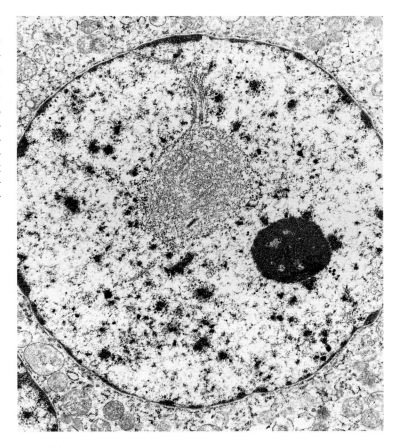

FIGURE 6.37
Radiograph of the femur from a patient with Paget's disease shows an expanded lytic area which seemed to indicate the development of a sarcoma, however biopsy showed that this area was entirely formed of reactive tissue.

FIGURE 6.38 An electron photomicrograph of one of the nuclei containing an eosinophilic inclusion illustrated in Figure 6.36 demonstrates microtubular structures—the image associated with the myxoma virus (original magnification x 20,000).

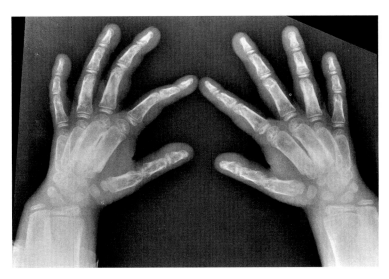

FIGURE 6.39 Radiograph of the hands of a child with Camurati-Engelmann disease illustrates the cortical sclerosis and fusiform enlargement of the metacarpals typical of this disease.

endosteal new bone formation (Figs. 6.40 and 6.41). However, periosteal new bone formation is sometimes observed. In children, the enlargement of the cortex of the bone produces a narrowed medullary cavity which, if narrowing is severe enough, may lead to extramedullary hematopoiesis and eventual hepatosplenomegaly.

The serum chemistries in patients with Camurati–Engelmann disease are usually normal, although an increase in the level of alkaline phosphatase (of bone origin) is sometimes observed. The disorder is of obscure etiology, but the pain may be relieved by the administration of steroids.

In 1962, Van Buchen and his associates reported

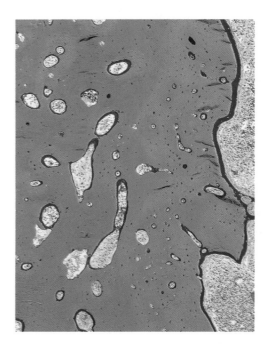

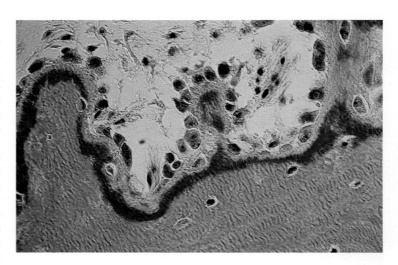

FIGURE 6.40 Photomicrograph of a cortical biopsy from a patient with Camurati—Engelmann disease. Bone surfaces are covered by a thin layer of osteoid, indicating increased bone formation. The endosteal surface (right) appears hypercellular with respect to osteocytes. The bone is lamellar with no increase in cement lines, differentiating this from Paget's disease (undecalcified bone, Goldner stain, x 4 obj.).

FIGURE 6.41 A photomicrograph taken at a higher power from the tissue shown in Figure 6.40 to demonstrate the prominent osteoblasts lining the endosteal surface of the bone together with a moderately thick layer of unmineralized osteoid (undecalcified section, Goldner stain, x 25 obj.).

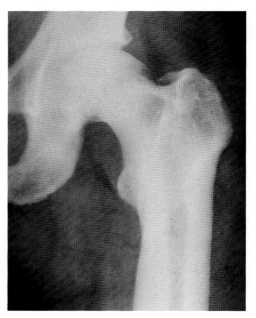

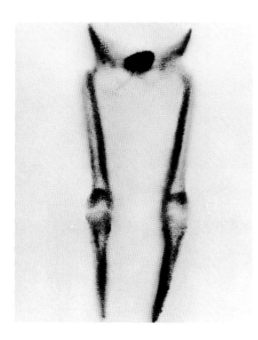

FIGURE 6.42 Radiograph of a 49-year-old man with a 3-year history of bone pain. Note the markedly thickened, dense cortex, which is more clearly defined than the thickened but pumice-like bone of Paget's disease. In this patient the serum calcium and phosphate levels were within normal limits, although the alkaline phosphatase level was persistently elevated (up to 1600 mU/ml).

FIGURE 6.43 Bone scan demonstrates increased diaphyseal uptake over the femurs and tibias bilaterally in a case of hyperostosis generalisata.

seven cases of a disease that was similar in many ways to Camurati–Engelmann disease but differed in that there was prominent skull involvement and a suggestion of autosomal recessive transmission (hyperostosis corticalis generalisata).

Other obscure entities with diaphyseal cortical bone thickening include hyperostosis generalisata with pachyderma, in which the diaphysis, metaphysis, and epiphysis are significantly involved (Figs. 6.42 and 6.43).

OSTEOPENIC CONDITIONS

GENERALIZED OSTEOPOROSIS

Decreased density of the skeleton (osteopenia) is a nonspecific condition that may result from any of a number of causes, including mineral and collagen disturbances, hematologic and endocrine abnormalities, neoplastic disorders, or immobilization (Fig. 6.44). The amount of

---

FIGURE 6.44

CAUSES OF OSTEOPOROSIS

Disuse	Prolonged bed rest		**Neoplasms**	Metastatic cancer
	General inactivity			Bone marrow tumors
	Prolonged casting or splinting localized osteoporosis			myeloma
				lymphoma
	Angiodystrophy			leukemia
	Paralysis			mast-cell
	paraplegia, quadriplegia, hemiplegia, lower motor neuron disease		**Endocrine Abnormalities**	Pituitary
	Space travel			hypersecretion
	weightlessness			tumor
Diet	Deficiency of calcium, protein, vitamin C			Adrenal cortex glucocorticoid excess (hyperplasia, tumor, iatrogenic)
	Anorexia nervosa			Ovary estrogen deficiency (postmenopausal, genetic, ovariectomy)
Drugs	Heparin			Testis testosterone deficiency (genetic, castration)
	Methotrexate			Parathyroid hyperparathyroidism (primary, secondary)
	Ethanol			
	Glucocorticoids			Thyroid hyperthyroidism
Idiopathy	Adolescent (10-18 yrs)			
	Middle-aged male			
Genetic Disorders	Osteogenesis imperfecta		**Postmenopausal**	Type I osteoporosis
	Homocystinuria			
			Age - related	Type II osteoporosis (male or female)
Chronic Illness	Rheumatoid arthritis (juvenile, adult)			
	Cirrhosis			
	Sarcoidosis			
	Renal tubular acidosis			

bone tissue in the skeleton also decreases with age, more significantly in women than in men, and to a greater extent in whites and Asians than in blacks (Fig. 6.45). Age-related osteopenia that results in fracture (usually vertebral crush fractures, Colles' fractures, or femoral neck fractures) is generally referred to as senile osteoporosis and is twice as common in females as in males. (Carter and Hayes have shown that the compressive strength of trabecular bone is proportional to the square of its apparent density. Thus, if the density decreases by a factor of 2, the compressive strength decreases by a factor of 4.)

Clinically significant osteoporosis related to the menopause may also develop in a significant number of women. These two common types of osteoporosis, postmenopausal and senile, have been classified by Riggs and his colleagues on the basis of their different clinical findings as Type I osteoporosis (postmenopausal) and Type II osteoporosis (senile or age-related). In postmenopausal osteoporosis, bone loss is rapid and associated with increased osteoclastic activity. It appears that estrogen deficiency increases the sensitivity of the osteoclasts to parathyroid hormone. In senile osteoporosis, bone loss is slow but relentless, and has been associated with decreased synthesis of bone matrix by the osteoblasts (Fig. 6.46).

It should be recognized that many other important factors affect bone tissue loss, particularly including physical activity level and diet. The maintenance of skeletal mass is especially affected by activity level. Daily weight-bearing activity is essential to the health of the skeleton, and mechanical weight-bearing stress is perhaps the most important exogenous factor affecting bone development and bone modeling. An interesting example of this process has been observed in astronauts. The marked reduction in gravitational field that results in the weightless environment of space flight leads to profound and rapid loss of skeletal and muscle mass. In everyday terms, a sedentary person is more likely to become osteoporotic than a person who engages in some form of weight-bearing exercise.

An adequate and balanced diet is also essential, and lack of it is an important contributor to disease. Chronic calcium deficiency in the diet leads to increased secretion of both parathyroid hormone and the hormonally active form of vitamin D, $1,25(OH)_2D$ (see Chapter 7), both of which stimulate osteoclastic activity. Excessive alcohol consumption also contributes to osteoporosis.

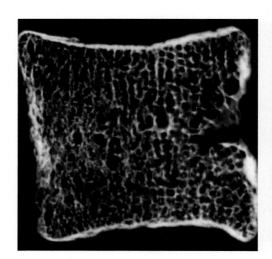 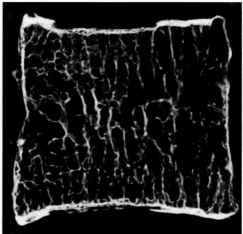 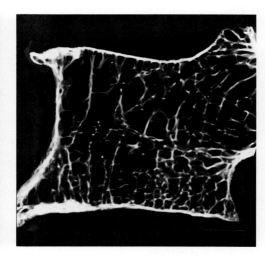

FIGURE 6.45 Specimen radiographs of 2-mm slices through the vertebral body of T-2. *(left)* The first specimen represents normal bone texture, density, and pattern. *(center)* The second specimen shows a moderate degree of osteopenia, with accentuation of the vertical trabeculae and selective loss of the horizontal trabeculae. *(right)* The third specimen shows severe osteoporosis, with irregular thin trabeculae and partial central collapse of the superior end plate.

FIGURE 6.46

INVOLUTIONAL OSTEOPOROSIS

	Postmenopausal (Type I)	Age - related (Type II)
Epidemiologic Factors		
Age	55 to 75	>70 (F); >80
Sex Ration (F/M)	6:1	2:1
Bone Physiology or Metabolism		
Pathogenesis of uncoupling	Increased osteoclast activity; ↑ resorption	Decreased osteoblast activity; ↓ formation
Net bone loss	Mainly trabecular	Cortical and trabecular
Rate of bone loss	Rapid/short duration	Slow/long duration
Bone density	>2 standard deviations below normal	Low normal (adjusted for age and sex)
Clinical Signs		
Fracture sites	Vertebrae (crush), distal forearm, hip (intracapsular)	Vertebrae (multiple wedge), proximal humerus and tibia, hip (extracapsular)
Other signs	Tooth loss	Dorsal kyphosis
Laboratory Values		
Serum Ca^{++}	Normal	Normal
Serum P_i	Normal	Normal
Alkaline phosphatase	Normal (↑ with fracture)	Normal (↑ with fracture)
Urine Ca^{++}	Increased	Normal
PTH function	Decreased	Increased
Renal conversion of $25(OH)D$ to $1,25(OH_2D$	Secondary decrease due to ↓ PTH	Primary decrease due to decreased responsiveness of $1\text{-}\alpha\text{-}OH_{ase}$
Gastrointestinal calcium absorption	Decreased	Decreased
Prevention		
High-risk patients	Estrogen or calcitonin supplementation; calcium supplementation; adequate vitamin D; adequate weight-bearing activity; minimization of associated risk factors	Calcium supplementation; adequate vitamin D; adequate weight-bearing activity; minimization of associated risk factors

The characteristic radiologic features in patients with osteoporosis are thinning of cortical bone and generalized rarefaction of the skeleton (Fig. 6.47). In postmenopausal osteoporosis, bone loss is mainly of cancellous bone, with less cortical bone loss, whereas in senile, age-related osteoporosis both cancellous and cortical bone loss are present. As the cortex becomes thinner, the overall diameter of the bone tends to increase to maximize mechanical efficiency. In the vertebral column, one sees thinning and eventual disappearance of the transverse trabeculae and subsequent thickening of the vertical trabeculae followed later by the thinning of these trabeculae also (Fig. 6.48). Compression fractures occur, giving rise to the widening of the intervertebral disc, the so-called "codfish" appearance (Fig. 6.49). In general, the lower thoracic and upper lumbar vertebrae are most affected. In a radiological survey reported in the *Journal of the American Medical Association* (Vol. 153: 625, 1953), 20 percent of men and 29 percent of women over the age of 60 showed compression fractures of the vertebral bodies. Therefore, back pain associated with loss of height due to vertebral compression and increased thoracic kyphosis are common manifestations.

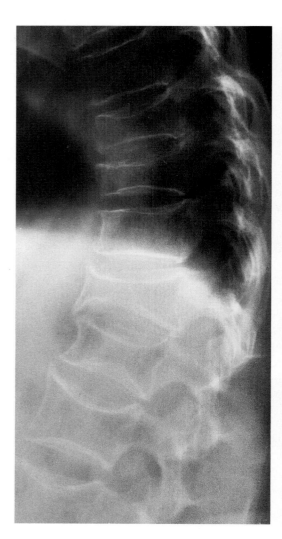

FIGURE 6.47 Biconcavity or "codfish vertebrae," seen here on the lateral view of the thoracolumbar spine in an 80-year-old woman with osteoporosis, results from weakness of the vertebral endplates and intravertebral expansion of nuclei pulposi.

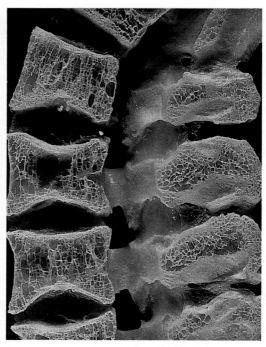

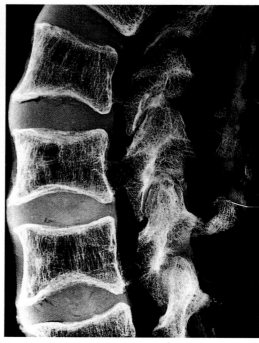

FIGURE 6.48 Photograph *(top)* of a sagittal section through the macerated spine of an elderly patient with severe osteoporosis. Note the central collapse of the end plates in the four lumbar vertebrae, along with accentuation of the vertical trabeculae and marked central porosity of the vertebral bodies. A specimen radiograph *(bottom)* of this patient emphasizes the uniform biconcavities of the end plates as well as the patchy nature of the osteoporosis.

Because vertebral bone loss has been calculated to approximate 30 percent before it can be radiologically detected, radiologists have long sought special techniques for the evaluation of bone mass, density, and calcium content. Three methods are widely available for assessing the bone tissue mass based on measurements of bone mineral content. Single-photon absorptiometry, performed for the assessment of cortical bone in the appendicular skeleton, uses the isotope iodine $125(^{125}I)$ as a source of photons, which are then passed through the forearm. The attenuation of the beam is measured by a scintillation counter. Dual-photon absorptiometry uses gadolinium $153(^{153}Gd)$ which emits photons of two distinct energies, making it possible to distinguish between soft tissue and mineralized tissue. This also allows measurements to be made over the spine and hip where there is considerable soft tissue. When measuring the spine, it is important to realize that aortic calcification, degenerative arthritis of the spine, or both, may contribute to falsely high readings, as may vertebral compression fractures, where the porosity may be masked owing to compaction of the trabeculae and formation of fracture callus. Quantitative CT scanning allows densitometric measurements of cross-sections of a vertebral body, which are then compared with a phantom.

Other techniques involving radionuclide uptake and neutron activation are still in the developmental stage. It is important to note that at the present time only a bone biopsy can adequately evaluate the cell activities of osteoclasts and osteoblasts—factors that are critical in assessment of osteoporosis and determination of a suitable mode of treatment.

In morphologic terms, osteoporosis is defined as a decrease in bone mass sufficient to result in spontaneous fracture, with the bone itself having a normal biochemical makeup (Figs. 6.50 to 6.52). Severe osteoporosis can develop only if there is a net uncoupling of bone formation and bone resorption. Morphometric analyses of the cell parameters, the amount of bone present, and the degree to which osteoid is present on the surfaces of the trabecular and cortical bones have led to the characterization of some of the types of osteoporosis (Figs. 6.53 and 6.54). Although cell activity, ie, relative and absolute osteoblast and osteoclast counts, is usually low in senile osteoporosis, indicating a relatively "inactive" state, it may sometimes be high. In more than 15 percent of patients this increased activity is associated with normocalcemic, normophosphatemic hyperparathyroidism. An additional subgroup of patients is noted to have increased osteoid surfaces. In disuse osteoporosis, the most dramatic initial finding is an increase in the number of resorptive surfaces. In steroid-induced osteoporosis osteoclastic activity is high, with relatively normal bone formation.

The treatment of osteoporosis should, insofar as possible, be directed toward the underlying etiology. Long-term corticosteroid therapy, excessive alcohol in-

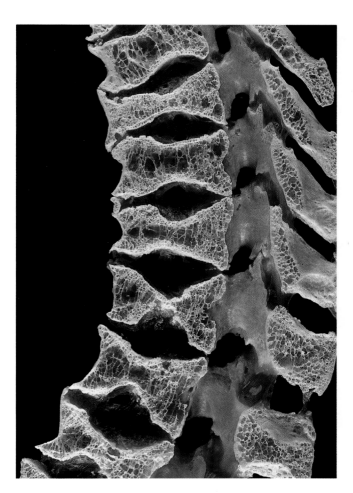

FIGURE 6.49 Photograph of a sagittal section of a macerated thoracic spine to demonstrate the various patterns and degrees of collapse that may be seen within the vertebral bodies. In the upper part of the segment, flattening of the vertebral bodies with some anterior wedging is seen. In the lower part of the segment, the more typical biconcave compression fractures of the central end plates are seen, which give rise to so-called fish-mouth vertebrae.

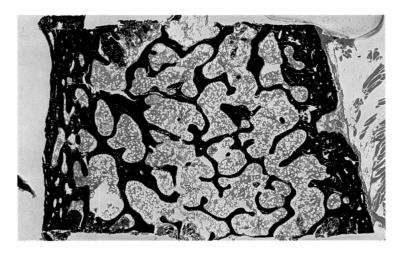

FIGURE 6.50 Transilial biopsy of normal bone demonstrates a cortical bone volume of 20.3% and a trabecular bone volume of 37.2% (undecalcified bone, von Kossa stain, x 1.5 obj.).

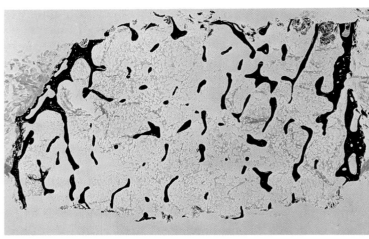

FIGURE 6.51 Transilial biopsy of a patient with moderate to severe osteoporosis. Morphometric analysis shows a cortical bone volume of 7% and a trabecular bone volume of 13% (undecalcified bone, von Kossa stain, x 1.5 obj.).

FIGURE 6.52 Photomicrograph taken from a vertebral body in a patient with osteoporosis shows a microfracture of one of the trabeculae. Surrounding the fractured trabecula is a small microcallus. In patients with osteoporosis such microfractures are abundant in the vertebral bodies (H & E, x 4 obj.).

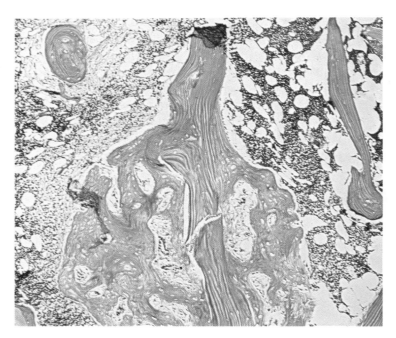

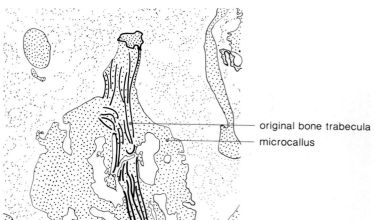

FIGURE 6.53 Photomicrograph of a histologic section obtained from a patient with inactive (senile) osteoporosis demonstrates the flat, inactive osteoblasts lining the bone, together with an inactive resorption surface (undecalcified section, Goldner stain, x 4 obj.).

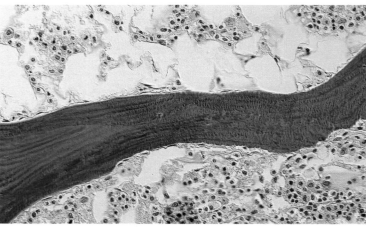

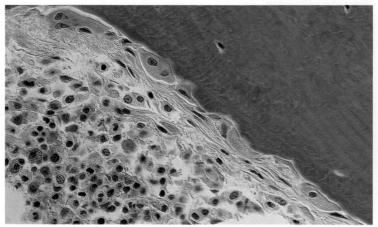

FIGURE 6.54 Photomicrograph of a histologic section obtained from a patient with active postmenopausal osteoporosis demonstrates active surface resorption (undecalcified section, Goldner stain, x 10 obj.).

take, and endocrinopathies such as hyperthyroidism account for a significant number of cases of osteoporosis and should be corrected medically. In patients with idiopathic osteoporosis, a number of therapeutic agents have been used with various degrees of success. Exercise is crucial in maintaining skeletal integrity. Calcium supplementation corrects the relative calcium deficiency in the postmenopausal state. The use of sodium fluoride as a stimulant to bone formation has been a popular treatment, but its use has recently been questioned. At present, more emphasis is placed on the suppression of osteoclastic activity (eg, by the use of calcitonin) and the stimulation of osteoblastic activity (eg, by the use of oral phosphates or parathormone).

Although estrogen replacement therapy is theoretically sound, its link with atypical endometrial changes has limited its widespread use.

LOCALIZED (TRANSIENT) OSTEOPOROSIS

In 1900, Sudeck described a transient yet painful osteoporosis of the lower extremity that occurred without obvious cause, though possibly related to trauma (Figs. 6.55 and 6.56). This syndrome, usually known as Sudeck's atrophy, has been related to a reflex sympathetic dystrophy. The symptoms, often involving the entire extremity, include pain, hyperesthesia, and tenderness. The pain varies in severity and character and

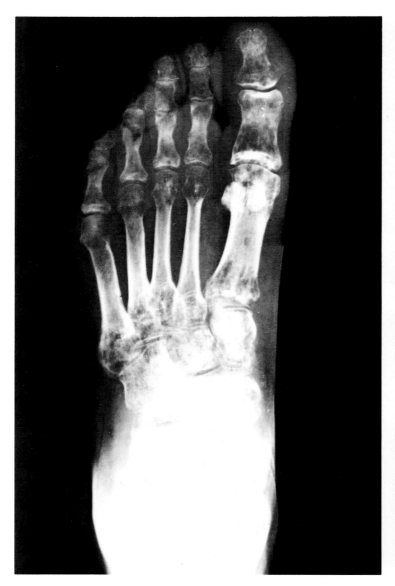

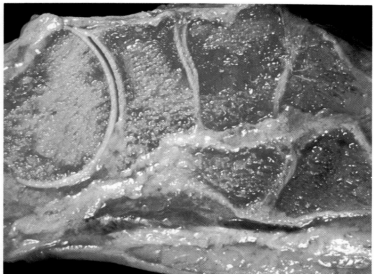

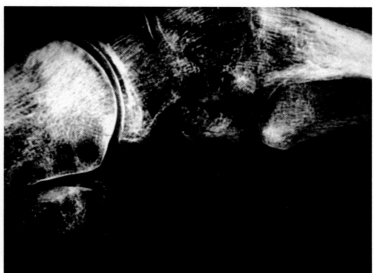

FIGURE 6.55 Radiograph of a foot in a patient with painful osteopenia localized to the foot and ankle following trauma. Note the juxta-articular location.

FIGURE 6.56 *(upper)* Gross specimen of a section through the foot shown in Figure 6.55 reveals marked hyperemia in patches, but particularly juxta-articularly. Radiograph of a slice of the specimen *(lower)*.

is associated with swelling and a decreased range of motion in neighboring joints. The skin may be clammy, cyanotic, cool, moist, or painful, the pain being burning or aching in nature. In 1959, Curtiss and Kincaid reported a number of cases of localized and transient osteoporosis which involved the hip joint of pregnant women (Fig. 6.57). Since that time it has become apparent that middle-aged men are also frequently affected by a similar condition. A related form of transient osteoporosis is migratory, and rather than being restricted to the hip it may affect the knee as well as the foot and ankle. This form is associated with swelling of the affected part, and is called regional migratory osteoporosis. In all these syndromes, the lesions tend to be juxta-articular.

Patients with transient osteoporosis characteristically have acute, localized pain that is often debilitating. Laboratory findings are unremarkable. The involved areas show an increased uptake of isotope on technetium bone scanning, and this increased uptake may predate the radiologic evidence of osteopenia by some months. Histopathologic findings have been only infrequently reported; however, microscopic examination of histologic sections has shown thinned-out bone trabeculae with evidence of osteoclastic bone resorption and hypervascularity of the marrow space (Fig. 6.58).

In some cases of transient osteoporosis, biopsy has demonstrated evidence of fat necrosis and fibrosis in the marrow, suggestive of an episodic ischemic etiology. Possibly, the osteoclasts and hyperemia are secondary events in these cases.

Because the lesions usually remit spontaneously within one year, the importance of this disorder rests in recognizing its benign nature. It should not be confused with diseases such as osteomyelitis or metastatic cancer, which it may mimic radiologically.

IDIOPATHIC OSTEOLYSIS

Primary idiopathic osteolysis is rare. It is characterized by the spontaneous onset of bone resorption without any obvious cause. Bones that previously appeared normal begin to undergo partial or complete resorption. This process may continue for years, until eventually it ceases spontaneously. The end result is severe deformity and serious functional disability.

Torg et al. have classified the osteolyses into four types: hereditary multicentric osteolysis with dominant transmission; hereditary multicentric osteolysis with recessive transmission; idiopathic nonhereditary multicentric osteolysis with nephropathy; and Gorham's massive osteolysis.

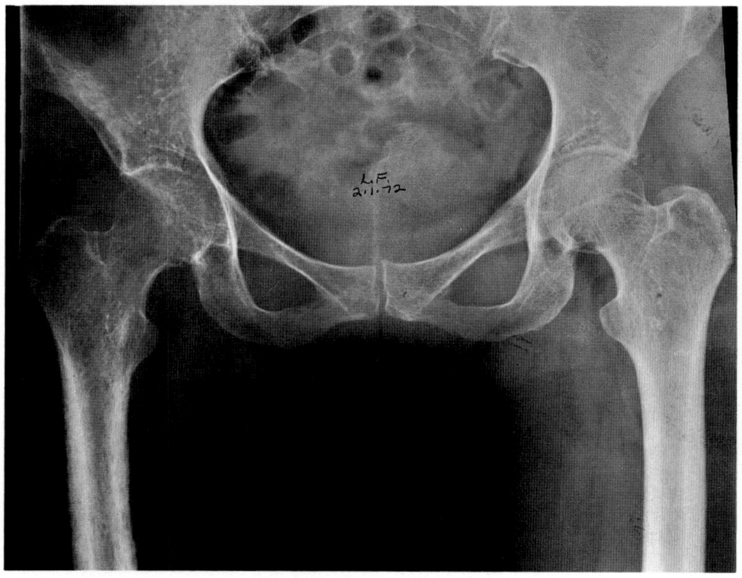

FIGURE 6.57 Radiograph of the pelvis of a woman with transient osteoporosis who had complained for some months of severe pain and weakness in the right hip. Note the osteolysis affecting both sides of the hip joint.

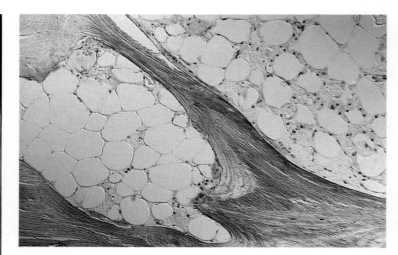

FIGURE 6.58 Photomicrograph showing early fat necrosis with foamy histiocytes in the marrow of a bone biopsy taken from a patient with transient osteoporosis. The adjacent bone trabeculae can be seen to be undergoing osteoclastic resorption (H & E, x 10 obj., Nomarski optics).

Type 1: Hereditary multicentric osteolysis with dominant transmission

The progression of this disease is characteristic. Between the ages of 2 and 7 years, spontaneous pain and swelling begin in the hands and feet. Over the period of a few years, partial or complete resorption of the involved bones occurs. In the majority of cases, the carpal and tarsal bones are affected. However, a high proportion of cases also have osteolytic involvement of the metacarpals, as well as the distal epiphyses of the radius and ulna which leads to shortening instability and ulnar deviation.

Type 2: Hereditary multicentric osteolysis with recessive transmission

The clinical appearance is similar to that described for the dominant form. However, in addition to the specific osteolysis, a generalized severe osteoporosis with cortical thinning and enlargement of the tubular bones is present.

Type 3: Nonhereditary multicentric osteolysis with nephropathy

This variety of idiopathic osteolysis is primarily characterized by a gradual disappearance of the carpus, with the tarsal bones involved to a lesser degree. The osteolysis crosses the epiphysial growth centers of the distal radius and ulna, resulting in growth disturbance and severe ulnar deviation. Concurrent with the onset of the osteolysis, a proteinuria reflecting pathologic renal function can also be observed. Death may occur in adolescence as a result of renal failure and malignant hypertension.

Type 4: Gorham's massive osteolysis

In 1955, Gorham and Stout reported 24 cases with a monocentric, massive osteolysis. This variety, known as Gorham's osteolysis, disappearing bone disease, or vanishing bone disease, is associated with angiomatosis. Unlike multicentric osteolysis, Gorham's disease may start at any age. It has neither a hereditary pattern nor an associated nephropathy.

Massive osteolysis is characterized radiographically by progressive and extensive reduction in bone density, and morphologically by the replacement of osseous tissue with fibrous tissue and thin-walled dilated vascular channels. Generally detected initially in children or in young adults, the disorder usually affects the peripheral skeleton, and is often confined to a single bone or to two or more bones centered around a joint. The shoulder and hip are the most common sites of involvement. The clinical course is protracted but rarely fatal, with eventual stabilization the most common outcome. Patients may complain of a dull aching pain or the insidious onset of progressive weakness. Radiographic examination reveals initial intramedullary and subcortical ill-defined lucent areas, with a subsequent loss of density extending from one end of the bone to the other. Reactive bone formation is not evident. Characteristic shrinkage or tapering of the long bones may occur (Fig. 6.59).

Reported descriptions of whole surgical specimens have featured thin, tapered, soft bone, and in specimens in which the mineralized bone has entirely disappeared, a fibrous band may be seen to replace the original bone. Biopsies of earlier lesions have revealed hypervascular fibrous connective tissue replacing bone; the proliferative vessels may be capillary, sinusoidal, or cavernous (Figs. 6.60 and 6.61).

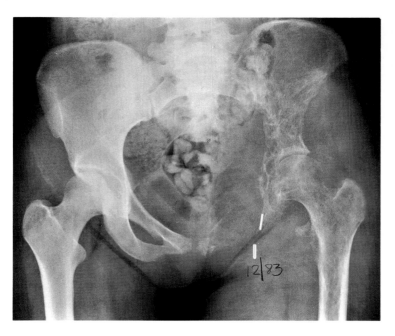

FIGURE 6.59 Radiograph of the pelvis of a young woman complaining of weakness of the hip. As can be seen from the radiograph, extensive bone loss involves most of the hemipelvis. The upper femur is also severely porotic.

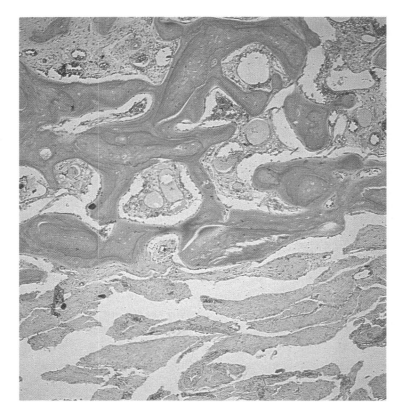

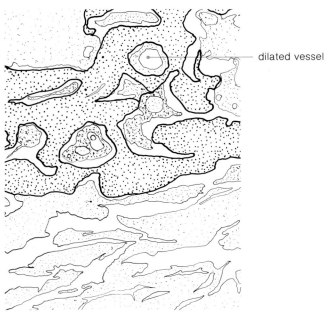

FIGURE 6.60 Bone biopsy from a patient with disappearing bone disease, adjacent to the site of involvement. Note the presence of large dilated vessels in the marrow spaces (H & E, x 4 obj.).

— dilated vessel

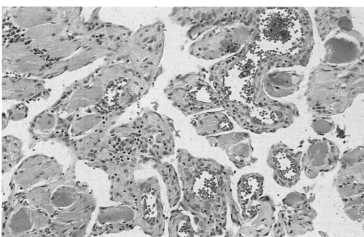

FIGURE 6.61 Photomicrograph of tissue obtained from a bone involved by Gorham's disease shows hypervascular tissue with an angiomatous appearance. No residual bone is present in this section (H & E, x 4 obj.).

Bone disease resulting from disturbances in mineral homeostasis

Calcium and phosphate play a crucial role in the biologic processes of both humans and higher animals. Calcium is essential to a number of physiologic mechanisms. Among the most important of these are neuromuscular function, cardiac function, and the blood clotting process. Calcium also acts as an obligatory co-enzyme in many processes, and assists in maintaining the integrity of membranes and normal skeletal function.

Calcium homeostasis is under the control of the endocrine system, involving a combination of interactions among parathyroid hormone (PTH), vitamin D, and calcitonin. In addition to endocrine mechanisms, however, it is also dependent on normal functioning of the target organs, ie, the intestines, kidneys, and bone cells.

Two principal patterns of disease associated with disturbed calcium homeostasis are recognized in the bone tissue: osteitis fibrosa cystica (Fig. 7.1) and hyperosteoidosis (as in osteomalacia and rickets) (Fig. 7.2). Osteitis fibrosa cystica results from hyperactivity of the parathyroid glands, which may be caused by a tumor of the parathyroids (ie, primary hyperparathyroidism) or by disease elsewhere (secondary hyperparathyroidism). Because of the important role of glomerular filtration and renal tubule reabsorption in serum calcium and

phosphorus metabolism and in maintenance of acid-base equilibrium, as well as in the important mechanism of intermediary vitamin D metabolism in the kidney, chronic renal disease is the most important cause of secondary hyperparathyroidism and may give rise to marked skeletal abnormalities. However, secondary hyperparathyroidism may also be caused by phosphate deficiency or by any disease that strongly stimulates bone formation (eg, Paget's disease) or retards mineralization of osteoid (eg, aluminum-induced bone disease).

Disturbances in calcium and phosphorus homeostasis may also lead to soft tissue calcification, as occurs with metastatic calcification in secondary hyperparathyroidism. In addition, soft tissue calcification may also be secondary to trauma or to abnormalities in the complicated feedback mechanisms that regulate calcification at the local level.

This chapter first considers normal calcium and phosphorus homeostasis, followed by a discussion of the effects of abnormal parathyroid activity, disturbances in vitamin D metabolism, disturbed phosphate metabolism, and renal disease. Finally, various forms of soft tissue calcification not covered by the preceding are considered.

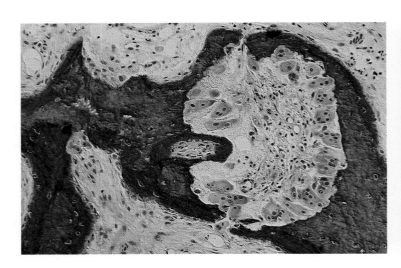

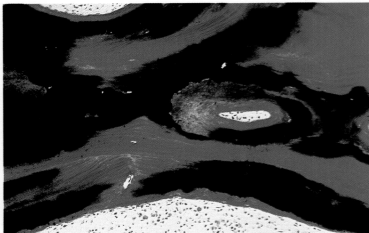

FIGURE 7.1 Photomicrograph of a bone biopsy from a patient with hyperparathyroidism secondary to renal failure. The most characteristic histologic feature is the osteoclastic cancellous bone tunneling, known as tunneling resorption. Note also the increased osteoblastic activity and marrow fibrosis (Goldner, x 10 obj.).

FIGURE 7.2 Photomicrograph of bone to demonstrate the lack of mineralization that occurs in vitamin D deficiency. A thick band of unmineralized bone, in this preparation stained red, covers all of the bony surfaces. The mineralized bone, stained black, has an irregular border with the unmineralized osteoid which is characteristic of osteomalacia (von Kossa stain, x 4 obj.).

CALCIUM AND PHOSPHORUS HOMEOSTASIS

Optimal functioning of the organism requires maintenance of the extracellular calcium ion concentration within normal limits, even under conditions of dehydration, starvation, or disease. Most laboratory determinations of blood calcium levels measure total calcium, which includes ionized calcium, protein-bound calcium, and calcium complexed to other organic ions. However, only the ionized fraction of calcium is physiologically important. Changes in serum calcium that are associated with, for example, hypo- or hyper-proteinemia, usually have no pathophysiologic significance.

Figure 7.3 illustrates the mechanism of calcium and phosphorus homeostasis in a healthy adult male with an adequate calcium and phosphorus intake. As this diagram shows, calcium and phosphorus are present in three principal pools: the bone tissue, the intracellular fluid, and the extracellular fluid. New calcium and phosphorus are added to the system from the gut, and both are lost through the gut, the kidneys, and by sweating. It should be noted that most of the blood calcium and phosphorus lost by glomerular filtration are

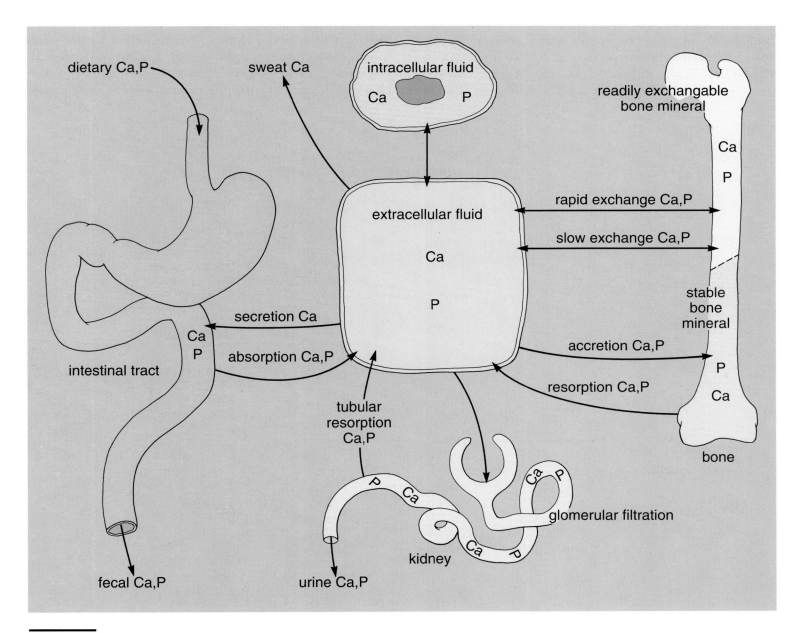

FIGURE 7.3 A schematic model of calcium and phosphorus metabolism.

reabsorbed through the renal tubule epithelium. Also noteworthy is that most of the bone mineral is not available for rapid exchange with the extracellular fluid.

Figure 7.4 illustrates the interactive and interdependent endocrine control of calcium and phosphorus homeostasis. Parathyroid gland activity is largely regulated by the level of Ca^{++} in the extracellular fluid; an increase in serum Ca^{++} suppresses PTH release, and vice versa. Once in the circulation, biologically active PTH has a short half-life, probably on the order of less than 5 minutes. It is degraded by enzymatic cleavage, mainly in the liver but also in the kidney and within the parathyroid gland itself. Conventional laboratory assays for measurement of PTH are focused primarily on biologically inactive fragments. The level of PTH in the blood regulates the conversion of 25-hydroxyvitamin D (25-OH-D) in the kidney to its active form, 1,25 dihydroxyvitamin D ($1,25(OH)_2D$). PTH acts on the renal tubules to increase the reabsorption of calcium while decreasing the reabsorption of phosphorus. It also directly stimulates the osteoblasts to synthesize new bone and, through activation of a second messenger, stimulates osteoclastic resorption of bone, and hence the release of Ca^{++} into the extracellular fluid.

Figure 7.5 shows the vitamin D hormone pathway. The principal natural source of vitamin D is the conversion of 7-dehydrocholesterol in the skin, through the action of ultraviolet irradiation, to vitamin D_3, which can then be stored in fat and muscle cells. Another form of vitamin D is vitamin D_2. This form, commercially produced by ultraviolet irradiation of plant sterols, is biologically equipotent to D_3; in the United States it is added extensively to milk, certain other foods, and vitamin supplements. Vitamins D_2 and D_3 circulate together in the body, are biologically interchangeable, and are usually referred to in the aggregate

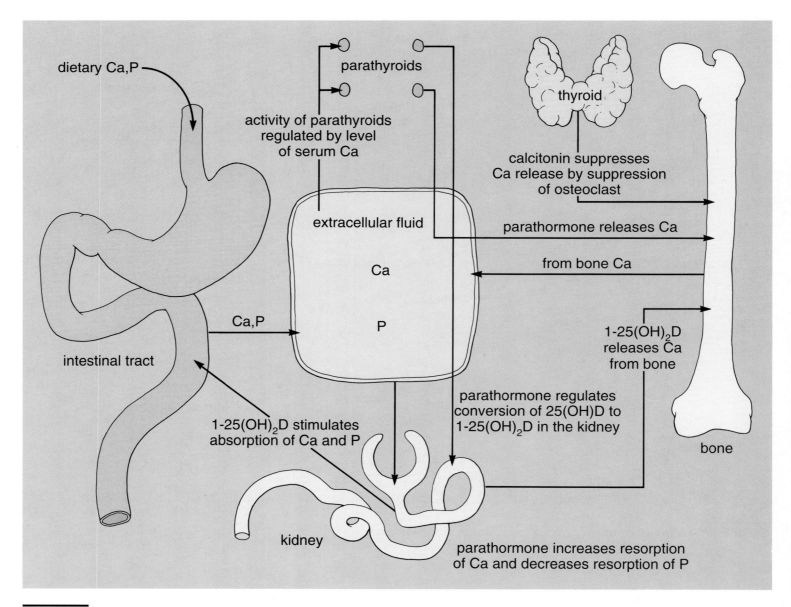

FIGURE 7.4 Endocrine regulation of calcium and phosphorus homeostasis.

as vitamin D. Exposure to sunlight of no more than 10 to 15 minutes can provide the body with the amount of vitamin D required for the next 3 days. Only a small part of the skin needs to be exposed for adequate production of vitamin D. Therefore, dietary vitamin D supplements are probably unnecessary except in children, pregnant women, old people with poor nutrition who are confined indoors, and a few other exceptional instances. However, there is evidence that the chronic use of sunscreens, especially by the elderly, can decrease circulating concentrations of 25-OH-D and cause frank vitamin D deficiency.

The further conversion of vitamin D to 25-OH-D takes place in the liver. Although 25-OH-D has only minimal physiologic activity, in pharmacologic dosage it can promote both gut absorption of calcium and bone mineralization. The hepatic conversion of vitamin D to 25-OH-D can be disturbed by liver disease or by administration of anticonvulsant drugs, such as phenytoin. Among other deleterious actions, phenytoin may accelerate the hepatic oxidation of 25-OH-D into more polar, inactive metabolites.

There is also a pathway for enterohepatic recirculation of 25-OH-D and its metabolites excreted in the bile. Therefore, intestinal malabsorption or anatomic loss of intestinal absorptive area can interfere with the reabsorption of these substances and inexorably deplete the systemic pool of vitamin D. In this way, severe vitamin D deficiency can develop even though exposure to sun and to dietary sources of vitamin D is adequate.

The adequacy of vitamin D status is determined by measuring the serum level of 25-OH-D. In the kidney,

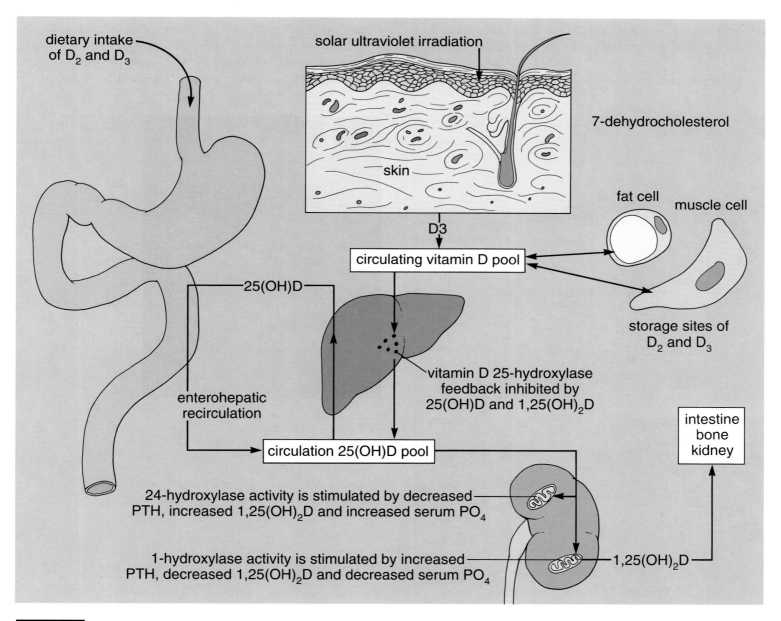

dietary intake of D_2 and D_3

solar ultraviolet irradiation

7-dehydrocholesterol

skin

fat cell   muscle cell

D3

circulating vitamin D pool

25(OH)D

storage sites of D_2 and D_3

vitamin D 25-hydroxylase feedback inhibited by 25(OH)D and 1,25(OH)$_2$D

enterohepatic recirculation

intestine bone kidney

circulation 25(OH)D pool

24-hydroxylase activity is stimulated by decreased PTH, increased 1,25(OH)$_2$D and increased serum PO$_4$

1-hydroxylase activity is stimulated by increased PTH, decreased 1,25(OH)$_2$D and decreased serum PO$_4$

1,25(OH)$_2$D

FIGURE 7.5 Regulation of vitamin D metabolism is shown from points of entry into the body pool: via solar irradiation of cutaneous 7-dehydrocholesterol, which produces vitamin D_3, and via ingestion of vitamins D_2 and D_3. The major part of the vitamin D pool is stored in fat and muscle. A portion is continually converted in the liver to 25-hydroxyvitamin D, the predominant circulating form; 25(OH)D is then converted in the kidney to the major active metabolite, 1,25(OH)$_2$D.

under the control of specific 1-alpha hydroxylases, 25-OH-D is converted to either $24,25(OH)_2D$ or $1,25(OH)_2D$. Therefore, patients with advanced renal disease become deficient in both of these vitamin forms, which is probably the primary reason for the frequency and severity of bone disease in this population.

The actions of $24,25(OH)_2D$ on bone metabolism are largely unknown. Although it only weakly accelerates the absorption of calcium by the gut, some important role in bone cell differentiation is suspected. By contrast, $1,25(OH)_2D$ is the most biologically potent form of vitamin D known and has multiple and profound actions on osseous metabolism. It accelerates the gut absorption of calcium and phosphorus, promotes bone cell differentiation and mineralization of osteoid, and enhances the sensitivity of bone to PTH-induced resorption to maintain serum calcium. Perhaps most important for patients on maintenance renal dialysis, it directly suppresses overactive parathyroid cells and enhances parathyroid suppression by ambient calcium levels.

In addition to its effects on bone metabolism,

$1,25(OH)_2D$ also has other biologic actions, including inhibition of the production of PTH, interleukin 2, and immunoglobulins, and stimulation of insulin and TSH secretion. With respect to its effect on cell proliferation and differentiation, it is of great interest that $1,25(OH)_2D$ induces monocytes to become multinucleated giant cells which act in vitro as osteoclast-like cells.

The physiologic importance of human calcitonin (CT) is unknown, but current theories are focused on the possibility that it is a regulator of skeletal homeostasis. In pharmacologic doses, CT inhibits osteoclastic resorption of bone, suggesting that it might act in vivo to conserve skeletal mass. It has been reported that women have lower whole plasma immunoreactive CT (iCT) concentrations than men, and that peak calcium-stimulated iCT concentrations decline with age. Although the data are controversial, some investigators have suggested that CT secretion decreases at the time of menopause and can be stimulated by estrogen replacement therapy. It is possible, therefore, that a relative, progressive deficiency of CT in postmenopausal women is a cause of age- and sex-related bone loss.

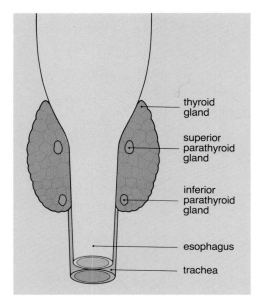

FIGURE 7.6
Posterior aspect of laryngeal junction with pharynx, and commencement of the esophagus and trachea. Note the position of the parathyroid glands, normally measuring no more than 4 to 5 mm.

thyroid gland

superior parathyroid gland

inferior parathyroid gland

esophagus

trachea

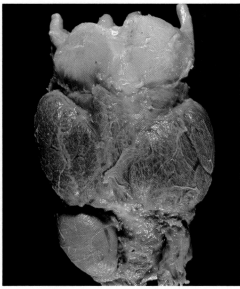

FIGURE 7.7
Parathyroid adenoma: large tan nodule measuring approximately 2 cm on the left side of the lower pole of the thyroid.

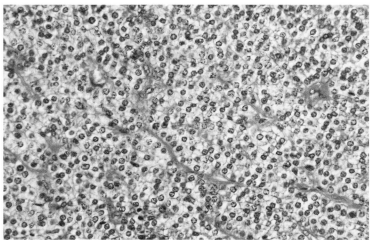

FIGURE 7.8 Photomicrograph of parathyroid adenoma shown in Figure 7.7. The cells are of one type, chief cells, partially arranged in small acini and cords. Characteristically no fat is visible in the adenomatous tissue (H & E, x 10 obj.).

HYPERCALCEMIC STATES

HYPERPARATHYROIDISM
(OSTEITIS FIBROSA CYSTICA;
VON RECKLINGHAUSEN'S DISEASE OF BONE)

Overproduction of parathyroid hormone may occur as either a primary or a secondary condition. In primary hyperparathyroidism, an adenoma, hyperplasia (of unknown etiology) or, rarely, carcinoma may lead to marked hypercalcemia, and usually to hypophosphatemia (Figs. 7.6 to 7.9). Patients are usually between the third and fifth decades of life. Although many are asymptomatic, others may present with a history of recurrent kidney stones despite minimal hypercalciuria. When hypercalcemia becomes more pronounced, nausea, vomiting, weakness, and headaches may appear. On rare occasions a patient presents with a hypercalcemic crisis. Nephrolithiasis is the most common clinical presentation of primary hyperparathyroidism; however, bone pain is present in a small percentage of patients. Surgical removal of the neoplastic gland is the treatment of choice.

When hyperparathyroidism is associated with chronic renal failure, the inevitable consequence is deranged mineral and bone metabolism. Such derangements can be identified even in patients with mild reductions of glomerular filtration rate (GFR). They become progressively more severe, with greater likelihood of significant clinical manifestations, as renal function declines further.

Secondary hyperparathyroidism dominates the pathophysiology of metabolic bone disease in chronic renal failure. It results from a fall in ionized calcium concentration as a consequence of phosphate retention, resistance of bone to the actions of PTH, and malabsorption of calcium through the gut. It is now understood that in addition to the loss of 1-alpha hydroxylat-

ing capacity as renal cell mass declines, there is also inhibition by phosphate of the renal production of $1,25(OH)_2D$ as an additional stimulus to hyperparathyroidism. Because $1,25(OH)_2D$ directly suppresses the parathyroid cells, loss of renal production of $1,25(OH)_2D$ encourages secondary hyperparathyroidism to develop more rapidly and severely.

The rise in plasma phosphate concentration as the GFR declines causes a reciprocal fall in ionized calcium and hence stimulates PTH secretion. PTH promotes phosphaturia and thus tends to normalize plasma inorganic phosphate. In addition, by its direct effect on bone and kidney and its indirect effect on the intestine through $1,25(OH)_2D$, PTH opposes the tendency of the serum calcium to fall. A new steady-state condition therefore develops, but only at the expense of the undesirable effects of secondary hyperparathyroidism. When PTH levels rise sufficiently, advanced bone resorption gives rise to hypercalcemia, bone pain, and fractures. The combined effects of hypercalcemia and hyperphosphatemia lead to severe metastatic calcification in blood vessels and at other sites. At this stage, subtotal parathyroidectomy is necessary.

In clinical renal disease, phosphate restriction can reverse the above sequence of events to a certain extent. In children with stable chronic renal failure, phosphate-restricted diets have been shown to increase $1,25(OH)_2D$ concentrations and to decrease PTH levels, thereby partially reversing the hormone imbalance. Conversely, phosphate supplementation exacerbates the abnormalities and leads to a reduction in $1,25(OH)_2D$ and an increase in PTH.

Medical treatment of secondary HPT in dialysis patients consists of phosphate restriction, administration of phosphate binders, the use of a high-calcium dialysate, and of oral or intravenous supplementation with $1,25(OH)_2D$. When adequate, such therapy usually obviates the necessity for subtotal parathyroidec-

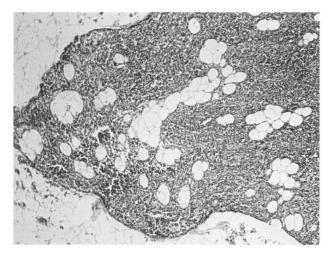

FIGURE 7.9 Photomicrograph of normal parathyroid gland shows glandular tissue admixed with fat (H & E, x 2.5 obj.).

tomy, which may be followed by significant postoperative hypoparathyroidism.

In a minority of patients with chronic renal failure, skeletal function is further disturbed by the accumulation of aluminum (derived from aluminum-contaminated dialysate and/or aluminium-containing phosphate binders) at the mineralization front, with resulting osteomalacia (Fig. 7.10).

Biochemically, hyperparathyroidism at a level advanced enough to cause bone disease is characterized by huge elevations in PTH and rises in serum alkaline phosphatase, the latter reflecting osteoblast stimulation.

The radiologic and pathologic features are similar in both primary and secondary hyperparathyroidism. Radiologic examination may reveal diffuse osteopenia and/or circumscribed lucent areas. However, the most characteristic changes include erosion of the tufts of the phalanges and subperiosteal cortical resorption, especially on the radial side of the middle phalanges (Fig. 7.11). Other sites at which erosive resorption may be seen are the symphysis pubis (Fig. 7.12), the distal clavicles (Fig. 7.13), and the end plates of the vertebral bodies (Fig. 7.14), as well as the lamina dura (ie, the layer of the dense bone at the roots of the teeth) (Fig. 7.15). The skull may show a granular demineralization,

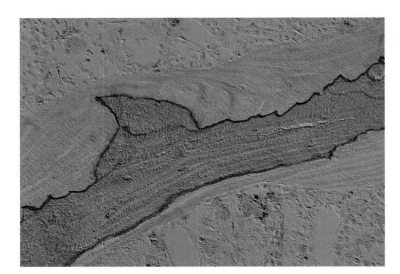

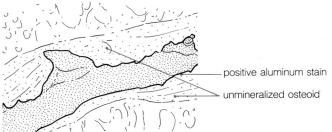

FIGURE 7.10 Photomicrograph of a section of bone with increased osteoid, stained with aurine tricarboxylic acid stain, which stains aluminum bright red. The red stain is seen to be concentrated at the mineralization front; it has been proposed that the presence of aluminum at this site blocks further mineralization of the bone (Nomarski optics, x 10 obj.).

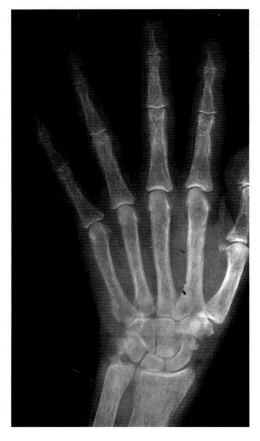

FIGURE 7.11 Clinical radiograph of the hand shows resorption of the tufts of the terminal phalanges and characteristic subperiosteal resorption of the middle and proximal phalanges. This resorption is more marked on the radial side of the phalanges.

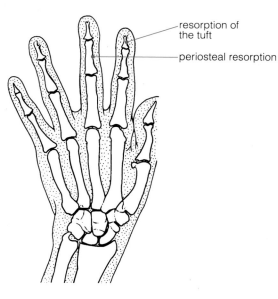

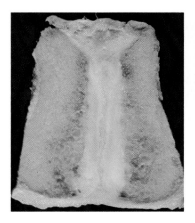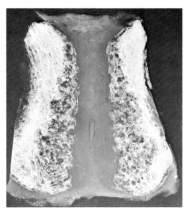

FIGURE 7.12 *(left)* Gross appearance of the symphysis pubis shows hyperemia and resorption of the bone on each side of the symphysis. Radiograph of the specimen *(right)*.

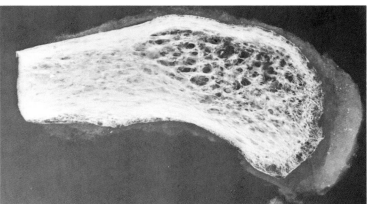

FIGURE 7.13 A characteristic anatomic site in which to note erosion in hyperparathyroidism is the distal clavicle. In this specimen radiograph resorption is clearly seen, with loss of the smooth cortex and replacement by a lacy irregular outline.

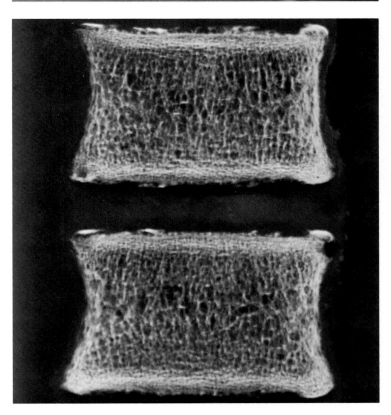

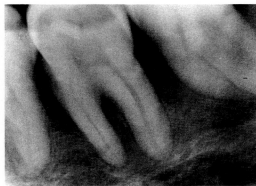

FIGURE 7.15 Radiograph of the lower second molar tooth in a patient with primary hyperparathyroidism shows loss of the lamina dura around the tooth socket.

FIGURE 7.14 Specimen radiograph of a slice taken through the vertebral bodies in a young person with hyperparathyroidism shows the irregularity and resorption of the cortical bone, particularly in the end plates of the vertebral bodies.

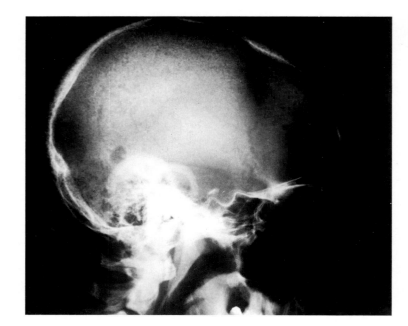

FIGURE 7.16 Hyperparathyroidism: clinical radiograph of a skull showing salt and pepper appearance.

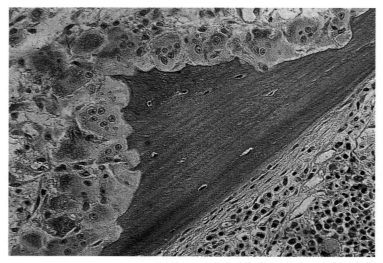

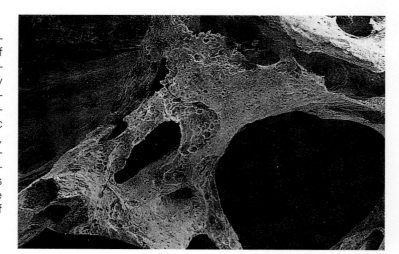

osteoclasts

peritrabecular fibrosis

FIGURE 7.17 Photomicrograph to show severe osteoclastic bone resorption in a patient with primary hyperparathyroidism. Note the mild peritrabecular fibrosis on the inferior bone surface (H & E, x 25 obj.).

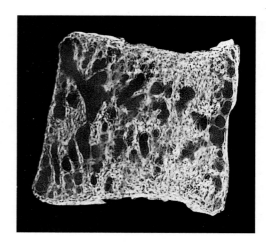

FIGURE 7.18
In a specimen radio-graph of a slice of vertebral body af-fected with primary hyperparathy-roidism, the trabec-ulae contain lytic lines within them, due to the dissect-ing resorption char-acteristic of this condition. Note the partial resorption of the end plates.

FIGURE 7.19 A scanning electron micrograph of the cancellous bone demonstrates numerous irregular erosions on the bone sur-face, due to osteoclastic resorption (x750 magnifications).

the so-called "salt and pepper" appearance (Fig. 7.16).

Microscopic examination demonstrates an increased number of osteoclasts on the bone surfaces (and even on periosteal surfaces), and a characteristic "tunneling" or "dissecting" resorption of trabeculae (Figs. 7.17 to 7.19). Other findings include resorption of pericellular bone by osteocytes (osteocytic osteolysis), increased amounts of woven bone, and marrow fibrosis, especially abutting trabecular surfaces (Fig. 7.20). (The latter finding should be distinguished mi-

croscopically from the more generalized fibrosis seen in association with myelofibrosis.)

Occasionally, patients with hyperparathyroidism present on radiologic examination with a lytic lesion which suggests a tumor (Fig. 7.21). Such lesions are particularly evident in the diaphysis of long bones, the jaw, or the skull. This entity is the so-called "brown tumor" (brown because of old and recent hemorrhage), and on microscopic examination it is composed of many clustered giant cells in a fibrous cellular stroma (Fig. 7.22).

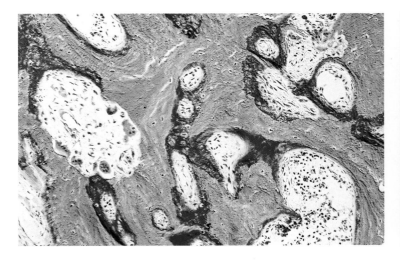
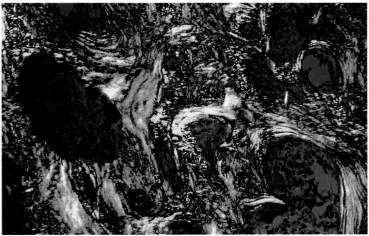

FIGURE 7.20 Photomicrograph of a biopsy from a patient with hyperparathyroidism *(left)* shows the overall pattern of marrow fibrosis, dissecting resorption and increased amounts of unmineralized bone, seen here in the Goldner stain as red seams on the bone surface. The increased amounts of osteoid are secondary to increased bone formation. The polarized light picture, *(right)*, shows extensive woven bone present in this section (Goldner, x 5 obj.).

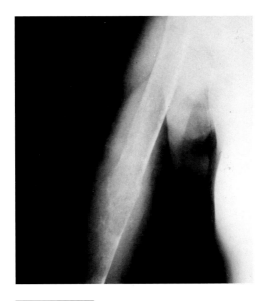

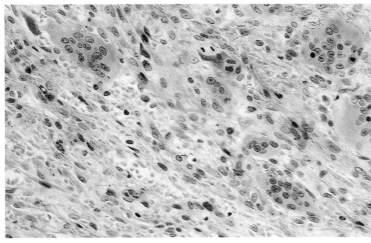

FIGURE 7.22 Photomicrograph of biopsy obtained from a lytic lesion in a single bone of a patient with hyperparathyroidism shows numerous giant cells in a fibrous stroma. Scattered hemosiderin-laden histiocytes and focal interstitial hemorrhage and clustering of giant cells are characteristic of a brown tumor (H & E, x 10 obj.).

FIGURE 7.21 Clinical radiograph shows large destructive lesion in lower end of the humerus. The patient presented initially with pain in the arm, and the radiologic examination suggested the presence of primary of secondary neoplasm. Further investigation revealed hypercalcemia and other radiologic changes consistent with hyperparathyroidism.

The "brown tumor" of hyperparathyroidism must be differentiated from giant cell reparative granuloma (see Chapter 15).

In many patients with chronic renal failure, increased density of the skeleton can be seen on radiographic examination. Histologically, this increased density appears as increased woven or immature bone superimposed on the usual characteristics of hyperparathyroidism (Figs. 7.23 to 7.25). Both the radiologic and histologic changes may be confused with those of Paget's disease.

Control of the hyperparathyroidism, whether surgical or medical, is followed by a dramatic regression of the histologic changes, and subsequent improvement of the radiologic abnormalities can be considerable. The serum alkaline phosphatase normalizes, and PTH falls to levels seen in dialysis patients who do not have HPT.

HYPERCALCEMIA NOT ASSOCIATED WITH HYPERPARATHYROIDISM (PSEUDOHYPERPARATHYROIDISM)

Hypercalcemia is common in patients with bone metastases and in multiple myeloma. On occasion, it is seen in cases of sarcoidosis or vitamin D intoxication. Yet another type of hypercalcemia is associated with certain rare tumors that secrete hormone-like substances which are presently referred to as parathyroid hormone-related protein (PTHrP) and "osteoclast activating factor" (OAF). The tumors most commonly associated with this type of humoral hypercalcemia are

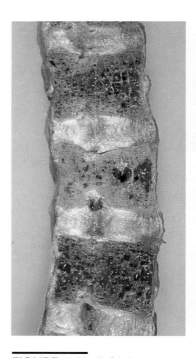 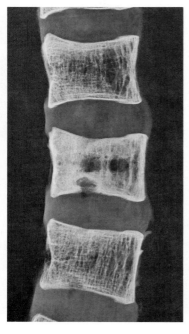

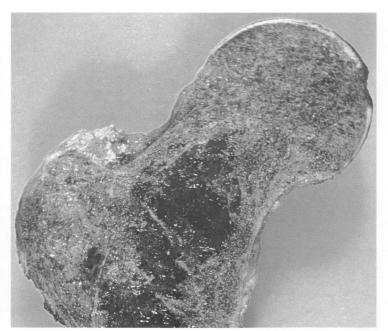

FIGURE 7.23 *(left)* A segment of the lower thoracic and upper lumbar spine from a patient with renal osteodystrophy shows loss of the normal trabecular appearance of the bone with increased sclerosis and some collapse. Radiograph of the specimen *(right)*.

FIGURE 7.24 Upper end of the femur from the patient shown in Figure 7.23. Again the disorganization of the bony architecture is apparent, and the cortex is seen to be hyperemic and irregular. These gross changes, both those seen in the vertebral bodies and in the femur, may suggest Paget's disease.

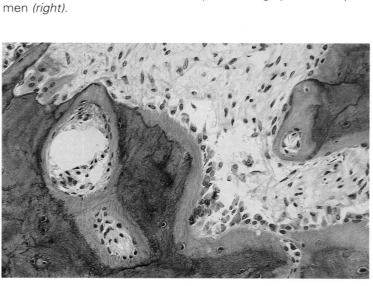

FIGURE 7.25 Photomicrograph of a bone biopsy from a patient with renal failure shows the stigmata of hyperparathyroidism. Note the markedly increased osteoblastic activity and widened osteoid seams (H & E, x 10 obj.).

squamous cell lung cancer, renal cell carcinoma, uro-genital tract carcinoma, and other squamous cell tumors. When a small occult tumor is at fault, localization of the malignancy may be delayed for some time. In cases of "humoral hypercalcemia of malignancy", the radiologic and microscopic appearance of skeletal tissue cannot be distinguished from that associated with primary hyperparathyroidism. Because PTHrP and OAF are usually not detected by conventional assays for PTH, PTH levels are profoundly depressed in most patients with this rare condition. This is the most important biochemical clue that the hypercalcemia is arising from a malignancy.

HYPEROSTEOIDOSIS

Hyperosteoidosis is a histologic term that describes an increase in the relative proportion of unmineralized to mineralized bone tissue. There are three basic causes of hyperosteoidosis. The first is an increase in the rate of bone formation, such that the osteoblasts form new bone matrix so quickly that a prominent band of

osteoid is present on the bone surface. In this case, labeling with tetracycline reveals a rather thick, granular, and dense mineralization front. A second cause is interference with calcium apposition at the unmineralized front as happens with aluminum toxicity and, to a lesser extent, with iron overload. In this case, a wide osteoid seam is observed, usually with flat, inactive osteoblasts (Fig. 7.26). The mineralization front is sharply demarcated and often at a reversal time (Fig. 7.27). Tetracycline labeling fails to show any uptake at the mineralization front. A third type of hyperosteoidosis is due to a lack of available calcium for mineralization of the bone, which is the principal subject of the following discussion.

As the industrial revolution swept across northern Europe, the cities became crowded and polluted. Because of poor dietary intake of vitamin D and little exposure to sun, the children in these cities commonly developed severe and debilitating rickets, which among the poor was almost universal. (Rickets and osteomalacia are clinical terms used to describe the disease that results from failure in the proper mineralization of the bone matrix.)

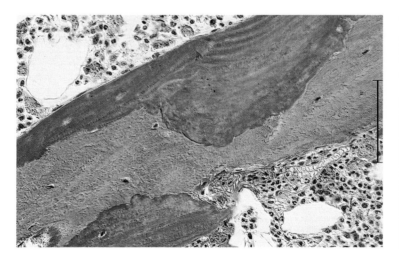

FIGURE 7.26 Photomicrograph of a bone biopsy from a patient with aluminum toxicity. The red staining is present where the bone is unmineralized. Note the sharp demarcation between the unmineralized (red) and the underlying mineralized bone (green). In contrast to other conditions where hyperosteoidosis is seen, here the overlying osteoblasts are flat and inconspicuous (undecalcified tissue, Goldner stain, x 10 obj.).

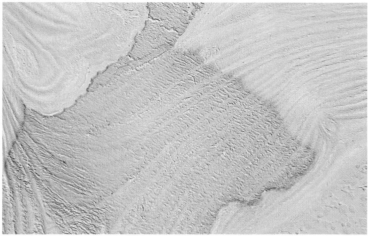

FIGURE 7.27 Photomicrograph of a section of a biopsy obtained from a patient with aluminum toxicity which has been stained to show the localization of the aluminum. In this section the aluminum is present at a reversal line, crossing the lamellar structure, and also at a mineralization front (aurine tricarboxylic acid, x 10 obj.).

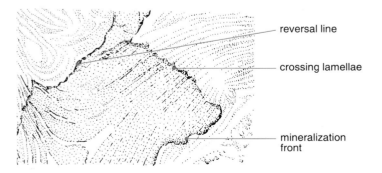

reversal line

crossing lamellae

mineralization front

OSTEOMALACIA

Osteomalacia may have a number of etiologies (Fig. 7.28). The availability of vitamin D may be decreased by poor nutritional intake, lack of sunlight, and by renal or hepatic disease. Calcium availability may also be disturbed by lack of calcium in the diet or by a malabsorption syndrome. In addition, congenital biochemical defects in the renal tubules, leading to deficient reabsorption of phosphate and calcium into the blood, may cause osteomalacia (hypophosphatemic rickets; see below).

The most common symptom of osteomalacia in adults is bone pain, often initially vague but gradually becoming severe, and sometimes localized. There may also be proximal muscle weakness, often profound. On biochemical assay, the serum calcium tends to be moderately low, the phosphate very low, and the alkaline phosphatase very high (released from stimulated osteoblasts). Serum 25-OH-D levels are extremely depressed, whereas $1,25(OH)_2D$ levels may be surprisingly maintained, although they too eventually fall. PTH levels tend to rise considerably, and in many instances are responsible for relative preservation of the serum calcium (although sometimes marked hypocalcemia may be noted).

Radiologic examination usually reveals generalized osteopenia; classically, multiple bilateral and symmetrical cortical lucent areas are present (Fig. 7.29). These lucent areas, which typically lie perpendicular to the long axis of the bone, are often referred to as Looser's zones. Microscopic examination shows them to be cortical fractures filled in with poorly mineralized callus and fibrous tissue. In general, the axial skeleton, with its higher rate of turnover (eg, the vertebrae, pelvis, ribs, and sternum), is more often affected clinically than the peripheral skeleton. Isotope uptake studies are useful to demonstrate the severity of the problem (Fig. 7.30).

FIGURE 7.28

CAUSES OF OSTEOMALACIA

Vitamin D Disturbances
  Inadequate endogenous production
    Deficient exposure to sunlight
  Dietary deficiency of vitamin D
  Inadequate intestinal absorption of vitamin D
    Malabsorption syndrome
    Postgastrectomy
    Celiac disease
    Inflammatory bowel disease
  Aberrant metabolism of vitamin D
    Liver
      Cirrhosis
      Dilantin therapy
    Renal disease

Kidney Disease
  Chronic renal failure
  Renal tubular disorders
    Acidosis
    Hypophosphatemia

Familial Errors in Metabolism
  Familial hypophosphatemia
  Hypophosphatasia

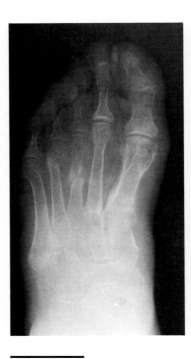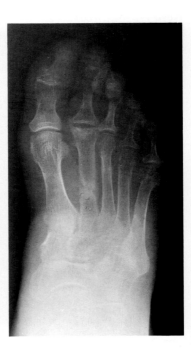

FIGURE 7.29 Radiograph of the feet of patient with osteomalacia shows bilateral fractures of the metatarsals.

Microscopic examination of diseased bone reveals a marked increase in the amount of nonmineralized matrix (osteoid) on the surfaces of the bone trabeculae and lining the haversian canals of the cortical bone (Fig. 7.31). Determination of the extent of osteomalacia requires quantitative histomorphometry (see Chapter 2). In patients with osteomalacia, most, if not all, of the trabecular and cortical bone surfaces are typically covered by osteoid, and on quantification reveals that at least 10 percent of the bone mass consists of nonmineralized bone matrix. Tetracycline uptake studies show patchy, blurred uptake (Fig. 7.32). Specific therapy depends on the etiology of the condition.

RICKETS

Rickets is the childhood manifestation of a defect in mineralization. (Classical rickets, resulting from a deficiency of vitamin D, is only rarely seen in Western societies. The most common cause of rickets in the United States is renal tubule dysfunction.) The disease is characterized by widespread skeletal deformities principally affecting the foci of most rapid growth, hence the typical epiphyseal changes.

Rickets may be observed in patients as young as 6 months of age, at which time thinning and softening of the calvaria and bulging fontanelles may be evident.

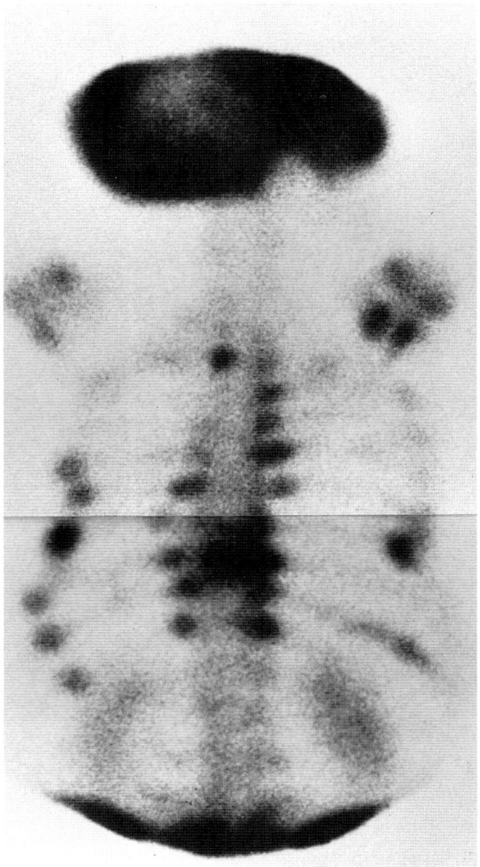

FIGURE 7.30 A gamma-camera image that shows the pattern of uptake of T^{99} diphosphonate in a patient with osteomalacia. There are multiple rib fractures as well as fractures at the neck of the scapula.

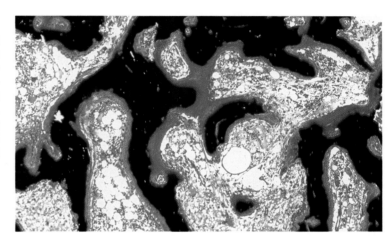

FIGURE 7.31 Low power photomicrograph of a specimen from a patient with osteomalacia demonstates that all the bone surfaces are covered by a thick layer of osteoid, which constitutes more than 10% of the total bone volume (von Kossa, x 4 obj.).

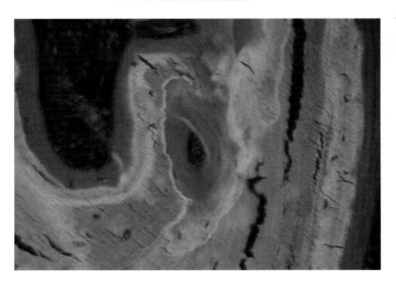

FIGURE 7.32 Photomicrograph taken using ultra-violet light shows fluorescence of a broad smudged band of tetracycline which marks the irregular calcification front in a section of bone obtained from a patient with osteomalacia (tetracycline labelled, U.V. incident light, x 10 obj.).

These cranial changes usually diminish by 2 years of age but are followed by other dramatic skeletal changes, including beading of the costochondral junctions of the ribs (the so-called rachitic rosary) (Fig. 7.33 and 7.34), a depression along the line of the rib–diaphragm attachment (Harrison's groove), and a chicken breasted appearance. In particular, the wrists, knees, and ankles may be enlarged owing to widening of the epiphysis consequent to failure of primary spongiosa to mineralize (Fig. 7.35). Eventually curvature of the long bones, especially anterior curvature, develops. Spinal abnormalities, including dorsal kyphosis, scoliosis, and lumbar lordosis, may diminish height.

Radiologic examination reveals a markedly widened and irregular growth plate zone, often with a cup-shaped concavity and flaring of the metaphyseal end of the bone (Fig. 7.36). These changes correlate microscopically with the presence of irregular, disorderly columns of proliferating cartilage in the growth plate and tongues of proliferating irregular cartilage extending into the adjacent bone (Figs. 7.37 and 7.38). These findings are associated with absence of the calcified zone of the cartilage and a poorly formed primary spongiosa.

The most striking histologic change is the presence of large amounts of nonmineralized bone throughout the skeleton. Pseudofractures, similar to those seen in osteomalacia, may also be noted.

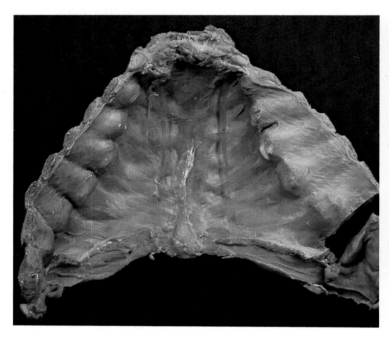

FIGURE 7.33 Rickets dissected specimen of the rib cage shows marked prominence of the costochondral junctions which gives rise to the so-called rachitic rosary.

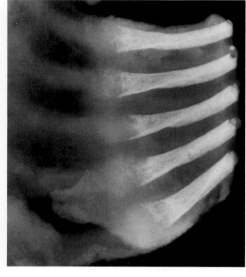

FIGURE 7.34 Radiograph of a portion of this specimen demonstrates the irregularity and poor mineralization of the metaphysis of the rib.

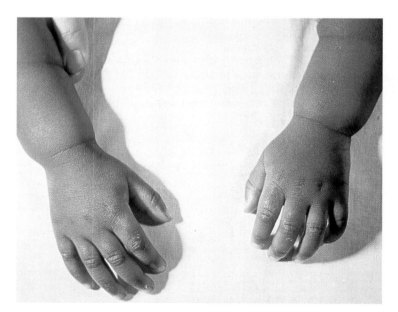

FIGURE 7.35 Rickets. Hand and forearm of a young child show prominence above the wrist, consequent upon the flaring and poor mineralization of the lower end of the radius and ulna.

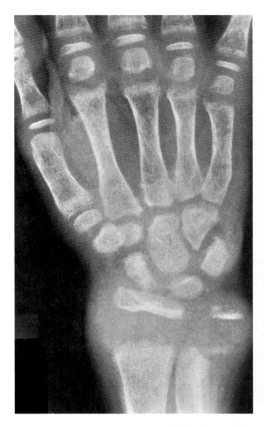

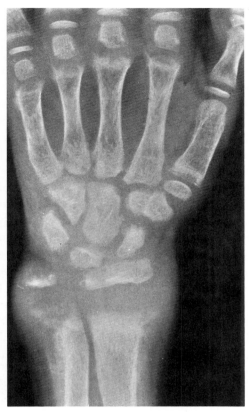

FIGURE 7.36 Dorsovolar view of both hands of an 8-year-old boy from India with untreated dietary rickets shows osteopenia of the bones and widening of the growth plates of the distal radius and ulna, with flaring of the metaphyses—typical features of this condition.

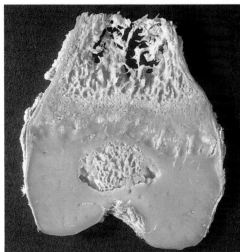

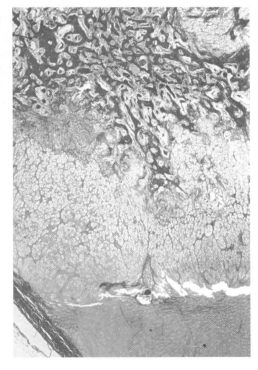

FIGURE 7.38 Photomicrograph of the costochondral junction in a patient with rickets shows widening of the growth cartilage region with irregularity at the cartilage-bone interface and poorly mineralized, disorganized primary spongiosa.

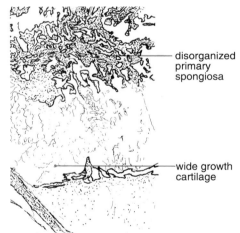

disorganized primary spongiosa

wide growth cartilage

FIGURE 7.37 Rickets. Section through the lower end of the femur in a young child shows widening of the epiphyseal growth plate region, together with irregularity of the metaphysis tongues of cartilage, which are seen penetrating into the metaphyseal bone.

HYPOPHOSPHATEMIA

Phosphate is a significant physiologic buffer and also plays a major role in calcium homeostasis. We have already discussed the process by which phosphate retention leads to hyperphosphatemia and secondary hyperparathyroidism. Because 85 percent of total body phosphorus is located in the skeleton, a decrease in the number of phosphate ions in the serum (hypophosphatemia) can also be expected to affect the skeleton.

It is now accepted that disorders of phosphate metabolism, particularly those associated with severe hypophosphatemia, can cause cell damage with potentially serious clinical consequences; examples, include erythrocyte hemolysis, leukocyte and platelet disorders, defects of the peripheral and central nervous system, myopathy, and rhabdomyolysis. In bone, however, the main consequence of hypophosphatemia is osteomalacia. Superficially, this impaired mineralization appears to be a purely extracellular problem arising from changes in the calcium and phosphate concentration product (Ca x Pi), which reflects the extent of saturation of extracellular fluid with respect to these ions.

Hypophosphatemia may result from any number of causes, either congenital or acquired. Among the latter are increased urinary phosphate loss caused by lowering of the renal tubule threshold for phosphate reabsorption (as seen in primary hyperparathyroidism) and therapeutic administration of diuretic agents. The condition may also be traced to decreased intestinal absorption, as seen in vitamin D deficiency, malabsorption syndromes, or starvation, or it may be induced by the excessive use of phosphate-binding antacids. The disorder also occurs after uptake of phosphorus from the serum into the cells, as seen after insulin administration, and in states of respiratory alkalosis, as in salicylate poisoning. Acquired hypophosphatemia is sometimes seen in association with a variety of benign or malignant mesenchymal tumors, fibrous dysplasia, metastatic carcinoma, and vascular tumors. The most outstanding feature of the disease is impaired renal tubule phosphate reabsorption, the mechanism of which is unclear. A marked reduction in serum 1,25(OH)$_2$D is usually observed. Complete excision of the tumor usually leads to resolution of the biochemical abnormalities and the osteomalacia.

Laboratory studies in patients with acquired hypophosphatemia reveal normal glomerular filtration rates, normal to high levels of serum calcium, a markedly lowered level of serum phosphorus, and elevated levels of alkaline phosphatase. PTH levels may be suppressed. 1,25-(OH)$_2$D levels should be elevated but frequently are not, and may even be low.

Familial Hypophosphatemia (Familial X-Linked Hypophosphatemic Rickets; Vitamin D Resistant Rickets; Refractory Rickets)

Familial hypophosphatemic rickets is a genetic disease which is transmitted as an X-linked dominant trait and is usually manifested by the second year of life. Typically, the patient's urinary excretion of phosphorus is increased. The disorder is clinically characterized by childhood rickets which is unre-

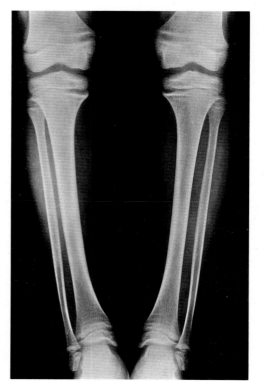

FIGURE 7.39 Radiograph of the legs of a young patient with hypophosphatemic rickets. Note the widening and cupping of the growth plates. Unlike the rickets secondary to vitamin D deficiency wich is illustrated in Figure 7.36, the metaphysis shows the sclerosis associated with dwarfing which occurs in these cases.

sponsive to physiologic doses of vitamin D, with associated growth retardation and poor dental development (Fig. 7.39).

In middle age, other clinical problems begin to appear: mineralization of the spinal ligaments and thickening of the neural arches. There is loss of mobility of the spine, shoulders, elbows, and hips. The lumbar spine remains flat and rigid so that flexion takes place entirely at the hip joints, and there is little rotation in the cervical region. Furthermore, reduction in the diameter of the spinal canal can lead to cord compression at more than one level.

The primary biochemical defect for this disorder of mineral metabolism remains unknown, although the site of the renal phosphate transport defect has been localized to the brush border membrane of the proximal-convoluted tubule.

X-linked hypophosphatemic rickets has long been recognized as different from any other form of rickets and osteomalacia in its clinical manifestations, pathogenesis, and difficulty of treatment. The disease is regarded primarily as a genetic defect of renal tubule phosphate transport, and this concept has led to treatment with phosphate supplements and large doses of vitamin D. However, successful therapy, particularly full

healing of the mineralization defects, usually requires that the phosphate therapy be combined with supraphysiologic dosages of $1,25(OH)_2D$.

Most hypophosphatemic states can be corrected medically and do not progress to development of severe skeletal aberrations. However, uncorrected hypophosphatemia may lead to severe skeletal sequelae, especially in growing children.

Bone biopsy specimens reveal characteristics of osteomalacia indistinguishable from those caused by vitamin D deficiency.

FANCONI'S SYNDROME (RENAL GLYCOSURIC RICKETS)

Fanconi's syndrome is a recessively transmitted genetic disorder characterized by marked aminoaciduria, glycosuria, bicarbonaturia, and phosphaturia. The condition may be accompanied by an associated metabolic defect in cystine metabolism, the so-called Lignac–Fanconi disease. Patients with these disorders exhibit normal glomerular function, a decreased level of serum carbon dioxide, normal to low levels of serum calcium, low levels of serum phosphorus, and elevated levels of alkaline phosphatase.

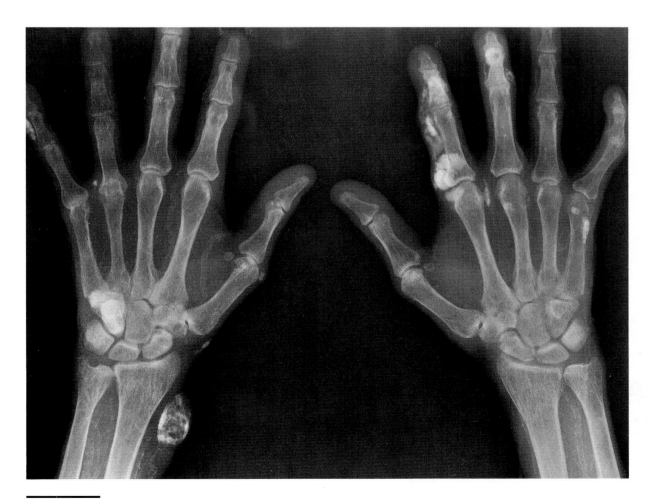

FIGURE 7.40 Posteroanterior view of the distal forearms and hands of a 48-year-old woman with secondary hyperparathyroidism shows evidence of soft tissue and vascular calcifications, characteristic findings in this condition.

Radiographic examination may reveal diffuse osteopenia and stress fractures. Irregular and widened epiphyseal cartilage zones are clearly seen in children, but the dramatic increase in nonmineralized bone observed in patients with rickets is not apparent. In patients with Fanconi's syndrome associated with cystinosis, cystine deposits are present in the bone and in the visceral organs.

The osteomalacia is believed to result principally from the severe hypophosphatemia caused by the renal tubule dysfunction. Amino acid deficiency may contribute to growth retardation.

SOFT TISSUE CALCIFICATION

METASTATIC CALCIFICATION

Metastatic calcification is caused by an increased calcium phosphate product in the blood, and therefore the condition can result from hypercalcemia and/or hyperphosphatemia (Fig. 7.40).

Deposition of calcium hydroxyapatite in soft tissues may occur as a complication of trauma, scleroderma, tumoral calcinosis, renal failure, hyperparathyroidism, sarcoidosis, metastatic disease, myeloma, or hyperme-

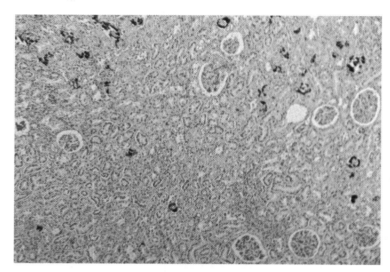

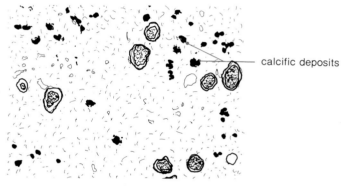

FIGURE 7.41 Photomicrograph of the kidney in a patient with prolonged hypercalcemia resulting from a parathyroid adenoma. Extensive calcium deposits are seen in relation to the glomeruli and the proximal tubules.

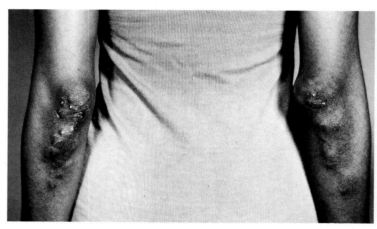

FIGURE 7.42 Photograph of a young black woman with extensive subcutaneous calcium deposits (tumoral calcinosis) around the elbows and along the extensor surfaces of the forearm.

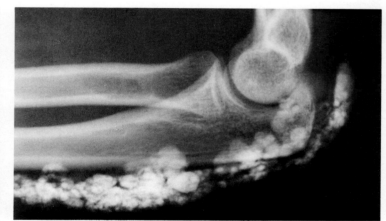

FIGURE 7.43 Radiograph of this patient's arm shows the extent of the calcified masses.

FIGURE 7.44 Cut surfaces of the excised specimen from the patient shown in Figures 7.42 and 7.43.

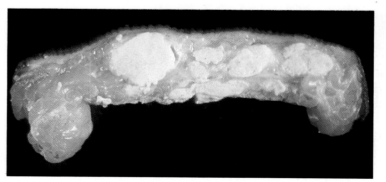

tabolic states. Metastatic calcification is a particular problem in patients with hypermetabolic states who have undergone prolonged periods of bed rest. This condition must be distinguished from gout and calcium pyrophosphate deposition disease, which will be discussed in Chapter 8.

The calcification is both intracellular and extracellular. Mineral deposition is particularly likely to occur in the kidneys (Fig. 7.41), alveolar walls of the lungs, cornea, conjunctiva, and gastric mucosa (ie, those areas subject to large pH changes), as well as in the media and intima of the blood vessels.

TUMORAL CALCINOSIS

Tumoral calcinosis is a rare condition which primarily but not exclusively affects black people in otherwise good health. The disease usually presents in the second decade of life and is characterized by deposition of painless calcific masses around the hips, elbows, shoulders, and gluteal area (ie, areas subject to movement and/or pressure) (Figs. 7.42 to 7.46). A familial incidence has been reported. In rare instances, intraosseous deposits may also occur (Fig. 7.47).

The lesions may be massive, are often bilateral, and

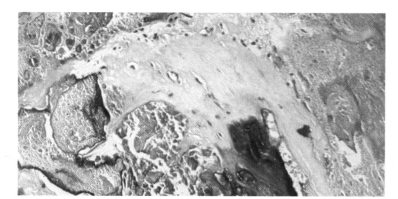

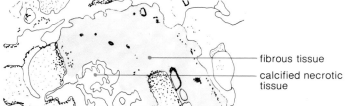

FIGURE 7.45 Microscopic appearance of the calcified tissue shown in Figure 7.44. Note that, although most of the tissue is necrotic and calcified, there is some viable fibrous connective tissue in the center of the field.

fibrous tissue

calcified necrotic tissue

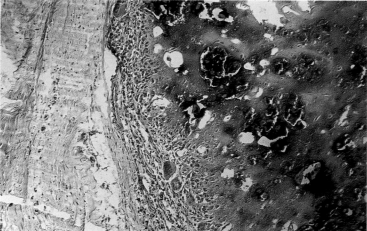

FIGURE 7.46 Photomicrograph of a calcium apatite deposit removed from a patient with tumoral calcinosis. Note the histiocytic and giant cell response at the edge of the calcified deposit (H & E, x 4 obj.).

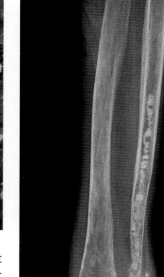

FIGURE 7.47
Radiograph of a 63-year-old woman with rheumatoid arthritis who, although normal with regard to $CaPO_4$-vitamin D chemistry, nevertheless presented with both soft tissue and intraosseous calcification as shown here. She was taking 1200 mg daily of $CaCO_3$ and 400 iu of vitamin D.

they affect multiple sites. The patient's serum phosphate level is usually elevated. Although the hyperphosphatemia should suppress $1,25(OH)_2D$ production, serum $1,25(OH)_2D$ levels tend to stay paradoxically normal. Surgical excision is the most successful form of treatment, although recurrences are common. Medical treatment to control the hyperphosphatemia (eg, a low phosphate diet and administration of oral administration of phosphate binders) is an important adjunct to surgical excision but is extremely difficult to effect in sufficient degree. We have recently seen an instance of correction of hyperphosphatemia and radiologically documented disappearance of a large tumor mass achieved by the combined use of the phosphaturic diuretics hydrochlorothiazide and furosemide.

Microscopic examination of tissues from these patients reveals calcific deposits which are surrounded by a mild infiltration at both histiocytes and chronic inflammatory cells. Some multinucleated giant cells may be present. X-ray diffraction studies have shown that the calcium deposits are mainly formed of hydroxyapatite crystals.

CALCIFICATION IN INJURED TISSUE

Dead tissue that does not undergo rapid absorption frequently becomes calcified. This type of calcification, which is not related to any disturbance in calcium homeostasis, is called dystrophic calcification. Calcification is common in areas of coagulation necrosis (eg, in cases of infarction). It is also common in caseous necrosis, which is seen in patients with tuberculosis, and in areas of fat necrosis (Fig. 7.48). Of particular interest to orthopedic surgeons is the calcification that is common in tendons, ligaments, and bursae (Figs. 7.49 to 7.52).

A common clinical presentation for patients with dystrophic calcification is a painful shoulder that corresponds anatomically to the insertion of the supraspinatus muscle onto the humerus. Gross examination reveals amorphous chalky white deposits or circumscribed gritty calcifications. These crystalline deposits have been shown by x-ray diffraction studies to be hydroxyapatite crystals. Histologic studies reveal that the calcium is isolated in fibrous or fatty tissue or may be present with chronic inflammatory cells including, at times, multinucleated giant cells.

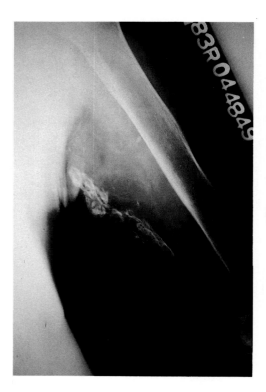

FIGURE 7.48 Radiograph of a middle-aged man who presented with swelling along the inner side of the left arm. The soft tissue calcification seen on x-ray was shown at operation to be both calcification and ossification within a large lobulated lipoma.

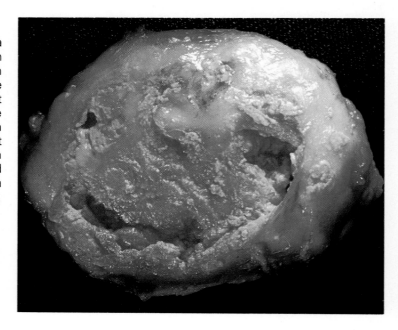

FIGURE 7.49 The cut surface of a grossly thickened achromial bursa with extensive calcium deposits.

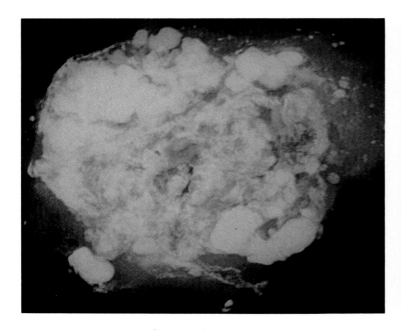

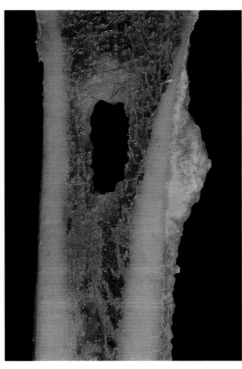

FIGURE 7.51
Photograph showing calcification occurring in the region of the linear aspera. Microscopically, the findings were similar to those found in association with tumoral calcinosis. In this case the lesion was mistaken radiographically for a neoplastic process.

FIGURE 7.50 Radiograph of the specimen shown in Figure 7.49 clearly reveals the extent of calcification.

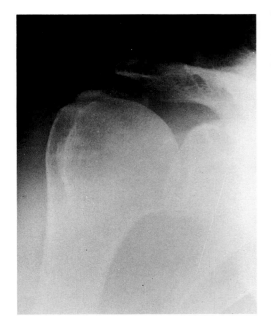

FIGURE 7.52
Radiograph of an antero-posterior view of the shoulder demonstrating calcific tendinitis.

CHAPTER 8

Accumulation of abnormal metabolic products and various hematologic disorders

keletal abnormalities may complicate a number of systemic metabolic disturbances that are characterized by accumulation of metabolic products in the tissues. In some of these diseases the skeleton shows the most obvious evidence of the condition, with the disease manifested primarily in the bone or in the joint. Conditions in which the joint is most commonly affected, such as gout and calcium pyrophosphate deposition, will be discussed in Chapter 10. The mucopolysaccharidoses have already been discussed in Chapter 5. The first part of this chapter covers the oxalic acid deposition, amyloidosis, and lipidoses. The second part discusses some of the effects of various hematologic disturbances.

OXALOSIS

Calcium oxalate crystals may be deposited in the connective tissues, including bone and cartilage, in either of two conditions. Primary (familial) oxalosis is characterized by excessive biosynthesis of oxalate, with subsequent nephrolithiasis and deposition of calcium oxalate crystals in the bone marrow. The latter is greatly accentuated by chronic renal failure and, in most patients with clinical disease from primary oxalosis, is widespread and severe. Primary oxalosis usually presents in childhood, although in a few cases its appearance may be delayed until adulthood. More commonly,

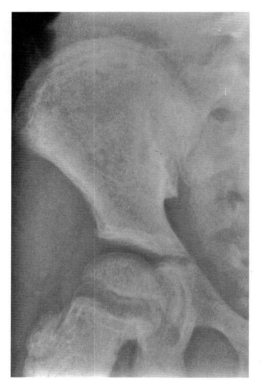

FIGURE 8.1
Radiograph of the right hip and pelvis from a child with primary oxalosis. Note the dense lines in the metaphysis of the femur as well as those paralleling the iliac crest.

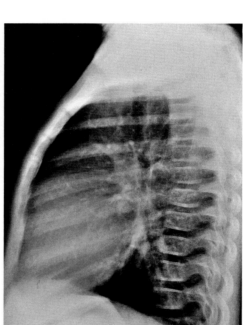

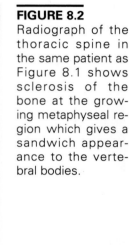

FIGURE 8.2
Radiograph of the thoracic spine in the same patient as Figure 8.1 shows sclerosis of the bone at the growing metaphyseal region which gives a sandwich appearance to the vertebral bodies.

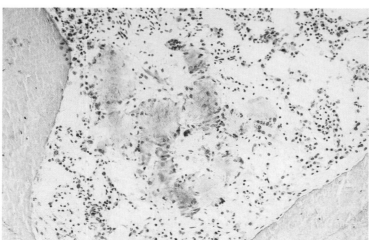

FIGURE 8.3 Photomicrograph of a section from a biopsy obtained from a patient with primary oxalosis. Faint greenish crystalline deposits can be seen in the marrow space (undecalcified section, H&E, x 4 obj.).

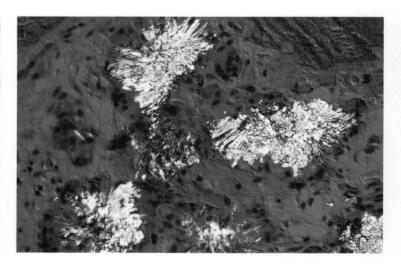

FIGURE 8.4 Photomicrograph of the crystalline material seen in Figure 8.3 examined by Nomarski optics and polarized light at a higher magnification. The starburst clusters of sharp needles of high refractility are typical of oxalosis. Around these crystalline deposits there is a histiocytic and giant cell response (undecalcified section, Normarski optics, polarized light, x 10 obj.).

patients are affected by secondary oxalosis, in which the setting is usually that of chronic renal failure and the degree of crystal deposition is generally much less severe.

The radiologic findings in patients with oxalosis depend on the severity of the disease. In general, however, radiodense areas in the metaphyseal region of the long bones are associated with this condition (Fig. 8.1); occasionally there is markedly increased density of the axial skeleton. In children, dense bands in the metaphysis may result from crystal deposition in growth arrest lines (Fig. 8.2).

Histologic examination reveals that the crystals from both primary and secondary oxalosis are deposited in mineralized bone, articular cartilage, and/or bone marrow. The crystals can be identified by polar-ized light microscopy, which reveals highly refractile needle-shaped crystals that form star-like clusters (Figs. 8.3 to 8.6). Positive identification of the crystals can be achieved by chemical analysis, x-ray diffraction, or electron diffraction. (The latter technique offers a precise method for identification of extremely small quantities of calcium oxalate in bone biopsy specimens.)

Microscopic examination of specimens from patients with oxalosis may reveal either lack of cellular response, a mononuclear cell reaction, or a giant cell reaction similar to that seen in patients with other crystal deposition disorders. (Although osteoclastic resorption of bone may be noted, this finding, as well as that of osteomalacia, is to be expected in the setting of chronic renal failure.)

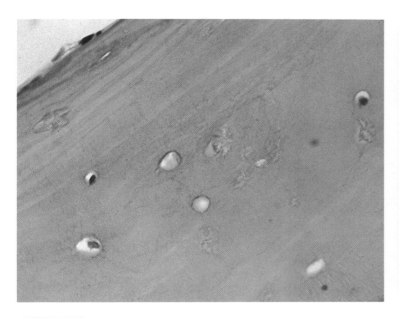
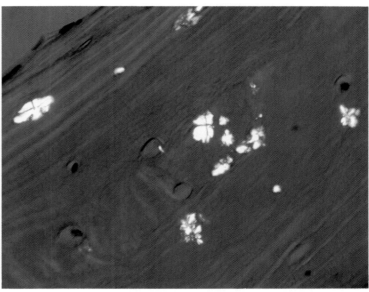

FIGURE 8.5 Oxalosis: photomicrographs of lamellar bone. Within the matrix of the bone and adjacent to the cells can be seen some indistinct deposits *(left)*. On examination with polarized light *(right)*, these deposits become evident as brightly refractile star-like clusters of crystallized material (H&E, x 50 obj.).

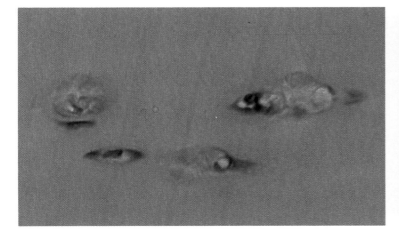
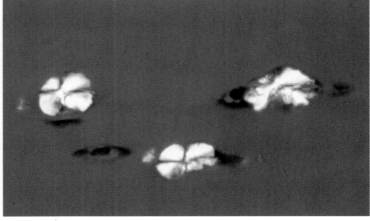

FIGURE 8.6 Oxalosis: photomicrograph of cartilage. Deposits of greyish-yellow material can be seen within the chondrocytic lacunae *(left)*, with the same field photographed using polarized light *(right)* (H&E, x 50 obj.).

AMYLOIDOSIS

Amyloid, a twisted, β-pleated fibrillary protein, appears histologically as a glassy eosinophilic deposit. It may be seen in bone and/or juxta-articular tissues, either as a manifestation of the primary form of amyloidosis or as a secondary amyloidosis resulting from multiple myeloma, rheumatoid arthritis, or other chronic disease. Skeletal involvement is not uncommon but is rarely observed clinically.

Clinically evident quantities of amyloid may be seen in the joints, as diffuse marrow deposits, or, in the rarest form, as localized destructive lesions (tumors). There is usually bilateral involvement of multiple joints (e.g., wrists, shoulders, elbows, and hips).

Radiologic examination may reveal juxta-articular osteoporosis, extensive swelling of the soft tissues, multiple well-defined subchondral cysts, pressure erosions from synovial hypertrophy, and relative preservation of the joint space (Fig. 8.7). Patients with diffuse marrow disease show a predominantly axial distribution of amyloid and may have painful compression fractures that mimic those of myeloma. The localized lytic form of amyloidosis affects the long bones, skull (Fig. 8.8), and ribs, and is usually manifest radiographically as one or more well-marginated lytic lesions. Patients often have aching bone pain and pathologic fractures (Figs. 8.9 and 8.10). Amyloid deposits in the wrist may

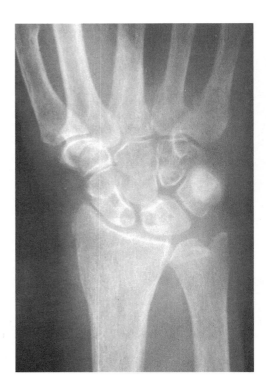

FIGURE 8.7 Radiograph of the wrist of a patient on long term dialysis shows tissue thickening and several lytic defects in the carpal bones due to pressure erosions from amyloid deposits in the synovial tissue.

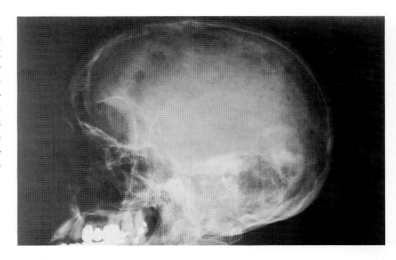

FIGURE 8.8 Radiograph of the skull in a patient with generalized primary amyloidosis shows osteoporosis and multiple lytic areas, which suggest the presence of a myeloma.

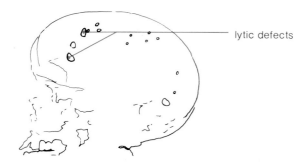

lytic defects

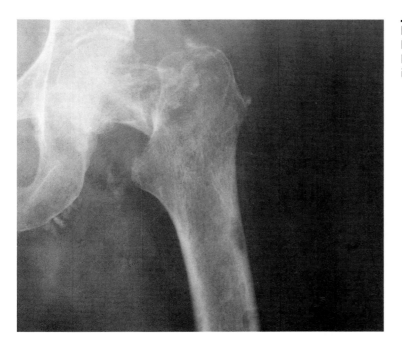

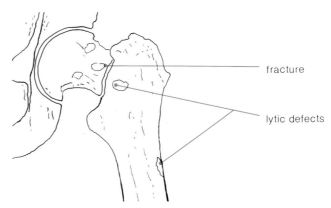

FIGURE 8.9 Radiograph of a portion of the pelvis and the right hip in the same patient illustrated in Figure 8.8. Again multiple lytic lesions can be seen in the neck and shaft of the femur, and, in addition, a fracture has occurred through the femoral neck.

fracture

lytic defects

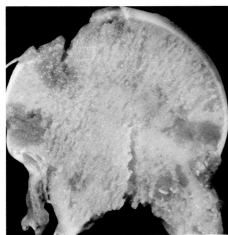

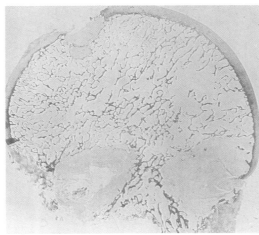

FIGURE 8.10 Cut surface of the femoral head removed from the patient with the pathologic fracture shown in Figure 8.9 *(left)*. The lytic areas are represented by sites of bone destruction filled by a glassy pink tissue. Histologic section *(right)* demonstrates that glassy areas are acellular deposits of amyloid. A higher power view *(below)* shows the dense eosinophilic amyloid deposits with admixed fibroblasts and vessels (H&E x 10 obj.).

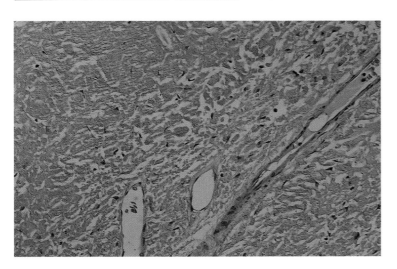

cause carpal tunnel syndrome, which is sometimes the presenting symptom of amyloidosis (Fig. 8.11).

Histologic sections stained with Congo red have a characteristic apple-green birefringence when examined under polarized light (Figs. 8.12 and 8.13). It may be difficult to recognize amyloid deposits when they occur in connective tissue matrix, because collagen produces a similar apple-green color when examined under polarized light.

GAUCHER'S DISEASE

The so-called "lipidoses" encompass a wide variety of disorders in which congenital enzyme deficiencies lead to the accumulation of complex lipid compounds. By far the most common of these disorders is Gaucher's disease, an autosomal recessively transmitted error of metabolism of the glucosyl ceramides (glucocerebrosides). These compounds accumulate in cells of the

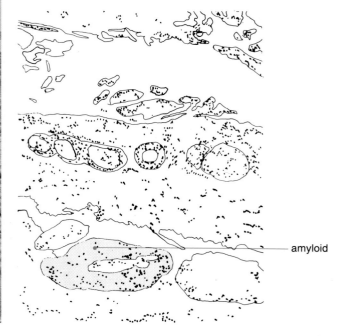

FIGURE 8.11 Tissue removed from the transverse carpal ligament in a patient with carpal tunnel syndrome. The amyloid deposit in the vessel wall has been stained by Congo red stain (x 10 obj.).

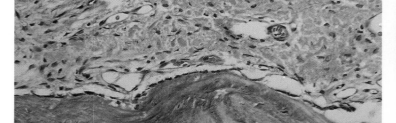

FIGURE 8.12 Photomicrograph of amyloid deposit in the bone marrow (H&E, x 10 obj.).

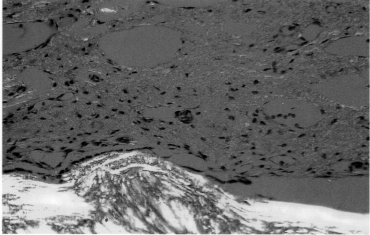

FIGURE 8.13 Photomicrograph of the same field as that shown in Figure 8.12 under polarized light. The amyloid deposits are birefringent and apple green (polarized light, x 10 obj.).

reticuloendothelial system, including the liver, spleen, lymph nodes, and bone marrow, as a result of a deficiency in the activity of glucosylceramide ∝–glucosidase. Splenomegaly may be dramatic. The disease is most common in Ashkenazic Jews.

Most patients have a chronic form of the disease that pursues a rather benign course. Other patients, however, develop many complications and, in rare cases, an acute neuropathic form of the disease occurs in which most of those affected die before the age of 3 years. Although the clinical course varies, patients who present with the disease in infancy or childhood usually have a poor prognosis.

On histologic examination the skeletal alterations in Gaucher's disease are seen to result from massive infiltration of the marrow space by typical large histiocytes that usually measure 40 to 80 μm in diameter and have a characteristic crumpled- or wrinkled-paper appearance of the cytoplasm (Figs. 8.14, 8.15 and 8.16). The tissue stains positively with PAS. Secondary morpho-

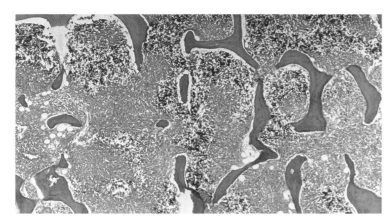

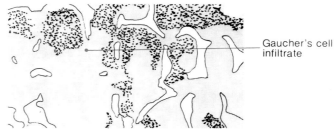

FIGURE 8.14 Gaucher's disease: photomicrograph shows replacement of the bone marrow by sheets of large pink cells. Some residual normal marrow is seen at the top of the frame (H&E, x 4 obj.).

Gaucher's cell infiltrate

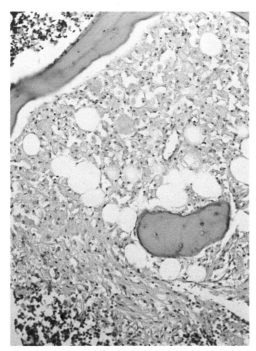

FIGURE 8.15 At higher power, the Gaucher cells are seen to be swollen histiocytes with a rather typical foamy cytoplasm and a crinkled appearance. This histiocytic infiltrate is replacing the normal bone marrow (H&E, x 25 obj.).

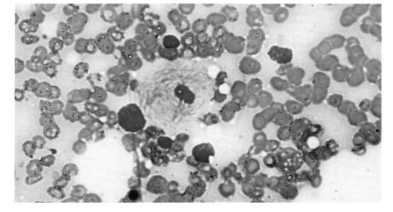

FIGURE 8.16 Photomicrograph of a Gaucher's cell seen here in a bone marrow aspirate. The size of the cell can be appreciated from the surrounding hematopoietic cells (Wright's stain, x 100 obj.).

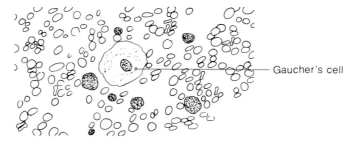

Gaucher's cell

logic changes induced by infiltrating Gaucher's cells include infarcts of bone, especially of the femoral head. Secondary infection may occur after biopsy (Fig. 8.17).

Radiologically, the long bones show irregular thinning of the cortices, which gives a trabeculated appearance. Frequently, the lower end of the femur, the upper end of the tibia, and the upper end of the humerus expand, which produces the "Erlenmeyer flask" deformity (Fig. 8.18).

The spine usually exhibits loss of density in this condition, and frequently one or more of the vertebrae show collapse with either a wedge-shaped deformity, platyspondyly, or occasionally fish-mouth deformities (Fig. 8.19). In addition to osteopenia, some osteosclerotic lesions are occasionally present. These are probably the result of infarction within the bone.

XANTHOMATOSIS (CHESTER-ERDHEIM DISEASE OF BONE)

Xanthomatosis refers to the tumor-like accumulation of lipid-laden histiocytes (foam cells, xanthoma cells) in the body. These tumor nodules may be noted in a broad range of clinical settings, including both familial and acquired disorders (such as biliary cirrhosis, pancreatitis, and diabetes mellitus) that result in hypercholesterolemia and/or hyperlipoproteinemia.

The most common presentation of xanthomatosis in the connective tissue is that of yellow nodular tumors in the Achilles tendon or the extensor tendons of fingers (Figs. 8.20 to 8.23). Patients thus affected often have bilateral involvement of other sites, including subcutaneous tissue. They also have hypercholesterolemia,

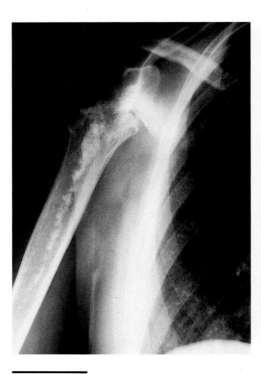

FIGURE 8.17 Radiograph of the humerus of a patient with Gaucher's disease complicated both by osteomyelitis and infarction.

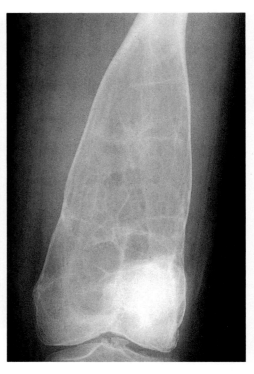

FIGURE 8.18 Radiograph of the lower femur of a patient with Gaucher's disease shows flaring of the metaphyseal region and distal diaphysis with a bubbly osteolysis of the affected bone.

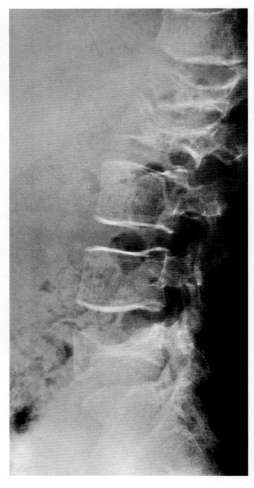

FIGURE 8.19 Lateral radiograph of a patient with Gaucher's disease. Osteopenia and collapse of L-1, L-2, and L-5 are seen. There is a kyphotic deformity in the thoracolumbar region.

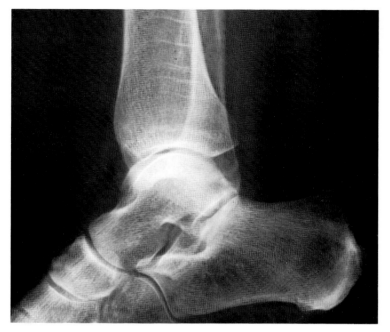

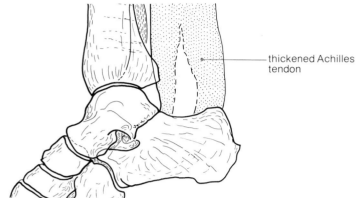

FIGURE 8.20 Radiograph of the heel in a 25-year-old woman who had bilateral thickening of the Achilles tendon owing to xanthomas. She also had xanthomas of the patellar tendon and xantholasmas of the skin. The patient had hypercholesterolemia. Several members of the family suffered from the same condition.

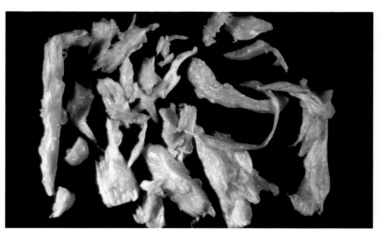

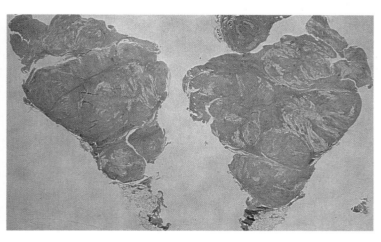

FIGURE 8.21 Tissue removed from the thickened heel cord shown in Figure 8.20. The yellowish color results from the lipid accumulation.

FIGURE 8.22 Lower power photomicrograph of tissue shown in Figure 8.21 shows extensive fatty replacement and cyst formation (H&E, x 1.5 obj.).

FIGURE 8.23 Photomicrograph at a higher power of cyst seen in Figure 8.22 shows lipid-filled foamy histiocytes and cholesterol clefts in the wall of the cyst (H&E, x 10 obj.).

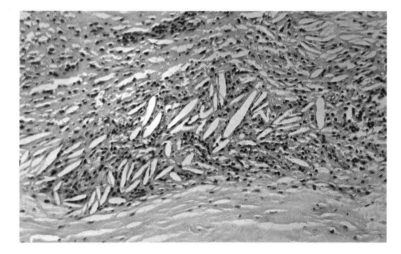

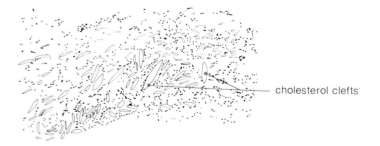

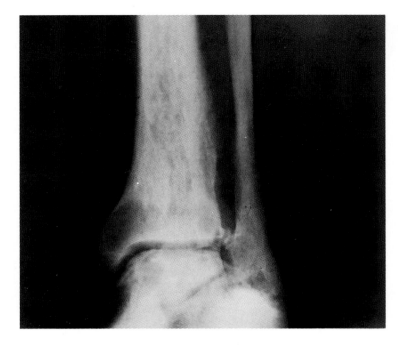

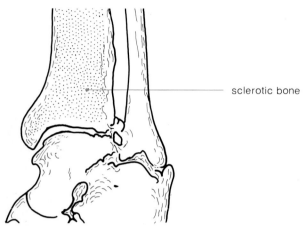

FIGURE 8.24 Radiograph of the lower leg in a patient with lipogranulomatosis of the bone (Chester-Erdheim disease). Note the patchy sclerosis with coarsening of the trabeculae.

sclerotic bone

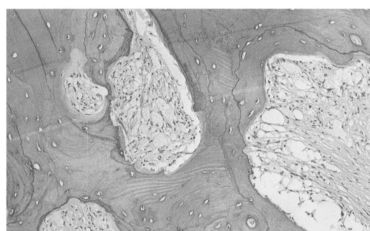

FIGURE 8.25 Photomicrograph of a biopsy obtained from the patient shown in Figure 8.24. In addition to thickening of the bone trabeculae, there is replacement of the fatty marrow by foamy histiocytes, fibroblasts, and occasional inflammatory cells (H&E, x 10 obj.).

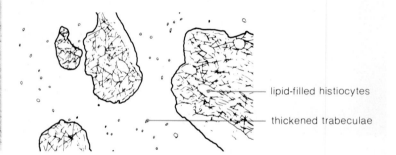

lipid-filled histiocytes

thickened trabeculae

FIGURE 8.26 Radiograph of the skull in a child with eosinophilic granulomas. Several lytic lesions are evident; within the largest, one can appreciate the beveled edge that is typical of this presentation of eosinophilic granuloma.

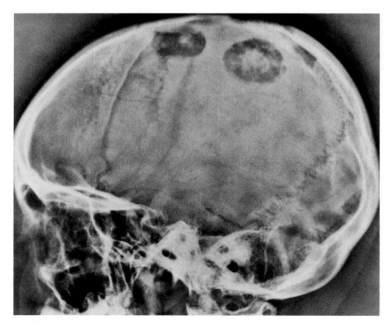

manifested as Type II hyperbetalipoproteinemia on lipoprotein electrophoresis.

Involvement of the skeleton is decidedly rare. On radiologic examination, the bone lesions show patchy sclerotic change accompanied by coarsened trabeculae, often with focal lytic destruction (Fig. 8.24). The cortical bone may be thinned by endosteal erosion, and ischemic necrosis may follow. Curettage has revealed yellow fragmented tissue due to replacement of the marrow elements by foamy histiocytes (Fig. 8.25). These cells have been found to contain intracytoplasmic cholesterol, phospholipids, and/or triglycerides. The amount of inflammation and fibrosis is variable.

EOSINOPHILIC GRANULOMA

The entity known as eosinophilic granuloma may appear as a unifocal lesion or as multifocal osseous lesions, sometimes with systemic involvement. Classically, eosinophilic granuloma presents in males in the first decade of life. Patients may complain of pain or local tenderness. Laboratory tests are usually unremarkable, although the erythrocyte sedimentation rate may be elevated. The most commonly affected parts of the skeleton are the proximal femoral metaphysis, the skull, mandible, ribs, and vertebral column. Eosinophilic granuloma may also occur in soft tissue, including the skin, oral mucosa, lymph nodes, and lungs. When the lung is affected, patients may develop progressive fibrosis with impaired pulmonary function.

On radiologic examination, one or more sharply circumscribed lytic defects may be evident in the bone (Fig. 8.26). These defects usually lack sclerotic rims. In the spine collapse of a vertebral body is a common presentation (Fig. 8.27). Sometimes a more destructive permeative lesion with periosteal new bone formation can be seen (Fig. 8.28).

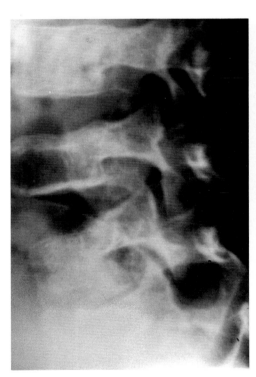
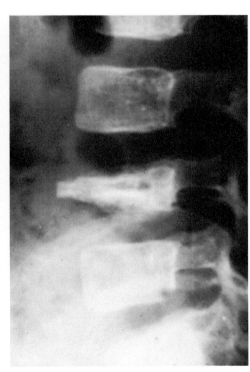

FIGURE 8.27 Lateral radiograph *(left)* of the lumbar spine in an 8-year-old child, showing a lytic lesion of L-3, with partial collapse. A lateral radiograph *(right)* of the same patient, one month later, shows that the vertebral body has now collapsed down to a thin sclerotic wafer, which is somewhat increased in AP diameter. This appearance is characteristic for Calve's disease.

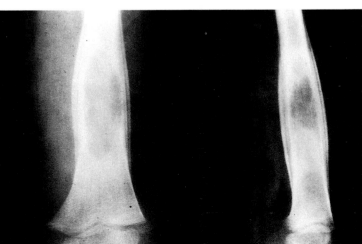

FIGURE 8.28 Radiograph of a child who presented with slight fever, and pain and swelling in the right lower femur. Biopsy proved the lesion to be an eosinophilic granuloma. The radiologic differential diagnosis might include Ewing's sarcoma or osteomyelitis.

Specimens for pathologic examination are usually in the form of multiple curetted tissue fragments, typically consisting of glistening reddish tissue with flecks of opaque yellow material throughout (Fig. 8.29). Eosinophilic granuloma is characterized microscopically by a mixture of eosinophils, plasma cells, histiocytes, and peculiar large mononuclear and multinucleated giant cells (Langerhans cells) with abundant pale-staining cytoplasm (Figs. 8.30 to 8.32). Many of the large mononuclear cells have indented or cleaved nuclei. A variable degree of necrosis and fibrosis may be evident, as may reactive cells such as foamy macrophages. Mitotic activity is minimal. On electron microscopy the Langer-

hans cell displays peculiar racket-shaped inclusion bodies in the cytoplasm (Birbeck granules) (Fig. 8.33).

Patients with unifocal lesions may show spontaneous regression, or they can be treated with minimal chemotherapy. In general, the prognosis is good if a second lesion does not appear within 1 year. In patients who present with a more systemic illness characterized by fever, organomegaly, and multiple osseous lesions, the course of the disease is likely to be protracted. Both the clinical course of this disease and its histopathology indicate that it is not neoplastic in nature. The presence of eosinophils and occasional skin lesions suggest that this is a peculiar immunoallergic phenomenon.

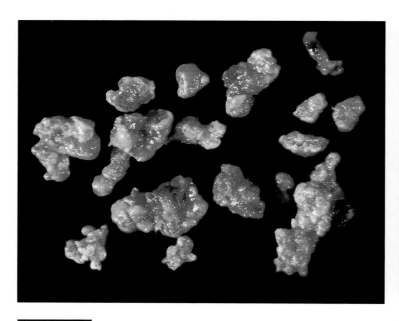

FIGURE 8.29 Gross photograph of curetted tissue obtained from a patient with an eosinophilic granuloma shows typically scant reddish-gray fragments of tissue flecked with dense yellow areas. These yellow areas represent loci of lipid accumulation or necrosis.

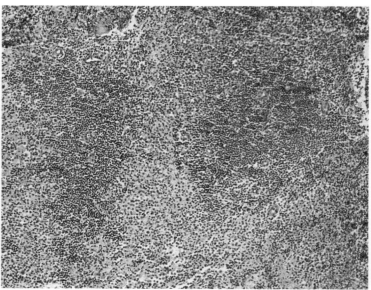

FIGURE 8.30 Low power view of tissue curetted from a patient with an eosinophilic granuloma demonstrates the lesion's variegated hypercellular appearance. One should not confuse this tissue with inflammatory tissue from a patient with osteomyelitis (H&E, x 10 obj.).

FIGURE 8.31 In this photomicrograph, the mixed cellular appearance of an eosinophilic granuloma can be appreciated. In addition to plasma cells and eosinophils, large histiocytes and giant cells are present. Occasionally, especially if the tissue is scarred, confusion with Hodgkin's disease may be a problem (H&E, x 40 obj.).

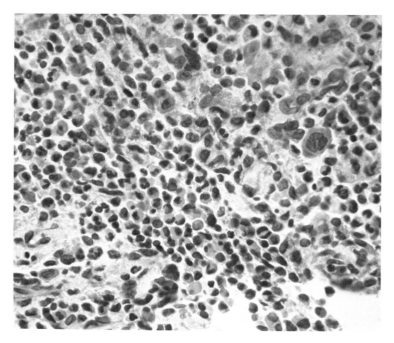

Eosinophilic granuloma has been considered as one of a group of disorders known as the histiocytoses, which include (in addition to eosinophilic granuloma) Hand-Schuller-Christian disease and Letterer-Siwe disease. However, the former is probably better thought of as multiple eosinophilic granuloma, and Letterer-Siwe disease (a rare disease of infants with a characteristically fulminant course) is probably an unrelated neoplastic condition.

SYSTEMIC MASTOCYTOSIS

Systemic mastocytosis is a rare condition characterized by infiltration of various organs by mast cells. Two clinical manifestations are known. The first is an infiltrative process characterized by osteoporosis or osteosclerosis, hepatosplenomegaly, lymphadenopathy, and/or mast cell infiltration in the skin (urticaria pigmentosa), gastrointestinal tract, heart, and lungs. This form may be accompanied by anemia, leukocytosis, leukopenia, eosinophilia, basophilia, or hypocholesterolemia. A second form is characterized by pharmacologic effects secondary to release of chemicals following degranulation of mast cells. The cells secrete a variety of pharmacologically active agents, including histamine, heparin, prostaglandins, serotonin, and mucopolysaccharides. Among these effects are flushing, pounding headache, bronchospasm, hypotension, diarrhea, rhinorrhea, urticaria, palpitation, dyspnea, peptic ulcer, and gastrointestinal bleeding. Various combinations and clinical syndromes are seen.

In patients with skeletal involvement, radiographs typically show diffuse, poorly demarcated sclerotic and lucent areas which involve predominantly the axial skeleton (Fig. 8.34). However, circumscribed lesions

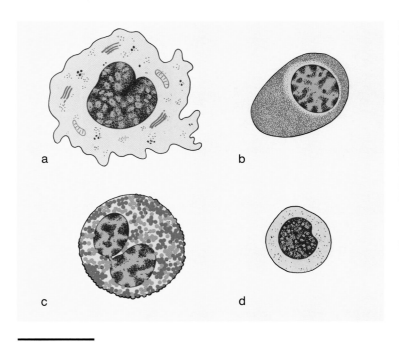

FIGURE 8.32 Diagram of the various cells seen in eosinophilic granuloma (drawn to scale). *(a)* Histiocyte, *(b)* plasma cell showing a cartwheel nucleus, *(c)* eosinophil, *(d)* lymphocyte.

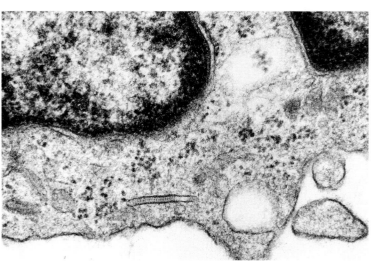

FIGURE 8.33 Electron micrograph of a histiocytic giant cell from a patient with eosinophilic granuloma shows a typical Birbeck granule in the cytoplasm (x 100,000).

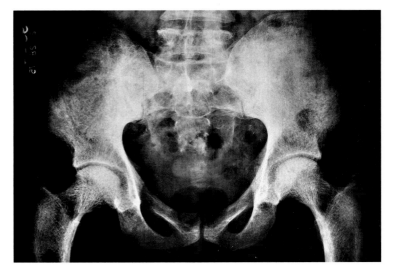

FIGURE 8.34 Radiograph of the pelvis of a patient with patchy mastocytosis shows diffuse bone sclerosis with patchy osteolysis. In other cases the sclerosis may be more obviously nodular suggesting a diagnosis of metastatic disease.

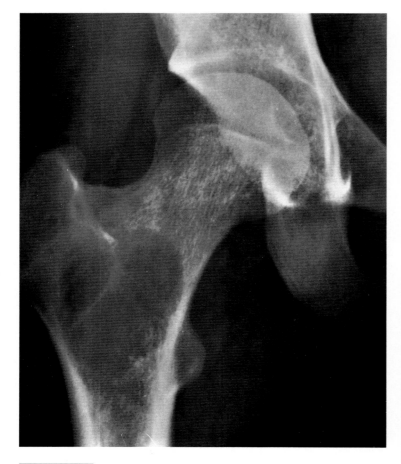

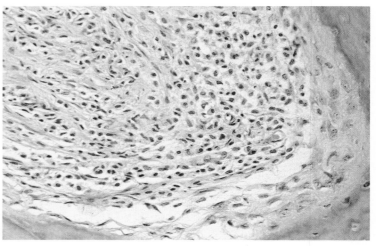

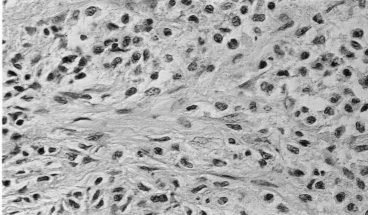

FIGURE 8.35 Radiograph of a 14-year-old girl with a 6 month history of pain in the hip which proved histologically to be caused by a mastocytoma (see Figure 8.38). (Courtesy of Dr. Ed McCarthy, Baltimore, MD)

FIGURE 8.36 *(top)* Photomicrograph of a biopsy obtained from a patient with generalized mastocytosis. Within the marrow space there is fibrosis with a mixed round cell infiltration (H&E, x 25 obj.). *(bottom)* A higher power of the same field. A few cells with granules are present but identification requires special stains (see Figure 8.37) (H&E, x 50 obj.).

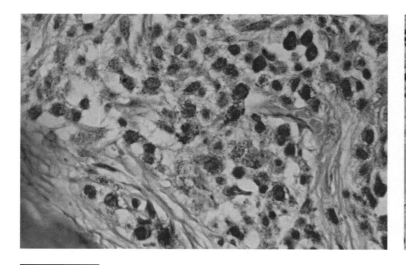

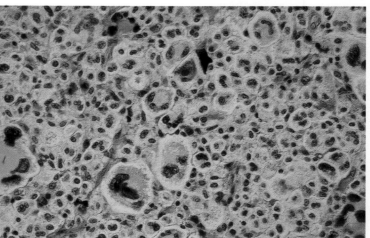

FIGURE 8.37 Photomicrograph of the same tissue shown in Figure 8.36 stained with a Giemsa stain shows the metachromatic granules in the cytoplasm of the mast cells (Giemsa stain, x 40 obj.).

FIGURE 8.38 Photomicrograph of tissue obtained from the case demonstrated in the radiograph in Figure 8.35. The rounded bizarre cells with abundant cytoplasm and many giant cell forms suggested a malignancy although careful searching showed no mitotic figures. However, electron microscopic studies in this case confirmed the presence in the cells of typical mast cell granules (H&E, x 25 obj.).

can occur, especially in the skull and in the extremities. These focal lesions may be mistaken for metastatic disease (Fig. 8.35).

Because the lesion may appear to be permeative and occasionally sclerotic, and because in a child it may be mistaken for a Ewing's sarcoma, isotope bone scanning is useful. Technetium and gallium scans demonstrate diffuse generalized uptake (Ensslen, Jackson and Reid 1983); gallium is particularly taken up by the mast cells.

Microscopic examination of tissue removed from the bone of patients with mastocytosis shows diffuse or focal replacement of the bone marrow, usually with a mixture of cells including lymphocytes, eosinophils, plasma cells, fibroblasts and, of course, mast cells (Fig. 8.36). The latter, however, may be easily overlooked unless a metachromatic stain (Fig. 8.37) or electron microscopy is done. Occasionally the cellular infiltrate is composed predominantly of mast cells.

Histologically, mastocytosis may closely mimic a malignant lymphoma or histiocytosis (Fig. 8.38).

SKELETAL MANIFESTATIONS OF HEMATOLOGICAL DISEASES

Hematologic diseases such as the hemoglobinopathies, hemolytic anemias, or bleeding diatheses may lead to severe bone and joint damage. Among the causes of skeletal changes are secondary erythroid hyperplasia following chronic states of anemia (as seen in patients with thalassemia and sickle cell disease); vascular thrombosis with subsequent infarction, and often infection (as seen in patients with sickle cell disease); and joint destruction secondary to chronic bloody synovial effusions (as seen in patients with hemophilia, which will be considered in Chapter 10.)

The severity of these skeletal diseases depends, to a certain extent, on the age of the patient. Children are dramatically affected because of the effect of blood disorders on the growing skeleton. In patients who manifest chronic hematologic disease during infancy, the hands and feet show marked skeletal alterations, whereas in slightly older children the skull may be the predominant site of involvement. In the mature skeleton of an adult the most dramatic changes usually affect the pelvis and in the spine.

HEMOCHROMATOSIS

Excessive iron accumulation in the tissues (especially of the visceral organs and in particular, the heart and liver) may be caused by severe chronic anemia that requires protracted courses of transfusion therapy or by massive oral iron intake. The resulting disease is known as *secondary hemochromatosis*. When a pathogenic mechanism is not apparent, the condition is called *idiopathic hemochromatosis*.

In general, the bone and joint changes in hemochromatosis are nonspecific and are best characterized as a noninflammatory arthropathy, classically with involvement of the metacarpophalangeal joints, especially the second and third (Fig. 8.39); less commonly, large

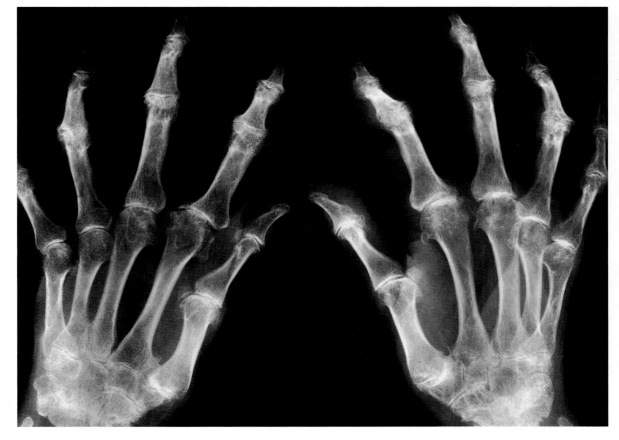

FIGURE 8.39
Dorsovolar view of both hands of a 53-year-old woman with hemochromatosis arthropathy shows beaklike osteophytes arising from the heads of the second and third metacarpals on the radial aspect. The interphalangeal, metacarpophalangeal, and carpal articulations are also affected.

joints, such as the shoulder and elbows (a distribution that is atypical for classic osteoarthritis), are involved. There may be regional osteoporosis, as well as peculiar cysts and erosions around the affected joints. Of interest is the associated high incidence of chondrocalcinosis in patients with this condition, which is usually attributed to interference by iron with the enzymatic degradation of pyrophosphates. Treatment should be directed at the underlying disorder that is causing the accumulation of iron.

The brown discoloration of the synovial tissue classically seen in patients with this disorder may be confused by the orthopedic surgeon with local iron deposition from extravasated blood, as seen in patients with rheumatoid synovitis, pigmented villonodular synovitis, or hemophilic arthropathy (Fig. 8.40).

SICKLE CELL DISEASE

A number of hematologic conditions are caused by the formation of abnormal hemoglobin; these conditions are known collectively as the hemoglobinopathies. In sickle cell disease, a substitution of one of the amino acids in the β-hemoglobin chain leads to increased hemolysis under conditions of low oxygen tension and to crystallization of the hemoglobin molecule, which results in formation of abnormal sickle-shaped erythrocytes. The hemolytic anemia leads to bone marrow hyperplasia.

Radiologic examination may reveal generalized os-teoporosis, sometimes associated with vertebral collapse, wedge-shaped deformities, and kyphoscoliosis. Characteristic radiographic changes may also be observed in the hands and feet following infarcts that develop in infancy (Fig. 8.41).

On macroscopic examination the bones show a congested, dusky red appearance, indicative of marked erythroid hyperplasia of the marrow (Figs. 8.42 and 8.43). The erythrocytes themselves are deformed and often crescent-shaped, which gives rise to the term sickle cell (Fig. 8.44). There may be profound osteoporosis because of marrow impingement on the adjacent trabecular bone structure. However, the most severe problem in sickle cell disease is the development of infarcts, which may cause sudden severe pain. The infarcts may be located anywhere, although they are most frequent in the femoral heads or in the spine (usually the lower spine), which may awaken the sleeping patient. Initial radiographs are normal, with infarct-related changes developing only after some months (see Chapter 10). In addition to compression fractures and wedging fractures, the spines of affected children may also exhibit a double concavity resulting from collapse of the central portion of the vertebral body under the hyaline growth plate (Fig. 8.45). Rather than being compression fractures caused by mechanical failure, it has been suggested that these lesions are the result of relative ischemia in this region of the vertebral body.

Osteomyelitis is a well-recognized complication of

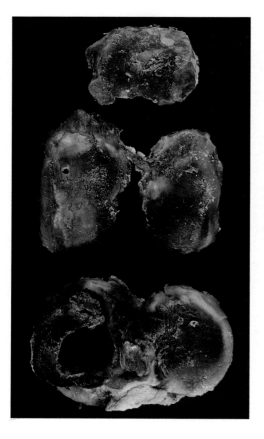

FIGURE 8.40
Photograph of the articular surfaces of the knee joint of a patient with hemochromatosis. The black-green staining of the cartilage results from the accumulated blood pigment which eventually interferes with chondrocyte function and hence cartilage matrix metabolism. (Note: the gross and microscopic changes in hemochromatosis are similar to those seen in hemosiderosis.)

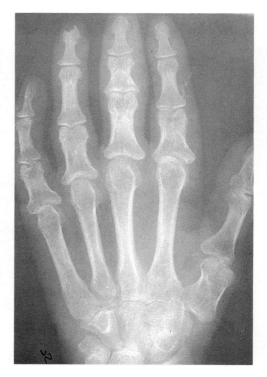

FIGURE 8.41
Radiograph of the hand of a patient with sickle cell disease. The shortening of the first metacarpal and of some of the phalanges is secondary to growth disturbances due to infarctions following sickle cell crises in infancy.

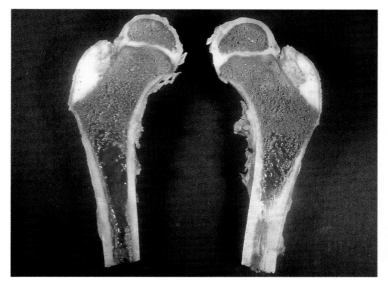

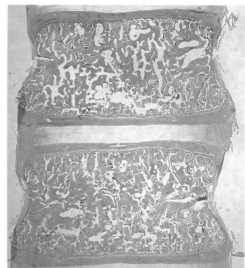

FIGURE 8.43
Histologic section of two vertebral bodies from a child with sickle cell disease. The marrow space is entirely filled with hematopoietic tissue and there is no fat evident. (Normally the marrow is 50% fat and 50% hematopoietic tissue.) Osteoporosis is also present.

FIGURE 8.42 Photograph of a frontal section through the femur of a child who died from the complications of sickle cell disease. Note the dusky red appearance of the hyperplastic packed marrow.

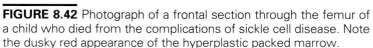

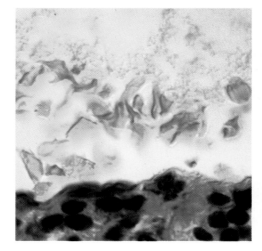

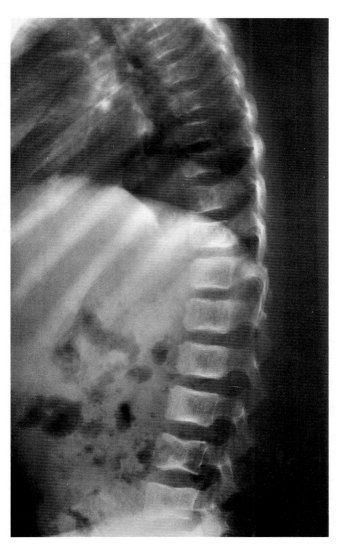

FIGURE 8.44 Photomicrograph of "sickled" red cells within the lumen of a blood vessel. (Normarski differential interference contrast microscopy, H&E, x 100 obj.).

FIGURE 8.45
Lateral radiograph of an adolescent male with sickle cell disease. Note the osteopenia, with accentuation of the vertical trabeculae, and the central collapse of the vertebral bodies in the upper and midthoracic spine.

sickle cell disease, and may be due to infection with the *Salmonella* organism (Fig. 8.46). In the past, this complication often necessitated amputation of the involved extremity (Fig. 8.47).

THALASSEMIA

The several types of thalassemia are characterized by a hemoglobin abnormality resulting from deletion of one of the amino acid chains. Patients with thalassemia major exhibit profound anemia and very severe marrow hyperplasia (mainly erythroid hyperplasia) associated with profound osteoporosis. These changes are evident mainly in the skull, long bones, and metacarpals and metatarsals. Although osseous changes may be observed in patients with thalassemia minor, they are usually less severe. In general, as the patient matures, there is less involvement of the peripheral skeleton.

On radiographic examination the long bones show medullary widening with cortical thinning, often involving the humerus and femur with development of "saber shins." Involvement of the spine is usually manifested as kyphosis or scoliosis, which results from vertebral collapse. There may be a dramatic widening of the diploetic space of the skull, with thinning and displacement of the trabeculae, producing a "hair on end" appearance (Figs. 8.48 and 8.49). The hands and feet may exhibit medullary widening and cortical thinning of the metacarpals and metatarsals, which appear on radiography as a honeycomb pattern (Fig. 8.50). Involvement of the maxillary bones and sinuses may lead to a peculiar "rodent" facies.

Grossly, the bones appear dusky red, and radiographically bones may reveal severe osteoporosis (Figs. 8.51 and 8.52). Microscopic examination of tissue from severely affected patients often reveals dramatic hyper-

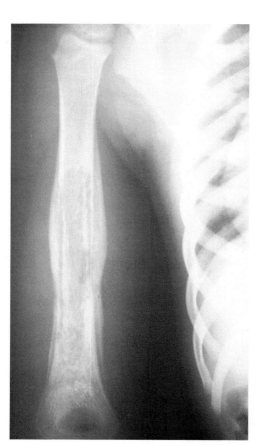

FIGURE 8.46
Radiograph of the right arm of a patient with sickle cell disease who has developed a diaphyseal osteomyelitis due to infection with a *Salmonella* organism.

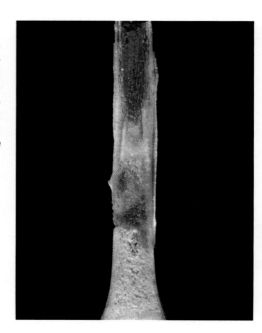

FIGURE 8.47
Section taken through the tibia from a patient with sickle cell disease who developed osteomyelitis. The specimen shows extensive necrosis, seen as an opaque yellow coloration of the bone towards the ankle joint, and between the necrotic bone and the living bone above there is a focus of infected tissue.

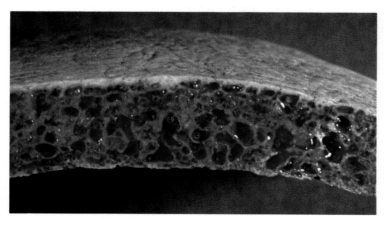

FIGURE 8.48 Thalassemia: section through the skull shows marked thinning of the cortices and an open porotic cancellous bone. The mahogany brown color results from extensive iron deposition in the marrow.

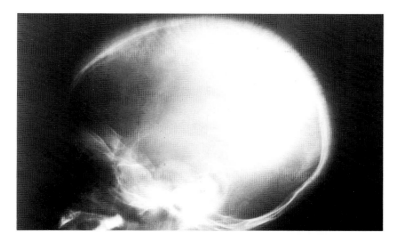

FIGURE 8.49 Radiograph of the skull of a patient with thalassemia major shows characteristic "hair on end" appearance.

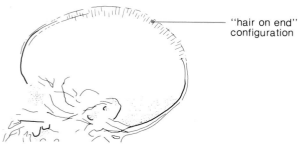

"hair on end" configuration

FIGURE 8.50 Radiograph of the hands in a patient with thalassemia shows severe osteoporosis with a "honeycomb" and cystic cancellous pattern.

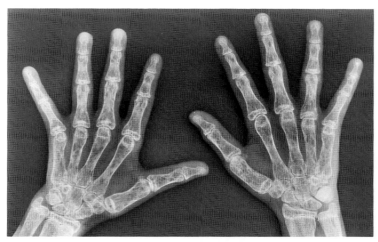

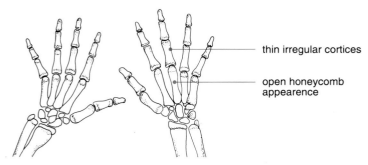

thin irregular cortices

open honeycomb appearence

FIGURE 8.51
Segment of the vertebral column from a young patient with thalassemia major. The bone marrow is mahogany brown.

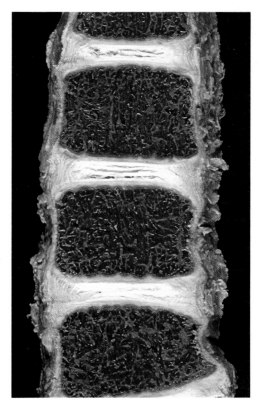

FIGURE 8.52
Radiograph of the specimen shown in Figure 8.51 reveals marked osteoporosis.

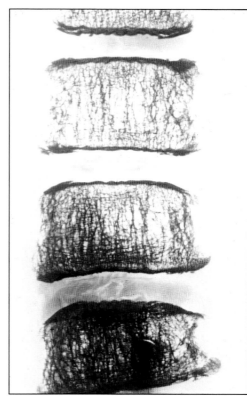

plasia of the marrow and erythroid components. In histologic sections of bone, Perls' Prussian blue staining demonstrates iron deposition in the zones of mineralization and cement lines (Fig. 8.53).

Occasionally thalassemia is seen in association with sickle cell disease, and in such cases infarcts may be superimposed on the other symptoms.

MYELOFIBROSIS

Myelofibrosis, a relatively uncommon disease, is characterized by fibrosis of the bone marrow and extramedullary hematopoiesis. In approximately 50 percent of cases the bones, particularly of the axial skeleton, show radiographically a diffuse but occasion-

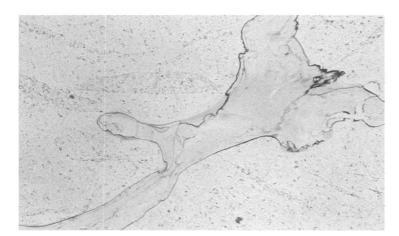

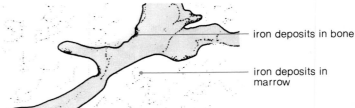

FIGURE 8.53 Thalassemia: photomicrograph of a section of bone stained with Perl's stain for iron, which stains a Prussian blue color. It can be appreciated that, on the surface of the bone and also running through the cement lines, there is much iron deposition, as well as extensive deposits throughout the bone marrow (iron stain, x 4 obj.).

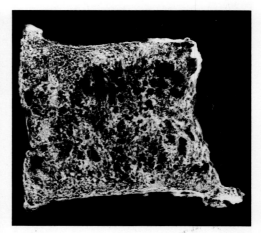

iron deposits in bone

iron deposits in marrow

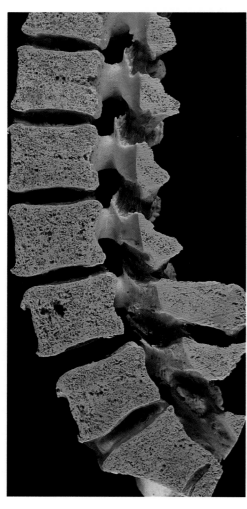

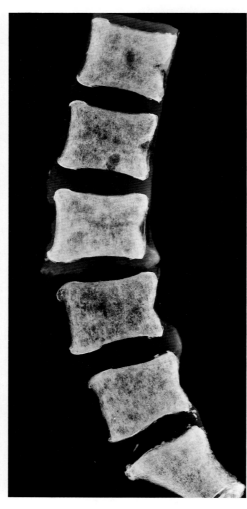

FIGURE 8.54 Photograph *(left)* of a sagittal section through the macerated lumbar spine of a patient with myelofibrosis. Note the extremely sclerotic bone associated with this condition. A radiograph *(center)* of the same specimen shows patchy osteosclerosis, with a complete loss of the normal trabecular pattern. A specimen radiograph *(right)* of a 2-mm slice through one of the vertebrae demonstrates the sclerosis and loss of trabecular pattern seen in this condition.

ally patchy sclerosis. The disease occurs with about equal frequency in men and women, and is more common among older individuals. On radiography it may be characterized by profound bony sclerosis which, in combination with the marrow fibrosis, accounts for the frequency of "dry taps" when marrow aspiration is attempted (Fig. 8.54). Approximately one half of all adult patients exhibit dramatic involvement of the spine, pelvis, ribs, sternum, proximal humerus, and femur (the common sites of adult hematopoiesis). The skull is rarely involved. The involved bones are not expanded, and there is no change in their contour (Fig. 8.55). The differential diagnosis is usually not difficult because of the diffuse sclerosis that occurs in this condition. Rarely, it may be closely mimicked by some cases of metastatic carcinoma and the rare osteosclerotic form of myelomatosis. Rare cases of spinal cord compression resulting from an extradural mass of hematopoietic tis-

sue have been reported. Many patients with myelofibrosis eventually develop myelogenous leukemia.

Microscopic examination of the marrow shows obliterative fibrosis in the late stages. In early stages, marked marrow hyperplasia with bizarre cell types may be seen, as well as an increase in reticulum fiber production. When viewed with polarized light, the thickened bone is found to have a largely woven appearance (Fig. 8.56).

LEUKEMIA

Neoplastic conditions of the marrow and lymphoid system frequently manifest local or generalized skeletal involvement (Fig. 8.57). In most cases discrete tumors are present but in some instances only a diffuse osteoporosis is noted. In patients with leukemia, it is not unusual to find widespread infarcts of the bone and bone marrow at autopsy (Fig. 8.58) (see also Chapter 17).

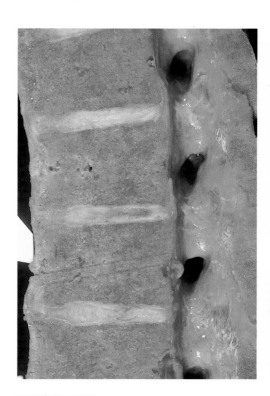

FIGURE 8.55 Close-up photograph of a portion of the lower thoracic spine to show the pale appearance due to the fibrotic replacement of the bone marrow. Note the lack of any deformity in the contours of the vertebral bodies.

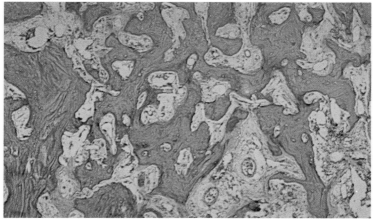

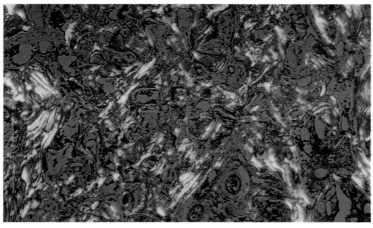

FIGURE 8.56
Photomicrograph *(top)* showing a section of bone from a patient with myelofibrosis. Note that there is extensive new bone formation, as well as fibrosis of the marrow space with displacement of the hematopoietic tissue. The same specimen photographed with polarized light *(bottom)* shows that the extensive new bone formation has an immature or woven pattern (H&E, x 10 obj.).

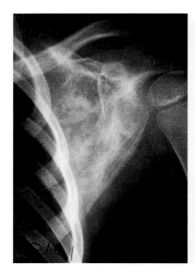

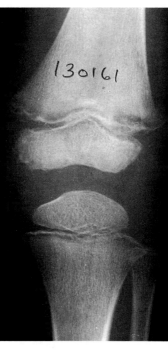

FIGURE 8.57 *(left)* Radiograph of a child who initially presented with a mass in the shoulder which on biopsy revealed a small cell sarcoma. *(right)* Further studies showed radiolucencies at the more rapidly growing epiphyses (knees, shoulders, wrists) typical of the diffuse involvement of the skeleton which characterizes most cases of leukemia.

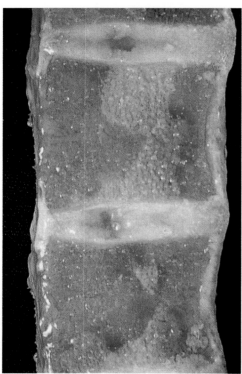

FIGURE 8.58 Photograph of a segment of the spine from a child who died from leukemia. Within the vertebral bodies, there are geographic areas of necrosis identified as yellow opacification of the bone and marrow. These are surrounded by a thin rim of hyperemic tissue. Note that the viable bone marrow has a fleshy tan color reflecting the leukemia infiltrate.

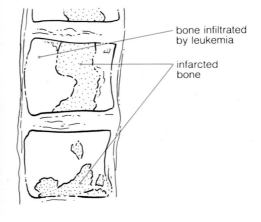

bone infiltrated by leukemia

infarcted bone

ARTHRITIS

A major part of the practice of orthopedics is concerned with the management and treatment of the diseases considered under the general heading of arthritis. In general, however, it can be said that arthritis still remains a fairly baffling disease. The causes of arthritis are many, including maldevelopment, infection, trauma, systemic immunologic disease, and crystal deposition. In a large number of patients the etiology of the arthritis is not apparent, and these are the cases usually diagnosed as idiopathic osteoarthritis (OA). However, as Dr. Paul Dieppe has stated, "it may (even) be unhelpful to regard osteoarthritis as a specific disease process or a distinct entity. It may be more analogous to heart failure—the state of an organ which can result from a number of different diseases or physiological changes."

The chapters that follow attempt to address the problem by first considering the function, anatomy, and physiology of the normal joint and relating them to the morbid anatomy and pathophysiology of the diseased joint. Subsequent chapters consider specific clinical states and arthritis as it affects the spine. Finally, a chapter is devoted to consideration of some of the problems and complications associated with total joint replacement.

CHAPTER 9

The pathophysiology of arthritis

ltered anatomy associated with a disease state is referred to as morbid anatomy; the alteration in the dynamic function of the organ is referred to as its pathophysiology. Joint dysfunction (ie, arthritis) can be understood only when the process of normal function has been comprehended.

NORMAL JOINT FUNCTION

Normal joint function is characterized by: freedom of the opposed articular surfaces to move painlessly over each other within the required range of motion; correct distribution of load across joint tissues, which might otherwise be damaged by overloading or might become atrophied because of habitual underloading (disuse); and maintenance of stability during use.

NORMAL JOINT ANATOMY

The three interdependent aspects of joint function referred to above depend themselves on the following three features of joint design.

• *The Geometry of the Opposed Articulating Surfaces of the Joint*

Perhaps the most obvious feature of any joint is its shape. In general, one joint surface is convex, whereas the other is concave. The convex or "male" side of the joint usually has a larger articular surface than the concave or "female" side. These complementary shapes of the joint surfaces are necessary to permit the range of motion required, to provide stability, and to ensure the most equitable loading during use (Fig. 9.1). In some joints (for example, the hip and the ankle) the articular surfaces appear at first sight to fit very exactly (ie, they appear congruent). However, in other joints (eg, the knee and finger joints) it is readily apparent that the surfaces are quite incongruent. For a long time it was believed that precise fit or congruence was a normal feature of a joint. However, the concept of congruence implies that the joint surfaces are perfectly spherical, which they obviously are not, and therefore no normal joint is congruent.

In many joints, of which the knee is a notable example, the gross incongruencies of the opposed surfaces are partially compensated for by the interposed, pliable intra-articular fibrocartilaginous menisci. [These latter structures constitute an important component contributing to joint shape and cannot be removed without significant consequences (Fig. 9.2).]

Because the tissues of the joint undergo elastic deformation under load (particularly the cartilage but also the bone), as the load increases the surfaces of the joint come into increasing contact, thereby distributing the load equitably (Fig. 9.3). In addition, the incongruence and the deformation of the joint space under load provide for circulation and mixing of the synovial fluid, both of which are essential to the metabolism of the chondrocytes.

• *The Mechanical Properties of the Extracellular Matrices of Bone, Cartilage, and Other Connective Tissues*

The mechanical properties of the connective tissues are determined by the extracellular matrices. In each of the different connective tissues, as well as in each

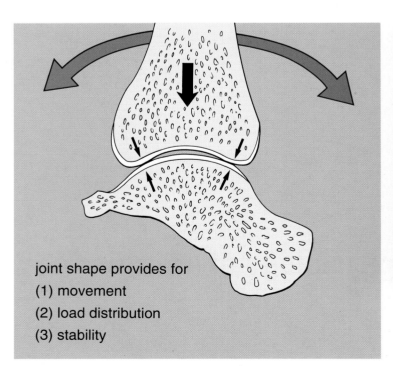

joint shape provides for
(1) movement
(2) load distribution
(3) stability

FIGURE 9.1

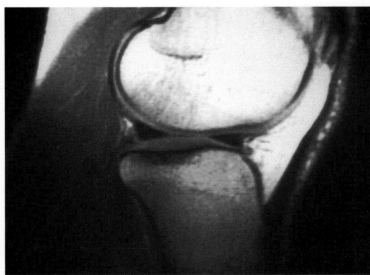

FIGURE 9.2 A lateral MRI of a normal knee shows the gross incongruity of the cartilaginous surfaces partially corrected by the interposed meniscus which acts as a load-bearing structure.

particular structure, the matrices have a unique composition and organization which provide for mechanical function at that locus. Some of this organization has already been discussed in Chapter 1.

Most investigators since William Hunter have recognized the articular cartilage as the key to understanding the mechanism of arthritis. As Hunter noted in 1743, "the articulating cartilages are most happily contrived to all purposes of motion in those parts. By their uniform surface, they move upon one another with ease; by their soft, smooth and slippery surface, mutual abrasion is prevented; by their flexibility, the contiguous surfaces are constantly adapted to each other and the friction diffused equally over the whole; by their elasticity, the violence of any shock, which may happen in running, jumping, etc. is broken and gradually spent; which must have been extremely pernicious, if the hard surfaces of bones had been immediately contiguous." However, as previously mentioned, the joint is an organ system that includes the bone beneath the cartilage, and alterations in the mechanical properties of bone may have equally disastrous effects on joint function as alterations in cartilage properties.

The connective tissue matrices are both synthesized and broken down by their intrinsic cells (eg, osteoblasts, osteocytes, osteoclasts, chondrocytes). In maintaining the physicochemical and mechanical properties of tissues, the function of these cells must be subject to highly sensitive feedback systems which are only now beginning to be understood (Fig. 9.4).

• *The Integrity of the Ligaments, Muscles, and Tendons Supporting the Joint and of Their Neuromuscular Controls*

Functional joint anatomy must include a consideration of the ligamentous conjoining of the articulating surfaces as well as of the neuromuscular control of joint motion. Sensory feedback monitors our movements through the perception of touch, temperature, pain,

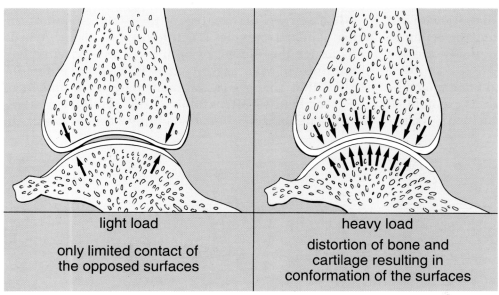

light load

only limited contact of the opposed surfaces

heavy load

distortion of bone and cartilage resulting in conformation of the surfaces

FIGURE 9.3

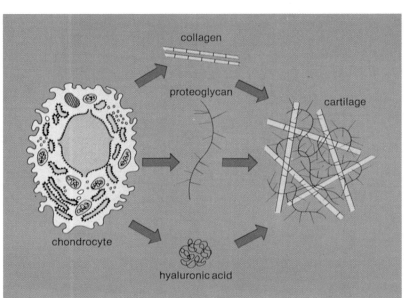

FIGURE 9.4 Diagrammatic representation of a chondrocyte showing its metabolic functions.

and position. During childhood we explore, learn, practice, and perfect skills that will eventually become automatic. The fact that some of us develop better athletic skills than others is perhaps not as dependent on strength and endurance as it is on optimization of the sensory modulation of movement. Correct joint function is thus dependent on intact ligaments and neuromuscular coordination. As recognized by Charcot in the nineteenth century, a breakdown of neuromuscular coordination can lead to profound arthritis (Fig. 9.5).

NORMAL JOINT PHYSIOLOGY

Anatomy is concerned with the structure of living things; physiology, with their normal dynamic phenomena. Wolff's law states that bone density and bone architecture correlate with the magnitude and direction of applied load. In the articular end of a bone, this implies that the subchondral bone trabeculae must also undergo a self-regulated modeling which maintains a joint shape capable of optimal load distribution. In other words, the shape of bones, including the articular ends, reflects a dynamic state that also incorporates a feedback dependent on mechanical stress.

One mechanism for both growth and bone modeling is endochondral ossification. This process is exemplified in the epiphyseal growth plate where calcified cartilage is invaded by blood vessels from the subchondral bone and is replaced by bone tissue synthesized by osteoblasts lying close to the blood vessels (see Chapter 1).

Studies of adult joints have shown that replacement of the calcified layer of articular cartilage by bone tissue involves the same process (Fig. 9.6). Replacement of the calcified layer of cartilage by new bone might be expected to result in thinning and eventual disappearance of the cartilage. However, histologic study of articular cartilage from subjects of various ages shows that this does not happen. Calcified cartilage remains much the same thickness throughout life because the calcification front continues to advance into the noncalcified cartilage at a slow rate which is in equilibrium with the rate of absorption of the calcified cartilage from the subchondral bone. Therefore, it can be postulated that articular cartilage is not a static tissue, as it was long believed to be. The extracellular matrix and the chondrocytes are replaced throughout life, and thus the joint undergoes continuous remodeling (see also Fig.1.43 in Chapter 1).

The extracellular matrix of the cartilage and of the other connective tissues is synthesized by their intrinsic cells under the control of both local and systemic factors. Both in vivo and in vitro studies have demonstrated that changes in the immediate environment of the joint lead to alterations of the cartilage matrix. Thus, immobilization or unloading of a joint results in

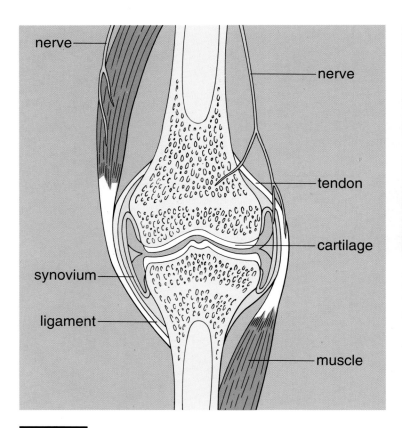

FIGURE 9.5 A joint not only consists of the articular cartilage and synovial lining, but is also a mechanical system which includes all the surrounding ligaments, tendons, sensory and motor nerves, and muscles.

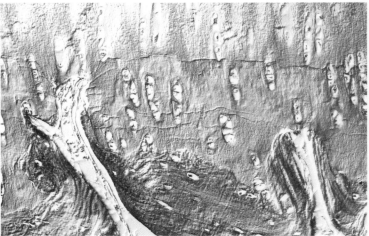

FIGURE 9.6 Photomicrograph demonstrating vascular invasion with subsequent bone formation in the calcified region of normal articular cartilage (H&E, x 10 obj.).

decreased synthesis of glycosaminoglycans (Figs. 9.7 and 9.8). Conversely, exercise appears to increase synthesis. These experimentally induced variations are in agreement with naturally observed topographic variations in joints which have been ascribed to normally occurring patterns of loading that affect the joints. In general, it seems that low levels of mechanical stress (ie, below the physiologic range) are associated with enhanced catabolic activity, whereas stress within the physiologic range is associated with increased anabolic activity. Under conditions of supraphysiologic stress the chondrocytes are unable to adapt. In other words, there is a window of physiologic stress above or below

which the chondrocytes cannot maintain an adequate functional matrix (Fig. 9.9).

Although a number of substances have been implicated in the transduction of mechanical stimuli to metabolic events, the exact mechanism still remain unclear.

THE ARTHRITIC JOINT

Clinical arthritis is the consequence of a breakdown in the joint's normal function which in turn is associated with anatomic and physiologic alterations. These

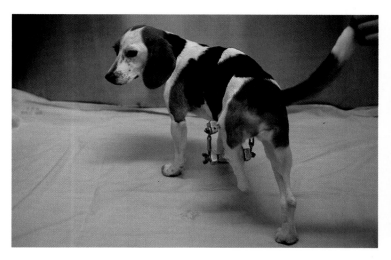

FIGURE 9.7 This dog has had a distraction device placed across the left knee joint to produce unloading of the joint.

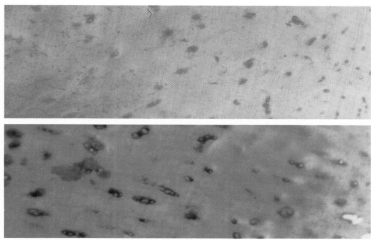

FIGURE 9.8 Photomicrograph of articular cartilage harvested from the unloaded joint shown in Figure 9.7 demonstrating diminished proteoglycan staining *(upper)*. In the lower half of the photograph a portion of normal control cartilage from the right knee is shown for comparison (Alcian blue stain, x 4 obj.).

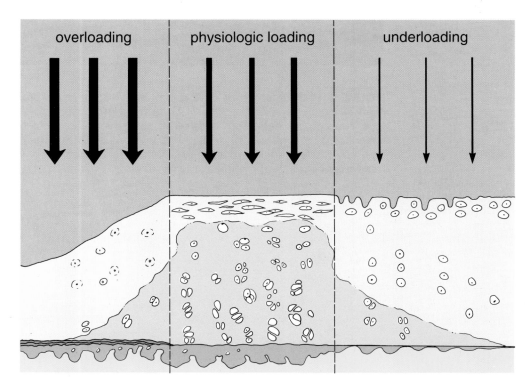

FIGURE 9.9 The continued optimal functional integrity of connective tissue depends on balanced rates of matrix production and breakdown by the cells. Healthy tissue *(center)* results from a physiologic range of stress that maintains optimal cell activity. If this range of stress is exceeded *(left)*, the result is cell injury and eventual necrosis (in cartilage, this is called chondrolysis). If the stress is inadequate *(right)*, disuse atrophy, ie, lack of adequate matrix production by the cells, may occur. In cartilage, this is associated with increased water content and superficial fibrillation of the collagen.

include loss of capacity for the articulating surfaces to move over one another easily, loss of joint stability, and, almost always, pain. The loss of freedom of motion is associated with a change in the tissues which affects their mechanical properties, a change in joint shape which results in severe incongruities, and alterations in ligamentous support and neuromuscular control. Pain may have a variety of sources: it may originate in the bone, as a result of maldistribution of load; from the synovium, as a result of reactive synovitis; or from muscle spasm.

Malfunction of a joint can be caused by acute or chronic injuries that produce either anatomic alterations in the shape of the articulating surfaces, eg, a fracture (Fig. 9.10); loss of integrity of the support structures around the joint, eg, inflammatory destruction of ligaments or capsular tissue; or alterations in the mechanical properties of the tissue matrices making up the joint, eg, ochronosis.

On the basis of their characteristic individual clinical presentations and their morbid anatomy, during the past century several types of arthritis have been well delineated. These include the infectious arthritides,

both granulomatous and pyogenic; metabolic arthritis (eg, gout and ochronosis); and the arthritis that complicates many cases of aseptic subchondral bone necrosis. The various "rheumatic syndromes" have been classified according to their clinical and immunologic characteristics; histologically, these inflammatory arthritides show a destructive pattern but are difficult to differentiate from each other solely by microscopic examination. In some cases, blood chemistry investigations, cell counts, and various immunologic tests may help to indicate the specific etiology.

Even when these various etiologies have been considered, there remain an enormous number of cases of arthritis affecting especially certain small joints of the hands and feet and some larger joints, of which the hip and knee are particularly commonly involved. These cases, which run a chronic course, are essentially noninflammatory and usually occur in older individuals. The clinical presentation and morbid anatomy in these cases are similar enough for all of them to be classified under the general appellation of osteoarthritis. In the majority of cases the etiology is at best unclear.

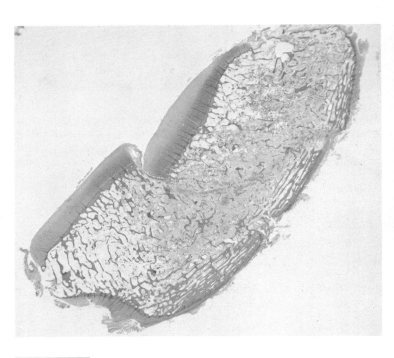

FIGURE 9.10 A section through a patella which has sustained a transarticular fracture. Such a change in the contour of an articular surface will lead rapidly to degenerative arthritic changes (H&E, x 1 obj.).

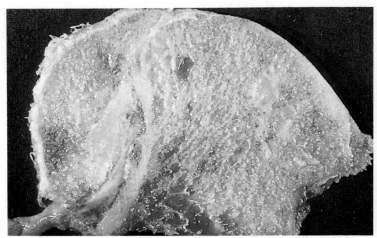

FIGURE 9.11 Photograph of a slice through an arthritic femoral head in which, despite the loss of bone from the superior surface, the contour has been restored to something approaching sphericity by a large medial osteophyte, which is seen to extend well down the medial femoral neck. Note also the increase in transverse diameter of the head, a typical finding in osteoarthritis.

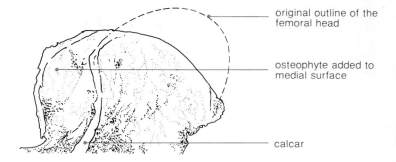

original outline of the femoral head

osteophyte added to medial surface

calcar

MORBID ANATOMY

Shape

A change in joint shape, resulting from cartilage and bone loss, is characteristic of most forms of arthritis. In osteoarthritis, however, although bone and cartilage loss play an important part in the process, it is the addition of new bone and cartilage in the form of osteophytes, particularly at the joint periphery and sometimes beneath the articular surface, that forms one of the characteristic features of the disease (Fig. 9.11).

Tissue

Before describing the gross and microscopic findings in the cartilage, bone, and synovial tissues of arthritic joints, it is necessary to preface these descriptions with some general remarks.

Regardless of the cause, joint injury is characterized by certain basic cellular and tissue responses. There is usually macroscopic and microscopic evidence of both degeneration and repair. There are alterations both in the cells and in the extracellular matrix. (Those in the extracellular matrix may result from direct physical injury, from alteration in the cellular synthesis of the matrix, or from its enzymatic breakdown.)

In the vascularized tissues, injury is followed by an acute and then by a chronic inflammatory response. As a result, the necrotic injured tissue is removed and replaced by proliferative vascular tissue (granulation tissue). The inflammatory response results in "repair" of injured tissue by fibrous scar. Independently of scarring, a second mode of repair involves regeneration of tissue similar to that which was injured originally.

In nonvascularized tissue, such as cartilage, an inflammatory response and subsequent scarring cannot occur, but this does not preclude tissue regeneration. (Note that joint injury always invokes an inflammatory response, since some vascularized tissues, ie, bone and/or synovium, are inevitably involved.)

Cartilage Injury and Repair

Gross evidence of injury to cartilage is evident only in the extracellular cartilage matrix, mainly the collagenous component. One of the earliest findings is a disruption of the surface which, instead of having the normal smooth appearance of articular cartilage, becomes rough and/or eroded.

Three patterns of macroscopic alteration involving the cartilage surface and to a variable degree, the underlying cartilage tissue, have been identified: fibrillation, erosion (ulceration) and cracking.

The term fibrillation is used to describe replacement of the normally smooth, shiny surface by a surface similar to cut velvet (Fig. 9.12). This type of transformation can be observed both on very thick cartilage, such as the patella, and on very thin cartilage, such as that found in the interphalangeal joints. The "pile" of the fibrillated area may be short or shaggy. The junction between the fibrillated area and the adjacent normal appearing cartilage is usually well defined and generally distinct.

There appear to be two patterns of fibrillation. Well-defined areas of fibrillation affect particular locations in certain joints and are present in everyone from an early age. It is suggested that these areas may be related to underloading of the cartilage. In osteoarthritic joints there are areas of fibrillation which appear in different areas of the joint than those previously alluded to, and which appear to be secondary to prior erosion of the cartilage surface. The microscopic characterization of these two distinct types of fibrillation is incomplete, but perhaps the latter is distinguished by deeper clefts and a greater tendency to form cartilage clones (see below).

Cartilage erosion, or solution of the surface, is

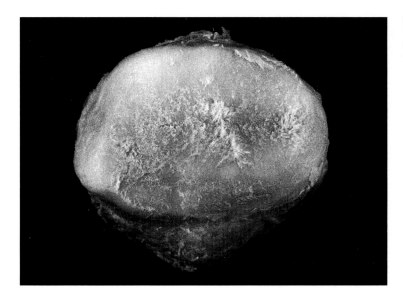

FIGURE 9.12 Photograph of the articular surface of a patella obtained from a young individual at autopsy shows fibrillation of the superficial cartilage (photographed using ultraviolet light).

characteristic of progressive degenerative changes in the joint. The base of the erosion appears initially to be either contoured or smooth (Fig. 9.13). Tissue damage may eventually be so extensive as to completely denude the bone surface of its cartilage cover (eburnation).

The last form of structural lesion in this group, which is distinctly less common than either fibrillation or ulceration, is cracking of the cartilage. These cracks extend vertically deep into the cartilage and microscopically often have a deep horizontal component (Figs. 9.14 and 9.15).

In considering the pathogenesis of these three histologic types of cartilage matrix damage, it is important to recognize that in the early stages of osteoarthritis, more often than not they affect only one of the opposed articular surfaces (Figs. 9.16 and 9.17). This is in marked contrast to eburnation, in which both of the opposed surfaces are affected. It therefore appears that in many cases fibrillation and other cartilage alterations cannot be ascribed simply to abrasion.

An increase in the ratio of water to the proteoglycan in the cartilage matrix leads to softening of the cartilage (chondromalacia) (Figs. 9.18 and 9.19). Chondromalacia and fibrillation usually occur together, but chondromalacia may be present before there is any evidence of fibrillation.

Injury at a cellular level may be recognizable only under a microscope. Necrosis can be identified when only the ghost outlines of the chondrocytes remain. This ghosting, usually scattered but focal in distribution, is a common finding in arthritis (Fig. 9.20). Less often, all of

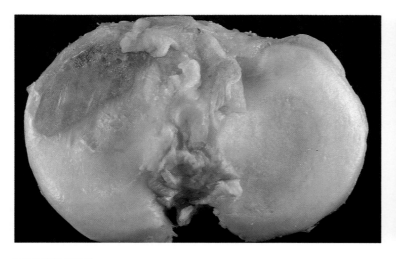

FIGURE 9.13 Photograph of a tibial plateau demonstrates deep cartilage erosion with exposed subchondral bone.

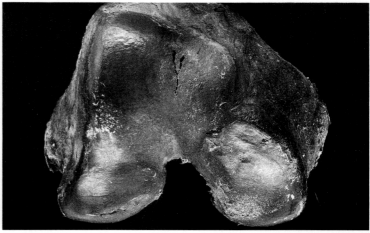

FIGURE 9.14 Photograph of the femoral articulation of the knee shows cracking of the cartilage in the patello–femoral joint (photographed using ultraviolet light).

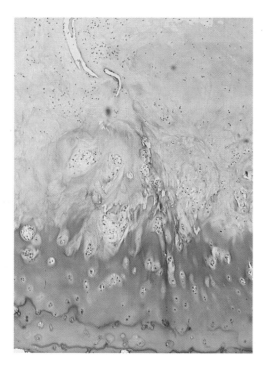

FIGURE 9.15 Photomicrograph of a section taken through a crack in the articular surface, showing the defect extending deep into the cartilage with focal degenerative changes in the surrounding tissue (H&E, x 4 obj.).

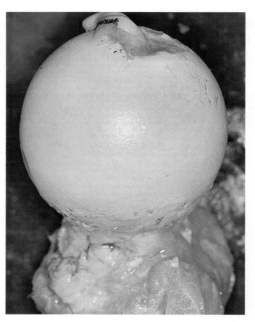

FIGURE 9.16 Photograph of the superior surface of the right femoral head removed from an 86-year-old male. Note the smooth, intact articular surface. This should be compared with Figure 9.17.

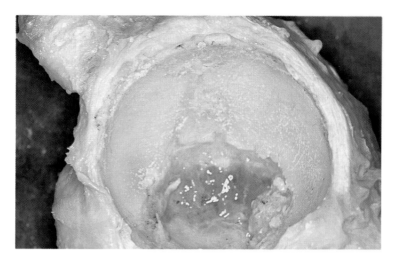

FIGURE 9.17 The acetabulum of the hip joint shown in Figure 9.16 demonstrates superficial erosion and fibrillation of the articular cartilage in the superolateral portion. Degenerative changes in this portion of the acetabulum are present in all adults, probably as a result of disuse atrophy.

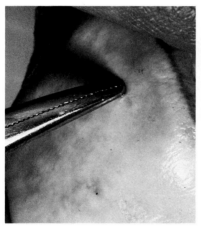 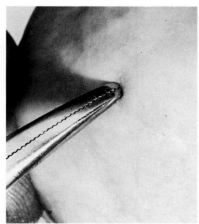

FIGURE 9.18 *(left)* Normal cartilage is firm but resilient and can be compressed with some degree of pressure (exerted here by a hemostat). However, as the cartilage softens or becomes chondromalacic it also becomes palpably softer *(right)*.

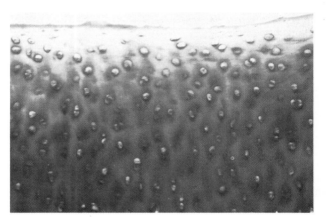 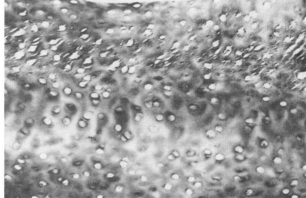

FIGURE 9.19
Intense staining of proteoglycan is seen in this photomicrograph of normal cartilage *(left)*. However, in chondromalacic cartilage, proteoglycan loss in the matrix is seen by the decreased intensity of staining *(right)* (Safranin O, x 10 obj.)

FIGURE 9.20 Photomicrograph demonstrates areas of cartilage with no chondrocytes, a consequence of focal cell necrosis (H&E, x 10 obj.).

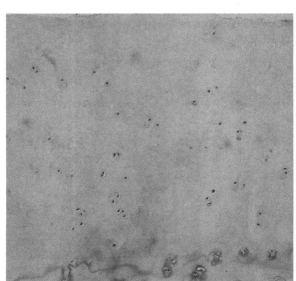 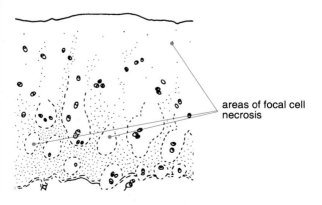

areas of focal cell necrosis

the chondrocytes are seen to be necrotic (Fig. 9.21).

Just as the effect of injury to the articular cartilage is reflected by the histologic response of both matrix and cells, so too is the effect of subsequent cartilage regeneration. In the cellular component, one sees microscopic evidence of focal cell proliferation and clumps, or clones, of chondrocytes (Fig. 9.22). There is often intense metachromasia around these clumps of proliferating chondrocytes when the tissue is stained with toluidine blue. This response is evidence of increased proteoglycan synthesis.

In a damaged joint, repair of cartilage may be initiated from either or both of two possible sites. It may come from the damaged cartilage itself, in which case

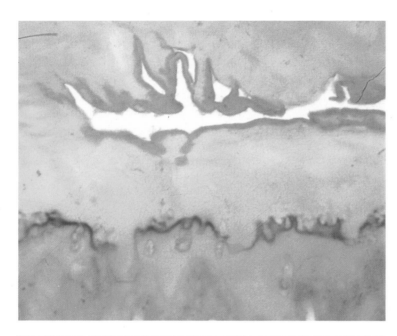

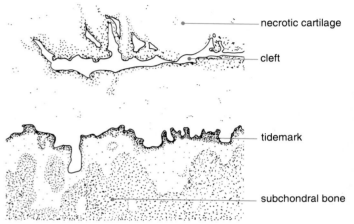

FIGURE 9.21 Photomicrograph demonstrates total cartilage necrosis. Note also the horizontal cleft resulting from failure of the cartilage matrix to resist shear forces within its substance (H&E, x 25 obj.).

FIGURE 9.22 Photomicrograph of a portion of degenerate cartilage demonstrates a large nest of proliferating chondrocytes in the deep zone (H&E, x 10 obj.).

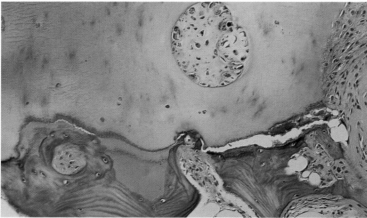

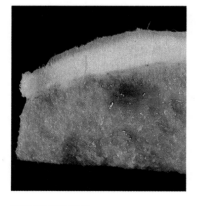
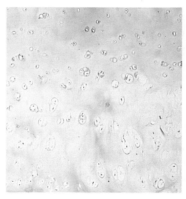
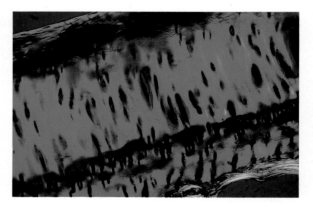

FIGURE 9.23 Gross specimen *(left)* demonstrates intrinsic cartilage repair, as evidenced by a white, wedge-shaped opaque area between the normal surface and the normal deeper cartilage. Photomicrograph of this area *(center)* shows proliferating cells, cell clumping, and disarrayed collagen. Under polarized light *(right)*, one can more easily see the disarrayed collagen in the central area of the cartilage (x 4 obj.).

the repair takes the form of cell proliferation and synthesis of new matrix, as already discussed. This process can be thought of as "intrinsic" repair. Extrinsic cartilage repair may originate either in the joint margin or in the subchondral bone. Extrinsic repair of cartilage, which develops from the joint margin, can be seen as a cellular layer of cartilage extending over, and sometimes dissecting into, the existing cartilage (Fig. 9.23). This extrinsically repaired cartilage is usually much more cellular than the preexisting articular cartilage, and the chondrocytes are evenly distributed throughout the matrix (Fig. 9.24). On microscopic examination this type of repair cartilage can easily be overlooked. However, examination under polarized light will clearly demonstrate the discontinuity between the collagen network of the repair cartilage and that of the preexisting cartilage. Many cases of arthritis reveal both intrinsic and extrinsic repair of cartilage (Fig. 9.25).

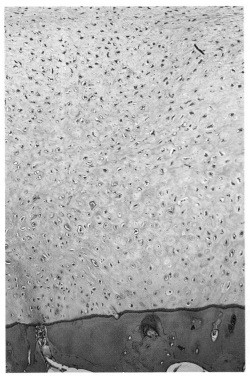
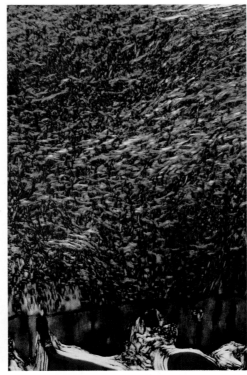

FIGURE 9.24 *(left)* A section through the articular surface of an arthritic joint demonstrates extrinsic reparative fibrocartilage, which extends to the tidemark of the original articular hyaline cartilage (H&E, x 4 obj.). *(right)* The same field photographed with polarized light shows the discontinuity of the collagen between the calcified zone and the reparative cartilage above.

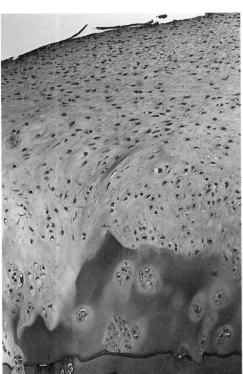
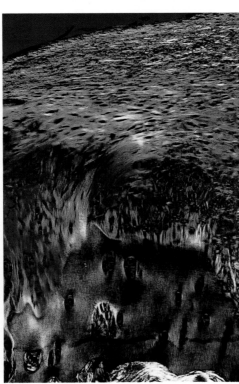

FIGURE 9.25 *(left)* Photomicrograph of a section through the articular surface of an arthritic joint demonstrates extensive fibrocartilaginous repair overlying residual hyaline cartilage (H&E, x 4 obj.). *(right)* The same field photographed with polarized light.

In arthritic joints in which loss of the articular cartilage has denuded the underlying bone, and especially in cases of osteoarthritis, there are frequently small pits in the bone surface, from which protrude small nodules of firm white tissue (Fig. 9.26). On microscopic examination these nodules have the appearance of fibrocartilage and arise in the marrow spaces of the subchondral bone (Fig. 9.27). They may extend over the previously denuded surface to form a more or less continuous layer of repair tissue (Figs. 9.28 and 9.29).

INJURY AND REPAIR OF BONE

Arthritis is a disease that affects not only the articular cartilage but also the underlying bone and the structures around the joint.

As the articular cartilage is eroded from the articular surface, the underlying bone is subjected to increasingly localized overloading. In subarticular bone that has been thus denuded, there is proliferation of osteoblasts and formation of new bone (Fig. 9.30), which occurs both on

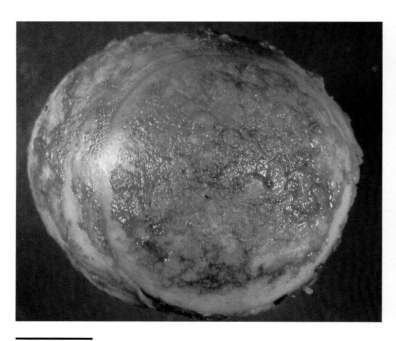

FIGURE 9.26 Gross photograph of the femoral head removed from a patient with advanced osteoarthritis. Most of the superlateral surface of the femoral head is with an irregular layer of tissue, which seems to be growing in the form of small tufts from many focal areas in the bone.

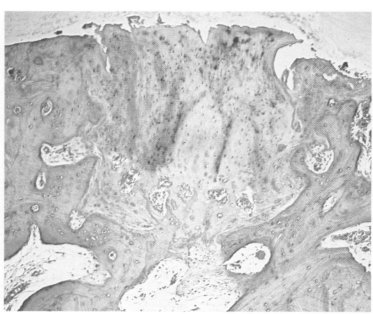

FIGURE 9.27 Photomicrograph of one of the tufts shown in Figure 9.26. The tuft is formed of fibrocartilaginous tissue extending from the marrow onto the joint surface. On either side is eburnated bone (H&E, x 10 obj.).

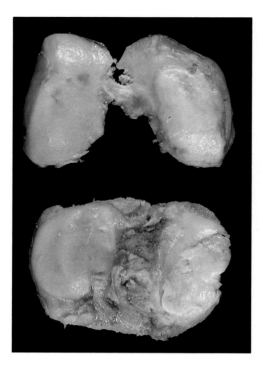

FIGURE 9.28 Photograph of a knee joint showing a layer of reparative cartilage covering most of the femoral condyle and the apposed tibial plateau. In some cases of osteoarthritis treated by osteotomy, and even in untreated cases, the damaged joint surfaces may be entirely recovered by a layer of fibrocartilaginous tissue, as seen in this example.

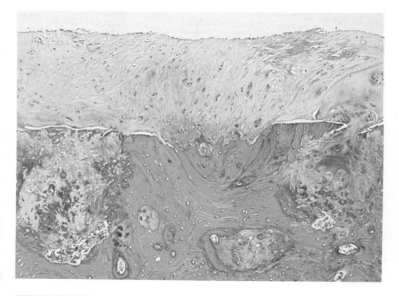

FIGURE 9.29 Photomicrograph of the fibrocartilage seen in Figure 9.28 reveals extension of cartilaginous tissue over the previously eburnated bone, presumably derived from the underlying subchondral bone (H&E, x 4 obj.).

the surfaces of existing intact trabeculae and around microfractures. In x-rays of arthritic joints, this new bone may appear as increased density or sclerosis.

A further result of increased local stress is that the surface bone is likely to undergo focal pressure necrosis (Fig. 9.31). [This superficial necrosis is different from that associated with "primary" subchondral avascular necrosis, which may of its own accord lead to sec-

ondary osteoarthritis, both in its etiology and pathogenesis. However, in clinical practice differentiation between the two may be difficult, especially in the late stages of primary subchondral avascular necrosis. (see Chapter 10).]

Subarticular cysts are usually seen only where the overlying cartilage is absent (Figs. 9.32 and 9.33). Such cysts are common in cases of osteoarthritis and are be-

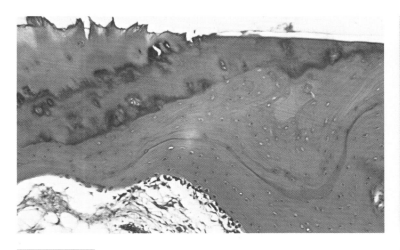

FIGURE 9.30 Photomicrograph shows increased osteoblastic activity and trabecular thickening underlying an area of cartilage erosion. (Section taken from the edge of a denuded and eburnated area) (H&E, x 10 obj.).

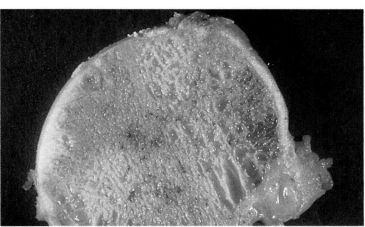

FIGURE 9.31 A portion of the eburnated surface of an osteoarthritic joint demonstrates focal superficial bone and bone marrow necrosis, which is seen macroscopically as an opaque yellow area.

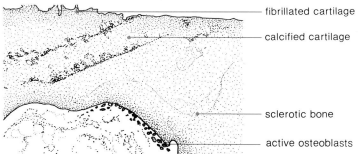

fibrillated cartilage

calcified cartilage

sclerotic bone

active osteoblasts

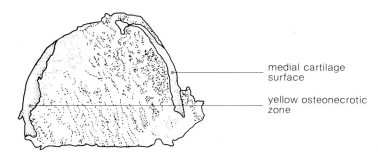

medial cartilage surface

yellow osteonecrotic zone

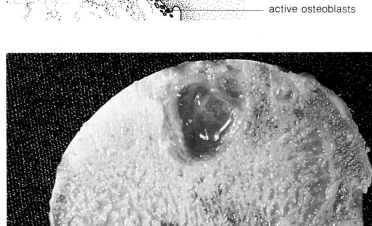

FIGURE 9.32 An area of cystic deneration in the subchondral bone of the superior surface of a femoral head. Such cysts are usually seen only in the absence of the overlying articular cartilage. Note the large, flat osteophyte on the medial surface.

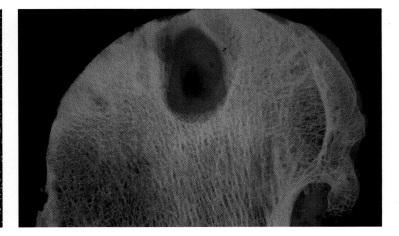

FIGURE 9.33 A radiograph of the specimen shown in Figure 9.32.

lieved to result from transmission of interarticular pressure through defects in the articulating bony surface into the marrow spaces of the subchondral bone (Fig. 9.34). The cysts increase in size until the pressure within them is equal to the intra-articular pressure. Cysts may also occur because of focal tissue necrosis. In cases of arthritis due to rheumatoid disease or gout, periarticular radiologic "cysts" may be associated with erosion of the marginal subchondral bone by the diseased synovium.

Separated fragments of bone and cartilage from a damaged joint surface may become incorporated into the synovial membrane and digested, or may remain free as loose bodies in the joint cavity (Fig. 9.35).

Under certain circumstances, proliferation of cartilage cells occurs on the surface of these loose bodies and consequently they grow larger (Fig. 9.36). As they grow, their centers become necrotic and calcified. In histologic sections it is possible to visualize periodic extension of this central calcification in the form of concentric rings which increase in number as the loose body grows larger (Fig. 9.37). Sometimes the bodies reattach to the synovial membrane, in which case they are invaded by blood vessels. Endochondral ossification then occurs and the loose bodies become bony (Figs. 9.38 and 9.39).

There is some degree of loose body formation in many cases of arthritis. Occasionally, in cases of os-

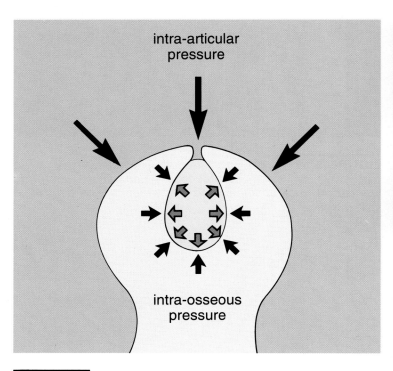

FIGURE 9.34 With the intrusion of synovial fluid into the subchondral bone the bone becomes resorbed, and a cyst is formed which will increase in size until the intra-osseous pressure is equal to the intra-articular pressure.

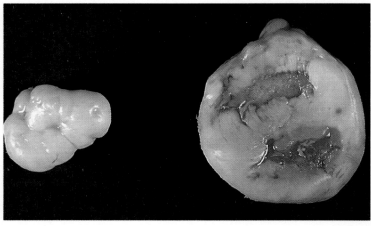

FIGURE 9.35 Traumatic arthritis of the elbow. A loose body (left) has arisen from the portion of the articular surface that is missing from the radial head (right).

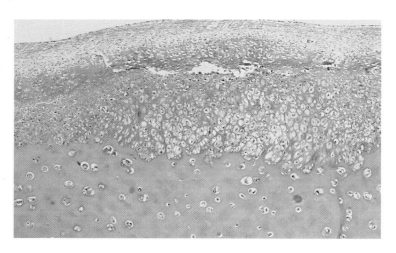

FIGURE 9.36 Photomicrograph shows the proliferation of immature cellular cartilage on the surface of a loose body; the original cartilage is seen in the lower part of the picture. Through this process of cartilage cell proliferation, loose bodies may grow to an enormous size (H&E, x 4 obj.).

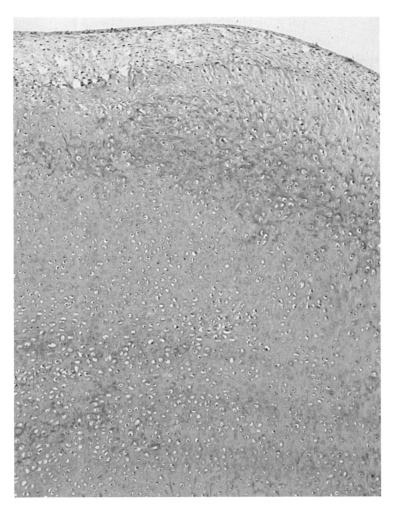

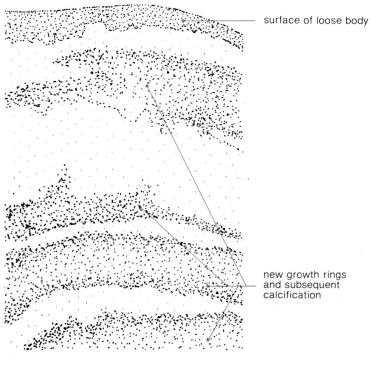

FIGURE 9.37 Photomicrograph of a section through a loose body. One can discern the concentric rings of growth. The tissue towards the center of the loose body is calcified (H&E, x 4 obj.).

surface of loose body

new growth rings and subsequent calcification

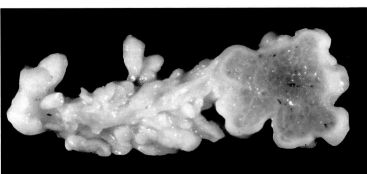

FIGURE 9.38 The photograph shows a loose body (right) that has become attached to the synovium (left). The specimen has been bisected and shows a viable osseous center which has resulted from vascular invasion and endochondral ossification of the cartilaginous loose body.

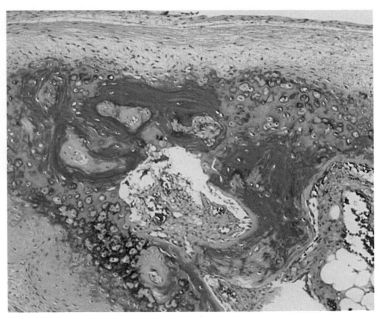

FIGURE 9.39 Photomicrograph of a portion of the loose body shown in Figure 9.38 demonstrates formation of the osseous core by the process of endochondral ossification (H&E, x 10 obj.).

teoarthritis, the loose bodies are so numerous that they must be distinguished from those that occur in primary synovial chondromatosis (Fig. 9.40) (see Chapter 16).

Ligaments

Microscopic evidence both of lacerations and of repair by scar tissue is common in the ligamentous and capsular tissue around an arthritic joint. Whether these preceded the arthritic process or whether they are a consequence of it cannot usually be determined by microscopic examination.

Injury of the Synovial Membrane

Even when cases of arthritis in which the disease is primary in the synovium have been excluded, microscopic examination of the synovium still demonstrates some degree of synovitis.

Injury and breakdown of cartilage and bone result in increased amounts of breakdown product and particulate debris within the joint cavity. The debris is removed from the synovial fluid by phagocytic cells (the "A" cells) of the synovial membrane. In consequence, the membrane becomes both hypertrophic and hyperplastic (Fig. 9.41). In addition, the breakdown prod-

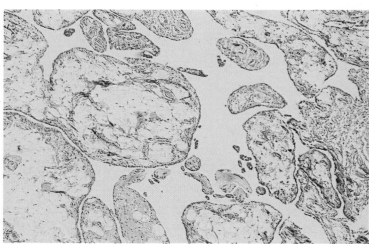

FIGURE 9.41 Photomicrograph of proliferative synovium from a patient with osteoarthritis (H&E, x 4 obj.).

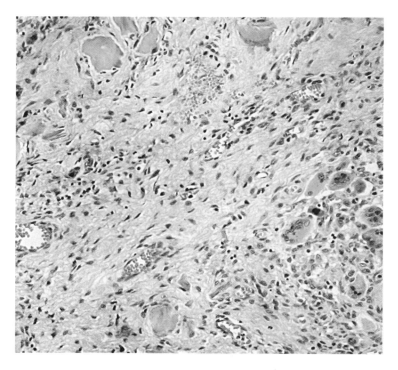

FIGURE 9.40 Photograph of multiple osteocartilaginous loose bodies removed from an osteoarthritic hip joint. This large number of loose bodies is uncommon and may be mistaken for synovial chondromatosis.

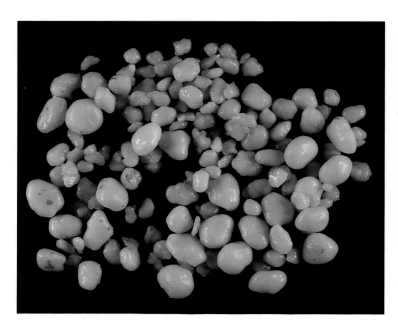

FIGURE 9.42 Photomicrograph of the synovium from a patient with rapidly destructive joint disease. Fragments of bone and cartilage, as well as foci of histiocytes and phagocytic giant cells, are present (H&E, x 25 obj.).

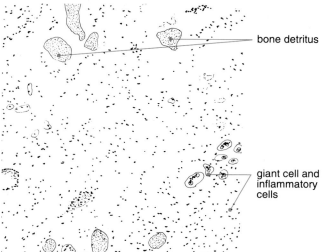

bone detritus

giant cell and inflammatory cells

ucts of cartilage and bone matrix evoke an inflammatory response. For this reason some degree of chronic inflammation can be expected in the synovial membrane of the arthritic joints, even when the injury has been purely a mechanical one. Inflammation is especially prominent where there has been rapid breakdown of the articular components as evidenced by the presence in the synovium of bone and cartilage detritus (Fig. 9.42). Histologic studies have shown that there may be a similarity between the degree of inflammatory response as seen in some cases of severe osteoarthritis and that of rheumatoid arthritis. However, in osteoarthritis the synovial inflammation is likely to be the result of cartilage breakdown, whereas in rheumatoid arthritis the synovial inflammation is the cause of the cartilage breakdown.

Extension of the hyperplastic synovium onto the articular surface of the joint (ie, a pannus) is a common finding even in osteoarthritis, particularly in the hip. However, the extent and the aggressiveness of this pannus with respect to underlying cartilage destruction is much less marked in osteoarthritis than in rheumatoid arthritis (Fig. 9.43).

Under normal conditions, the synovial membrane is responsible for the nutrition of articular cartilage. In this regard, it might be expected that the chronically inflamed and scarred synovial membrane of an arthritic joint would function less effectively than that of a normal joint. Disturbance in synovial nutrient function, as well as increased enzymatic activity, may contribute to the chronicity of the arthritic process. The hypertro-

phied and hyperplastic synovium is also likely to be traumatized as it extends into the joint cavity. Evidence of bleeding into the joint, with subsequent hemosiderin staining of the synovial membrane, is a common histologic finding and may occasionally be marked. When this is the case, and despite their similar color, the orange-brown staining of the fine villous synovium seen at operation should not be confused with the swollen papillary synovium of pigmented villonodular synovitis (Fig. 9.44).

The Synovial Fluid in an Injured Joint

Normal synovial fluid, a dialysate of plasma to which hyaluronic acid produced by the "B" cells of the synovial lining is added, is viscous, pale yellow, and clear. Even in large joints the volume is small.

Examination of synovial fluid is extremely helpful in the diagnosis of arthritis for determining both the cause and the stage of the disease. Whatever the cause of arthritis, the synovial fluid is altered (Figs. 9.45 through 9.47).

In cases of inflammatory arthritis there is an increased volume of synovial fluid while the amount of hyaluronic acid is markedly diminished. This leads to a typical decrease in viscosity. However, in degenerate forms of arthritis the amount of hyaluronic acid is increased, resulting in an extremely viscous fluid. Often there is also an increase in volume, although not to the same degree as that which is seen in the inflammatory arthritides.

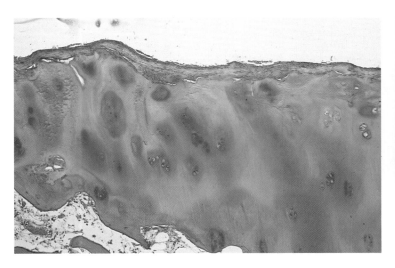

FIGURE 9.43 Photomicrograph of a portion of the articular surface of a femoral head in a case of osteoarthritis, demonstrating a fibrous pannus extending over the articular surface (H&E, x 4 obj.).

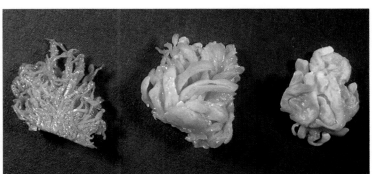

FIGURE 9.44 Hemophilia (left), pigmented villonodular synovitis (center), and rheumatoid arthritis (right). In this photograph the synovial membranes from individuals with three different conditions are compared. In patients with hemophilia, the hemosiderin staining of the synovium results from excessive bleeding into the joint, but in individuals affected by the other two conditions, the hemosiderin staining is probably secondary to trauma to the hypertrophic synovium. The plump papillary appearance of the synovium in pigmented villonodular synovitis (PVNS) and rheumatoid arthritis (RA), as opposed to the villous appearance of the synovium in hemophilia, reflects the considerable cellular infiltration of the subsynovium in patients with PVNS or RA.

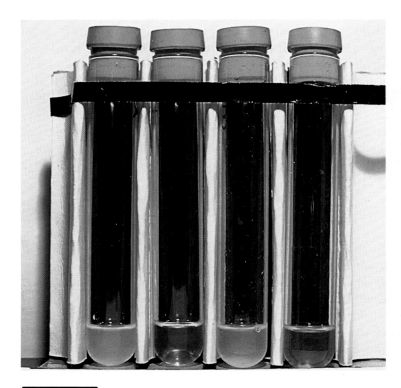

FIGURE 9.45 The examination of synovial fluid can provide valuable information concerning the etiology of a patient's condition. Samples of synovial fluid from four patients (from left to right):
  Chondrocalcinocic—cloudy white fluid
  Normal—clear white/amber fluid
  Rheumatoid arthritis—cloudy yellow fluid
  Traumatic arthritis—clear blood-stained fluid

FIGURE 9.46

NORMAL SYNOVIAL FLUID

PHYSICAL DATA	AVERAGE	RANGE
Amount in knee (ml)	1.1	0.13–3.5
Specific gravity (20°C)		1.0081–1.015
Viscosity (37°C) relative to water	235	5.7–1160
Cell count per mm³	63	13–180
Differential %		
Lymphocytes	24.6	0–78
Monocytes	47.9	0–71
Polymorphonuclear leukocytes	6.5	0–25
Macrophages	10.1	0–26
Synovial lining cells	4.3	0–12
pH	7.434	7.31–7.74

INORGANIC SUBSTANCES

Electrolytes (Na, K, Cl, CO_2)	Approximately the same as plasma
Calcium, phosphate, sulfate	Approximately the same as plasma

ORGANIC SUBSTANCES

Hyaluronic acid (mg/ml)	4.0	
Nonprotein nitrogen		Approximately the same as plasma
Glucose		Approximately the same as plasma
Total lipid (mg/ml)	0.2	
Mucin nitrogen (mg/ml)	1.04	0.68–1.35
Mucin glucosamine (mg/mg)	0.74	0.12–1.32
Uric Acid		Approximately the same as plasma

Source: Paget S, Bullough PG: Synovium and synovial fluid. In Owen R et al. (eds.) Scientific Foundations of Orthopaedics and Traumatology. Saunders, Philadelphia, 1980.

FIGURE 9.47

EXAMINATION OF SYNOVIAL FLUID

	CONDITION			
	Normal	**Noninflammatory**	**Chronic Inflammatory**	**Septic**
Clinical example		Osteoarthrosis	Rheumatoid arthritis	Bacterial infection
Cartilage debris	0	+	0	0
Volume (ml) (knee)	<3.5	>3.5	>3.5	>3.5
Color	Clear	Clear yellow	Opalescent yellow	Turbid yellow to green
Viscosity	High	High	Low	Low
WBCs per mm^3	200	200–2000	2000–100,000	>100,000
Polymorphonuclear leukocytes (%)	<25	<25	50% or more	75% or more
Culture	Negative	Negative	Negative	Positive
Mucin clot	Firm	Firm	Friable	Friable
Fibrin Clot	None	Small	Large	Large
Glucose (% of blood glucose)	~100	~100	75, may be less than 50	50
Total protein		Equal to normal joint	Elevated	Elevated

Source: Paget S, Bullough PG: Synovium and synovial fluid. In Owen R et al. (eds.) Scientific Foundations of Orthopaedics and Traumatology, Saunders, Philadelphia, 1980.

CHAPTER 10

The noninflammatory arthritides

The noninflammatory arthritides are certainly the most commonly encountered form of arthritis in the Western world, and osteoarthritis is the most commonly encountered condition in orthopedic practice. The other form of arthritis discussed in this chapter, that following subchondral bone infarction, is also common although often overlooked clinically.

OSTEOARTHRITIS (DEGENERATIVE JOINT DISEASE)

CLINICAL CONSIDERATIONS

There is as yet no generally accepted definition of osteoarthritis, but for the purposes of this discussion the following definition is offered: "Osteoarthritis is a functional disorder of joints, characterized by altered joint anatomy, especially by the loss of articular cartilage. Unlike many other forms of arthritis, it is essen-tially noninflammatory."

There are four generally recognized patterns of clinical presentation. The first three of these include osteoarthritis presenting as disease limited to a single large joint, usually the knee or hip, sometimes with bilateral involvement (Fig. 10.1); a generalized process involving the distal and proximal interphalangeal joints of the hand, the first carpometacarpal joint, knees, hips and metatarsophalangeal joints (Fig. 10.2); and extreme cases of osteoarthritis seen in association with a neurologic deficit (known as Charcot's joints.) The underlying neurologic disorder in the latter may be peripheral neuropathy in association with pernicious anemia and diabetes mellitus, spinal cord degeneration as in tabes dorsalis, or syringomyelia. In these patients one characteristically observes a rapidly destructive osteoarthritis, complicated by the production of multiple loose bodies, severe subluxation, and even dislocation of the joint (Figs. 10.3 to 10.5). The fourth pattern, which is much more rare, is that of an erosive inflam-

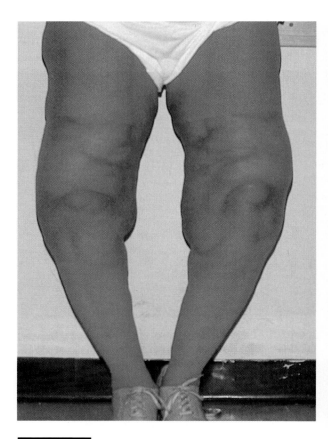

FIGURE 10.1 The obese patient above has a marked genu varus deformity of both knees associated with severe bilateral osteoarthritis.

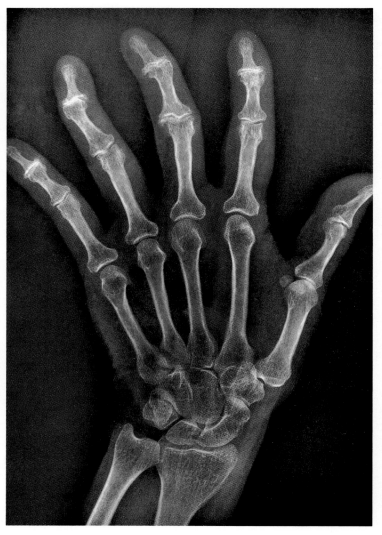

FIGURE 10.2 Radiograph of a patient with primary generalized osteoarthritis shows the characteristic wavy appearance of the third and fourth digits. Irregular erosions at the articular surfaces usually affect the ulnar aspect of the joint.

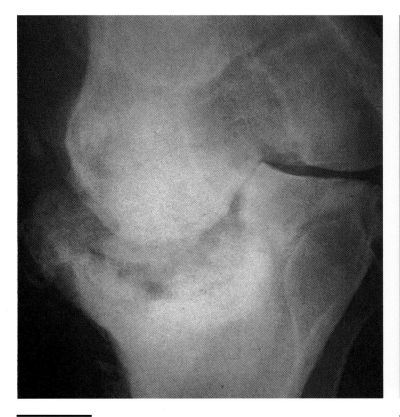

FIGURE 10.3 Radiograph of the knee in a patient with diabetes and a history of pernicious anemia. The patient presented with grossly deformed and unstable knees; however, the condition was painless. Note extensive destruction of the medial compartment of the knee and the multiple loose bodies.

FIGURE 10.4 Coronal section through a grossly deranged knee joint (Charcot's joint). Subluxation and severe destruction of the joint surfaces are evident. The synovium is markedly hypertrophic and hyperplastic.

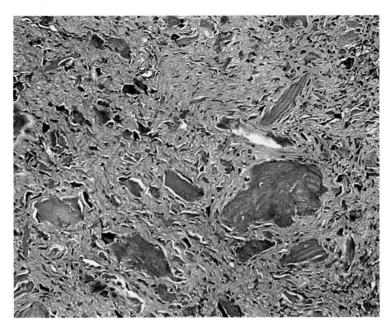

FIGURE 10.5 Photomicrograph of a portion of the synovium in a Charcot's joint. The scarred and chronically inflamed synovium is filled with multiple irregular fragments of bone and cartilage. The finding of bone and cartilage detritus in the synovial membrane usually denotes a rapid breakdown of the joint. In patients with osteoarthritis it is rare to find any significant degree of detritus (phloxine and tatrazine, x 10 obj.).

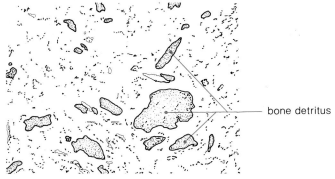

bone detritus

matory osteoarthritis which usually affects the distal or proximal interphalangeal joints of the hand (Fig. 10.6) but may occasionally involve large joints (Fig. 10.7).

A patient with clinical osteoarthritis typically presents with complaints of pain and usually of stiffness. On examination, movement of the affected joint may be limited, and the patient often lacks the capability for full flexion or extension. The most characteristic radiologic finding in patients with osteoarthritis is loss of the joint space. In the majority of patients, bony osteophytes are also seen around the periphery of the joint. The bone on both sides of the joint exhibits increased density, and cystic lesions can frequently be noted in the subchondral bone.

PATHOLOGIC FINDINGS

In examination of a joint removed at surgery or autopsy, the most significant features of an osteoarthritic joint are alterations in the shape of the articular surfaces and damaged cartilage. In the weight-bearing areas of the joint the cartilage may be entirely absent, and the exposed subchondral bone has a dense, polished appearance like that of marble (eburnation) (Fig. 10.8).

When the affected joint in the areas without cartilage is sectioned, the bone usually appears markedly thickened (sclerotic); adjacent to the surface, cystic defects filled with loose fibromyxoid tissue (or sometimes with a thick fluid) may be found (Fig. 10.9). The superficial bone in the eburnated areas may be necrotic. In areas of the joint that do not bear weight, and around its margins, bony and cartilaginous overgrowths (osteophytes or exostoses) develop.

In each joint the location of the osteophytes is characteristic. In the distal interphalangeal joints the osteophytes (Heberden's nodes) are prominent on the dorsal and palmar aspects of both articulating surfaces. In the metatarsophalangeal joint of the big toe, the osteophyte is on the medial joint margin (hallux valgus) (Fig. 10.10). In the hip joint, although osteophytes are usually present around the entire joint margin, there is characteristically a large flat osteophyte on the medial articular surface, extending to the fovea (Figs. 10.11 and 10.12). Despite the loss of bone and cartilage in some parts of the joint, which is assumed to be the result of overloading and mechanical abrasion, the net ef-

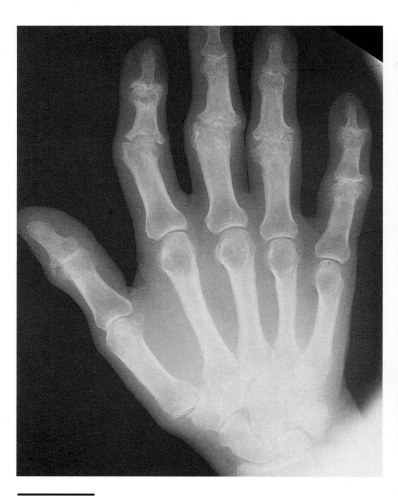

FIGURE 10.6 Radiograph of the hand of a 45-year-old woman with erosive osteoarthritis, showing the typical involvement of the proximal and distal interphalangeal joints.

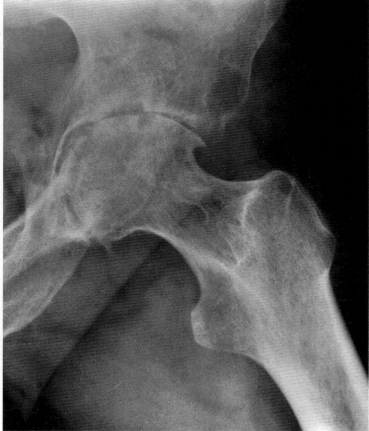

FIGURE 10.7 Radiograph of the hip of a 55-year-old woman with recent complaints of pain and stiffness, showing concentric narrowing of the joint space and erosive changes in both the femoral head and acetabulum. Testing for rheumatoid factor was negative in this case, which was clinically diagnosed as erosive osteoarthritis.

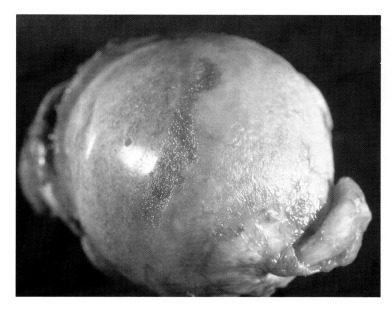

FIGURE 10.8 Gross photograph of the femoral head removed from a patient with osteoarthritis. Note the absence of the articular cartilage on the superior and lateral aspect of the femoral head, and the polished appearance of the exposed bone (eburnation). The remaining surrounding cartilage has a somewhat yellow color and a roughened surface.

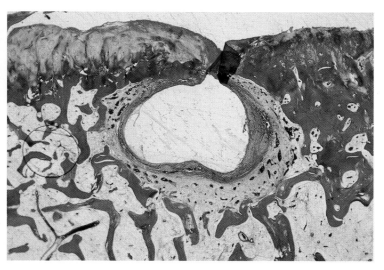

FIGURE 10.9 Photomicrograph of a portion of the articular surface in an osteoarthritic joint, showing focal absence of the articular cartilage. An underlying cyst connects via a short neck with the joint space (phloxine and tartrazine, x 2.5 obj.).

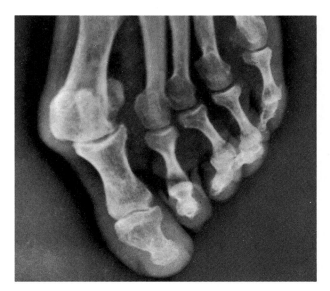

FIGURE 10.10 Hallux valgus deformity. Radiograph of the foot shows marked angulation of the first phalanx. Note the bone hypertrophy of the medial aspect of the head of the first metatarsal bone.

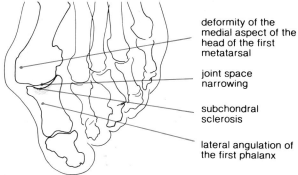

deformity of the medial aspect of the head of the first metatarsal

joint space narrowing

subchondral sclerosis

lateral angulation of the first phalanx

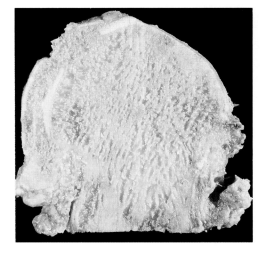

FIGURE 10.11 A large, flat, medial osteophyte associated with subluxation of the femoral head in a patient with osteoarthritis of the hip. The osteophyte extends from the joint margin to the region of the fovea. The residual cartilage of the medial surface of the femoral head can still be seen.

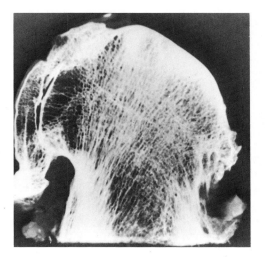

FIGURE 10.12 Radiograph of the tissue slice shown in Figure 10.11 again illustrates the large medial osteophyte. Note that the loss of bone on the superior and lateral surfaces seems to equate with the gain of bone on the medial surface, so the femoral head retains its sphericity.

fect of the productive new bone formation is an overall increase in joint size: in general, an osteoarthritic joint is larger than its normal counterpart.

Osteophytes form through the process of endochondral ossification in one of two ways. The first involves vascular penetration into existing cartilage. In these areas the cartilage overlying the bone overgrowth is usually hypercellular, and the process histologically resembles the epiphyseal growth plate in the growing individual (Fig. 10.13). In the base of the osteophyte there are often remnants of the original tidemark and zone of calcified cartilage. In some cases these remnants are themselves undergoing ossification not only from the region of the original subchondral bone but also from the osteophyte itself (Fig. 10.14). Osteophytes may also form from foci of cartilaginous metaplasia at the joint margins. These foci of metaplasia occur at the capsular and ligamentous insertions and may be the result of traction injuries.

Microscopic examination of the cartilage that remains on the joint surface reveals many clefts in its substance, most but by no means all of which are verti-

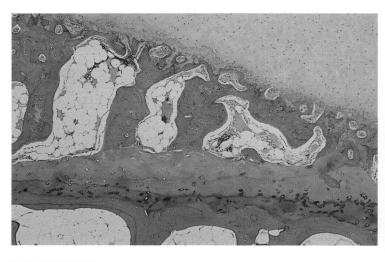

FIGURE 10.13 Photomicrograph of a section through a marginal osteophyte shows a wedge of bone formation dissecting into the cartilage. The cartilage on the articular side of the osteophyte is cellular, and there is more active endochondral ossification on this surface than on the lower surface that faces the bone (H&E, x 4 obj.).

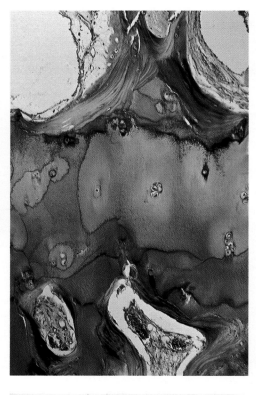

FIGURE 10.14 Photomicrograph of a portion of cartilage and calcified cartilage trapped under an osteophyte (H&E, x 10 obj.).

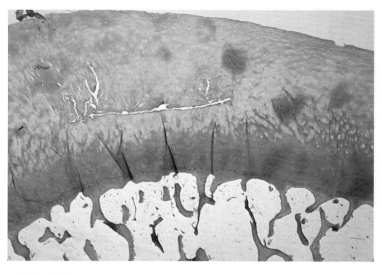

FIGURE 10.15 Section through the articular cartilage of the patella demonstrates a horizontal failure with cleft formation in a patient with chondromalacia patellae. In patients with this condition, a soft blister on the surface of the cartilage may indicate structural failure within the substance of the cartilage (H&E, x 1.25 obj.).

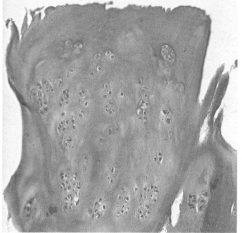

FIGURE 10.16 Photomicrograph of fibrillated cartilage away from the eburnated area shows a considerable proliferation of chondrocytes within the cartilage matrix. Many of the chondrocytes are seen to form cell nests or clones (H&E, x 10 obj.).

cally oriented (Fig. 10.15). The cartilage cells far from the areas of eburnation may show considerable cell replication, with formation of prominent cell nests (Fig. 10.16). However, cell replication does not usually occur adjacent to the eburnated areas (Fig. 10.17). Proteoglycan staining of the matrix is usually diminished, although, as discussed in the previous chapter, there is evidence from radioactive SO_4 uptake studies that the amount of proteoglycan produced by the chondrocytes in osteoarthritis may be increased.

In areas of residual cartilage on the articular surface of a diseased joint there is often marked duplication and irregularity of the tidemark (Fig. 10.18). Histologic evidence of increased endochondral ossification, which expands the subchondral bone periphery without actually forming an osteophyte is seen as increased irregularity of the bone cartilage junction, increased vascular penetration of the calcified cartilage, and deposition of woven (immature) bone at the bone-cartilage interface (Figs. 10.19 and 10.20).

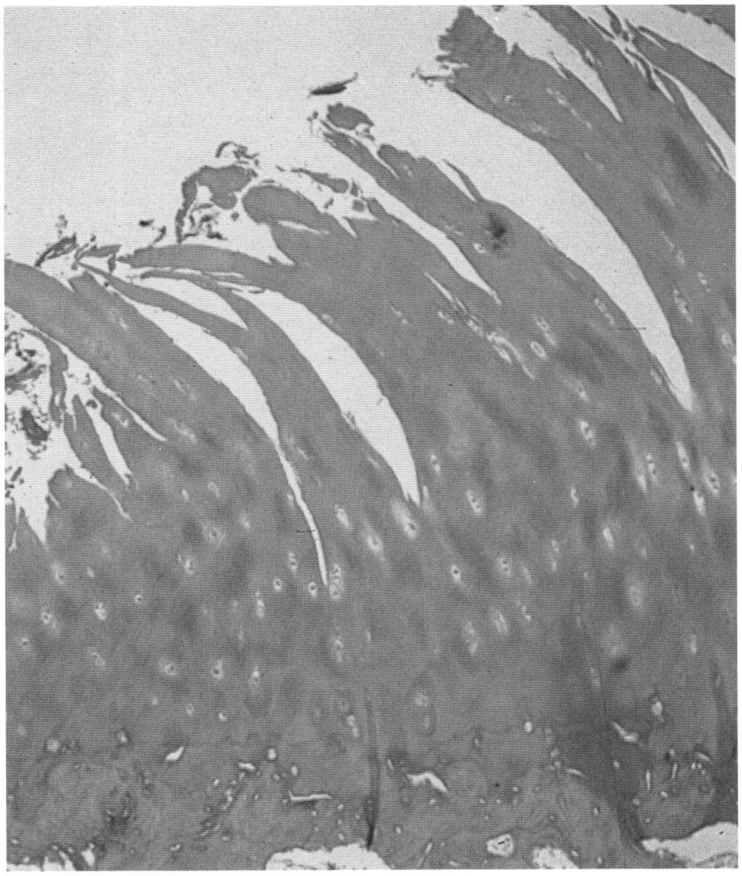

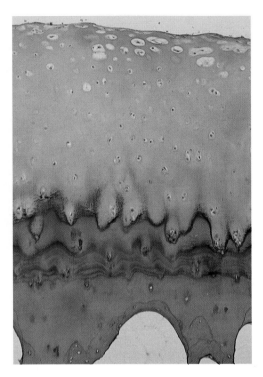

FIGURE 10.17 Low-power photomicrograph of the articular surface adjacent to an eburnated area. The articular cartilage contains vertical clefts resulting from fraying and splitting of the collagen fibers at the surface of the cartilage, but no obvious chrondocyte replication (H&E, x 10 obj.).

FIGURE 10.18 Photomicrograph of a portion of the articular cartilage in a patient with osteoarthritis, showing irregularity and duplication of the tidemark (H&E, x 4 obj.).

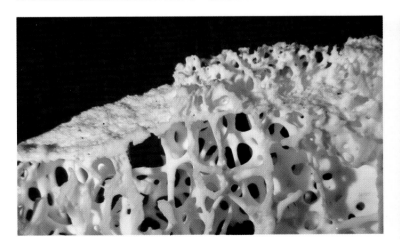

FIGURE 10.19 Photograph of a macerated specimen of a portion of an osteoarthritic joint surface, showing accelerated bone growth (right side) extending beyond the subchondral bone plate (left side).

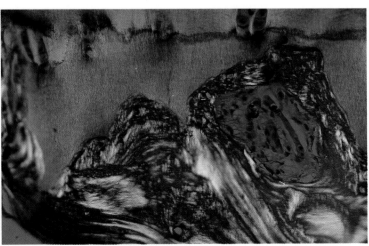

FIGURE 10.20 Photomicrograph taken with polarized light shows woven bone formation in the subchondral region. This is an indication of accelerated modeling in a case of osteoarthritis (x 25 obj.).

The synovial membrane shows villous proliferation and slight hyperplasia of the lining cells. A mild chronic inflammation may be noted (Figs. 10.21 to 10.23). Small osteochondral loose bodies are commonly found in the synovium and in the joint.

NATURAL HISTORY

A wide variety of questions have been asked about osteoarthritis (OA). Is OA a single disorder or a family of disorders? What are the roles of acute and chronic trauma in pathogenesis? Is OA an inevitable consequence of aging? How do the anatomic, physiologic, biochemical, and mechanical alterations in cartilage matrix interrelate in the pathogenesis of OA? What roles do extracartilaginous structures play in OA? Under what circumstances does inflammation develop in OA? Does articular cartilage undergo repair in OA?

The answers to these questions have, in part, been addressed in the preceding chapter. Osteoarthritis appears to comprise a family of disorders. In about one fifth of the patients, it is evident to the clinician that an

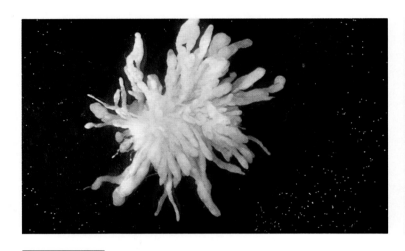

FIGURE 10.21 The synovium from a patient with osteoarthritis exhibits a marked villous pattern. The villi are fine and delicate, an appearance that grossly reflects the lack of any significant cell infiltrate in the subsynovium.

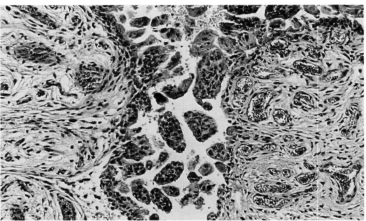

FIGURE 10.22 Photomicrograph of the specimen shown in Figure 10.21 demonstrates the overgrowth of the synovial lining cells without significant cell infiltration of the subsynovial tissue (H&E, x 10 obj.).

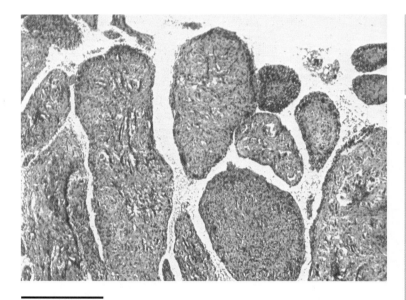

FIGURE 10.23 Photomicrograph of the synovial membrane in a patient with osteoarthritis. The villous pattern of the synovium and hyperplasia of the synovial lining cells are evident. In this patient, as in many patients with osteoarthritis, one may also note a mild chronic inflammatory infiltrate in the synovial tissue. (This inflammation can be quite severe in some individuals.) (H&E, x 4 obj.).

FIGURE 10.24

CONDITIONS THAT MAY PRECEDE OSTEOARTHRITIS (SECONDARY OSTEOARTHRITIS)

Hip dysplasia

Congenital dislocation or subluxation of the hip

Legg–Calvé–Perthes disease

Slipped capital femoral epiphysis

Intra-articular fracture; traumatic dislocation

Radiation damage

Infection

Metabolic diseases (eg, gout, CPPD, ochronosis)

Unrecognized avascular necrosis

"**B**urnt-out" rheumatoid arthritis

Paget's disease

antecedent condition is causally related to the OA, which can therefore be considered secondary osteoarthritis (Fig. 10.24). Individuals affected by secondary OA are likely to be about 10 years younger than those with primary (idiopathic) OA, who are usually over 60 years of age.

Both acute and chronic trauma play a role in the pathogenesis of OA. It is not necessarily the consequence of aging per se, since many joints remain essentially normal even into extreme old age. The pathogenesis of osteoarthritis can be understood only in terms of the interdependence of anatomy, physiology, biochemistry, and mechanical function. All components of the joint play a role in both the etiology and the pathogenesis of the disease, not just the cartilage. Tissue breakdown results in inflammation, which must play a role in disease processes. Finally, articular cartilage does undergo repair in OA.

A number of autopsy studies have demonstrated the incidence of osteoarthritis in various joints, as well as its progression from mild to severe disease. The availability of a large volume of tissue specimens from hip replacement arthroplasty, together with the availability of these patients' clinical radiographs and case histories, makes it possible to gain further insights into the natural history of osteoarthritis of the hip.

One of the problems with most classifications of the radiographic changes in osteoarthritis is that they tend to miss the dynamic progressive nature of the disease which, as already discussed, involves mechanical wear, cell injury, and repair. It is possible to stage the disease not only on the basis of horizontal comparisons of radiographs in different patients' hips but also in longitudinal studies of serial x-rays of the same patient.

Radiographic stage I is characterized by narrowing or absence of the joint space, with preservation of the subchondral bone contours of the femoral head and of the acetabulum. In this early stage of the disease, migration of the femoral head has not occurred beyond the distance caused by the loss of the cartilage (Fig. 10.25). Radiographic stage II is characterized by complete absence of the superior joint space, with incomplete or complete loss of the subchondral bone contour. In this stage bone loss may be marked, and subchondral sclerosis and cystic changes in the bone on both sides of the joint are prominent. Migration of the joint, in most cases superiorly and laterally, has also occurred relative to the bone loss (Fig. 10.26).

The final stage, radiographic stage III, is characterized by some reappearance of the joint space after maximal bone loss and migration have occurred. The bone contours again become relatively well defined. Sclerosis has diminished, and cysts have become indistinct (Fig. 10.27).

This radiologic staging corresponds well to the du-

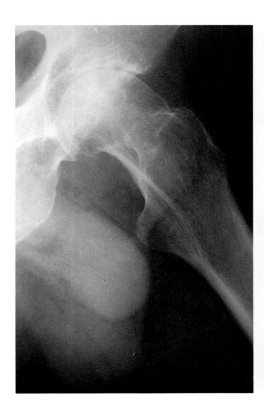 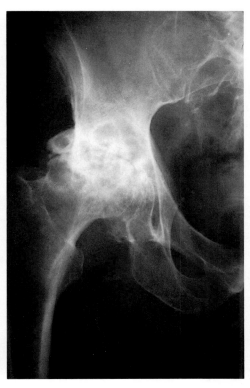 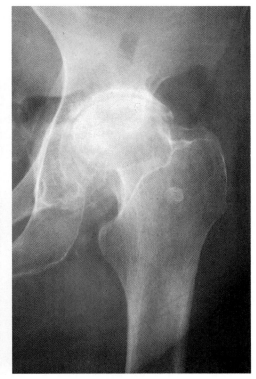

FIGURE 10.25 Radiograph demonstrating the characteristics of stage I osteoarthritis. There is narrowing of the superior joint space, with some subchondral sclerosis and subchondral cyst formation in the acetabulum.

FIGURE 10.26 Radiograph demonstrating the features of stage II osteoarthritis. There is marked subluxation of the joint, with distortion of the femoral head, and severe sclerosis and cyst formation on both sides of the joint.

FIGURE 10.27 Radiograph showing the features of stage III osteoarthritis. Maximal subluxation of the joint is associated with diminished sclerosis, absence of subchondral cyst, and reappearance of the joint space.

ration of symptoms. A number of correlations can be made between this system of radiographic staging and the pathological appearance of the resected specimens. The most striking of these correlations is that reparative cartilage is much more prominent in radiographic stage III than in stage I (Figs. 10.28 through 10.30). Subchondral cysts are most prevalent in stage II and tend to decrease in number in stage III.

When the changes of injury and repair within cartilage, bone, and synovium are considered, it is important not to lose sight of a significant fact. Joint function depends on the anatomy of the entire joint structure. If the repair processes observed in the various tissues are not directed towards restoration of the shape of the joint, as well as restoration of stability and of an equitable loading pattern over the joint surfaces, then they serve no useful purpose (Fig. 10.31).

The most easily recognized evidence of the attempt at functional restoration is the production of new bone, in the form of osteophytes, at various sites along the joint surface, particularly at the joint margins. Such remodeling of bone occurs early in the process of osteoarthritis. The degree of remodeling by this process can be considerable, and its efficiency is reflected clinically. The presence of osteophytes in the knee and hip by no means always heralds the development of progressive symptomatic OA. Radiographic studies have shown that two thirds of knees that exhibit evidence of osteophyte formation, even when followed up for as long as 17 years, do not develop other degenerative changes.

ETIOLOGY

The term "osteoarthritis" was first introduced by Sir Archibald E. Garrod in the 1890s. In 1909, Nicholas and Richardson, on the basis of anatomic features, distinguished the two major categories of chronic arthritis by separating inflammatory arthritis from degenerative arthritis: "These joint lesions can be divided with great definiteness into two pathological groups: 1) those which arise from primary proliferative changes in the joints, chiefly in the synovial membrane and in the perichondrium, and 2) those which arise primarily as a degeneration of the joint cartilage. These two pathological groups are characterized by distinct gross and histological differences." Nicholas and Richardson went on to state that "the earliest change to be observed in hypertrophic arthritis is a roughening of the cartilage, which begins near the center of the articular surface, ie, at the point where pressure and friction between the ends of the bones is greatest."

Since the time of that report, most authors on the subject have concluded that the earliest changes are found in "those areas in which weight bearing is pre-eminently concentrated, and which are the most severely subjected to shearing and twisting types of stress."

The wear-and-tear theory of causation has had a stultifying effect on medical opinion with regard to its views concerning the prevention and treatment of osteoarthritis. It is more helpful to regard clinical arthritis as the consequence of a breakdown of the normal functional and physiologic pathways; the etiology of arthritis can be defined, in general terms, as any condition that changes the shape of the articulating surface, changes the joint support, or alters the tissue matrices. It is not an inevitable disease resulting from wearing out of the joint by long use. Rather, osteoarthritis is a disease of multiple etiologies, and searches for a single, all-encompassing cause of osteoarthritis are fruitless. Although dysfunction may begin in any of the structures that make up the joint, by the time the disease comes to the attention of a clinician most structures of the joint are involved. Because of this overall involvement it is usually impossible for the pathologist to determine the etiology in a given case of arthritis; this is especially true in later stages of the disease.

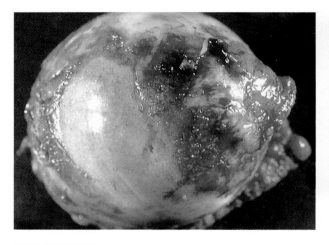

FIGURE 10.28 Gross superior view of a femoral head from a patient with radiographic stage I shows an area of complete cartilage loss, with polishing or eburnation of the underlying bone.

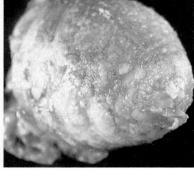

FIGURE 10.29 In this gross specimen of a deformed femoral head from a patient with radiologic stage III disease, the weight-bearing surface has been recovered with an irregular, cobblestoned layer of cartilage.

SUBCHONDRAL AVASCULAR NECROSIS (SAVN)

CLINICAL CONSIDERATIONS

Necrosis in the subchondral region of a bone, usually on the convex side of the joint, is a common cause of arthritis, accounting for approximately 18% of surgery for total hip replacement. The three joints most commonly affected are the hip, knee and shoulder. Although circulatory disturbance is assumed to be the principal mechanism of necrosis in the ends of bones, the cause of the disruption usually cannot be demon-strated by anatomic dissection. Because of this, a large number of names have been applied to this condition. Among these are segmental subchondral infarction, osteonecrosis, ischemic necrosis, idiopathic avascular necrosis, aseptic necrosis, steroid necrosis, and many eponymic designations (eg, Legg-Calvé-Perthes disease, Freiberg's disease, Kienböck's disease), depending on the anatomic location and the joint involved.

The overall incidence of SAVN in any population is difficult to determine because the lesion may be clinically silent in a significant proportion of cases. However, certain groups of people demonstrate a predilection for the condition. Some of these risk groups likely

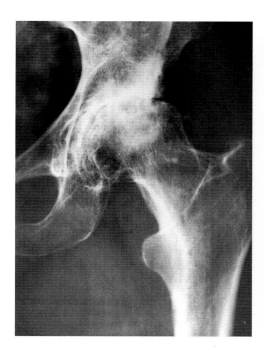

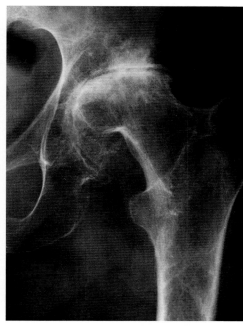

FIGURE 10.30 The radiograph shown on the right was taken 8 years after that on the left. It demonstrates the improvement that may occur in the radigraphic appearance of a case of osteoarthritis even without treatment.

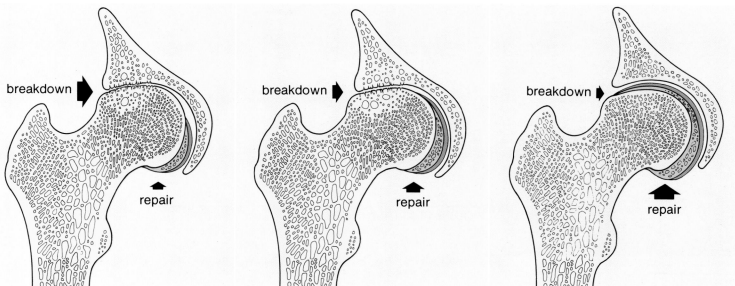

FIGURE 10.31 The radiographic and clinical signs of arthritis depend, to some extent, on the balance between injury to the joint and repair of the joint. *(left)* Deterioration is taking place because breakdown (ie, loss of cartilage, bone, and bone shape, as well as bone necrosis) is proceeding more rapidly than repair (ie, regeneration of cartilage and formation of new bone). *(center)* Both injury and repair are proceeding at about the same pace, and the joint is stabilized. *(right)* Repair is proceeding more rapidly than injury, leading to morphologic and perhaps clinical improvement.

to be encountered in clinical practice are alcoholics, those taking corticosteroids, Blacks with sickle-cell disease, and Jews with Gaucher's disease. Approximately 60 percent of the cases exhibit bilateral involvement, indicating the systemic nature of the disease. The mean age of patients with SAVN of the hip is 55 years, as compared with the mean age of 67 in patients with primary osteoarthritis.

The primary presenting complaint in SAVN of the hip is pain experienced on weight bearing and, in two thirds of the cases, also pain at rest. In most respects the symptoms of SAVN and osteoarthritis are similar. However, most patients with SAVN report a sudden onset of acute pain, whereas in osteoarthritis the onset is usually more gradual.

MORBID ANATOMY

Stage One

In this stage the shape of the joint is unaltered, and external examination of the joint reveals no abnormalities. However, on cut section the necrotic zone, a somewhat wedge-shaped region in which the marrow is dull-yellow, chalky, and opaque, can be seen in an immediately subarticular location. This region is well demarcated and is separated from the surrounding bone marrow by a thin, red "hyperemic" border (Figs. 10.32 and 10.33). At this stage changes in the trabecular architecture are not appreciable, either by gross inspection or on specimen radiographs, which typically

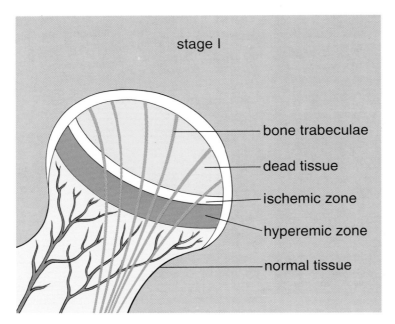
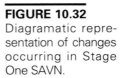

stage I

— bone trabeculae

— dead tissue

— ischemic zone

— hyperemic zone

— normal tissue

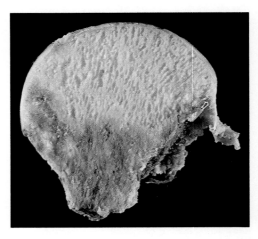

FIGURE 10.32 Diagramatic representation of changes occurring in Stage One SAVN.

FIGURE 10.33 Femoral head excised from a patient approximately a week after a subcapital fracture exhibits extensive bone necrosis.

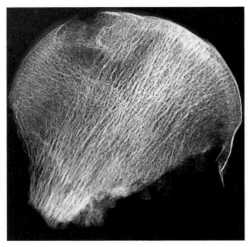

FIGURE 10.34 Radiograph of the specimen shown in Figure 10.33.

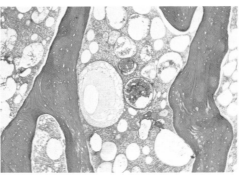

FIGURE 10.35 Photomiograph of infarcted bone and bone marrow reveals the acellular nature of the tissue and large fat cysts characteristic of infarcted bone marrow (phloxine & tartrazine, x 4 obj.).

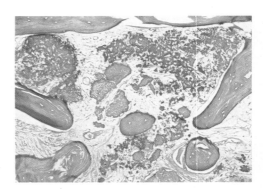

FIGURE 10.36 Calcification is sometimes a prominent feature in infarcted bone marrow, and may on occasion give rise to increased density on radiographs (H&E, x 4 obj.).

show no abnormality (Fig. 10.34).

On microscopic examination, the overlying articular cartilage appears viable down to the calcified zone. However, the bony end plate is necrotic. The subchondral bone, corresponding to the opaque yellow region seen grossly, is characterized by necrotic bone and bone marrow. The marrow elements are replaced by granular, eosinophilic material lacking cellular elements except for occasional ghosts of disrupted fat cells (Fig. 10.35). There may also be cysts of lipid material together with extensive calcification (Fig. 10.36). The osteocytic lacunae in the bone may be empty, may contain cellular debris, or may have a pale-staining nucleus. At the margin of the infarct there is increased osteoclastic activity and an infiltration of proliferating fibroblasts and capillaries into the marrow space. This zone corresponds to the thin red rim seen in the gross specimen. Beyond this hypervascular zone the bone and bone marrow are unchanged by the necrotizing process and reflect the state of the marrow before the necrotizing event.

Stage Two

As in Stage One, the overall shape of the bone is preserved and the articular surface is intact (Fig. 10.37). However, on sectioning, a rim of bony sclerosis can be seen at the periphery of the necrotic zone, at the boundary between the necrotic zone and the unaffected marrow. This feature is best seen on specimen radiographs (Figs. 10.38 and 10.39). The central region of necrosis is unchanged from Stage One, but the hyperemic zone is generally thicker and may now contain a mixture of tan and white tissue.

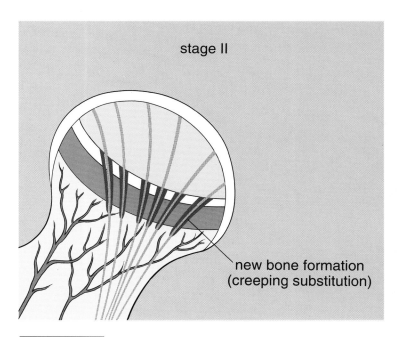

stage II

new bone formation (creeping substitution)

FIGURE 10.37 Diagramatic representation of the changes that occur in Stage Two SAVN.

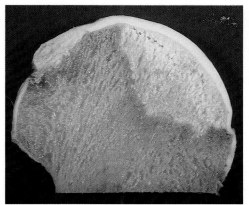

FIGURE 10.38 Gross photograph from a patient with Stage Two SAVN shows a well-demarcated hyperemic border.

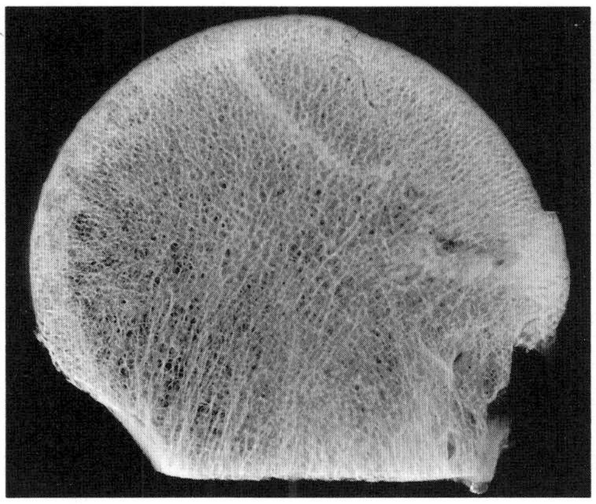

FIGURE 10.39 Specimen radiograph of a femoral head with Stage Two SAVN showing a line of bone sclerosis which corresponds to the zone of hyperemia seen in the gross photograph.

On microscopic examination, an advancing front of granulation tissue composed of lipid-laden macrophages, proliferating fibroblasts, and capillaries can be seen at the periphery, extending into the central region of the necrotic zone (Fig. 10.40). Following closely behind this "clean-up" front is a second front at a variable distance; limited amounts of both the old dead bone and new living bone are being removed by osteoclasts. The overall effect of these combined processes is removal of the necrotic marrow and bone while the structural integrity of the bone is maintained. This series of processes has been called "creeping substitution" by Phemister (Fig. 10.41). The increased osteoblastic activity and the layer of new bone contribute to the clinical radiographic appearance of

bone sclerosis and to the increased uptake of the radiographic technetium diphosphonate isotope on bone scanning.

Stage Three

Alteration of the shape of the bone is first encountered in this stage. It is caused by collapse within the necrotic region, and may be apparent on external examination of the bone as a buckling or fragmentation of the articular cartilage (Fig. 10.42).

On cut section, it becomes apparent that the reason for collapse is fracture of trabecular bone with associated fracture of the end-plate itself (Figs. 10.43 and 10.44). Fracture of the trabeculae occurs either just

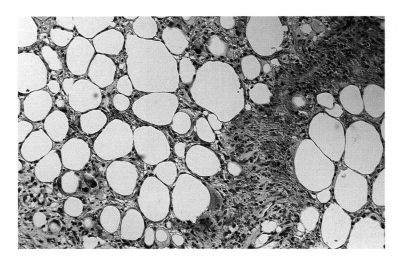

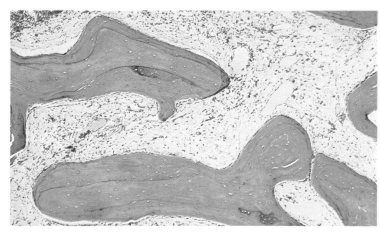

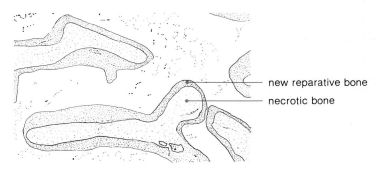

new reparative bone
necrotic bone

FIGURE 10.40 Photomicrograph demonstrating focal fat necrosis as well as fibroblastic and vascular proliferation at the margin of the infarcted area seen grossly in Figure 10.38.

FIGURE 10.41 In the process of healing an infarcted area of bone, a layer of living bone is deposited on the surface of the necrotic bone. This process, referred to as creeping substitution, gives rise to increased radiodensity at the healing margin of the infarct. Note also the vascularized fibrous tissue in the marrow spaces (H&E, × 10 obj.).

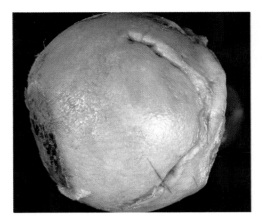

FIGURE 10.42 Gross photograph of a femoral head removed surgically after clinical signs and symptoms of avascular necrosis were detected. On the articular surface of the femoral head there is a linear dimpling of the articular cartilage, marking the site of an underlying fracture.

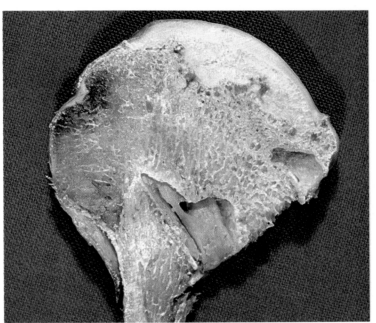

FIGURE 10.43 Photograph of a slice through the femoral head shown in Figure 10.42. The area of infarction is seen as a triangular, opaque yellow area lying immediately beneath the articular surface. Also seen in this photograph is the track of the nail that was used for fixation of the subcapital fracture that preceded the necrosis.

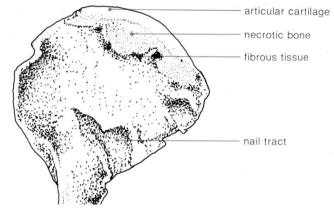

articular cartilage

necrotic bone

fibrous tissue

nail tract

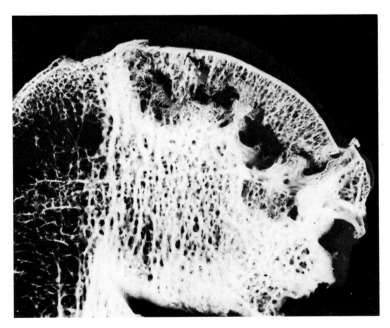

FIGURE 10.44 Radiograph of the specimen shown in Figure 10.43. Note the unaltered trabecular pattern of the infarcted bone. The lucent area at the base of the infarction results from fibrous granulation tissue eroding the necrotic bone. The collapse of the necrotic segment is well demonstrated by the fracture through the subchondral plate, which is seen at both edges of the infarct. In contrast to the appearance of the infarct, the viable bone is dense, resulting from the formation of new bone in this area by the process of creeping substitution (see text).

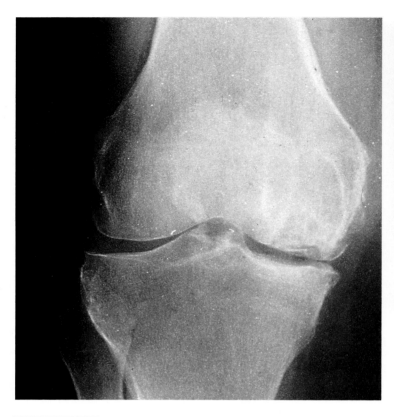

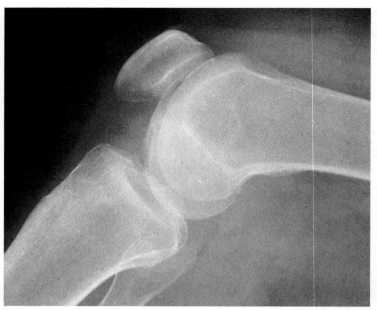

FIGURE 10.46 Lateral view of the same knee shown in Figure 10.45 reveals a subchondral fracture of a portion of the articular surface of the femoral cartilage.

FIGURE 10.45 Anteroposterior radiograph of the knee in a 58-year-old woman who complained of sudden onset of pain in the knee. Irregularity of the articular surface of the medial femoral cartilage is evident.

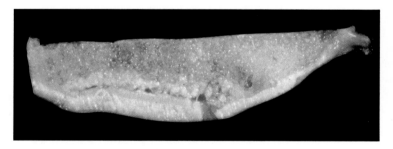

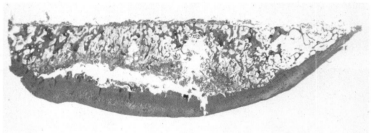

FIGURE 10.47 Frontal slice taken through the medial condyle of a patient with osteonecrosis of the knee. The zone of bone necrosis lies immediately under the articular surface and is characterized by an opaque yellow appearance. Immediately beyond the necrotic zone is a band of hyperemia. Separating the necrotic bone from the overlying cartilage is a gap created by collapse of the bone trabeculae in the necrotic segment.

FIGURE 10.48 Radiograph of the specimen illustrated in Figure 10.47. The subchondral bone end plate remains attached to the articular cartilage, and around the margin of the infarct the fracture extends through the bone end-plate, producing deformity of the articular surface.

FIGURE 10.49 Photomicrograph of a histologic section through the specimen illustrated in Figures 10.47 and 10.48 (H&E, x 1 obj.).

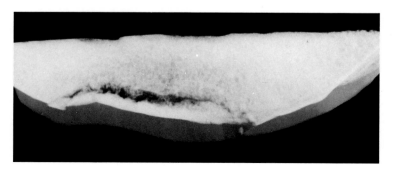

below the bony end-plate, deep within the necrotic region, or on the necrotic side of the advancing sclerosis in the reparative front (Figs. 10.45 to 10.49).

The fracture of the trabeculae may result from any of three causes: the cumulative effect of fatigue-induced microfactures within the necrotic zone; weakness of trabeculae in the reparative front due to osteoclastic activity; or focal concentrations of stress at the junctions between the thickened sclerotic trabeculae of the reparative zone and the necrotic trabeculae. This last cause may be associated with the bioengineering concept of "stress risers" (Fig. 10.50).

The linear fracture beneath the end-plate corresponds to the radiolucent zone, referred to as the "crescent sign," seen on clinical radiographs (Figs. 10.51 to 10.56).

Microscopically, the fractured trabeculae in the necrotic region are fragments of pulverized bony and cartilaginous detritus. The overlying cartilage may still appear viable. Fractures within the reparative zone have abundant fibrous tissue, cartilaginous tissue, and reactive woven bone, and have the usual appearance of non-united, unstable fractures elsewhere in the skeleton.

Stage Four

The major feature of this stage is the appearance of morphologic changes usually associated with osteoarthritis. Depending on the degree of the osteoarthritic changes, it may no longer be possible on the clinical radiographs to recognize the initial events as those of SAVN. However, in most cases there is sufficient evidence on gross and microscopic examination to allow proper diagnosis (Figs. 10.57 to 10.60).

In general, as is best seen in the femoral head, formation of osteophytes is not pronounced and areas of cartilaginous erosion and bone eburnation surround the collapsed infarcted segment. Because of this col-

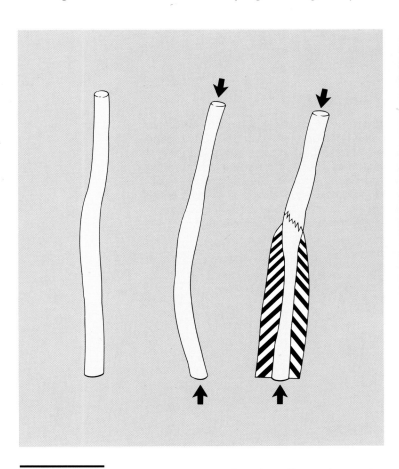

FIGURE 10.50 Diagram demonstrating the effect of creeping substitution. Increased stiffening of the bone causes focal stress concentration at the junction between the existing bone and the sclerotic bone. When a bending force is applied to the bone, fracture is likely to occur at this point.

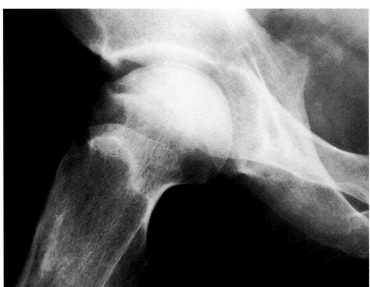

FIGURE 10.51 Radiograph of a young patient who complained of sudden onset of pain in the hip. Although the joint space is normal, in this frog-lateral view, a crescentic lucent zone outlining the articular surface can be seen on the superior aspect of the femoral head. This crescent sign is often an early radiologic manifestation of avascular necrosis and is best appreciated in the frog-lateral view.

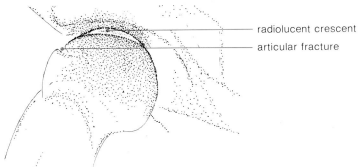

radiolucent crescent
articular fracture

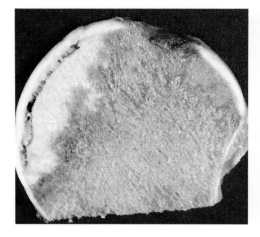

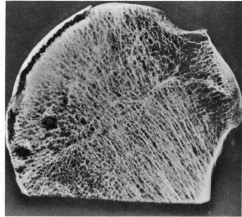

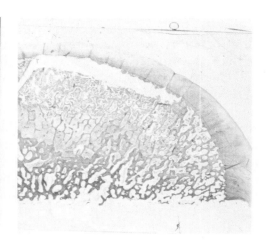

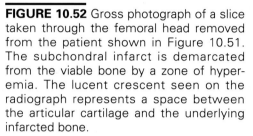

FIGURE 10.52 Gross photograph of a slice taken through the femoral head removed from the patient shown in Figure 10.51. The subchondral infarct is demarcated from the viable bone by a zone of hyperemia. The lucent crescent seen on the radiograph represents a space between the articular cartilage and the underlying infarcted bone.

FIGURE 10.53 Radiograph of the specimen slice shown in Figure 10.52. Again the crescent sign is clearly seen. The dense lucent line evident on the superior surface of the femoral head is an image of the subchondral bone end-plate and the calcified cartilage, which remain adherent to the articular cartilage after the collapse of the infarcted area. After such a collapse the articular surface probably springs back like a ping-pong ball, giving rise to this radiologic phenomenon.

FIGURE 10.54 Photomicrograph of a histologic preparation of the femoral head shown in the previous three figures. The thickened trabeculae of the viable bone can be clearly appreciated (H&E, x 1 obj.).

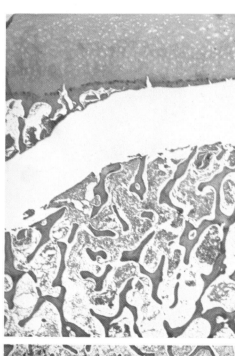

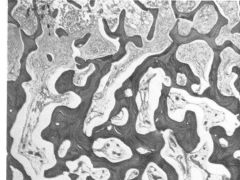

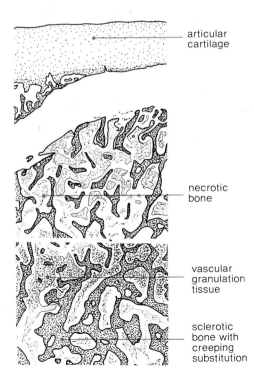

FIGURE 10.55 Photomicrograph of the specimen shown in Figure 10.54. At the top can be seen the necrotic bone and bone marrow of the infarcted area, together with the subchondral crescent; the lower portion of the frame shows the junction between the necrotic and viable bone. At the bottom the thickened trabeculae of viable bone are evident. This thickening is the result of new bone deposition on the trabecular surfaces, which occurs as part of the healing of the infarct (H&E, x 4 obj.).

articular cartilage

necrotic bone

vascular granulation tissue

sclerotic bone with creeping substitution

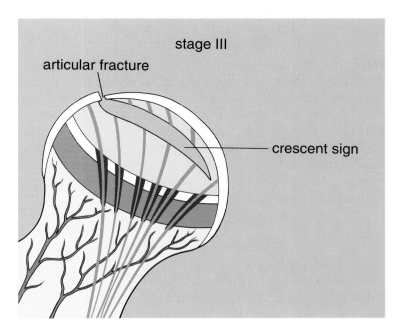

FIGURE 10.56 Diagram illustrating the associated tissue changes with the crescent sign in Stage Three SAVN.

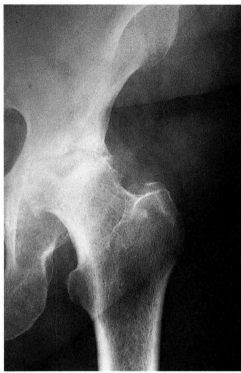

FIGURE 10.57
Radiograph of a patient with severe hip disease secondary to SAVN shows marked deformity of the superior margin of the femoral head secondary to collapse.

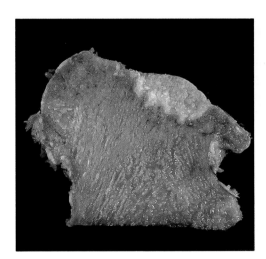

FIGURE 10.58
A frontal section through the femoral head resected from the patient illustrated in Figure 10.57.

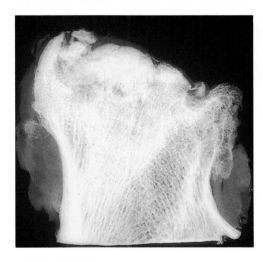

FIGURE 10.59
Specimen radiograph of the case illustrated in Figures 10.57 and 10.58.

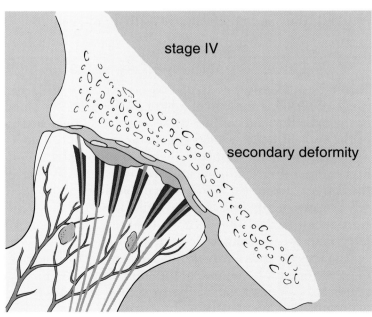

FIGURE 10.60 Diagramatic representation of Stage Four SAVN.

lapse, fragmented cartilage may persist in the region. When the changes of osteoarthritis are marked, the only clue that the initial event may have been SAVN is that the femoral head has a deep, saddle-shaped deformity.

The cut surface in this stage of SAVN may show residual fragments of articular cartilage and dense fibrous connective tissue in the infarcted area, surrounded at the surface by a margin of densely sclerotic bone which represents the eburnated articular surface. In markedly destructive cases, the "articular surface" may be composed of pulverized bony detritus.

In more advanced cases, two useful clues to the diagnosis of SAVN are the absence of clearly eburnated bone at the articular surface and the presence of bony and cartilaginous debris in the accompanying synovial and capsular tissue.

Arthritis secondary to osteonecrosis is rarely detected in joints other than the hip, the knee, and the shoulder. However, osteonecrosis may occasionally be the cause of disease at three other sites: the carpal lunate bone (Kienböck's disease); the head of a metatarsal bone, usually the second (Freiberg's disease); and the tarsal navicular bone (Kohler's disease).

IMAGING MODALITIES

The radiographic diagnosis of SAVN is based on four main imaging modalities: plain radiographs, radionuclide scintigraphy, computed tomography, and magnetic resonance imaging. As with all advances in medical technology, the more modern methods have been touted as replacements for their predecessors. However, none of the newer methods has proven infallible for diagnosis of SAVN, and a combination of techniques is still often necessary.

Plain Radiographs

Plain radiographs are limited by their inability to demonstrate the early changes of the disease at a time (in Stage One) when therapeutic intervention has the greatest chance to prevent further development of arthritis. The earliest plain radiographic finding in an end of a bone affected by SAVN is the presence of a poorly defined region of sclerosis which does not usually reach to the subchondral end-plate. This sclerosis corresponds to the deposition of bone in the process of "creeping substitution" during Stage Two.

In Stage Three where collapse has occurred, the plain radiograph demonstrates the alteration in the shape of the joint. The characteristic finding of the crescent sign, best seen in the frog lateral view of the femoral head, is easily recognizable in plain radiographs. After collapse in Stage Four, changes of osteoarthritis may supervene and obscure or even obliterate the features characteristic of SAVN.

Radionuclide Scintigraphy (Bone Scanning)

Bone scanning is used in the diagnosis of SAVN because of its ability to identify skeletal regions at which bone deposition and mineralization are occurring. Early in Stage Two the presence of an incorporated radioactive isotope can be detected well before the plain radiographs demonstrate increased sclerosis (Fig. 10.61). An important feature of the bone scan is that it is capable of demonstrating multiple sites of involvement without increasing the exposure of the patient to ionizing radiation.

Computed Tomography

The advantage of the computed tomography (CT) scan over plain radiographs is its ability to obtain "slices" through the bone, thereby reducing or eliminating overlap and providing a clearer image of the necrotic zone without interference from surrounding structures such as soft tissues and regional cortical bone (Fig. 10.62).

Magnetic Resonance Imaging

Magnetic resonance imaging (MRI) offers the considerable advantage of being able to identify chemical changes in necrotic bone marrow well before changes in the bone can be detected by the other methods. It is also useful in demonstrating other clinically silent foci of SAVN in patients who already have a clinically evident focus.

The earliest finding of SAVN as demonstrated by MRI is a decrease in the usual high signal associated with marrow fat on the T1-weighted image (Fig. 10.63). This decreased signal results from a chemical alteration in the fat which causes the opaque, yellow, and "soapy" appearance apparent on gross examination. However, in some conditions, such as sickle-cell disease and Gaucher's disease, the marrow signal may already be reduced, thus making the image difficult to evaluate.

ETIOLOGY AND PATHOGENESIS

Regardless of any predisposing conditions, the final cause of SAVN is the loss of adequate perfusion of blood in the articular ends of bones. Several anatomic features of the ends of bones render them susceptible to compromise in their blood supply. Subchondral bone has a limited collateral circulation, and this is especially true of the convex side of the joint, where the subchondral vessels are essentially end arteries (Fig. 10.64). The perfusion pressure and blood flow of the epiphyses and of fatty marrow, in comparison with those of red diaphyseal marrow, are relatively low. Finally, and possibly most important, bone, unlike the soft tissues, is rigid and nondistensible, and can neither expand nor collapse to maintain adequate perfusion pressures.

Necrosis of subchondral bone results from either an

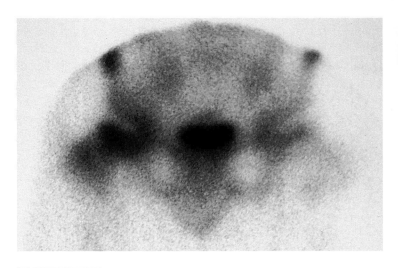

FIGURE 10.61 Scintigram of the pelvis of a patient with symptoms suggestive of SAVN, but without radiographic changes, shows increased uptake of isotope in the affected femoral head.

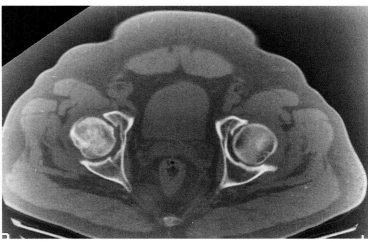

FIGURE 10.62 CT scan through the region of the femoral heads shows increased density in the right femoral head associated with Stage Two SAVN.

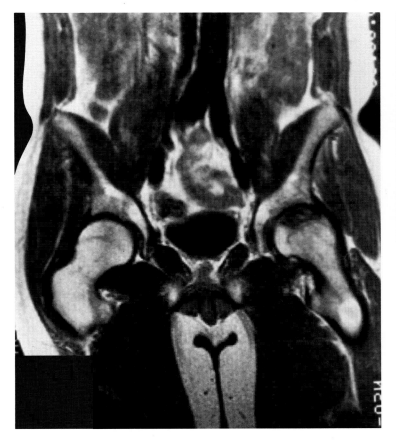

FIGURE 10.63 MRI of the pelvis of a patient with recent acute pain in the left hip. Plain radiograph and isotope examinations were normal in this case. However, in this T1-weighted image the lack of signal is suggestive of Stage One SAVN.

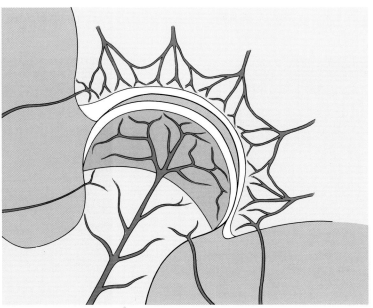

FIGURE 10.64 Diagramatic representation of the blood supply around the hip joint.

intravascular or an extravascular disturbance.

Intracapsular fracture of the femoral neck, with its concomitant physical disruption of blood vessels, causes clinical symptoms resulting from SAVN in more than 20 percent of fracture cases. Extracapsular fractures of the proximal femur are much less likely to result in SAVN.

Necrosis of bone may also be caused by the direct toxic effects on the vessels of high-dose radiation, chemotherapy, thermal and electrical injury, and freezing.

Approximately 90 percent of patients with nontraumatic bone necrosis have disorders involving disturbances in fat metabolism or associated with fat embolism. The two most common predisposing conditions are hypercortisolism and alcoholism, which account for about two thirds of the cases and frequently give rise to multiple joint involvement (Figs. 10.65 and 10.66). Both steroid therapy and alcoholism lead to alterations in the fat content of the liver, and in both conditions fat microemboli have been found in many parenchymal organs at autopsy. Other theories suggest that the in-

creased fat deposits in turn increase marrow pressure, leading to venous stasis. An alternative possibility is that the alteration in fat metabolism affects cell function, with subsequent osteopenia and cumulative microfractures.

SAVN in dysbarism (caisson workers' disease, or "the bends") is caused by the release of nitrogen dissolved in the tissues; bubbles of nitrogen accumulate in the extracellular, extravascular space leading to compression of the capillary network. The infarcts are extensive and are seen on both sides of the joint (Fig. 10.67).

In Gaucher's disease and other storage diseases in which the normal marrow constituents are replaced, accumulations of storage cells pack the marrow space and constrict the vascular network, with subsequent compromise in venous return.

In sickle-cell disease, occlusion of the small vessels most likely occurs because of the increased viscosity of the blood caused by clumping of the affected red cells in response to hypoxia.

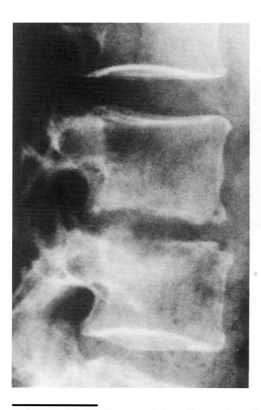 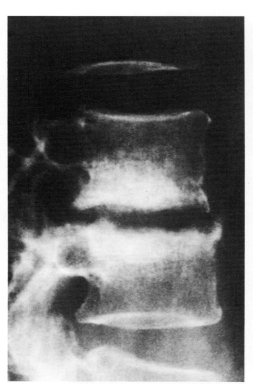 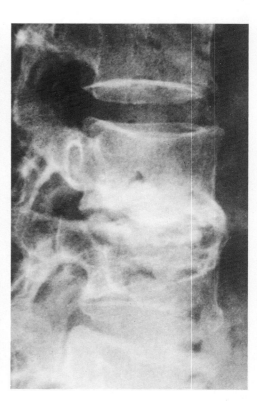

FIGURE 10.65 Sequential radiographs of a 50+-year-old man receiving cortisone therapy for a chronic skin condition. The time interval between the first and second films is 8 months and the time between the second and the third films is 2 years. At the time of the second examination the patient began to complain of pain in the shoulder. (Radiograph of the shoulder is shown in Figure 10.66.) The changes at the joint surfaces resulted from osteonecrosis secondary to cortisone therapy, although at first the radiologic changes were considered to be caused by tuberculosis.

LEGG–CALVE–PERTHES DISEASE

Osteonecrosis of the femoral head occurs in children, usually between the ages of 5 and 9 years. The disease is more likely to affect boys, and in about 13% of patients the condition is bilateral. In some instances a familial predisposition has been noted.

Because the growth plate of the femoral head lies above the insertion of the capsule of the hip joint in children, and because the epiphyseal plate acts as a firm barrier to blood flow between the metaphysis and epiphysis, the femoral head is therefore dependent on vessels that track along the surface of the neck of the femur to enter the epiphysis above the growth plate. Injection studies have demonstrated that the most important vessels supplying the epiphysis are the lateral epiphyseal vessels. These vessels are vulnerable to interruption of blood flow by trauma or by increases in intra-articular pressure (Fig. 10.68). It is possible that in this condition the ischemic events are episodic in nature and result from increased intra-articular pressure.

One of the earliest radiologic signs of Legg-Calvé-Perthes disease is widening of the joint space. This is probably caused by the cessation of endochondral ossification and resultant failure of cartilage to be converted to bone. Therefore, on the radiologic film the continuous growth of the cartilage will be appreciated as an increase in the width of the joint space (Fig. 10.69). Although the necrotic bony epiphysis may undergo collapse and subsequent deformation, deformity may also result from the irregular growth of new bone on the surface of the necrotic secondary center of ossification (Fig. 10.70). Characteristic radiologic findings in patients with Legg-Calvé-Perthes disease include enlargement of the femoral head and sometimes alterations in the epiphysis of the femoral neck. Since the growth plate is dependent upon the epiphyseal vasculature for growth and nutrition, it can be expected that secondary changes will occur in the growth plate after necrosis of the epiphysis. In the early stages of the disease lytic lesions are often present in the metaphysis, whereas as a late consequence there is widening and shortening of the neck of the femur because of cessation of growth.

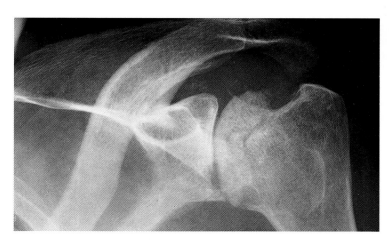

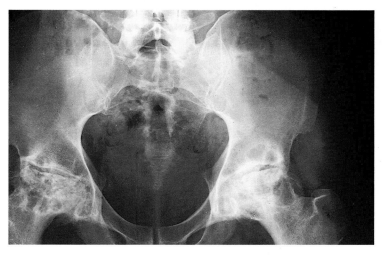

FIGURE 10.66 Radiograph of the shoulder from the patient in Figure 10.65 shows collapse of the humoral head secondary to SAVN.

FIGURE 10.67 Radiograph of the pelvis of a patient with bilateral infarcts affecting both femoral heads and acetabula. This patient was previously a caisson worker.

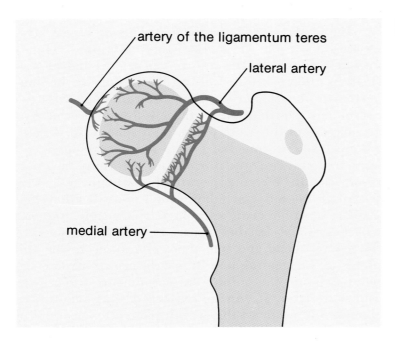

FIGURE 10.68 Blood supply to the femoral head in a child.

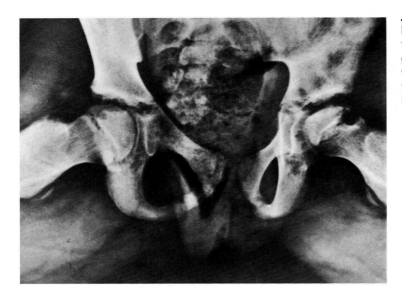

FIGURE 10.69 In the early stage of Legg–Calvé–Perthes disease, there is cessation of growth in the bony epiphysis with continued growth of the cartilage. Therefore, radiographic studies reveal widening of the joint space. Interference with the vascular supply to the growth plate results in defects in the metaphysis, seen here as a lytic area on the lateral side of the left femoral head.

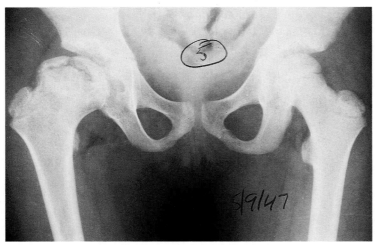

FIGURE 10.70 Radiograph of a patient with Legg–Calvé–Perthes disease after revascularization of the necrotic femoral head shows enlargement of the head, with the original necrotic ossification center seen as a "head within a head." Alterations in the growth plate vasculature have resulted in decreased growth at the upper end of the right femur.

The inflammatory arthritides

Bacterial infections of the joint may lead to severe and rapid breakdown of the joint tissues, with resultant severe arthritis (see Chapter 4 under "Joint Infection"). The acute inflammatory infiltrate produces proteolytic enzymes which rapidly break down the articular cartilage and intra-articular structures (Fig. 11.1). Aspiration of the joint in such cases reveals a predominance of polymorphonuclear leukocytes, with a count usually well over 100,000/mm^3 (see Figs. 9.46 and 9.47).

Since both acute gout and acute rheumatoid joint disease, two of the principal topics of this chapter, may present with fever and hot, tender joints accompanied by a high polymorphonuclear leukocyte count, on occasion the correct diagnosis is difficult to make. Infection may also complicate preexisting joint disease, further adding to the diagnostic difficulties.

INFLAMMATORY ARTHRITIS ASSOCIATED WITH DIFFUSE CONNECTIVE TISSUE DISEASE

Generalized polyarticular arthritis (or rarely monarticular arthritis) is often the presenting symptom in patients with a variety of diffuse connective tissue diseases such as rheumatoid arthritis, systemic lupus erythematosus, and Sjögren's syndrome. Rheumatoid arthritis is the most common of these conditions and is most typically characterized by arthritis. Although the various rheumatic diseases differ markedly in clinical presentation, the histopathology of the associated joint disease tends to be similar. There are no specific diagnostic histologic findings in the synovium that distinguish rheumatoid arthritis from lupus erythematosus or from the arthritis associated with psoriasis or ulcerative colitis.

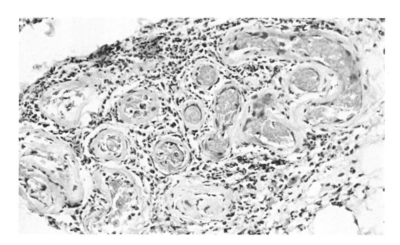

FIGURE 11.1 Acute synovitis in early septic arthritis. Interspersed between the hypervascular stroma of this synovium are many polymorphonuclear leukocytes, the hallmark of acute bacterial infection (H&E, x 4 obj.).

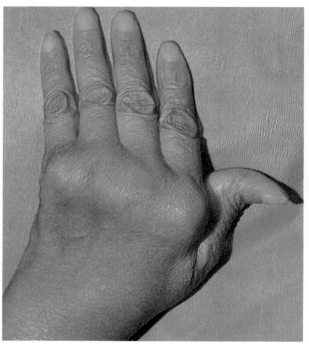

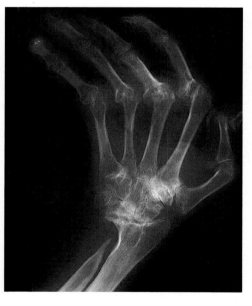

FIGURE 11.3 Radiograph demonstrating the destructive joint changes associated with advanced rheumatoid arthritis. Note especially the marked bone destruction at the wrist, the subluxation and ulnar deviation at the metacarpophalangeal joints, and the dislocation of the distal interphalangeal joint of the thumb.

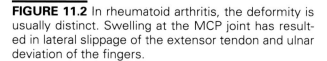

FIGURE 11.2 In rheumatoid arthritis, the deformity is usually distinct. Swelling at the MCP joint has resulted in lateral slippage of the extensor tendon and ulnar deviation of the fingers.

RHEUMATOID ARTHRITIS

Rheumatoid arthritis (RA) is a chronic systemic disease of unknown etiology which frequently involves the peripheral joints and ultimately causes joint deformities (Figs. 11.2 and 11.3). RA is two to three times more common in women than in men, and is characterized by spontaneous remission and exacerbation. Although it may occur at any age, the peak age of onset in women is the period from the fourth to the sixth decade. Seventy to 80 percent of all affected individuals test positive for histocompatibility antigen DW4 and/or DR4, a finding that implies a strong hereditary component. Extra-articular features, such as arteritis, neuropathy, pericarditis, splenomegaly, lymphadenopathy, and rheumatoid nodules occur with considerable frequency, indicating the systemic nature of the disease.

The affected patient is likely to complain of symptoms of general malaise, as well as pain and stiffness in the joints, characteristically pronounced in the morning. Although any joint can be involved, most commonly affected are the small joints of the hands and feet. In general, the disease is polyarticular, bilateral, and symmetrical.

Clinical examination reveals the acutely affected joint to be hot, swollen, and tender. The synovial effusion is milky and turbid (Fig. 11.4). Compared with septic arthritis, in which the synovial fluid usually contains more than 100,000 white blood cells/mm^3 at least 75 percent of which are polymorphonuclear leukocytes, the rheumatoid joint effusion contains 20,000 to 50,000 inflammatory cells/mm^3 only about 50 percent of which are polymorphonuclear leukocytes. Cultures of the synovial fluid and synovial membrane for various organisms, including viruses, are usually negative.

The principal morphologic feature of rheumatoid disease, seen both on x-ray examination and anatomically, is joint destruction (Fig. 11.5). Unlike the nonin-

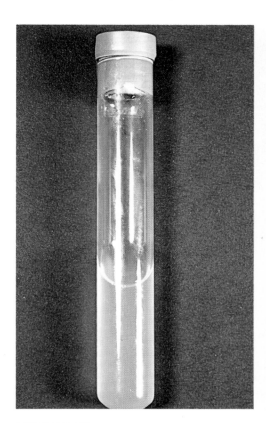

FIGURE 11.4 Synovial fluid aspirate from a patient with rheumatoid arthritis. Note the turbidity of this specimen.

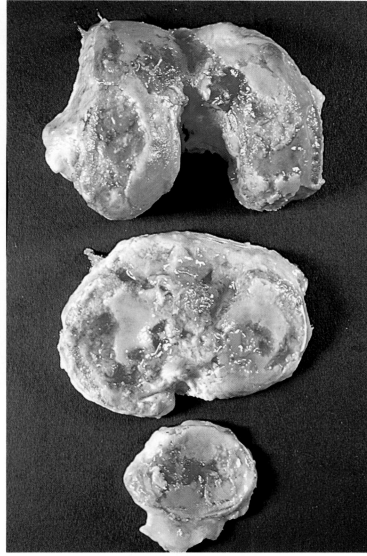

FIGURE 11.5
Gross photograph of the articular surfaces of a knee joint from a patient with rheumatoid arthritis. The articular cartilage is destroyed more at the periphery of the joint, whereas the central areas are spared. This finding is characteristic of the inflammatory arthritides, and should be contrasted with the findings in patients with osteoarthritis, in whom the central cartilage is usually destroyed first and the periphery is spared.

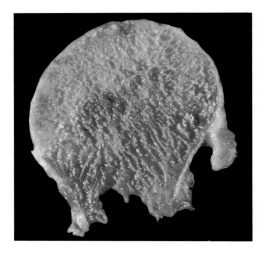

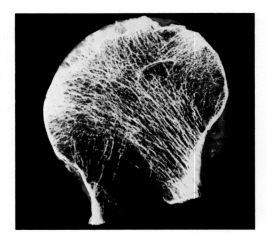

FIGURE 11.6 Frontal section through the femoral head in a patient with rheumatoid arthritis. The joint surface is destroyed but there is no evidence of osteophyte formation or bone sclerosis. The absence of these two features is in marked contrast to the morphologic findings in patients with osteoarthritis.

FIGURE 11.7 Radiograph of the specimen shown in Figure 11.6.

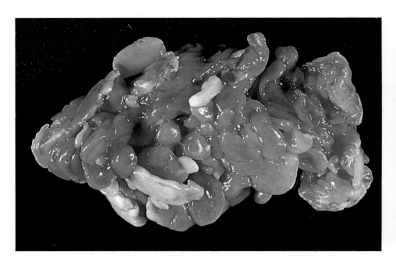

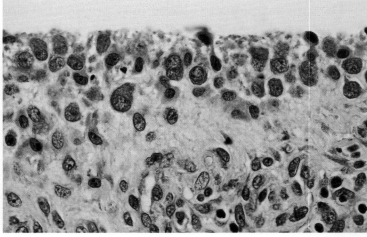

FIGURE 11.8 Gross photograph of synovium from a patient with rheumatoid arthritis. The cinnamon color is caused by posthemorrhagic hemosiderin deposits in the synovium. The plump papillae stem from the cellular overgrowth of the synovium, as well as from lymphoid infiltration of the subintimal layer. The irregular white nodules on the surface are fibrin, the product of vascular exudation in the inflamed tissue.

FIGURE 11.9 Photomicrograph demonstrating the hyperplasia of the synovial lining cells (H&E, x 40 obj.).

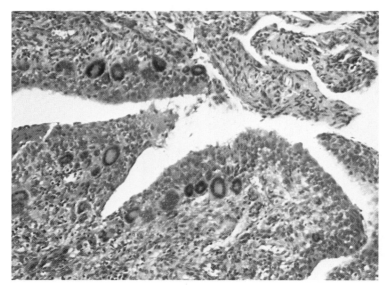

FIGURE 11.10 Photomicrograph of a section of synovial membrane from a patient with rheumatoid arthritis. The increased number of lining cells (hyperplasia) and their increased size (hypertrophy) are evident. Many giant cells are also present just below the surface. In the subintimal tissue one may note a chronic inflammatory infiltrate (H&E, x 10 obj.).

flammatory arthritides, there is little reparative activity, and osteophytes and new bone formation are not prominent (Figs. 11.6 and 11.7). Nonsuppurative chronic inflammation of the synovium is characterized by hypertrophy and hyperplasia of the synovial lining cells, resulting in a papillary pattern at the surface of the synovium (Figs. 11.8 and 11.9). Occasionally there are scat-

tered giant cells among the synovial lining cells (Fig. 11.10). Also typical is infiltration of the synovial membrane by lymphocytes and plasma cells (Fig. 11.11), the latter often containing eosinophilic inclusions of immunoglobulin (Russell bodies) (Figs. 11.12 and 11.13); lymphoid follicles (Fig. 11.14); and fibrinous exudation with admixed polymorphonuclear leukocytes at the sur-

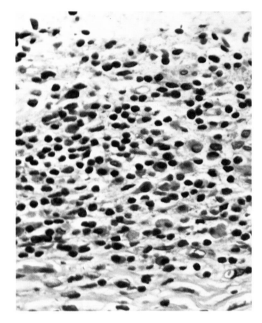

FIGURE 11.11
Photomicrograph of the subintimal region of the synovial membrane in a patient with rheumatoid arthritis shows infiltration of both lymphocytes and plasma cells (H&E, x 25 obj.).

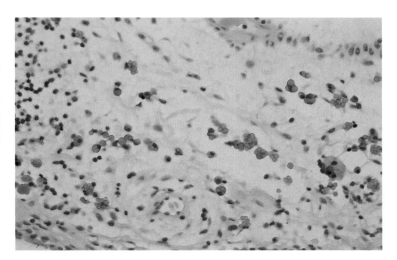

FIGURE 11.12 Photomicrograph of inflammatory infiltrate in rheumatoid synovium reveals eosinophilic cytoplasmic inclusions (Russell's bodies) in the plasma cells (H&E, x 10 obj.).

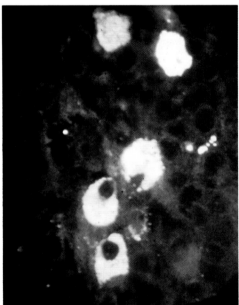

FIGURE 11.13
The plasma cells and Russell's bodies contain rheumatoid factor (immunoglobulin including IgM), demonstrated here by staining with fluorescein-labeled antibody to rheumatoid factor. This specimen is viewed with ultraviolet light.

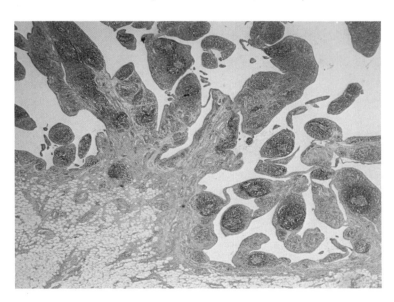

FIGURE 11.14 Low-power photomicrograph of synovium from a patient with rheumatoid arthritis demonstrates the distribution of lymphoid follicles (Allison–Ghormley bodies) in the subintimal tissue (H&E, x 4 obj.).

face of the synovium and within the synovial tissue (Figs. 11.15 to 11.18). Later in the course of the disease the hypertrophied, inflamed synovium extends over the articular surface (pannus) (Fig. 11.19) and destroys the underlying cartilage by interfering with chondrocyte nutrition and by enzymatic degradation of the matrix (Figs. 11.20 and 11.21). The end result of this inflammatory destruction of the articular surfaces is often fusion of the joint (ankylosis), either by fibrous granulation tissue or by bone (Fig. 11.22).

In addition to destroying the cartilaginous surface of the joint, the rheumatoid synovium may invade and destroy the joint capsule and other periarticular supportive tissues. This process can lead to marked instability of the joint, and frequently to subluxation or complete dislocation. The inflamed synovium also invades the bone

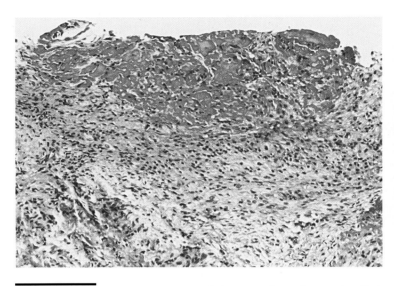

FIGURE 11.15 Photomicrograph of the synovium shows the fibrinous exudate on the inflamed synovial surface (H&E, x 10 obj.).

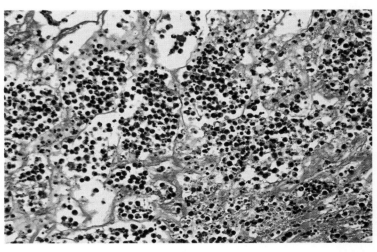

FIGURE 11.16 Photomicrograph showing polymorphonuclear leukocytes in the fibrinous exudate of a patient with an acute rheumatoid joint. With this severity of acute exudation, it is important to rule out an infection (H&E, x 10 obj.).

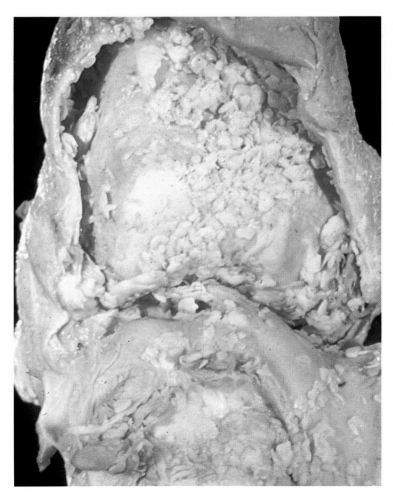

FIGURE 11.17 Gross photograph of the suprapatellar pouch and synovium of a knee joint demonstrates copious fibrinous exudate on the surface of the synovium.

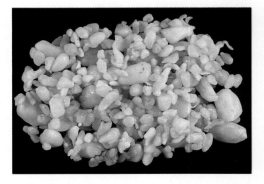

FIGURE 11.18 Photograph of fibrinous loose bodies or "rice bodies" recovered from the knee joint of a patient with rheumatoid arthritis.

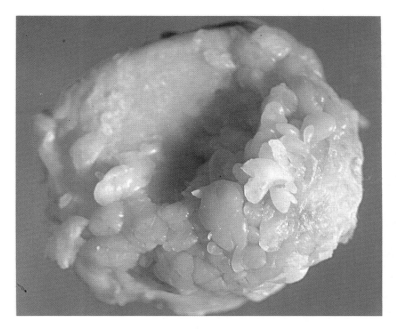

FIGURE 11.19 Gross photograph of the radial head from an elbow in a patient with rheumatoid arthritis. The hyperplastic papillary synovium extends onto and over the articular surface.

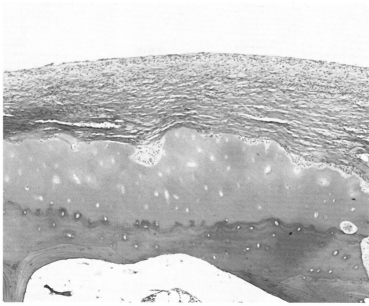

FIGURE 11.20 Low-power photomicrograph of a section of the synovium and underlying cartilage and bone from the specimen shown in Figure 11.19. The inflamed synovium forms a covering or pannus over the cartilage, which in turn is being eroded (H&E, x 4 obj.).

FIGURE 11.21 Close-up of the section shown in Figure 11.20. Not only is the cartilage being eroded from the surface but the chondrocytes are seen to be mostly necrotic, and lysis of the matrix around the chondrocytes has occurred (H&E, x 10 obj.).

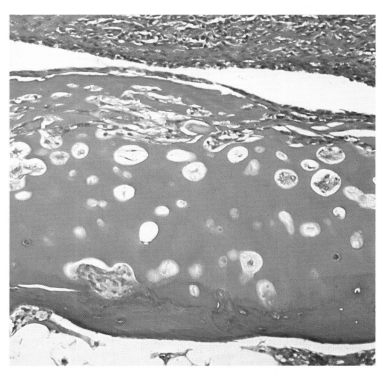

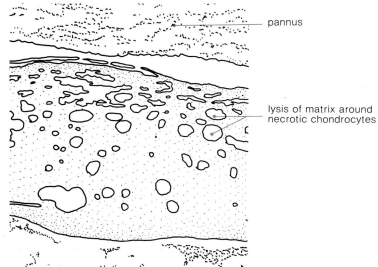

pannus

lysis of matrix around necrotic chondrocytes

FIGURE 11.22 Low-power photomicrograph of a metacarpophalangeal joint with a fibrous ankylosis (H&E, x 2.5 obj.).

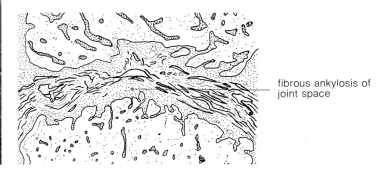

fibrous ankylosis of joint space

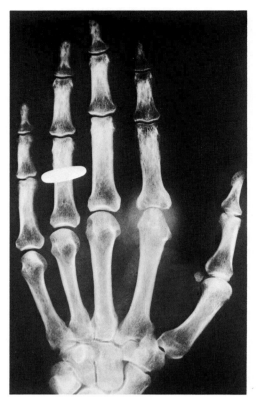

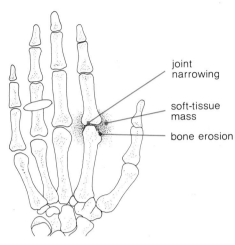

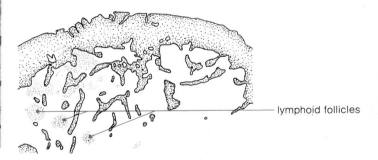

FIGURE 11.23 Radiograph of the hand in a patient with early rheumatoid arthritis. Note the soft-tissue swelling, the reduction in the width of the joint space, and the erosion that has taken place at the margin of the metacarpophalangeal joint of the index finger.

joint narrowing

soft-tissue mass

bone erosion

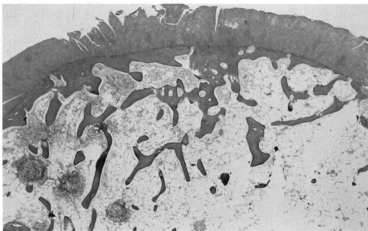

FIGURE 11.24 Low-power photomicrograph of a section through a joint in a patient with rheumatoid arthritis. Note the considerable chronic inflammatory infiltrate in the subchondral bone, as well as occasional lymphoid follicles (H&E, x 2.5 obj.).

lymphoid follicles

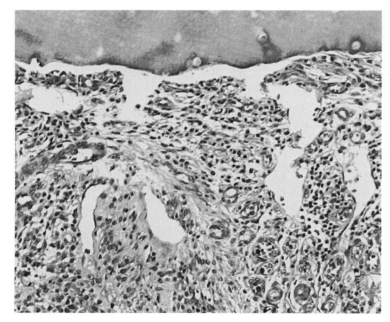

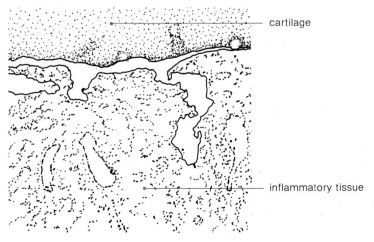

FIGURE 11.25 Photomicrograph demonstrates the erosion of the articular cartilage by subchondral inflammatory tissue (H&E, x 25 obj.).

cartilage

inflammatory tissue

at the articular margins, a change that appears on radiographs as marginal erosion (Fig. 11.23). Extra-articular synovitis may lead to carpal tunnel syndrome or "trigger finger," and in some cases these clinical syndromes herald more generalized articular disease.

In the subchondral bone not in contact with the articular margins, there may be considerable chronic inflammation and formation of lymphoid follicles (Fig. 11.24). This inflammation is confined to the subchondral bone and does not extend far into the underlying cancellous bone. In some cases, the inflammatory tissue destroys the articular cartilage from below (Fig. 11.25). Radiographs of affected joints usually reveal a juxta-articular osteopenia (Fig. 11.26), which is caused either by inflammation of the subchondral bone or by hyperemia secondary to the inflammation of the synovium.

About 25 percent of patients with rheumatoid arthritis have subcutaneous nodules, most commonly over the extensor surfaces of the elbow and forearm (Fig. 11.27). Nodules may also occur in other subcutaneous sites, as well as in the gastrointestinal tract, lungs, heart, and the synovial membrane (Fig. 11.28).

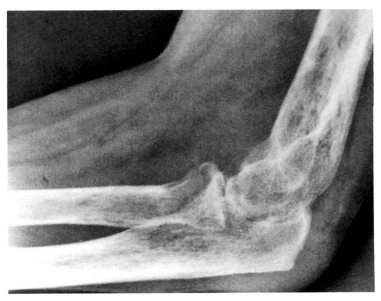

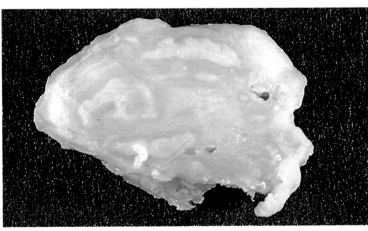

FIGURE 11.26 Radiograph of the elbow in a patient with polyarticular rheumatoid arthritis. Note the loss of joint space resulting from destructive inflammatory synovitis. Considerable osteoporosis has occurred around the joint, a finding in marked contrast to the bony sclerosis associated with noninflammatory osteoarthritis.

FIGURE 11.27 Photograph of the cut surface of a subcutaneous nodule removed from a patient with rheumatoid arthritis. Note the multiple well-defined areas of necrosis with their irregular "geographic" outlines.

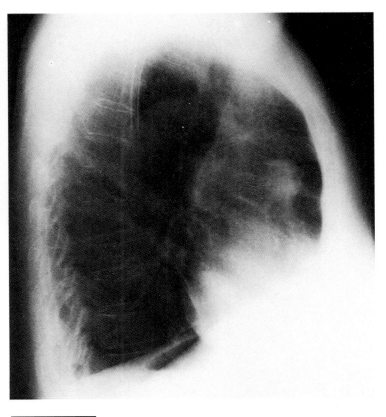

FIGURE 11.28 Radiograph of a lateral projection of the chest shows a well-defined nodule in the anterior lung field.

The nodules may appear before any other signs of rheumatoid disease. The rheumatoid nodule is characterized histologically by an irregular shape and a central zone of necrotic fibrinoid material surrounded by histiocytes and some chronic inflammatory cells (Figs. 11.29 and 11.30). The long axes of these histiocytes are frequently radially disposed or palisaded. The fact that generalized vasculitis is much more common in patients with rheumatoid nodules than in those without rheumatoid nodules is consistent with the belief that the nodules are caused by vascular damage.

Although the ultimate cause of rheumatoid disease is unknown, two important factors contribute to its pathogenesis: an immunologic reaction and an increased number of degradative enzymes. The serum and synovial fluid of most patients with RA contain a number of immunoglobulins, the most common of which is IgM. These immunoglobulins are known as rheumatoid factors; they are produced by plasma cells in the synovium and lymphoid system as antibodies to autologous IgG, which is believed to be altered in some way. These factors appear on microscopic examination, both within and in the vicinity of plasma cells, as dense, homogeneous, eosinophilic globules (or Russell's bodies). Approximately 70 percent of patients with RA have a positive rheumatoid factor, and high titers are usually associated with either severe or acute disease.

Rheumatoid factor complexes with IgG in a manner not unlike an antigen–antibody reaction. Leukocytes are attracted to the immune complexes which, along with fibrin, form deposits on the surface of the inflamed synovium. These cells, filled with particles of ingested fibrin and immune complex, may be found in the synovial fluid and are called "RA cells." After destruction of the polymorphonuclear leukocytes, lysosomal enzymes are released into the extracellular space, where they further provoke an acute inflammatory response and tissue necrosis. These lysosomal enzymes exist in large concentrations in both the synovial fluid and tissue of rheumatoid joints, and they play an important role in perpetuation of the tissue destruction that characterizes the disease.

In the late stages of rheumatoid arthritis the affected joint may show very little inflammation, and the disease may be anatomically indistinguishable from osteoarthritis.

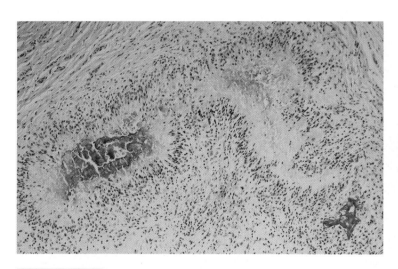

FIGURE 11.29 Photomicrograph of a rheumatoid nodule illustrates the serpiginous shape of the central geographic fibrinoid necrosis and the surrounding pallisaded cells (H&E, x 2.5 obj.).

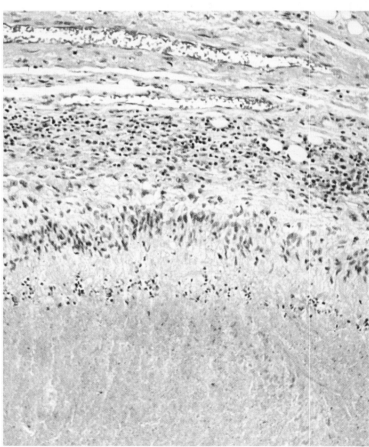

FIGURE 11.30 Photomicrograph of a portion of a rheumatoid nodule demonstrates well-defined zones of central fibrinoid necrosis surrounded by a layer of palisaded histiocytes, which in turn is surrounded by a layer of lymphocytes and dense fibrous connective tissue (H&E, x 25 obj.).

JUVENILE RHEUMATOID ARTHRITIS (JUVENILE CHRONIC POLYARTHRITIS; JUVENILE CHRONIC ARTHRITIS)

A chronic inflammatory arthritis is not unusual in children. About 20 percent of cases are polyarthritic, with systemic disease; 40 percent are polyarthritic without systemic disease; and 40 percent are pauciarticular, with few joints affected. Most patients test negative for rheumatoid factor. The few patients who are positive tend to pursue a more severe course and are more likely to end with a crippling arthritis. However, the outlook for most children with JRA is good. Although the disease is chronic, at least 75 percent of cases enter long remission with little or no residual disability. Synovial biopsies in children affected by JRA usually show much less severe disease than the typical rheumatoid arthritis of adult onset (Figs. 11.31 and 11.32).

DISEASES RESULTING FROM THE DEPOSITION OF METABOLIC PRODUCTS IN THE JOINT TISSUES

GOUT

Gout is characterized by episodic acute attacks of inflammatory, usually monarticular, arthritis, and by the development of chalky deposits of sodium urate around affected joints.

Uric acid is the end product of the catabolism of purines, and since humans lack the enzyme uricase, increased synthesis of uric acid or decreased secretion of uric acid by the kidneys leads to hyperuricemia. Uric acid is not very soluble and begins to precipitate as sodium urate at concentrations above 8.0 mg/dl. Pro-

longed hyperuricemia eventually leads to the deposition of monosodium urate crystals in both the joints and the visceral tissue, but especially in the kidneys, in which precipitates of urates and subsequent stone formation are seen in nearly all patients with gout. When crystals are precipitated in body cavities, such as a joint, they provoke an acute inflammatory response.

Primary hyperuricemia is an inherited error of metabolism that results from an enzymatic defect in purine synthesis and/or in the renal excretion of uric acid. However, hyperuricemia is most often secondary to disorders that increase the production of uric acid by cell breakdown or that decrease the excretion of uric acid (as in various forms of chronic renal disease). The former group includes the myeloproliferative disorders, in which there is an increased turnover of nucleic acid, and patients with cancer, in whom the breakdown of cells and the turnover of nucleoprotein is abnormally rapid.

Gout can be divided into three clinical stages: acute gouty arthritis, an intermediate stage called intercritical gout, and the chronic stage, in which diffuse deposits are seen (chronic tophaceous gout). Acute gouty arthritis is usually monarticular, with a particular predilection for the lower extremities. The first metatarsophalangeal joint (the great toe) is the most common site of initial involvement. Acute gout is characterized by the rapid onset of severe pain and swelling, often accompanied by a low-grade fever and leukocytosis. Acute attacks may be precipitated by trauma, intercurrent illness, or debauchery. Between attacks of acute gout, the patient may have long clinically asymptomatic periods, even though the hyperuricemia persists. Eventually the state of chronic tophaceous gout occurs, in which deposition of monosodium urate crystals occurs throughout the body but particularly in the kidneys and para-articular re-

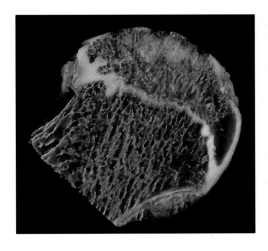

FIGURE 11.31 Photograph of a frontal section taken through the femoral head of a child with juvenile rheumatoid arthritis. Extensive destruction of the articular cartilage has occurred, with associated erosion of the subchondral bone.

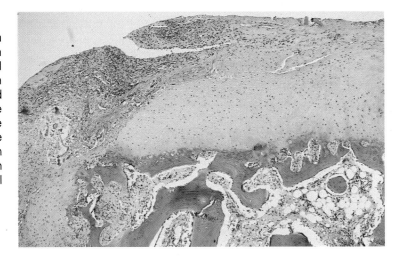

FIGURE 11.32 Photomicrograph of a section taken at the articular margin of the specimen demonstrated in Fig. 11.31 shows a destructive inflammatory pannus extending onto the articular surface (H&E, x 4 obj.).

gions (Figs. 11.33 to 11.35). Although the reason for the deposition of crystals is not understood, the process is known to be accelerated by the presence of a low pH, as seen in the joint spaces.

The radiographic features of gout include swelling of the soft tissues and subsequent erosion of the joint space, giving rise to the classic punched-out lesion in the periarticular bone. Radiologic examination reveals little reactive sclerosis and, in contrast to rheumatoid arthritis, there is no regional osteoporosis (Fig. 11.36). In acute gouty synovitis, microscopic examination of the synovial fluid reveals an inflammatory exudate, which may be mistaken for evidence of infection. However, further examination by polarized light using a

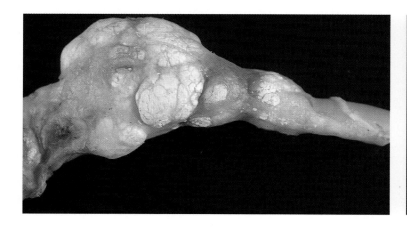

FIGURE 11.33 Photograph of a partially dissected finger amputated from a patient with gout. The large deposits of monosodium urate crystals are chalky white.

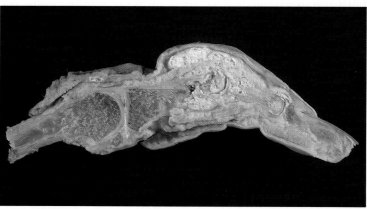

FIGURE 11.34 Photograph of a sagittal section through the finger illustrated in Figure 11.33, showing the extent of the tophaceous deposits and the bone destruction.

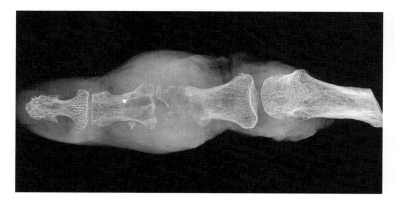

FIGURE 11.35 Radiograph of the specimen illustrated in Figures 11.33 and 11.34.

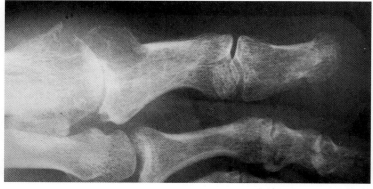

FIGURE 11.36 Radiograph of the great toe shows involvement of the first metatarsophalangeal joint. Overlying the joint there is soft tissue swelling, and at the joint margin a clear-cut bone erosion with a characteristic overhanging edge. There is no porosis of the surrounding bone, as would be seen in a patient with rheumatoid arthritis.

FIGURE 11.37 Low-power photomicrograph of a portion of the joint shown in Figure 11.36. The erosion of the bone and articular cartilage by an amorphous material is evident (H&E, x 2.5 obj.).

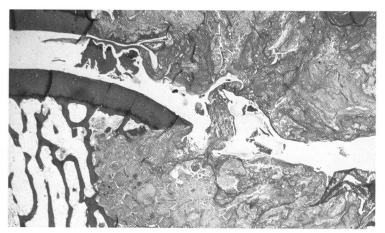

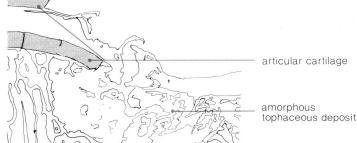

articular cartilage

amorphous tophaceous deposit

first order red filter reveals crystals with a strong negative birefringence. Characteristically the crystals are found in polymorphonuclear leukocytes.

The chalky tophi associated with the chronic phase of gout consist of large deposits of crystals surrounded by fibrous tissue and rimmed by both mononuclear histiocytes and giant cells (Figs. 11.37 to 11.40).

(It should be noted that preservation of the crystals for identification with polarized light microscopy requires the use of unstained sections since the aqueous dyes used in most staining techniques will dissolve the crystals. Crystal preservation is also improved by the use of alcohol rather than formalin fixative.)

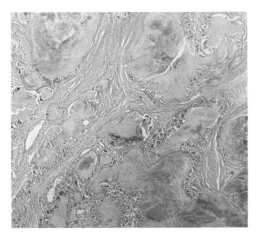
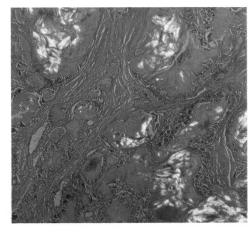

FIGURE 11.38 Low-power photomicrograph of a tophaceous deposit *(left)*. A bluish amorphous material is seen surrounded by bundles of dense collagenized tissue and inflammatory cells. The same field examined by polarized light *(right)*. The birefringence of the crystalline material is evident. (Preservation of the crystals is improved by fixation in alcohol) (H&E, x 4 obj.).

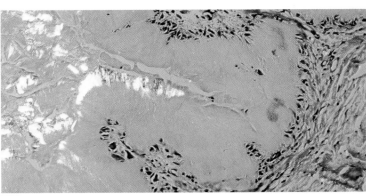

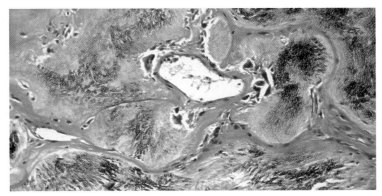

FIGURE 11.39 Photomicrograph shows a detail of the field shown in Figure 11.38. Surrounding the amorphous crystalline deposit is a thin layer of mononuclear and giant cells, with an occasional sprinkling of chronic inflammatory cells (H&E, x 25 obj., polarized light).

FIGURE 11.40 Photomicrograph of another section of tophaceous gout fixed in alcohol. This section has been stained by de Galantha's method for demonstration of monosodium urate crystals (x 25 obj.).

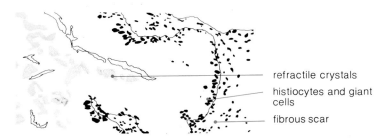

refractile crystals
histiocytes and giant cells
fibrous scar

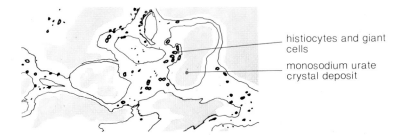

histiocytes and giant cells
monosodium urate crystal deposit

CALCIUM PYROPHOSPHATE DIHYDRATE DEPOSITION DISEASE (CPPD) (PSEUDOGOUT, CHONDROCALCINOSIS)

Disease resulting from the deposition of calcium pyrophosphate has been recognized only comparatively recently. Initially the term *chondrocalcinosis* was introduced to describe a familial condition with typical radiologic evidence of calcification within the cartilage. The term *pseudogout* came into use later because of the gout-like symptoms with which many of the patients present. Since the disease may clinically mimic many conditions, including rheumatoid arthritis, osteoarthritis, neuropathic arthritis, and ankylosing spondylitis, the term *calcium pyrophosphate dihydrate deposition disease* (CPPD) is perhaps a more appropriate name.

CPPD occurs as a hereditary condition, or occasionally as a sporadic condition (it is probable that patients with the sporadic form would demonstrate a familial history if they were more carefully investigated). In some cases it may be associated with some other metabolic dysfunction, such as hyperparathyroidism, hypothyroidism, gout, or hemochromatosis (Fig. 11.41). Reports in the literature on the incidence of this disease vary considerably. Because most affected individuals are asymptomatic, the incidence of CPPD found at autopsy is very much higher than that observed in clinical practice.

The initial manifestation of the disease is likely to occur in the patient's third or fourth decade. The most common clinical presentation of CPPD is similar to that of osteoarthritis. About 50 percent of symptomatic patients present with a progressive degeneration that

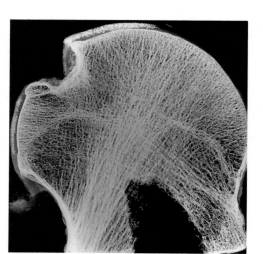

FIGURE 11.41 Radiograph of a slice taken through the femoral head of a patient with hemochromatosis shows extensive calcification of the articular cartilage.

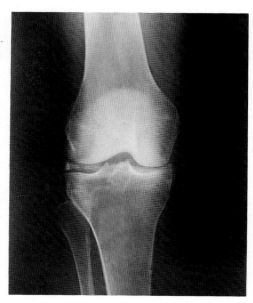

FIGURE 11.42 Radiograph of a knee joint in an elderly individual with extensive calcification of the menisci.

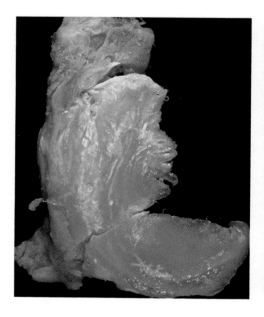
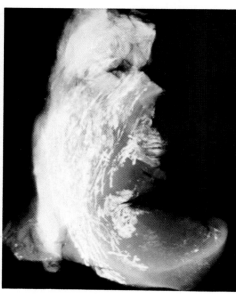

FIGURE 11.43 Gross appearance of a meniscus with extensive calcium pyrophosphate dihydrate deposition *(left)* and a radiograph of this specimen *(right)*.

often affects several joints. In order of frequency of involvement, the joints most likely to be affected are the knees, ankles, wrists, elbows, hips, and shoulders. Rarely, the metacarpals or metatarsals are involved.

Patients with pseudogout account for about 25 percent of those who present with CPPD. Like gout, pseudogout has an acute onset with marked inflammatory changes and swelling. However, it is likely to be less severe than gout, and often there are cluster attacks; that is, a single joint will first be affected, and then satellite joints around it will become involved. Pseudogout, like gout, may be provoked by an associated illness or by trauma (including surgery), and examination of the blood may on occasion show hyperuricemia, further complicating the diagnosis.

There are three other clinical presentations that may occur, and these include multiple symmetrical involvement of the joints in a rheumatoid-like fashion, rapidly degenerating joint conditions similar to Charcot's joints, and stiffening of the spine (usually a familial condition).

On radiographic examination the calcium deposits are characteristically seen in fibrocartilage (Figs. 11.42 to 11.44), but may also be present in hyaline cartilage. The deposits are punctate or linear, and in hyaline cartilage they usually parallel the subchondral

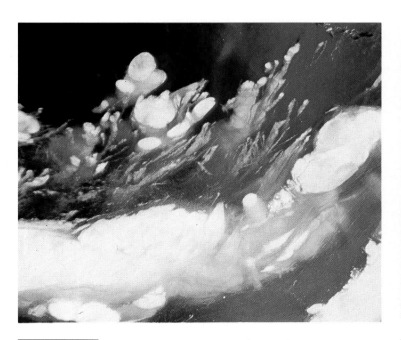

FIGURE 11.44 Detail of gross specimen shown in Figure 11.43.

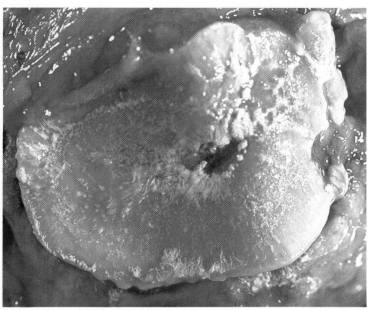

FIGURE 11.45 A degenerated patella with extensive deposits of chalky-white material both on the surface and in the deeper portions of the cartilage, as well as in the synovium.

FIGURE 11.46 In this cut surface of a femoral head, chalky-white deposits of calcium pyrophosphate dihydrate can be seen in the depths of the cartilage *(left)*. Radiograph of the specimen clearly demonstrates the calcific nature of the deposit *(right)*.

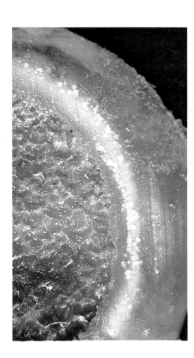
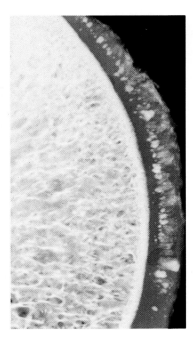

bone end-plate (Figs. 11.45 and 11.46). Punctate calcification may also be seen in the synovial tissue (Figs. 11.47 and 11.48). In addition to the diarthrodial joints, the intervertebral discs and symphysis pubis are often affected. Chondrocalcinosis may be associated radiographically with joint space narrowing and bony sclerosis similar to that seen in patients with degenerative joint disease, but differing in location in the joint. The radiocarpal compartment of the wrist, the glenohumeral joint, and the elbow are commonly involved.

On microscopic examination the chalky white deposits appear either crystalline or amorphous. In vascu-larized tissue they may be surrounded by a chronic inflammatory and giant-cell reaction (Fig. 11.49). In non-vascularized tissue no inflammatory reaction is present (Fig. 11.50). The crystals are distinguished from gout crystals by their shape (rhomboidal) and by their weakly positive birefringence (Figs. 11.51 and 11.52).

Most investigators who have studied chondrocalcinosis believe that the crystal deposition has a chondrocytic origin at least in the articular form. Unlike gout and ochronosis, the immediate changes involve the cartilage lacunae, which become enlarged and coalescent. The adjacent matrix is replaced by chondromucoid ma-

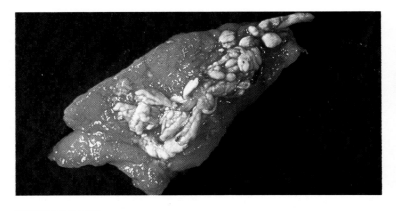

FIGURE 11.47 Synovial tissue with extensive calcific deposits immediately at the surface.

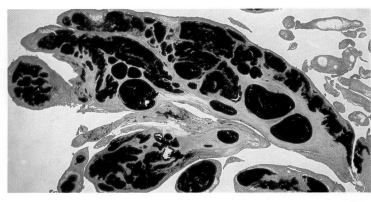

FIGURE 11.48 Histologic preparation of the tissue shown in Figure 11.47, which has been stained with a von Kossa stain to demonstrate the calcium deposits (x 1 obj.).

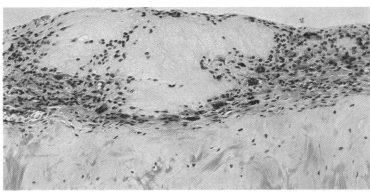

FIGURE 11.49 This photomicrograph shows a deposit of calcium pyrophosphate dihydrate on an articular surface. The deposit is surrounded by mononuclear histiocytes and giant cells, which gives the lesion an appearance very similar to that seen in patients with gout (H&E, x 10 obj.).

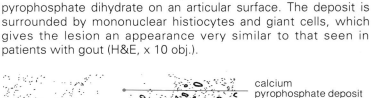
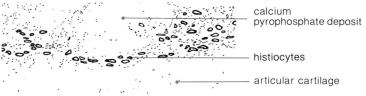

calcium pyrophosphate deposit

histiocytes

articular cartilage

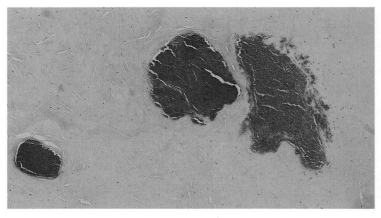

FIGURE 11.50 Photomicrograph of a deposit of CPPD in the meniscus. Note the absence of any inflammatory response (H&E, x 10 obj.).

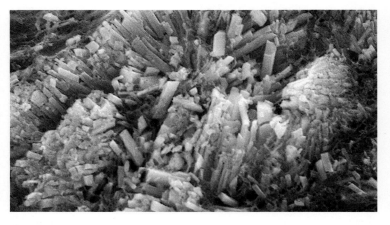

FIGURE 11.51 Scanning electron photomicrograph of a deposit of CPPD, showing the characteristic rhomboidal crystals (x 2400).

terial from which the cells ultimately disappear (Fig. 11.53). The characteristic calcified punctate lesions come about through the deposition of crystals in these chondromucoid pools. It is thought that the deposits are finally released into the joint, where they produce an inflammatory reaction.

EXAMINATION OF SYNOVIAL FLUID FOR CRYSTALS

An important diagnostic procedure for the clinical diagnosis of crystal synovitis is examination of synovial fluid for crystals and identification of these crystals by polarized light microscopy. This examination requires a polarizing microscope with a compensating first-order red filter. With the red filter in position, the crystals in the synovial fluid should be aligned so that their long axis is parallel to the line that is drawn on the compensating filter, which is the axis of slow vibration (Fig. 11.54). Sodium urate crystals are usually needle-shaped and exhibit strong negative birefringence; that is, they appear bright yellow when aligned parallel with

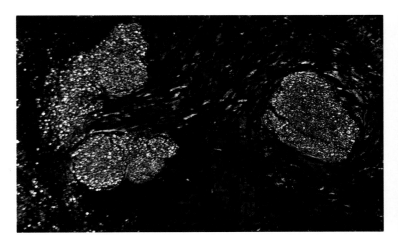

FIGURE 11.52 Photomicrograph of an unstained section taken using polarized light, showing the refractive properties of the CPPD crystals (x 10 obj.).

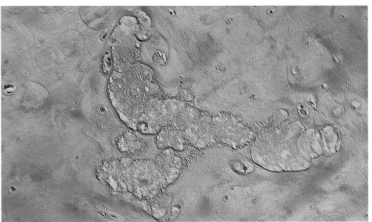

FIGURE 11.53 Photomicrograph of a portion of articular cartilage demonstrates the appearance of the mucoid pools associated with the deposition of CPPD (H&E, x 25 obj.).

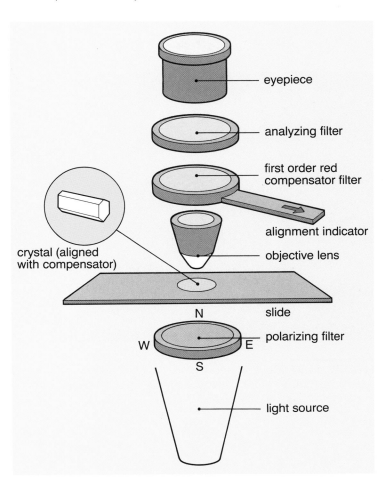

FIGURE 11.54 The light is first passed through a polarizing filter which is usually oriented east–west. The polarizing filter will lie somewhere between the light source and the object being examined. The analyzing filter will lie between the object being examined and the observer, and usually the analyzer is oriented north–south. A refractile body will usually show maximum refraction when the axis of the body is oriented at 45 degrees to the axis of the polarizing filter and the analyzing filter. When the axis of the body being examined is either parallel to or at right angles to the orientation marks on the polarizing filter, it does not refract, and these points are called the extinction points. The use of a first-order red compensator filter enables the observer to distinguish between positive and negative birefringence.

the line on the compensating filter. Calcium pyrophosphate dihydrate crystals are usually rhomboidal and they exhibit weakly positive birefringence, ie, when their long axis is aligned with the line on the compensating filter they appear blue and much less bright than urate crystals (Fig. 11.55). It is important to remember that when a crystal is oriented at 90 degrees to the line on the compensating filter, it will appear the opposite color to which it appears when parallel. Furthermore,

the shape of the crystal may be misleading, because pyrophosphate crystals are occasionally needle-shaped, and urate crystals may be broken up into short, squared-off fragments (Figs. 11.56 to 11.58).

OCHRONOSIS

The term *ochronosis* denotes a brownish-black pigmentation of connective tissue. The condition results from a

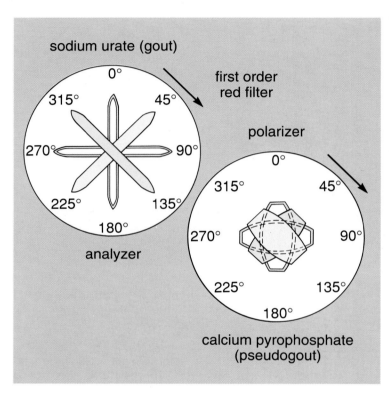

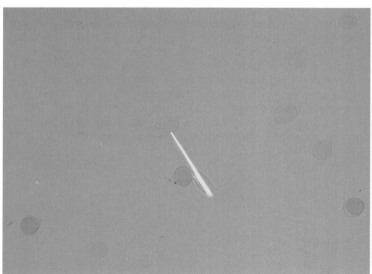

FIGURE 11.55 This illustration shows the effect of rotating a crystal of calcium pyrophosphate dihydrate or sodium urate through 90 degrees. With the crystal lying at 45 degrees to the orientation line on the polarizing filter, and parallel to the orientation line on the first-order red compensator filter, the calcium pyrophosphate dihydrate crystal appears faintly blue. This appearance is described as weak positive birefringence. However, when the crystal is observed perpendicular to the orientation line, rather than parallel to the orientation line, it appears pale yellow. In the case of sodium urate, when the crystal is parallel to the orientation line it appears bright yellow, and we speak of this appearance as strong negative birefringence. When the crystal is perpendicular to the orientation line of the first-order compensator filter, it appears bright blue.

FIGURE 11.56 Needle-shaped crystal in a synovial fluid sample. When this crystal was aligned with the indicator on the compensating filter, it appeared bright yellow and so was identified as a sodium urate crystal (x 100 obj.).

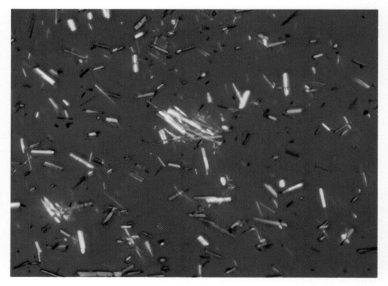

FIGURE 11.57 Multiple short pieces of crystalline material are seen in aspirated fluid. Despite their shape, these are sodium urate crystals (x 100 obj.).

from a rare hereditary disorder of tyrosine and phenylalanine degradation, in which the absence of the enzyme homogentisic acid oxidase leads to the accumulation of homogentisic acid in the body. The presence of excess homogentisic acid in the urine causes the condition known as alkaptonuria, characterized by darkening of the urine on exposure to air; this discoloration may be the only abnormality in children affected by ochronosis (Fig. 11.59). However, in time, the widespread deposition of dark oxidative products occurs in virtually all collagen-containing structures in the body, including the sclerae and the skin. The predominant deposition of homogentisic acid in cartilage (including the intervertebral discs and articular cartilage) causes brittleness and consequent breakdown of the cartilage, which in turn leads to spondylosis and arthropathy, in which the large joints are most severely involved (Fig. 11.60).

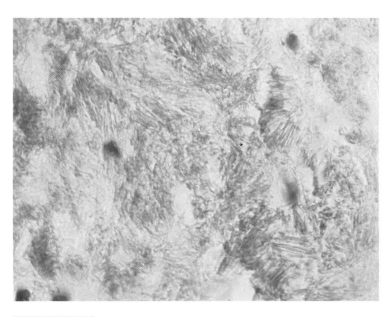

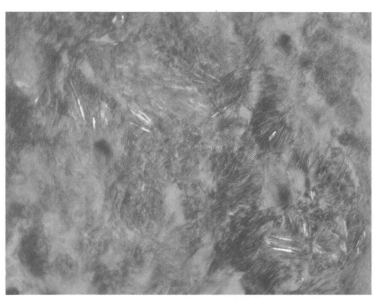

FIGURE 11.58 *(left)* Tissue removed from a patient with calcium pyrophosphate dihydrate deposition disease. The crystals are needle-shaped rather than rhomboidal; however, they are only weakly birefringent (x 100 obj.) *(right)* Same field viewed under polarized light (x 100 obj.).

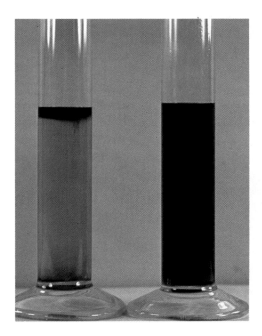

FIGURE 11.59
In the flask on the left is urine from a patient with ochronosis, which has been left to stand for 15 minutes. Some darkening, owing to oxidation of homogentisic acid, is apparent at the surface. After 2 hours the specimen is entirely black (flask on the right).

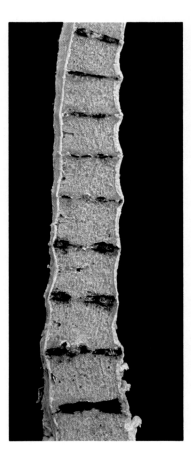

FIGURE 11.60
Section obtained at necropsy through the spine of a patient with ochronosis. Note the black discoloration of the intervertebral discs and the pronounced narrowing of the disc spaces.

Radiographic examination of the spine of patients with ochronosis reveals calcification of the intervertebral discs, with narrowing of the disc spaces (Fig. 11.61). The changes seen in the large diarthrodial joints may be indistinguishable on radiographs from "osteoarthritis" with osteophytosis and subchondral bone sclerosis (Fig. 11.62).

Gross examination of the affected tissues reveals a brownish-black discoloration, often with degenerative changes (Figs. 11.63 and 11.64). Histologic features of ochronosis include the intracellular accumulation of pigment and irregular fragments of pigmented cartilage that may be embedded in the synovium, a phenomenon that suggests a rapidly destructive arthropathy similar to that seen in a Charcot joint (Fig. 11.65). Ultrastructural study of the affected tissue reveals widening and fragmentation of collagen fibers in association with the deposition of the pigment in the matrix (Fig. 11.66).

The precise mechanism of the tissue injury is not yet understood, but the disruption of collagen crosslinking by metabolites of homogentisic acid is a probable explanation.

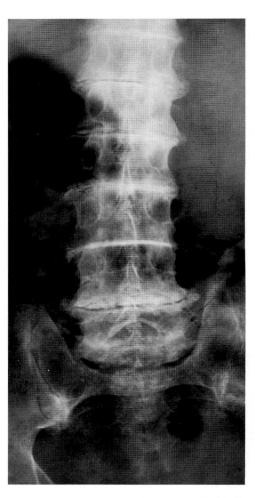

FIGURE 11.61 Radiograph of the vertebral column in a patient with ochronosis. There is marked narrowing of the intervertebral disc spaces, together with some calcium deposition.

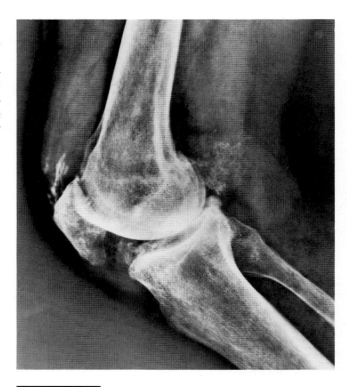

FIGURE 11.62 Radiograph of the lateral aspect of the knee in a patient with ochronosis. Note the joint space narrowing, together with irregular calcified material in the joint space both in the suprapatellar space and in the popliteal space.

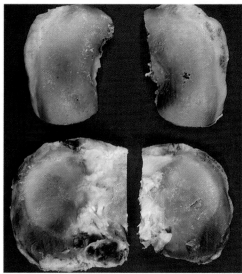

FIGURE 11.63 Photograph of the articular surfaces of a knee joint from a patient with ochronosis, showing discoloration of the cartilage and mild degenerative changes.

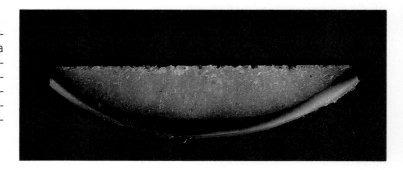

FIGURE 11.64 Section through the femoral condyle illustrated in Figure 11.63 shows that the pigmentation is mainly seen in the deep cartilage.

HEMOPHILIA

Hemorrhage into a joint space, resulting in a hot, painful, and swollen joint, is one of the commonly observed clinical complications of hemophilia. These bloody joint effusions can be precipitated by even minor trauma or stress, and typically involve the knees, elbows, and ankles. Chronic, even subclinical, bloody effusions into the joint spaces may lead to a destructive

arthropathy which is characterized on radiographic studies by a narrow joint space, cartilage destruction, bone erosion, multiple juxta-articular cysts and, if the lesion has progressed over a long period of time, osteophytes (Fig. 11.67). Radiographs may also reveal a peculiar juxta-epiphyseal osteoporosis (Fig. 11.68). Bleeding into the periosteum sometimes gives rise to a large, eccentric pseudotumor (Fig. 11.69).

In the tissues, hemophilia or other bleeding diathe-

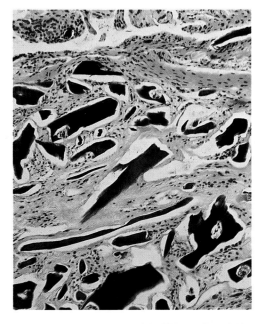

FIGURE 11.65 Photomicrograph of a portion of the synovial membrane from a patient with ochronosis demonstrates irregular fragments of pigmented cartilage, together with fibrosis and mild chronic inflammation in the subsynovial tissues (H&E, x 10 obj.).

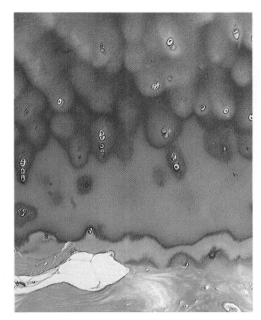

FIGURE 11.66 Photomicrograph of a portion of ochronotic articular cartilage shows the yellowish-black pigmentation of the cartilage matrix. Note the poor viability of the chondrocytes (H&E, x 10 obj.).

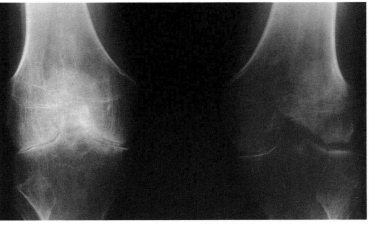

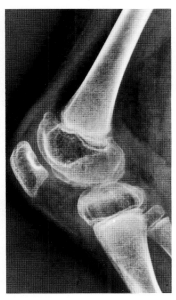

FIGURE 11.68 Radiograph of a young patient with hemophilia. Note the osteoporosis of the epiphyses, irregularity of the articular margins, and squaring-off of the patella.

FIGURE 11.67 Radiograph of the knees of a hemophilic patient shows destructive arthritis of both knees, with marked juxta-articular osteopenia.

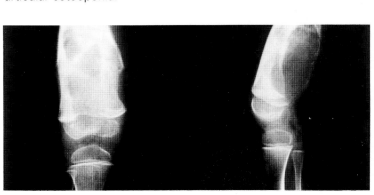

FIGURE 11.69 Radiograph of a large pseudotumor secondary to a subperiosteal hemorrhage in the distal femur of a hemophiliac.

ses are characterized by copious iron deposition and a markedly hyperplastic synovium (Fig. 11.70). The hyperplasia and the hemosiderin deposition are usually limited to the synovial lining cells, although proliferative changes in the subsynovial capillary bed may be dramatic. On the basis of gross examination of the synovium, the differential diagnosis includes rheumatoid arthritis and pigmented villonodular synovitis. However, microscopic examination of the synovium in hemophilia-related destructive joint disease does not reveal the striking lymphoplasmacytic infiltrate that characterizes rheumatoid arthritis, nor is there the

nodular proliferation of mononuclear and giant cells characteristic of pigmented villonodular synovitis (Figs. 11.71 and 11.72).

A characteristic finding in joints affected by chronic hemorrhage is a greenish-black discoloration of the articular cartilage (Fig. 11.73). Microscopic examination of the cartilage often reveals widespread necrosis of the chondrocytes, as well as hemosiderin deposits in the chondrocytic lacunae (Fig. 11.74). However, no iron pigment is seen in the extracellular matrix with the use of conventional light microscopy.

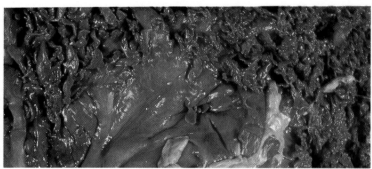

FIGURE 11.70 Photograph of the synovium removed from the knee of a patient suffering from hemophilia. The staining of the synovium with hemosiderin is apparent as a mahogany color. Also apparent is the papillary proliferation of the synovium.

papillary hemosiderin-stained synovium

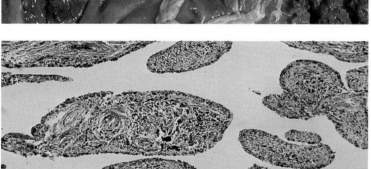

FIGURE 11.71 Photomicrograph of a portion of hemophilic synovium demonstrates hemosiderin deposition both within the synovial lining cells and in the chronically inflamed and fibrotic subsynovial tissue (H&E, x 10 obj.).

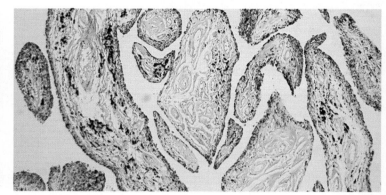

FIGURE 11.72 Photomicrograph of tissue similar to that shown in Figure 11.71, stained by the Prussian blue reaction to demonstrate the distribution of iron in the tissue (x 10 obj.).

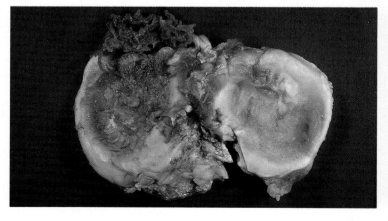

FIGURE 11.73 Photograph of the articular surface of the tibial plateau excised from a patient with hemophilia. Attached to the joint margin is a heavily pigmented papillary synovium. The articular cartilage has a greenish-black discoloration.

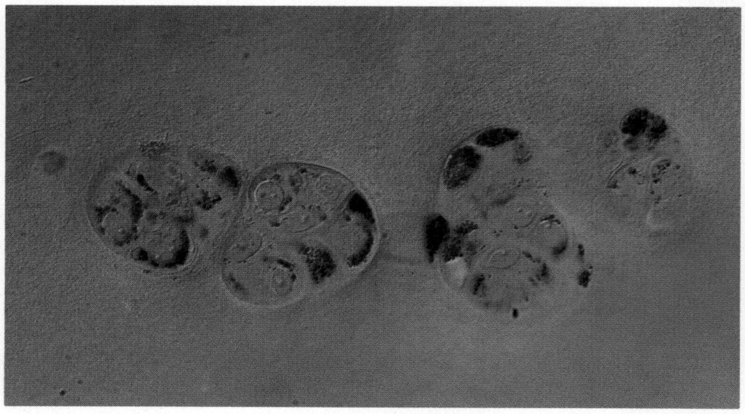

FIGURE 11.74 Photomicrograph demonstrating iron-containing particles within the chondrocytes of hemophilic cartilage (Gomori stain, x 50 obj.).

**Spinal arthritis and
degenerative disc disease**

he vertebral column plays a central role in static and dynamic motor functions, supporting the head, shoulders, arms, and thoracic and abdominal contents, and transmitting their weight to the pelvis. The vertebral column must simultaneously protect the spinal cord and nerves, participate in the locomotion of the entire body, and provide sensory orientation. Each component of the vertebral column—vertebrae, intervertebral discs, muscles, and ligaments—contributes in different ways to its biomechanical function.

Because the spinal column contains over 130 articulations, including the solid intervertebral discs and the synovial joints of both the posterior articular processes and the vertebral articulations of the ribs, many pathological conditions that affect the spine are arthritic in origin. Some diseases, such as disc tissue displacement, initially affect the discs, whereas others, such as rheumatoid arthritis, affect the diarthrodial joints. In general however, both the joints of the vertebral bodies and those of the arches are eventually involved by disease. This chapter discusses the different types of disc tissue displacement, followed by discussions of Scheuermann's disease and degenerative arthritis of the spinal column (facet joint arthrosis, spondylosis, degenerative spondylolisthesis, and Charcot spine). Finally, the effects of inflammatory arthritis and the ankylosing spondyloarthropathies will be examined.

DISPLACEMENT OF DISC TISSUE

The intervertebral disc comprises a nucleus pulposus consisting mainly of water and proteoglycan confined within an anulus of obliquely oriented collagen fibers (see Chapter 1). Because the water in the nucleus is incompressible, loads are transmitted hydrodynamically from one vertebra to the next through the cartilage and bony end plates, while radial forces are absorbed through the tension in the fibers of the anulus (Fig. 12.1). If normal intradisc pressure exists in the standing position, a 5 percent tilt of the spine increases the load on the vertebra by about 25 percent. Sitting increases it by about 40 percent, but lying supine reduces it by about half. Forward flexion of the disc, however, increases the intradiscal pressure by as much as 400 percent, demonstrating the importance of lifting with bent knees and a straight back (Fig. 12.2).

The disc of the young adult, with its bulging mucoid nucleus pulposus, dense collagenous anulus fibrosus, and well-defined cartilaginous end plates, can be clearly differentiated from that of the elderly person, with its shrunken, yellowed, and dehydrated nucleus pulposus (Figs. 12.3 and 12.4). In general, acute displacement of the disc tissue is a disease of people in their third and fourth decades. It is less likely to occur or to cause significant compromise of the neural canal or foramen in an older individual, in whom disc tissue, especially the nucleus pulposus, is shrunken and dehydrated.

Displacement of disc tissue (usually the nucleus pulposus) from the intervertebral disc space may occur anteriorly, posteriorly, superiorly, or inferiorly (Fig. 12.5). Displacement of disc tissue anteriorly usually produces spondylosis deformans, whereas displacement posteriorly produces pressure on the nerve roots or encroachment on the contents of the spinal canal. Displacement superiorly or inferiorly, into the adjacent

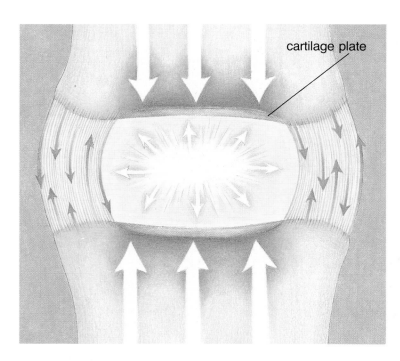

cartilage plate

FIGURE 12.1 Schematic drawing of the forces acting through the area of the vertebral body and intervertebral disc. Compressive forces are transmitted through a central layer of hyaline cartilage interposed between the nucleus and bone, whereas tensional forces generated in the anulus are transmitted to the bone through Sharpey's fibers attached around the periphery.

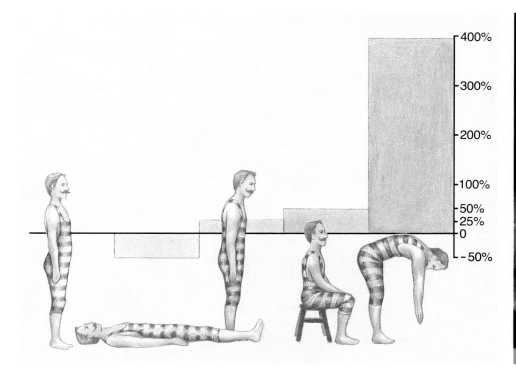

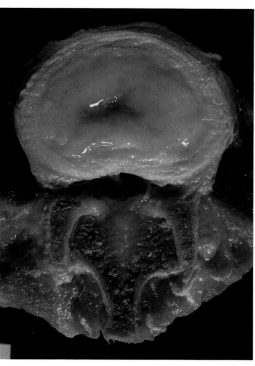

FIGURE 12.2 Schematic drawing showing the percentage change in load on the lower lumbar discs according to body position. The standing position is taken as the reference point. (Based in part on the original work of Dr. Alf Nachemson)

FIGURE 12.3 Transverse section through the L1–2 disc from an adolescent. Note the clear demarcation between the bulging mucoid nucleus pulposus and the laminated anulus fibrosus.

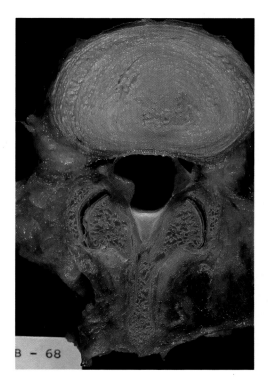

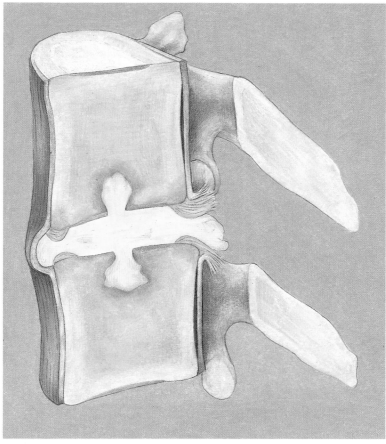

FIGURE 12.4 Transverse section through the lumbar disc of a 70-year-old. There is no clear distinction between the anulus and the shrunken, dehydrated nucleus.

FIGURE 12.5 Schematic drawing showing the several directions in which disc tissue displacement may occur: anteriorly, posteriorly, superiorly, or inferiorly.

vertebral bodies, will lead to the development of Schmorl's nodes.

The different forms of displacement include protrusion, prolapse, extrusion, and sequestration (Fig. 12.6). Protrusion is a bulging of the nucleus pulposus through a weakened anulus fibrosus, usually in a posterior or posterolateral direction; prolapse is a rupture of the nucleus pulposus through the anulus but not through the posterior or anterior longitudinal ligament; extrusion is a rupture of the nucleus pulposus through both the anulus and the ligament, usually the posterior longitudinal ligament; sequestration is a fragmentation of the extruded segment, occasionally with displacement of the free fragment into the spinal canal and often to a site far removed from the point of rupture. The general term "disc herniation" is used to describe either prolapse, protrusion, or extrusion. For displacement of the nuclear tissue to occur, there must be prior traumatic laceration of the anular fibers. Such tears are usually associated with torsion and compression injuries resulting from the sudden application of force.

Anterior protrusion (spondylosis deformans) is one of the most common forms of spinal disease seen radiographically and at autopsy. By the age of 50 it is present in at least 50 percent of women and more than 60 percent of men. The disease appears to occur more frequently in people engaged in occupations that require heavy physical labor. The lumbar spine is the site most commonly affected. Spondylosis deformans is initiated by tears that occur anteriorly in the periphery of the anulus, where the collagen bundles attach to the vertebral bodies by Sharpey's fibers (Fig 12.7). This leads to anterior herniation of nuclear disc tissue and is potentiated by weight bearing and by spinal motion. Because the anterior longitudinal ligament has only weak attachments to the anulus, continuous tearing of these attachments by prolapsed disc material stimulates the development of beak-like boney outgrowths or spurs (Figs. 12.8 and 12.9).

Posterolateral displacement is found at autopsy in approximately 50 percent of older individuals, mostly in the lumbar region of the spine. The basis for poste-

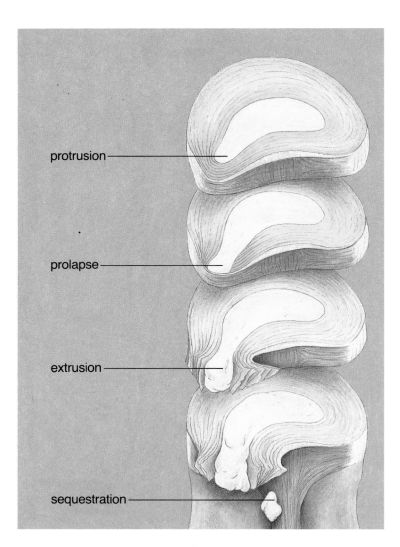

protrusion

prolapse

extrusion

sequestration

FIGURE 12.6 Schematic drawing illustrating the different types of disc tissue displacement: protrusion, prolapse, extrusion, and sequestration.

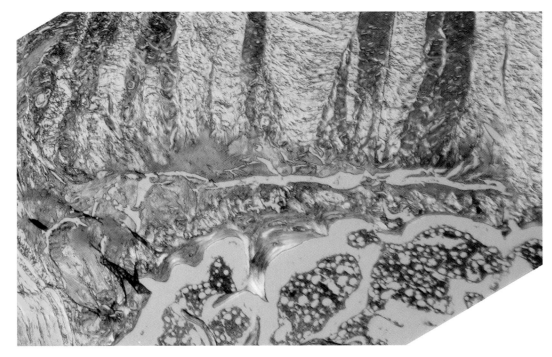

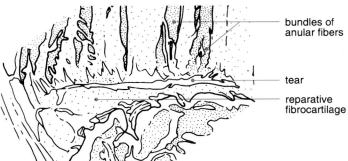

FIGURE 12.7 Polarized photomicrograph showing the early development of spondylosis deformans, taken at the junction of the anulus fibrosus, subchondral bone, and anterior longitudinal ligament. At the insertion of the anulus into the bone is a linear tear through Sharpey's fibers, providing a route for the herniation of nuclear material. The defect is partially filled with reparative fibrocartilage (polarized light, x 1.5 obj., approx. 12 magnifications)

bundles of
anular fibers

tear

reparative
fibrocartilage

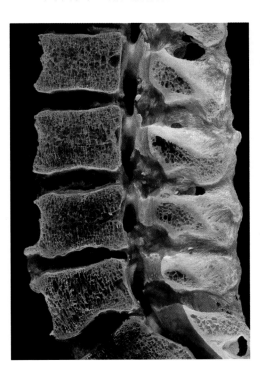

FIGURE 12.8
Photograph of a macerated sagittal section of the lumbar spine in spondylosis deformans. Note the narrowing at the L4–5 disc space, compared with the levels above, and an anterior traction osteophyte.

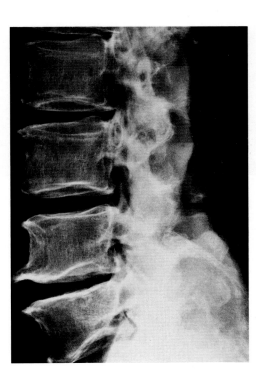

FIGURE 12.9
A specimen radiograph of this section shows the anterior osteophyte directed in a horizontal manner at the L4–5 disc space.

rior disc displacement is the small tears that accumulate in the anulus of the disc as a result of the stresses and strains of daily activities. These clefts, especially the radial ones, pave the way for displacement of the nucleus pulposus after acute trauma (Figs. 12.10 to 12.12). Disc material removed at the time of surgery usually displays evidence of degeneration, along with regenerative clones of chondrocytes (Fig. 12.13).

Displacement of disc tissue posteriorly and posterolaterally usually causes clinical symptoms, depending on the amount of disc tissue displaced and its proximity to neural structures. The typical presentation is that of nerve root compression with radiating pain, resulting from an acute inflammatory response to the displaced tissue. After a period of bedrest there is regression of edema and inflammation, and the pain usually subsides. Later recurrence of pain may result from further displacement of disc tissue or from scarring, which is sometimes accompanied by calcification and ossification. The relative infrequency of osteophyte formation in the posterior aspect of the vertebral body is due to the firm attachment of the disc to the posterior longitudinal ligament.

Herniation of disc substance through the cartilaginous end plate into the adjacent vertebral body leads to the formation of Schmorl's nodes (Figs. 12.14 and 12.15). These herniations, which are probably traumatic in origin, extend for variable distances into the cancellous bone of the adjacent vertebral body. When they are large and symptomatic, Schmorl's nodes may be misdiagnosed radiologically as tumors. Biopsy can lead to a histologic misdiagnosis of chordoma or a cartilaginous tumor (Fig. 12.16).

The clinical significance of Schmorl's nodes is that as disc tissue escapes into the vertebral bodies, the intervertebral disc becomes degenerated and thinned, thus placing strain on the facet joints and leading to spondylosis.

SCHEUERMANN'S DISEASE

Scheuermann's disease, which has its clinical onset in adolescence, is also known as juvenile kyphosis. It is characterized by an abnormal increase in the dorsal convexity of the thoracic spine (Fig. 12.17). Although the etiology of the disease is unknown, it is generally believed to be caused by an abnormality in the

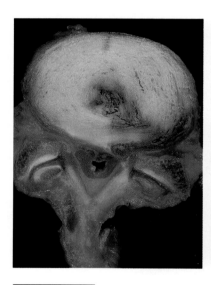

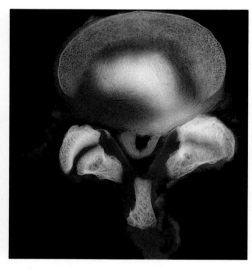

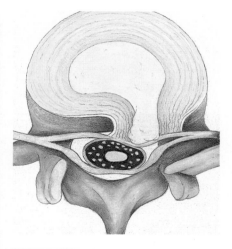

FIGURE 12.10 Photograph of the L4–5 disc in cross-section after injection of contrast medium into the nucleus pulposus. Note extension of the dye posterolaterally. It is dissecting between the disc and the posterior longitudinal ligament, which appears to be intact. There is a bulging that results in an impression upon the dura, with narrowing of the intervertebral foramen (lateral recess).

FIGURE 12.11 A CT scan of the same specimen shown in Figure 12.10 well illustrates the posterolateral bulging with encroachment on the lateral recess.

FIGURE 12.12 Schematic drawing shows posterolateral disc herniation, with encroachment on the nerve root as it goes through the intervertebral foramen.

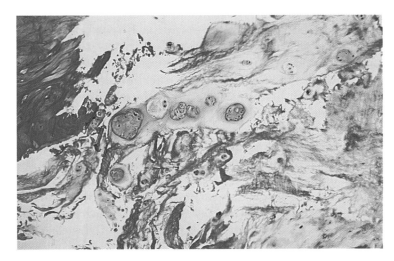

FIGURE 12.13 Photomicrograph of tissue removed at surgery from a herniated intervertebral disc. Note the irregular fibrillated matrix of the nucleus pulposus, which appears largely necrotic but has foci of proliferating cartilage cells (H&E, x 4 obj.).

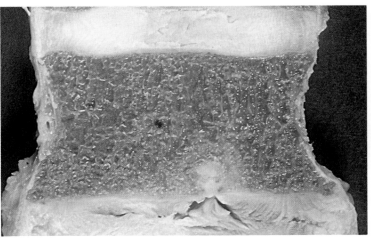

FIGURE 12.14 Photograph of a segment of spine removed at autopsy demonstrates herniation of the intervertebral disc into the adjacent vertebral body. Such herniations are commonly found at autopsy and are known as Schmorl's nodules.

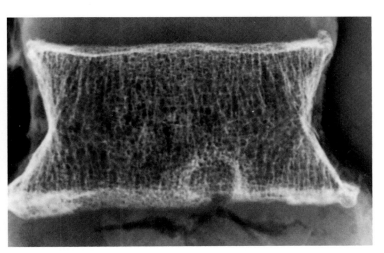

FIGURE 12.15 Radiograph of the specimen shown in Figure 12.14.

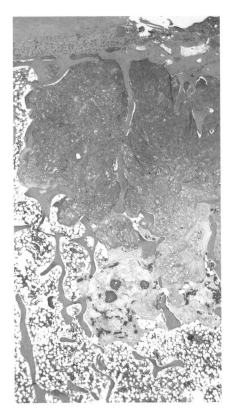

FIGURE 12.16
Photomicrograph of Schmorl's node. On microscopic examination alone this could be confused with a cartilaginous tumor (H&E stain, x 4 obj., approx. 30 magnifications). (Courtesy of Dr. Howard Dorfman)

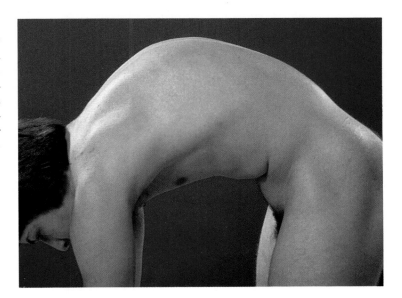

FIGURE 12.17 Clinical photograph of a 16-year-old boy with adolescent kyphosis. In this case, significant thoracic kyphosis has occurred as a result of Scheuermann's disease. (Courtesy of Dr. David S. Bradford)

cartilaginous end plate. The apex of the curve is usually around T7 to T9.

Lateral radiographs are most helpful in clinical diagnosis and classification. Anterior wedging of the thoracic vertebrae is characteristic, and irregularities of the vertebral end plates constitute a prominent feature (Fig. 12.18). Schmorl's nodes are characteristic, and narrowing of the intervertebral disc space occurs in the late stage of the disease. Concomitant with the above changes is an increase in the thoracic kyphosis (beyond 40 degrees).

Characteristic anatomic findings in Scheuermann's disease include intervertebral disc narrowing and irregularly thinned cartilaginous end plates, with focal attenuations through which herniations of the intervertebral disc tissue extend into the adjacent vertebral body (Fig. 12.19). Narrowing of the disc is usually more pronounced anteriorly than posteriorly, resulting in interference with growth of the vertebral ring epiphysis.

cumferential tearing in the anulus fibrosus, and replacement of normal disc tissue by fibrous tissue (Fig. 12.20). Calcification is also common. However, apatite crystal deposits can be easily overlooked in sections prepared with hematoxylin and eosin staining, and are clearly revealed only with the von Kossa stain. Large horizontal clefts develop in the central part of the disc tissue and can be seen on clinical radiographs, where they are often referred to by radiologists as the "vacuum phenomenon" (Fig. 12.21).

As disc tissue degeneration progresses, with subsequent narrowing of the disc space, formation of new bone takes place around the periphery of the disc, at the junction of the anulus and the vertebral body. New bone formation also occurs as a result of endochondral ossification of the cartilaginous end plate, which contributes to narrowing of the disc space (Fig. 12.22).

After vascular invasion, progressive breakdown of the disc tissue contents will lead to their resorption. Frequently, the final stage of the resorption process is a spontaneous fusion of adjacent vertebral bodies.

OSTEOCHONDROSIS

The term osteochondrosis describes the pathologic changes that occur in the intervertebral disc and in the adjacent bone of the vertebral bodies as a result of disruption in the region of the end plate of the disc.

After disruption of the cartilaginous end plate, the other disc components exhibit rapidly progressive degeneration, with focal necrosis, fissuring, radial or cir-

SPONDYLOSIS
(OSTEOARTHRITIS OF THE SPINE)

Anatomic evidence of osteoarthritis of the spinal articulations is rare before the age of 30. However, after the age of 45 osteoarthritis becomes more common, and is found at autopsy in more than 80 percent of spines from older individuals.

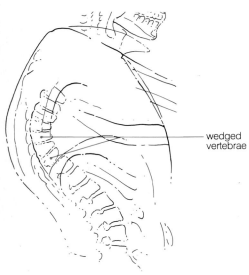

FIGURE 12.18 Lateral radiograph of a 13-year-old female with Scheuermann's kyphosis. Note the wedging of the vertebrae at the apex of the curve and the irregularities of the end plates.

wedged vertebrae

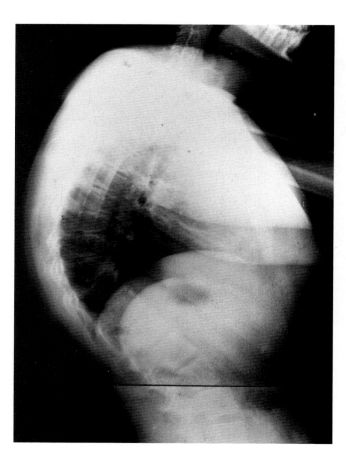

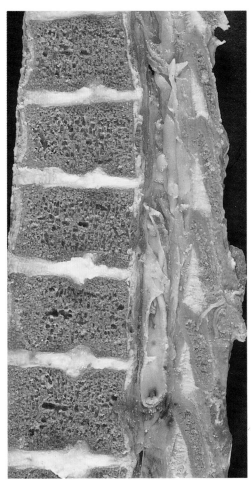

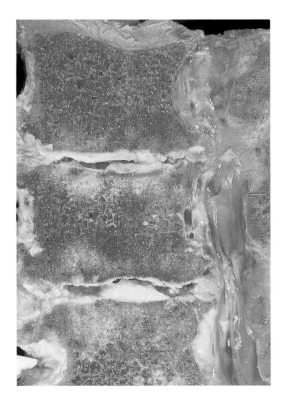

FIGURE 12.19
Photograph of a sagittal section through the thoracic spine removed from a patient with Scheuermann's disease. Note the multiple end-plate irregularities as well as herniation of the disc tissue into the adjacent vertebral bodies.

FIGURE 12.20 Photograph of a sagittal section through L3–5 of a 72-year-old male. Note severe disc degeneration, along with irregularity of the end plates and adjacent sclerosis of the bone.

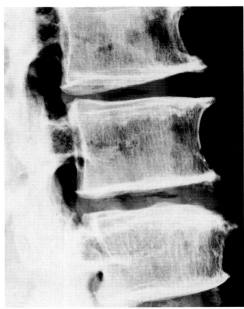

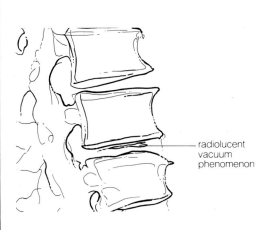

radiolucent vacuum phenomenon

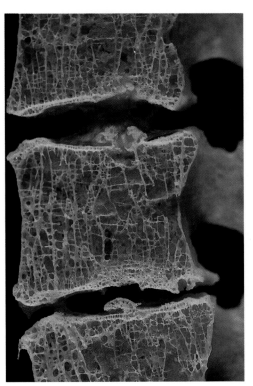

FIGURE 12.21 Specimen radiograph of the portion of spine illustrated in Figure 12.20. Note the radiolucent line, which corresponds to the cleft in the disc seen in the gross photograph. This line is usually referred to by radiologists as the "vacuum phenomenon."

FIGURE 12.22 Photograph of a sagittal section through a portion of the macerated spine of an 83-year-old female. Ossification extends into the disc space. Such ossification may eventually occlude the space entirely. In addition, note fractures through the end-plate and associated bony sclerosis.

The term *spondylosis* embraces the clinical disease resulting from degenerative disc disease (osteochondrosis), together with the associated vertebral osteophytosis, ligamentous disease, facet joint disease, and accompanying neurologic complications. In the older population, this condition is almost universally present and certainly it is one of the greatest single causes of loss of work, particularly among those who do heavy manual labor. Although spondylosis can occur in any spinal segment, it most often affects the more mobile segments of the spine (the cervical and lumbar segments).

The cervical portion of the vertebral column possesses the greatest mobility and thus has the greatest susceptibility to functional stress and trauma. Therefore, cervical spondylosis is very common and is often debilitating (Fig. 12.23).

Degenerative arthritis of the zygapophysial (or facet) joints of the cervical spine is usually progressive, leading to the formation of osteophytes which may pro-

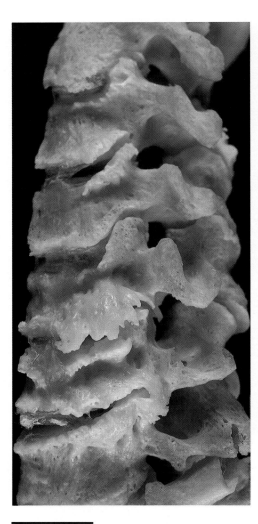

FIGURE 12.23 Photograph of the anterior oblique view of the macerated cervical spine of a 77-year-old female. There is marked osteophyte formation of the uncovertebral joints, particularly in the lower cervical region. Note encroachment of the osteophytes on the intervertebral foramina, particularly at C5–7.

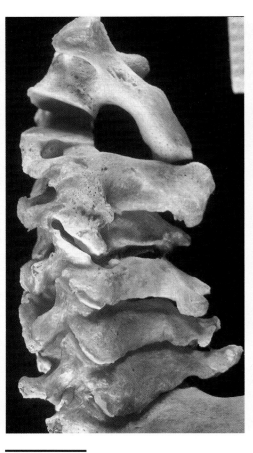

FIGURE 12.24 A macerated preparation of the cervical spine in a 74-year-old female is shown externally in lateral view. Note the marginal osteophytes, which affect all of the facet joints.

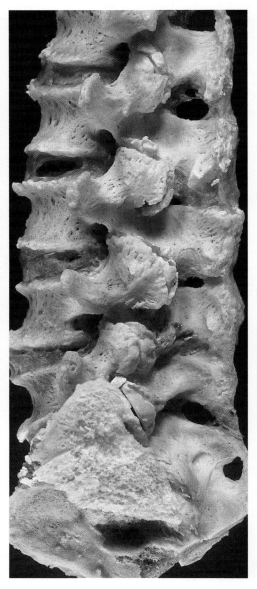

FIGURE 12.25 Posterior oblique view of the lumbar spine of an elderly male, revealing severe facet joint arthritis. Note the exuberant marginal osteophytes with their irregular, serrated margins.

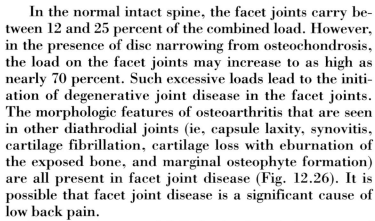

trude into the intervertebral foramina, causing vascular congestion and subsequent irritation of the spinal nerve roots (Fig. 12.24).

Vertebral artery insufficiency is yet another potential complication, as a result of osteophytes impinging on the vertebral artery within the transverse foramina of C2 to C6. This complication is usually compounded by the presence of atherosclerotic vascular disease.

Lumbar spondylosis, which occurs most often in males, particularly affects the lower lumbar spine, where it represents one of the most common causes of low back and leg pain. Lumbar disc degeneration follows a chronic course, with repeated injury playing a precipitating role. These degenerative changes cause alterations in the size and shape of the vertebral canal and its lateral recesses, with subsequent nerve root compression (Fig. 12.25). The clinical manifestations include sciatica and/or ischemia of the cauda equina, with pseudo- (neurogenic) claudication.

In the normal intact spine, the facet joints carry between 12 and 25 percent of the combined load. However, in the presence of disc narrowing from osteochondrosis, the load on the facet joints may increase to as high as nearly 70 percent. Such excessive loads lead to the initiation of degenerative joint disease in the facet joints. The morphologic features of osteoarthritis that are seen in other diathrodial joints (ie, capsule laxity, synovitis, cartilage fibrillation, cartilage loss with eburnation of the exposed bone, and marginal osteophyte formation) are all present in facet joint disease (Fig. 12.26). It is possible that facet joint disease is a significant cause of low back pain.

Degenerative spondylolisthesis, the displacement of a vertebral body on the one directly below it, is caused by degeneration of the facet joints, which in turn is caused by narrowing of the intervertebral disc space. The end result of degenerative spondylolisthesis is spinal stenosis (Fig. 12.27).

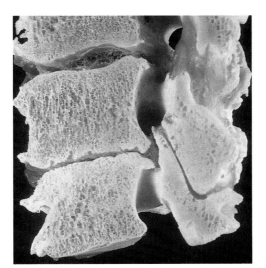

FIGURE 12.26
Macerated sagittal section through L4–5 of a 79-year-old male shows severe narrowing of the facet joint, with associated subchondral sclerosis and osteophyte formation. Note the associated disc narrowing, posterior osteophytes, and lateral recess stenosis.

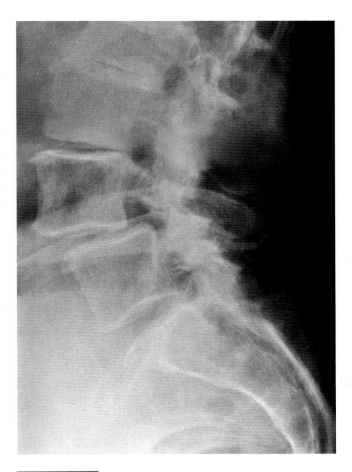

FIGURE 12.27 Lateral radiograph of the lumbar spine of a 58-year-old woman with back pain and pseudoclaudication. At L4–5, there is spondylolisthesis secondary to degenerative disc disease. Note the narrowing of the spinal canal at that level.

NEUROPATHIC (CHARCOT) SPINE

Trauma to the spinal articulations, with their ultimate destruction, may occur as the result of impaired perception of pain or of proprioception, and is generally referred to as neuropathic arthropathy. Tabes dorsalis (neurosyphilis), diabetes, syringomyelia, paraplegia, peripheral neuropathy, and congenital indifference to pain, as well as intra-articular steroid injections, are considered etiologic factors in the development of neuropathic arthropathy. Ten to 15 percent of patients with tabetic arthropathy of the peripheral joints also have involvement of the lumbar spine (Figs. 12.28 and 12.29). In advanced cases, the spine exhibits extensive disc destruction, with sclerosis and fragmentation of the vertebral bodies and massive osteophytosis. Histologic features include marked joint destruction, with bone debris in the synovial tissue and many loose bodies—changes similar to those seen with Charcot joints elsewhere (Fig. 12.30).

INFLAMMATORY SPONDYLITIS

Approximately 60 to 70 percent of all rheumatoid arthritis patients develop symptoms and signs relating to the cervical spine. Pain is the most common symptom. Vertebrobasilar artery insufficiency may also occur, leading to transient blindness, vertigo, loss of consciousness and, occasionally, sudden death.

Radiographically, bone erosion and apophysial joint space narrowing are common, and may be followed by fibrous ankylosis and occasionally by bony ankylosis (Fig. 12.31). Erosions of the odontoid process occur in one third of patients with rheumatoid arthritis. As a result of such erosions, three major complica-

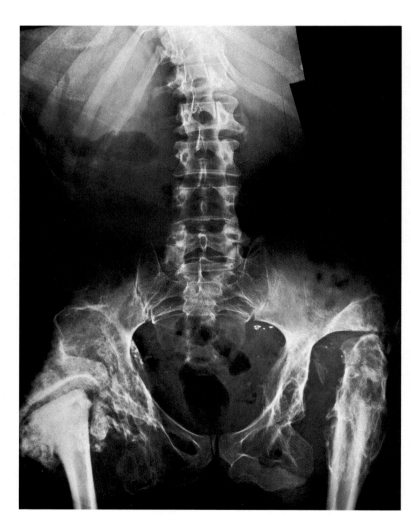

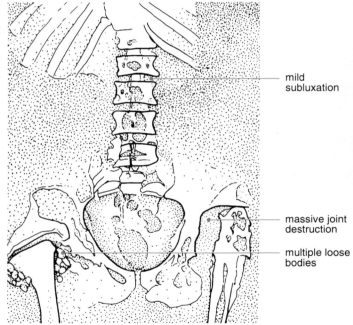

FIGURE 12.28 Radiograph of the pelvis and thoracolumbar spine in a 30-year-old male with congenital syphilis and severe bilateral hip disease. In the lumbar spine, at the level of L2–3, there is mild lateral subluxation.

mild subluxation

massive joint destruction

multiple loose bodies

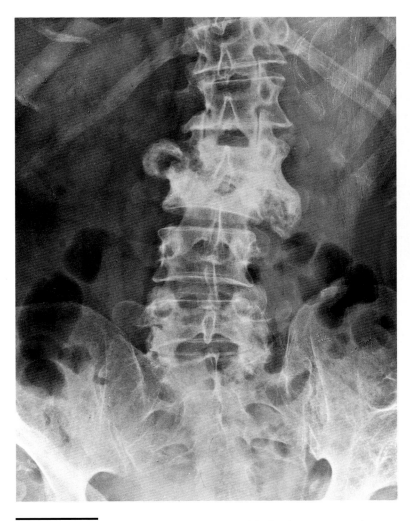

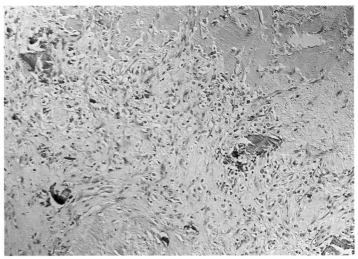

FIGURE 12.30 Photomicrograph of tissue obtained from around a Charcot joint. It is scarred and chronically inflamed with fibrinous exudation, and is filled with multiple irregular fragments of bone and cartilage. Such rapid breakdown of the joint is characteristic in patients with a Charcot joint.

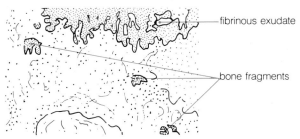

— fibrinous exudate

— bone fragments

FIGURE 12.29 The lumbar spine and pelvis in the same patient as shown in Figure 12.28, 11 years later. At L2–3, there is severe destruction and collapse of the bony elements, with large productive osteophytes characteristic of a Charcot joint.

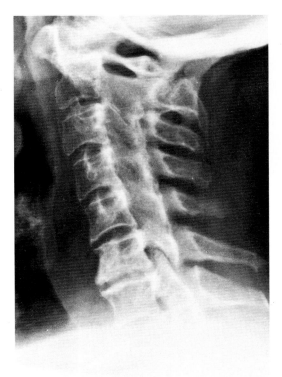

FIGURE 12.31 Lateral radiograph of the cervical spine of a 50-year-old woman with rheumatoid arthritis. Note the fusion of the facet joints in C-2 through C-6. There is narrowing of the spinal canal at the level of C1–2 due to anterior displacement of the atlas. The entire spine is osteopenic.

tions may occur: fracture of the odontoid after minimal trauma; disappearance of the odontoid if the erosion is severe enough; or atlantoaxial subluxation and/or basilar invagination (Figs. 12.32 and 12.33).

It is important to recognize that secondary infections are common in the rheumatoid patient, especially with the use of steroids and other immunosuppressive agents. It is not unusual for such infections to be clinically silent.

Inflammatory spondylitis is also frequently seen in patients who have tested negative for rheumatoid factor. Many of these patients have systemic disorders such as psoriasis or inflammatory bowel disease. Characteristically, the distribution and morphology of spinal articular lesions in these conditions are different from those of rheumatoid arthritis. Whereas in rheumatoid disease the lesions are most obvious in the cervical region, in the

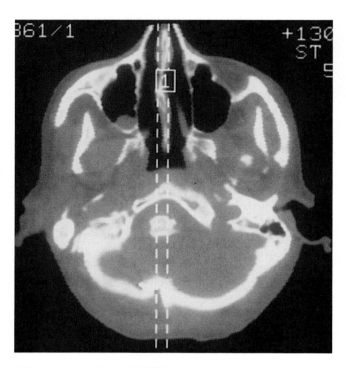

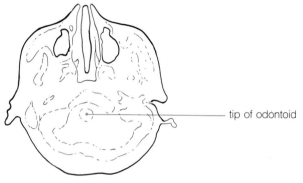

FIGURE 12.32 CT scans *(top and lower left)* of the base of the skull in a woman with rheumatoid arthritis and complaints of transient episodes of loss of consciousness. In both the sagittal reconstruction and the transverse section, displacement of the odontoid into the base of the skull is obvious. An MRI *(lower right)* of the same patient shows an encroachment of the odontoid on the medulla oblongata.

— tip of odontoid

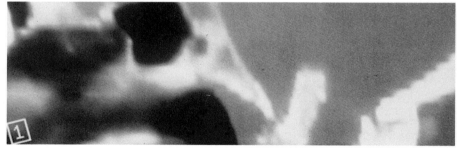

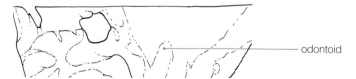

— odontoid

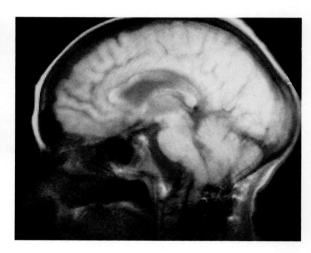

seronegative spondylitidies, sacroiliitis and involvement of the lumbar and lower thoracic spine are more common. Osteoporosis is not usually seen, and in marked contrast to rheumatoid disease, there is bony proliferation and occasionally intra-articular osseous fusion.

ANKYLOSING SPONDYLITIS

Ankylosing spondylitis is a systemic ankylosing arthropathy which primarily affects Caucasian men in their late adolescent or young adult years. Although the onset of the disease is usually insidious, its manifestations may evolve clinically in one of three patterns: in the axial skeleton, chiefly in the lumbar and sacroiliac joints; in the peripheral joints, predominantly in the hips, knees, and heels, especially among adolescents; or as recurrent iritis, aortic valvular disease, fatigue, and other systemic features, without obvious arthritis (Fig. 12.34).

The spinal disease may eventually progress in an ascending fashion to involve the thoracic and cervical vertebrae, along with other axial articulations such as the pubic symphysis and ribs. Either transient or chronic involvement of the peripheral joints has been reported in 50 percent of cases, especially in the hips and knees, but the small joints of the hands and feet are not commonly affected. The natural course of the disease is usually characterized by slow progression without periods of remission.

The antigen associated with ankylosing spondylitis (HLA B27) is present in 90 to 95 percent of patients with ankylosing spondylitis, compared to an incidence of 6 to 9 percent in the normal population. Other laboratory findings characteristic of the disease may include an elevated ESR, and mild hypochromic anemia (in less than one third of cases). Elevated levels of serum creatinine phosphokinase (CPK) of muscle origin are seen in about one third of patients with ankylosing spondylitis.

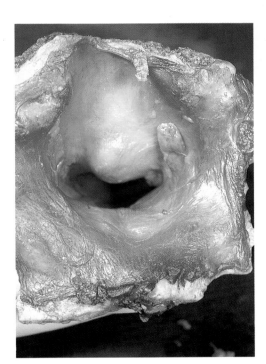

FIGURE 12.33 Photograph of the base of the skull, seen from above, in a patient with rheumatoid arthritis who died suddenly in a minor automobile accident. The odontoid process protrudes through and narrows the exit of the foramen magnum.

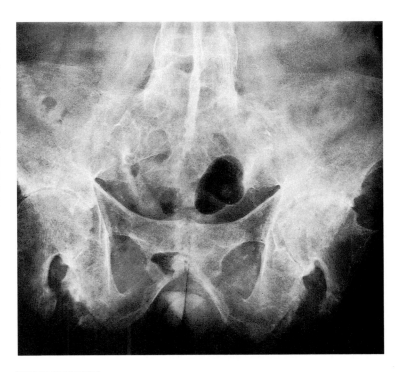

FIGURE 12.34 AP radiograph of the lower lumbar spine, pelvis, and hips of a man with advanced ankylosing spondylitis. Note generalized osteoporosis with fusion of the spinous processes, intervertebral discs, sacroiliac joints, and symphysis pubis, and severe concentric degeneration with partial fusion in both hips. Thus, the entire skeletal unit has been transformed into one continuous osseous mass.

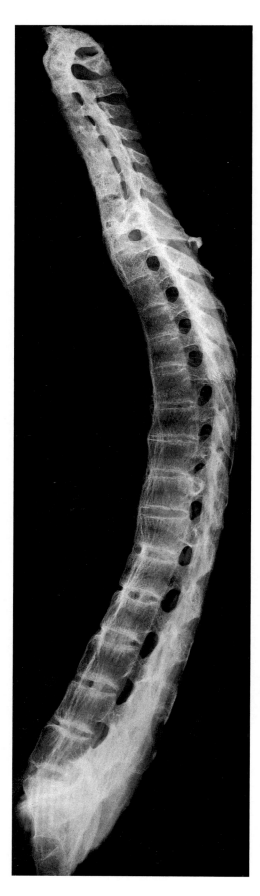

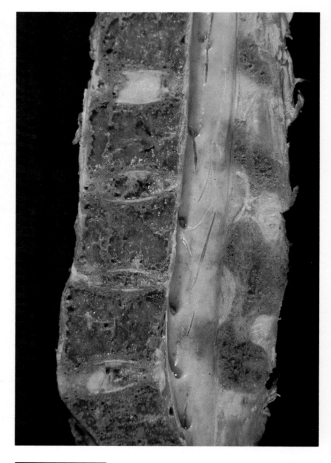

FIGURE 12.35 Radiograph of a sagittal section through the vertebral column of a patient with ankylosing spondylitis. There is complete fusion of the spine, and accentuated kyphosis and loss of lumbar and cervical lordosis. At the C-7 to T-1 level is an angular deformity of the spinal canal, resulting from a healed fracture at this site. Complete fusion of the apophysial joints, as well as fusion across the intervertebral disc spaces, is obvious.

FIGURE 12.36 Photograph of a sagittal section through the lumbar spine of the patient illustrated in Figure 12.35. Fusion of the intervertebral disc spaces, mainly peripherally, is apparent. The paravertebral ligaments are spared, both anteriorly and posteriorly.

Examination of the spine at autopsy of a patient with end-stage ankylosing spondylitis reveals fusion of the apophysial joints and intervertebral discs, resulting in a rigid, immobile vertebral column with accentuated kyphosis. However, unlike ankylosing hyperostosis or DISH (see below), ossification of the paravertebral ligaments is not a prominent feature (Figs. 12.35 to 12.37).

ANKYLOSING HYPEROSTOSIS OF THE SPINE

Ankylosing hyperostosis of the spine, also known as Forestier's disease or diffuse idiopathic skeletal hyperostosis (DISH), is an ankylosis of the vertebral column resulting from ligamentous ossification without significant disc disease. It usually is manifest in older men, without obvious clinical symptoms (Figs. 12.38 to 12.40).

The diagnostic radiographic criteria include the presence of focal spinal ankylosis, intact vertebral end plates, normal intervertebral disc height and, most important, flowing ossification of the anterior longitudinal ligament, especially along the right side of the thoracolumbar region. Absence of facet joint and sacroiliac joint sclerosis and fusion differentiates the disorder from ankylosing spondylitis.

Approximately one third of the older adult population has ankylosing hyperostosis at necropsy, more than half of these showing end-stage disease. The thoracic spine is involved twice as often as the lumbar spine, which in turn is involved twice as often as the cervical spine (Fig. 12.41).

A peculiar variant of cervical ankylosing hyperostosis has been described, particularly in the Japanese literature, in which ossification of the posterior longitudinal ligament (OPL) occurs, sometimes leading to cord compression (Figs. 12.42 and 12.43).

In patients who have undergone total hip replacement, a higher incidence of heterotopic bone formation after surgery has been found in patients with preexisting ankylosing hyperostosis (Figs. 12.44 and 12.45).

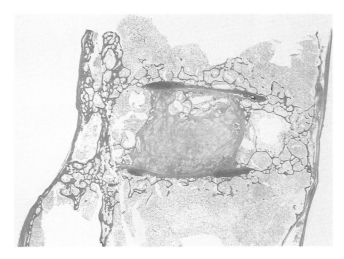

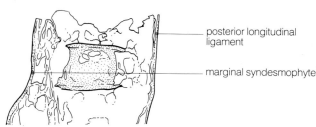

posterior longitudinal ligament

marginal syndesmophyte

FIGURE 12.37 Photomicrograph of a lumbar disc and adjacent vertebral bodies, in this case of ankylosing spondylitis, shows absence of ossification in the anterior and posterior longitudinal ligaments, with severe osteoporosis of the vertebral bodies. Fusion is confined to the intervertebral disc (H&E, x 1 obj.).

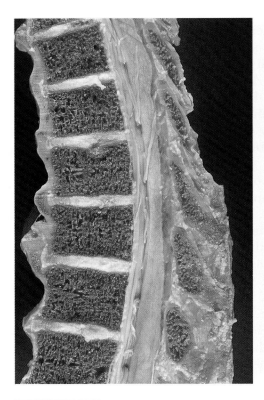

FIGURE 12.38 Photograph of a sagittal section through a segment of midthoracic and lower thoracic spine demonstrates ossification of the anterior longitudinal ligament, with consequent ankylosis of the anterior segment. Note that the disc spaces are relatively normal.

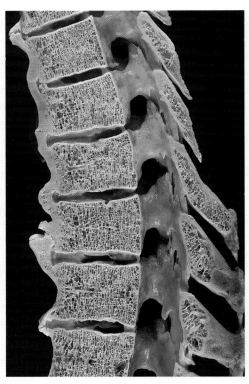

FIGURE 12.39 In the same specimen as shown in Figure 12.38, macerated, a thick plate of bone is seen lying along the anterior cortices of the vertebral bodies and extending in front of the intervertebral discs, like a layer of armor plating.

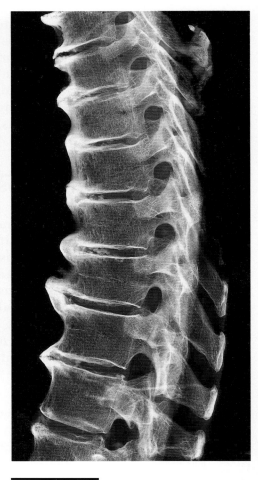

FIGURE 12.40 Radiograph of the macerated specimen shown in Figure 12.39 shows hyperostosis with intact vertebral end plates.

FIGURE 12.41 Lateral radiograph of the cervical spine of an elderly male who complained of difficulty in swallowing. There is an irregular severe anterior hyperostosis, which is largely the result of ossification of the anterior longitudinal ligament typical of DISH. Neither the disc spaces nor the facet joints appear fused and the bone is not osteopenic, thus ruling out a diagnosis of ankylosing spondylitis.

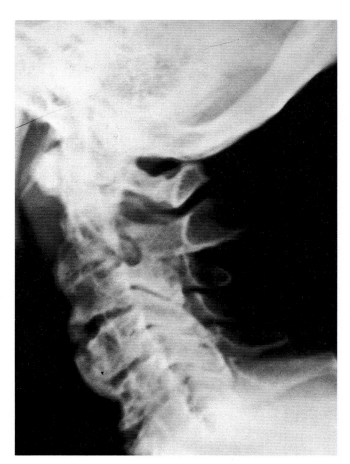

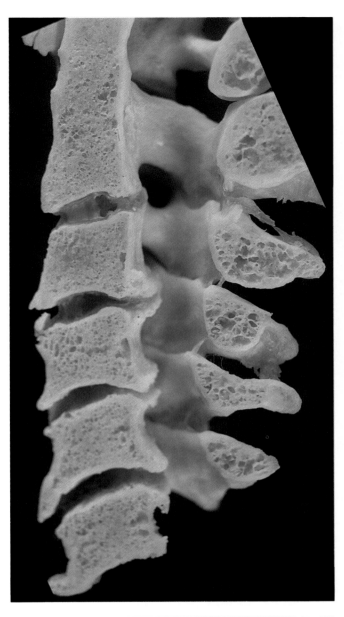

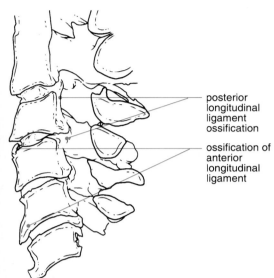

FIGURE 12.42 Photograph of a sagittal section through the cervical spine, which demonstrates ossification of the anterior longitudinal ligament (DISH) and severe ossification of the posterior longitudinal ligament (OPL).

posterior longitudinal ligament ossification

ossification of anterior longitudinal ligament

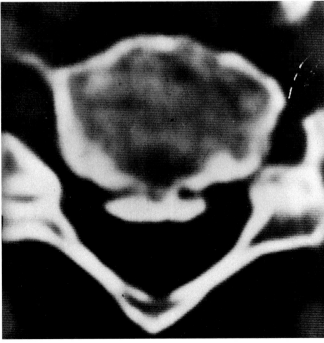

FIGURE 12.43 CT scan of the upper cervical spine of a patient with OPL and encroachment on the cervical canal. After minor trauma, this patient presented with myelopathy.

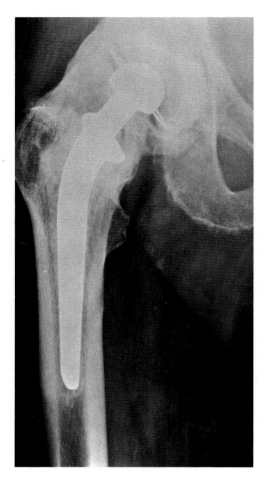

FIGURE 12.44
Post-operative radiograph of a 65-year-old male with total hip replacement 3 years previously. Total bony ankylosis of the joint from ectopic ossification is seen.

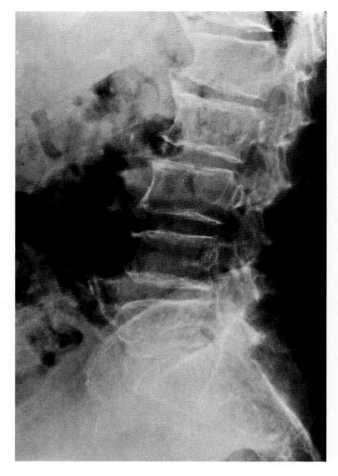

FIGURE 12.45 A lateral radiograph of the lumbar spine of the patient illustrated in Figure 12.44 shows the anterior cortical hyperostosis and nonmarginal syndesmophyte formation typical of ankylosing hyperostosis (DISH).

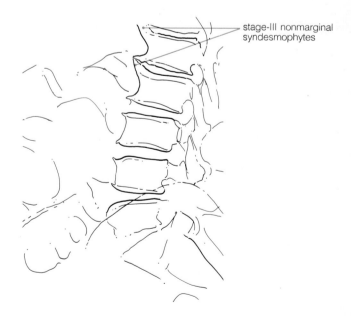

stage-III nonmarginal
syndesmophytes

Tissue response to implanted prostheses

Foreign materials, usually introduced into the human body by trauma, have long been known to cause damage and inflammation in the tissues. The need to design artificial replacements for lost or diseased anatomic parts has resulted in a search for materials that can be implanted into the body to restore the lost function while not causing a deleterious reaction. The search for such biologically compatible materials has a long history and many materials have been used, including gold, animal bone, ivory, and in the early attempts at bone replacement, lucite (Fig. 13.1).

Until comparatively recently the use of inorganic materials was restricted mostly to dentistry, although some metal was used for the internal fixation of fractures. With the advances in artificial replacement of the hip joint by Sir John Charnley in the late 1950s, the use of metals and plastics by orthopedic surgeons has vastly increased. Since that time millions of arthroplasties have been performed worldwide, and in the United States alone it is estimated that over 500,000 such procedures are performed each year. Despite the success of the procedure it is associated with some morbidity, in the form either of loosening of the implanted part or of infection around it. Most orthopedic research and development in recent years has been directed toward reducing this morbidity.

At the present time, prostheses for replacement of large joints, such as the hip and knee, usually employ metal for the convex side of the joint and polyethylene, with or without a metal backing, for the concave side of the joint. Implants manufactured of ceramics can be used by themselves or with metal backing. Polymethylmethacrylate (PMMA) can be used as a grouting material to secure fixation (Fig. 13.2). It is prepared from a mixture of its monomer, beads of fully polymerized PMMA, with a small amount of a radiodense substance,

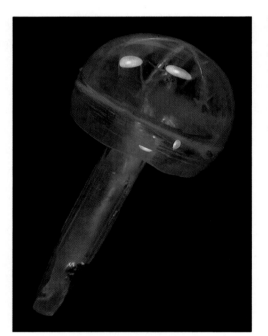

FIGURE 13.1
A Judet type prosthesis manufactured of lucite, which had been in place for many years before removal was necessary.

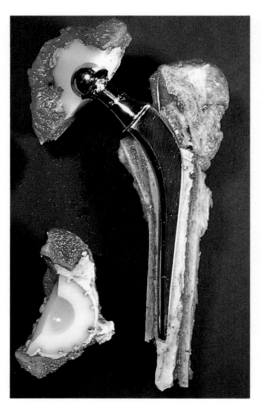

FIGURE 13.2
In this photograph the components of a total hip replacement are seen attached to the bone. A layer of cement is interposed between the prosthesis (the plastic acetabular component and the metal stem of the femoral component) and the bone to obtain a close, optimally immobile, fit of the prosthesis. Looseness of the prosthetic parts is a significant cause of failure in such operations.

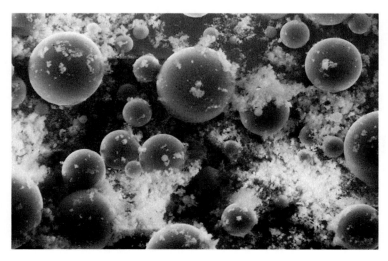

FIGURE 13.3 Scanning electron micrograph of the polymer beads and admixed barium sulfate powder. A monomer is added to this powder to make bone cement (x 350 magnification).

such as barium sulfate, for imaging purposes during postoperative follow-up (Figs. 13.3 and 13.4). Recently, for use with metallic implants, various porous surfaces to promote the ingrowth of tissues into the prosthesis have been developed (Fig. 13.5). Implants of silicone rubber are usually reserved for the small joints of the hand, wrist, and feet, and are not cemented in place.

Despite extensive searches for materials that are biologically inert, it has become clear that no material implanted in living tissues is truly inert. On the contrary, general experience indicates that there are essentially four types of response to implanted material: if the material is toxic, the surrounding tissues are damaged or destroyed; if the material is nontoxic but can dissolve, the surrounding tissues remove and replace it; if the material is nontoxic and biologically relatively inactive, as is the case with most materials used in prostheses, a capsule of fibrous tissue is formed around it (Figs. 13.6 and 13.7); and if the material is nontoxic but biologically active, a bond can form between it and the surrounding tissue.

The metals and other inorganic materials that have been used in orthopedic surgery abrade, corrode, or dissolve to variable degrees after implantation, produc-

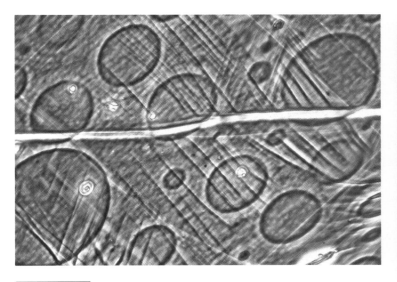

FIGURE 13.4 Histologic section of a piece of cement reveals the "two-phase" character of this material. The spherical objects are the microscopic equivalent of the bead-like polymer, and the material between is the polymerized monomer (unstained, x 40 obj.).

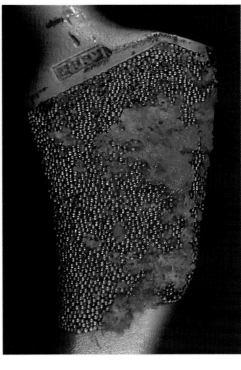

FIGURE 13.5 Portion of a femoral prosthesis covered with a layer of metal beads to provide for porous ingrowth. Fragments of attached bone and fibrous tissue are seen.

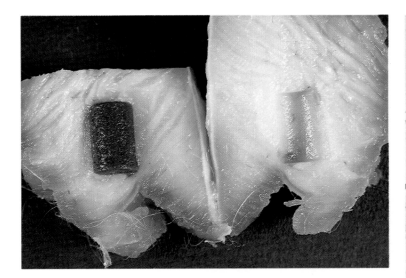

FIGURE 13.6 Photograph demonstrating the appearance after a cylinder of inert metal has been implanted in skeletal muscle for 6 weeks.

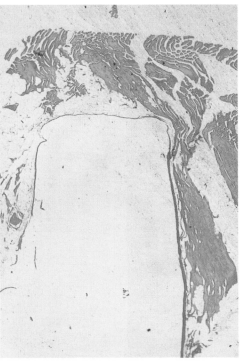

FIGURE 13.7 Photomicrograph of a histologic section prepared from the specimen illustrated in Figure 13.6 shows a very thin fibrous membrane around the space that was occupied by the metal implant (H&E, x 4 obj.).

ing both particulate debris and ionized constituents. With the use of moving parts, as in total joint replacement, the generation of particulate debris is of the greatest concern with respect to possible cytotoxic effects (Figs. 13.8 and 13.9).

The cytotoxic effects of the different metals used in orthopedic implants are varied. In cell culture using murine peritoneal macrophages, Rae studied the effects of particulate cobalt, chromium, molybdenum, nickel, titanium, and cobalt–chromium alloy on the release of lactate dehydrogenase (LDH) and the activity of glucose-6-phosphate dehydrogenase (G6PD). These investigations showed that cultures exposed to particulate molybdenum, chromium, or titanium did not produce elevations in extracellular LDH or reductions in intracellular G6PD. However, cultures exposed to particulate cobalt, nickel, or cobalt–chromium alloy produced elevations in LDH and reductions in G6PD. In addition, the cells that ingested particles of chromium or molybdenum showed no morphologic alterations, whereas those that ingested particles of cobalt or cobalt–chromium alloy showed morphologic features of toxicity, characterized by shrunken cytoplasm and nuclear pyknosis.

It has been suggested that the alterations in G6PD activity indicate decreased phagocytic capacity. This may possibly contribute to increased incidence of delayed infections.

Although there is little evidence that the fully polymerized MMA is toxic to host tissues, the monomeric form has been shown to have local and systemic toxic effects, which will be discussed later. It has been hypothesized that biomedical polymers as a group, and polyethylene in particular, are capable of significantly affecting macrophage activation and production of interleukin-1.

In addition to their composition, the size, shape, and the surface characteristics of implanted materials have important effects on the cell response, which ranges from barely observable alterations to destructive inflammatory processes leading to necrosis and even to carcinogenesis (Fig. 13.10).

USUAL TISSUE RESPONSE TO CLINICALLY NON-FAILED ARTICULAR IMPLANTS

CEMENTED IMPLANTS

At the time of initial fixation with PMMA, a rim of necrosis a few millimeters in thickness develops in the adjacent bone. It is likely that this rim of necrosis results from a combination of the effects of surgery with direct physical damage to the bone, disruption of the local blood supply, heat generated during polymerization, and possibly a toxic effect of any residual monomer. The repair process begins with the ingrowth of granulation tissue and localized osteoclastic removal of damaged bone, and may occur as early as 1 week after implantation. This process is usually complete within 2 years.

Implants recovered at autopsy show that securely fixed prostheses have a cement-bone interface of variable composition. Most of the interface consists of a thin fibrous membrane, which is usually thicker at surfaces that are subjected to compressive forces, such as those on the acetabular side of the hip and the tibial side of the knee (Fig. 13.11). Histologically, this membrane is composed of densely packed collagenized tissue, which in some areas may show fibrocartilaginous metaplasia. Small amounts of fragmented cement, with macrophages and chronic inflammation, may be pres-

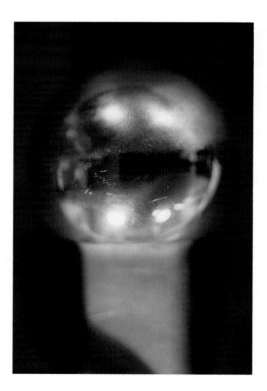

FIGURE 13.8
Photograph of the articular surface of the femoral component of a total hip replacement. This component, manufactured from titanium, shows severe burnishing of the articular surface.

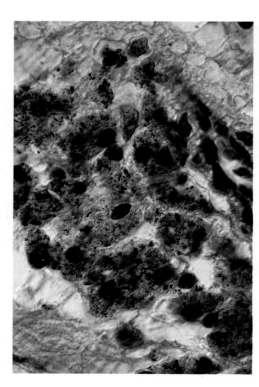

FIGURE 13.9
Photomicrograph of tissue obtained from the capsule around the joint illustrated in Figure 13.8. Large histiocytes filled with fine black metallic debris are seen (H&E, x 50 obj.).

ent in the membrane. Occasionally the membrane undergoes complete osseous replacement, so that bone comes into direct contact with the cement. This is most likely to occur at the more vertically oriented surfaces.

The surface appearance of the cement mantle varies according to the type of bone tissue with which it comes into contact. For example, proximally in the femoral neck, where cancellous bone predominates in the medullary canal, the cement mantle presents a nodular and papillary roughened surface, corresponding to the distribution of the bony trabeculae (Fig. 13.12). More distally in the femoral shaft, the cement comes into contact with the endosteal surface of the cortex, which is relatively smoother, and therefore the mantle has much less surface irregularity than the region of the neck.

NONCEMENTED IMPLANTS

In a similar way to the interface of a cemented implant, that of a noncemented implant has variable morphology, depending on whether the contact surface is vertically or horizontally oriented.

Along the more vertically oriented smooth surfaces of, for example, a Thompson–Moore prosthesis, the interface is composed of a dense, fibrous membrane which is usually a few millimeters thick. The collagen fibers in this membrane are oriented parallel to the implant surface (Fig. 13.13). Cellularity is sparse, and consists mostly of fibroblasts and occasional aggregates of chronic inflammatory cells. An ill-defined layer of cells may be present at the surface of the membrane in

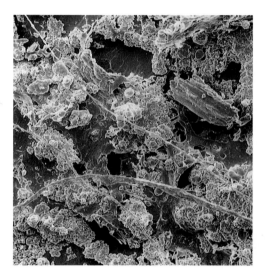

FIGURE 13.10 Scanning electron micrograph of the surface of a removed silastic prosthesis showing gross irregularities and fragmentation (x 100 magnification).

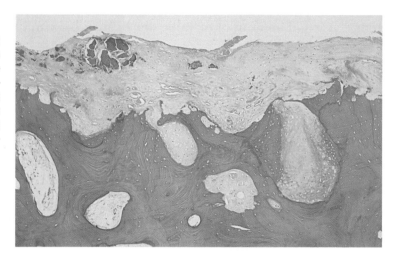

FIGURE 13.11 Photomicrograph showing the fibrocartilaginous membrane at the bone–cement interface of the acetabular component of a total hip replacement. Fragments of bone are present in the fibrous membrane (H&E, x 4 obj.).

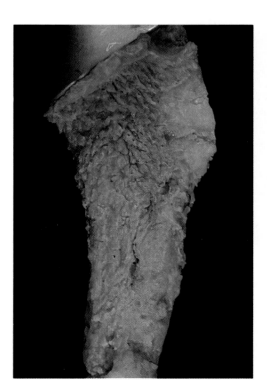

FIGURE 13.12 Photograph showing the cement mantle in a well-fixed femoral component. Note the irregularity of the surface of the cement as it interdigitates with the exposed cancellous bone.

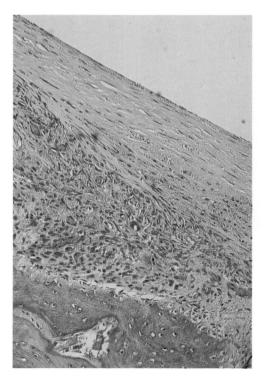

FIGURE 13.13 Photomicrograph of the fibrous membrane between the metal stem of a femoral prosthesis and the bone. Note at the surface the parallel arrangement of the collagen fibers. Adjacent to the bone there is histiocytic and mild chronic inflammatory response (H&E, x 10 obj.)

contact with the implant. Cells other than fibroblasts are not present in significant numbers in the membranes except in association with bone detritus, which is usually present in small amounts. When blood vessels are present, they are usually concentrated on the bone side and do not penetrate to the implant side of the membrane. Evidence of osteoclastic activity is not usually present on the bony surface of the membrane.

The interface membranes at implant surfaces that are more horizontally oriented, such as in the fenestration of interlocking femoral prostheses, differ from those at the vertically oriented surfaces. Thick fibrocartilage-containing chondrocytes in lacunae develop along the weight-bearing surfaces of the implant and are supported by a well-developed bony endplate which overlies cancellous bone. The fibrocartilage may be so well developed as to mimic the features of articular cartilage. A small amount of metallic debris may be seen in these membranes.

The appearance of the tissue reaction at the coated porous surfaces of an implant also depends on the vertical or horizontal orientation of the bone–implant interface. In the vertically oriented regions, osseous tissue normally grows into the roughened surface of the implant without a well-defined intervening fibrous membrane (Fig. 13.14). On horizontal surfaces a visible fibrous membrane is more likely to develop despite the roughened surface (Fig. 13.15).

MORBIDITY ASSOCIATED WITH TOTAL JOINT REPLACEMENTS

The overall long-term failure rate for hip and knee replacements in recent experience is around 5 percent. The most commonly reported types of morbidity following joint replacement are listed in Figure 13.16.

Some of the acute complications of total joint replacements represent familiar surgery-associated morbidity, eg, pulmonary embolism, and will not be discussed here. The complications that can be attributed to the joint replacement itself can be grouped into those that occur locally and those that are systemic.

LOCAL COMPLICATIONS

Infection

Deep infection complicating total joint replacement occurs in about 1.4 percent of cases and may be categorized according to the postoperative period in which it occurs. Acute, or early, infections (23 percent of cases) occur within 12 weeks of surgery. Subacute infections (27 percent of cases) occur within 1 year. Late infection (50 percent of cases) develops after 1 year of pain-free use. The most common pathogens in the acute infections are *S. epidermidis* (28 percent) and *S. aureus* (20

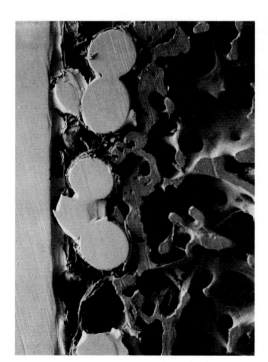

FIGURE 13.14
Scanning electron micrograph showing bone ingrowth on a porous metal surface. The cut surface of the metallic stem is seen at the left of the picture with the overlying cut metal beads. The bone trabeculae can be seen interdigitating between the metal beads.

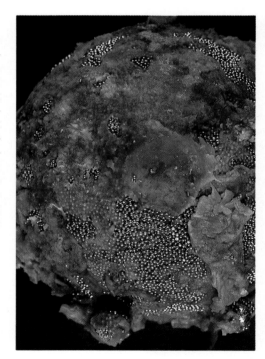

FIGURE 13.15
A photograph of the under surface of the tibial component shows a fibrous membrane and some bone attached to the porous metal surface.

percent). Gram negative bacilli predominate in the sub-acute and the late infections.

Since infection around an implant cannot usually be cured by antibiotic therapy alone, removal of the prosthesis and extensive local debridement may be required.

Technical Failure

Failure associated with alignment of the implant and the placement of the methylmethacrylate cement depends on surgical technique (Fig. 13.17). Improper cementing technique has been reported as the cause of such diverse complications as penetration of the medial wall of the acetabulum, obstruction of the small bowel caused by adhesions around a bolus of polymethylmethacrylate cement, unilateral ureteral obstruction, and postoperative hematuria. Other reported complications following total hip replacement include delayed

irritation of the sciatic nerve, false aneurysm of the external iliac artery, formation of various fistulas, and progressive dyspareunia.

Incorrect surgical alignment of the implant is a significant cause of fracture of the various components of the implant.

TUMORS AND PSEUDOTUMORS

Malignant Tumors

A small number of malignant tumors have been reported in association with orthopedic implants. The largest number have occurred in animals treated for fracture of long bones, osteosarcoma, fibrosarcoma, and undifferentiated sarcoma represent the tumor types. Isolated cases of malignancy developing near plates in humans have also been reported.

FIGURE 13.16

MORBIDITY OF TOTAL JOINT REPLACEMENTS

Time	Morbidity	Localization
Early	Intraoperative hypotension	Systemic
	Infection	Local
	Nerve disorders	Local
Late	Infection	Local
	Aseptic loosening	Local
	Hypersensitivity	Systemic
	Breakage of implant	Local
	Lymphadenopathy	Systemic
	Tumors	Local
	Pseudotumors	Local

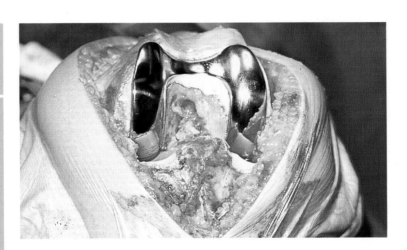

FIGURE 13.17 Total knee replacement seen at necropsy. A large amount of cement has extruded around the prosthetic parts. Such excess cement is likely to break up and be ground between the articular surfaces into a fine powder, which will eventually be incorporated into the synovium and will also cause wear between the articulating surfaces of the artificial joint. In joint replacement procedures, the use of cement should be kept to a minimum, and any extruded cement, particularly around the prosthesis, should be carefully cleared from the joint before closure.

A few cases of malignant tumor have been reported in patients who had undergone total hip or total knee arthroplasty. However, since several million implants are in place, the incidence of malignancies developing in these patients may not be above that normally expected in an aging population (Figs. 13.18 to 13.20).

Pseudotumors

In the context of implant reactions, a pseudotumor is a space-occupying lesion resulting from the tissue reaction to accumulated particulate debris at or near the site of the implant (Figs. 13.21 to 13.23).

The problem of pseudotumor formation plagued the early experience of Charnley with the use of teflon for the acetabular component of his total hip replacements. However, reports of extensive reactions to large amounts of polyethylene debris in both total hip and total knee arthroplasties, with subsequent loosening resulting from endosteal bone resorption caused by the mass effect of the accumulating debris and its accompanying cellular infiltration, still continue to appear in the literature.

Pseudotumors in the bones of the wrist after replacement of carpal bones or joints by silicone rubber implants have also been reported (Figs. 13.24 to 13.26).

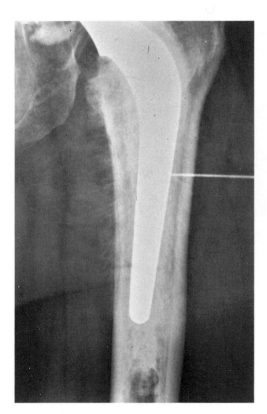

FIGURE 13.18
Radiograph of a 53-year-old female who underwent total joint replacement 8 years previously for secondary osteoarthritis following congenital disclocation of the hip. Recent pain in the hip prompted radiographic examination, which revealed the periosteal reaction seen here.

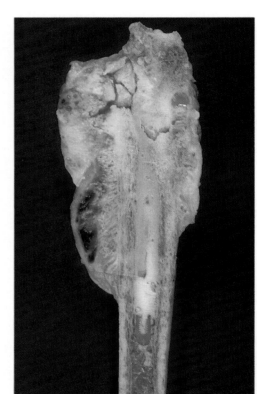

FIGURE 13.19
The resected specimen from the case illustrated in Figure 13.18 shows a large tumor around the upper end of the femur. The prosthesis has been removed.

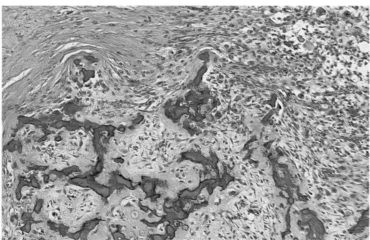

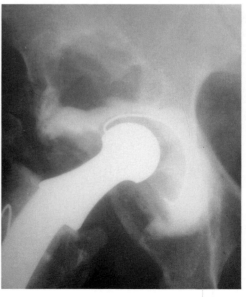

FIGURE 13.21
Radiograph of the pelvis in a patient with total joint replacement of some years' duration. Recent pain prompted radiographic examination, which shows a lytic defect in the ilium. Histological examination revealed an accumulation of polyethylene and cement, with an associated histiocytic response.

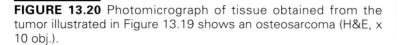

FIGURE 13.20 Photomicrograph of tissue obtained from the tumor illustrated in Figure 13.19 shows an osteosarcoma (H&E, x 10 obj.).

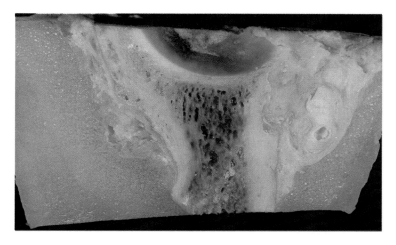

FIGURE 13.22 Section through the acetabulum of a dog several months after total hip replacement shows a juxta-articular tumor mass of yellowish-gray tissue.

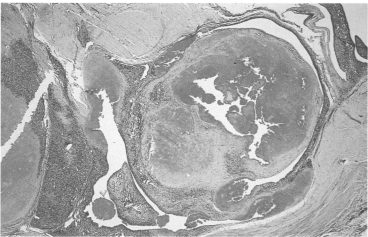

FIGURE 13.23 Photomicrograph of a section through the specimen shown in Figure 13.22 reveals large pink collections of fibrin, in which there was admixed cement and polyethylene debris, surrounded by histiocytes and chronic inflammatory cells (H&E, x 1.25 obj.).

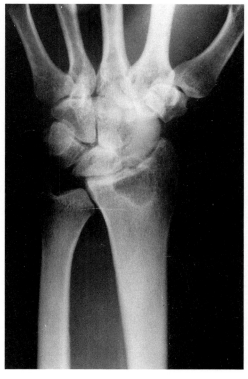

FIGURE 13.24 Radiograph of the wrist of a patient following a silastic replacement of the scaphoid. The large lytic defect in the lower end of the radius was found on microscopic examination to be secondary to a histiocytic and giant-cell reaction to particulate silastic.

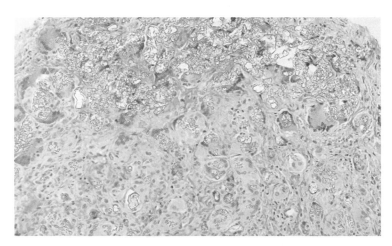

FIGURE 13.25 A lower-power photomicrograph of the synovium surrounding a failed silicone polymer prosthesis. A definite histiocytic and giant-cell reaction can be observed in the synovium, which is markedly cellular (H&E, x 10 obj.).

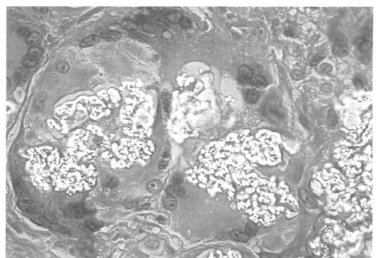

FIGURE 13.26 A high-power view of the giant cells from the tissue shown in Figure 13.25. Within the cytoplasm of the giant cells can be seen bosselated inclusion of yellowish-gray material. This microscopic appearance is typical of silicone breakdown, and similar inclusions may be found around silicone injections used in plastic surgery procedures (H&E, x 40 obj.).

SYSTEMIC COMPLICATIONS

Hypotension and Intraoperative Death

Hypotension developing as a reaction to monomeric methylmethacrylate is fairly common during the instillation of methylmethacrylate; however, death resulting from it is fortunately rare.

Allergy/Hypersensitivity

Tissue reactions due to hypersensitivity are difficult to evaluate in implant sites because of surgical scarring and the small amount of inflammation usually present in the tissues surrounding most types of implants during the early to intermediate postoperative time period. Such reactions are also very similar in appearance to those seen in association with low-grade infections which may not be identifiable in all cases.

Since the mid 1970s, attention has been drawn to the possibility that metals used in orthopedic implants may induce a hypersensitivity reaction. However, the importance of sensitivity to metals in patients who receive metallic joint implants is not clear. In reports that suggest hypersensitivity to have a causative role in loosening, the implants had already failed clinically and the timing of development of the sensitivity was not known. The sensitivity may be dose-dependent and therefore may result from the loosening rather than being its cause. Inflammation and necrosis, as will be discussed later, often accompany failure of an implant, and in these cases the effects of hypersensitivity on the tissues may not be distinguishable from other causes of inflammation.

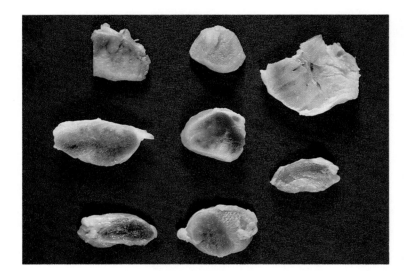

FIGURE 13.27 Sections taken through enlarged para-aortic lymph nodes from a dog which had a total hip replacement some months previously.

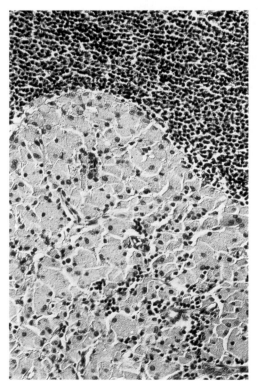

FIGURE 13.28 Photomicrograph of a section through one of the lymph nodes illustrated in Figure 13.27 shows a nodular collection of pale histiocytes (H&E, x 10 obj.).

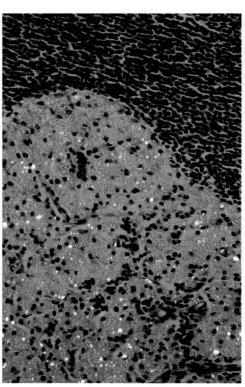

FIGURE 13.29 The same field as in Figure 13.28, photographed with polarized light, shows refractile inclusions of polyethylene within the histiocytes.

Lymph Node and Pulmonary Spread

Autopsy studies have shown that careful dissection of lymph nodes, draining sites of replaced joints, and adequate sampling of lung tissue usually reveals the presence of particulate debris originating from the joint components, whether metal, plastic, or ceramic (Figs. 13.27 to 13.29). The significance of these findings is not known; however, the presence of the implant material in lymph nodes may provide chronic stimulation to the lymphoreticular system, leading to various disturbances possibly including neoplasms.

TISSUES AROUND NONINFECTED, CLINICALLY FAILED ARTICULAR IMPLANTS

Fatigue at the implant–bone interface or in the metallic or plastic components, and wear and tear on the articulating surfaces, are clear causes of failure of an articular prosthesis (Figs. 13.30 and 13.31). Alterations in geometry and mechanics which result from fatigue and wear in the components can, in turn, potentiate and accelerate the process of failure.

All failed implants that have been cemented in place have particulate cement in the surrounding bone and soft tissues. It is usually possible to find particulate polyethylene in the tissues surrounding failed implants that have polyethylene components. Likewise, metallic debris can be found in many cases.

CEMENTED IMPLANTS

The surfaces of the cement mantle in failed implants are generally smooth, polished, and devoid of the surface irregularities that characterize the tight interlock with bone in stable implants. This smooth appearance is due to fragmentation at the interface and results in pulverization of both cement and bone, which then accumulate in the surrounding tissues (Fig. 13.32).

The most obvious feature observed after failure of a

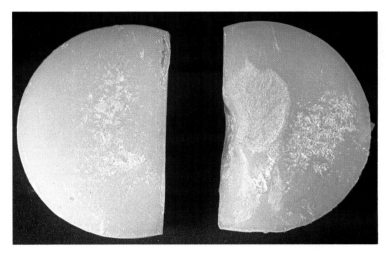

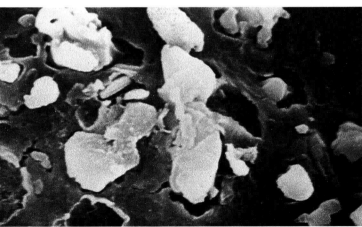

FIGURE 13.31 Scanning electron photomicrograph shows cement particles buried in the polyethylene surface of a total joint replacement (x 500 magnification).

FIGURE 13.30 The tibial components of a total knee prosthesis show extensive wear and scuffing on the articular surfaces by the polyethylene components. The material generated by this wear process is taken up by the synovium and causes a considerable synovial reaction. Significant wear results from fragments of cement that are caught between the articular surfaces and ground into the polyethylene.

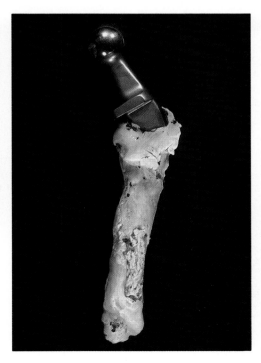

FIGURE 13.32 Photograph showing the surface of the cement mantle in a loose, failed prosthesis. Note the smooth, polished appearance of the cement surface, which should be compared with the rough surface of a well-fixed prosthesis shown in Figure 13.12.

cemented implant is the presence of a thickened membrane around the cement. This membrane may measure up to several millimeters in thickness; it usually has a granular surface and a grummous, friable consistency (Fig. 13.33).

The microscopic features of the membrane include fibrosis, necrosis, and infiltrates of macrophages (Fig. 13.34). Macrophages are usually concentrated at the surface adjacent to the cement and may form a layer which has been said to resemble a synovial lining. Fibrosis is usually concentrated on the bone side of the membrane. Necrosis may be distributed throughout the membrane but is frequently seen nearer the cement side.

NONCEMENTED IMPLANTS

Aseptically loosened noncemented implants also develop a thickened membrane which usually has a granular, roughened surface and is friable, generally tan, and usually also has regions of gray or black discoloration owing to metal debris. In our experience, failed implants made

of titanium usually have the blackest appearance (Fig. 13.35). Microscopic examination shows the presence of variable amounts of necrosis, fibrosis, and cellular infiltrates consisting mostly of macrophages.

METAL IN TISSUES

Metals are subject to chemical corrosion in the body, which results in coarsely granular brown-black debris. However, much more common are metallic particles produced as a result of wear at exposed surfaces and fractures of the metallic component (Figs. 13.36 to 13.38).

Microscopic examination of tissue sections from around metal implants, whether cemented or not, usually show small, irregular black fragments measuring from 1 to 3 micrometers in greatest dimension. These fragments are opaque, but because of diffraction at their edges they can be more clearly seen in polarized light (Figs. 13.39 and 13.40). Many of the fragments are present within macrophages. However, when there is heavy deposition, as in cases where a metal component

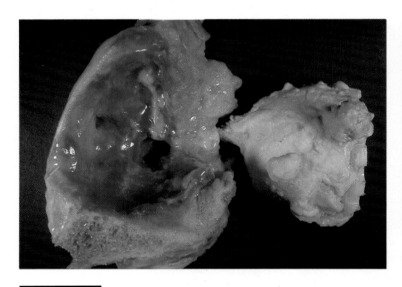

FIGURE 13.33 Photograph of the membrane lining the acetabulum in a patient with a failed prosthesis. The detached cement is shown on the righthand side of the photograph. Note the edematous and hyperemic appearance of the membrane.

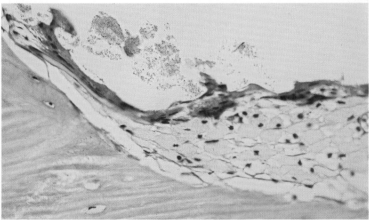

FIGURE 13.34 Photomicrograph showing the cellular response adjacent to cement. The upper part of the picture shows yellowish-gray granules of barium sulfate in the space formerly occupied by cement. Immediately adjacent to that is a giant-cell reaction, and between the cement and the bone is a layer of foamy histiocytes with abundant granular eosinophilic cytoplasm (H&E, x 10 obj.).

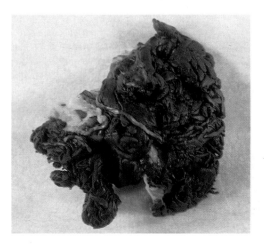

FIGURE 13.35 A portion of synovial tissue removed from around a failed prosthesis manufactured of titanium. Note the intense black discoloration of the synovial membrane.

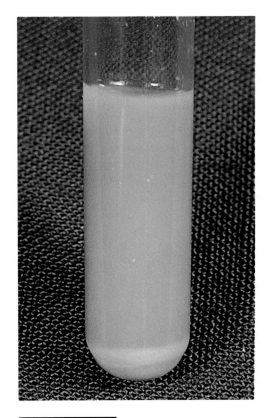

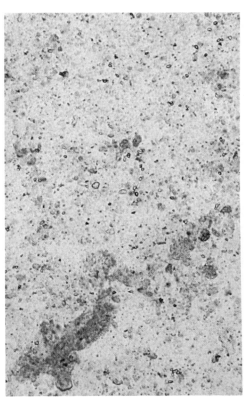

FIGURE 13.36 A synovial effusion removed from a patient with a metal-on-metal prosthesis may be quite turbid, giving the mistaken impression that one is dealing with an infection.

FIGURE 13.37 Microscopic examination of the fluid from the example in Figure 13.36 fails to reveal polymorphonuclear leukocytes, but does reveal many fragments of fine amorphous debris (x 100 obj.).

FIGURE 13.38 Viewed under polarized light, the fragments from the specimen in Figures 13.36 and 13.37 are seen to be refractile. This appearance results from refraction at the edge of the opaque metal particles.

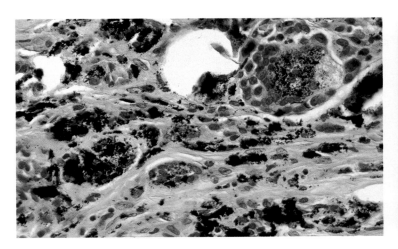

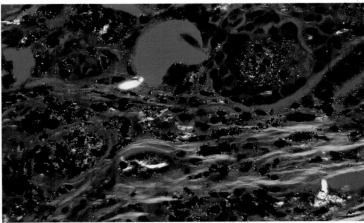

FIGURE 13.39 Photomicrograph of a section taken through the synovium shown in Figure 13.35. Particulate black debris is seen both intra- and extracellularly in a chronically inflamed fibrous tissue stroma (H&E, x 25 obj.).

FIGURE 13.40 The same field as in Figure 13.39 photographed with polarized light, which shows many refractile particles of polyethylene as well as small points of reflected light over the metal particles.

has fractured, where metal components articulate with each other, or where the prosthesis is manufactured of Ti-Al-V alloy, the metallic debris can also be seen free in the necrotic or fibrous tissue.

Ultrastructural studies demonstrate that most of the metal particles are in phagolysosomes and that many have a diameter of less than 0.5 micrometers, which is below the resolution of light microscopy (Fig. 13.41). The affected macrophages demonstrate a decrease in the endoplasmic reticulum and other distortions of cytologic ultrastructure.

POLYETHYLENE IN TISSUES

Polyethylene debris is generated at the articulating surfaces by a number of mechanisms, including direct abrasion, three-body wear (often from entrapped particles of cement as illustrated in Figs. 13.30 and 13.31), and fatigue surface damage which increases with time.

Microscopic examination shows a cellular infiltrate of macrophages and giant cells in a roughly granulomatous pattern, which may be confluent in some areas and appear as dense sheets of cells. The polyethylene, in the form of variably sized shards of glassy, refractile mate-

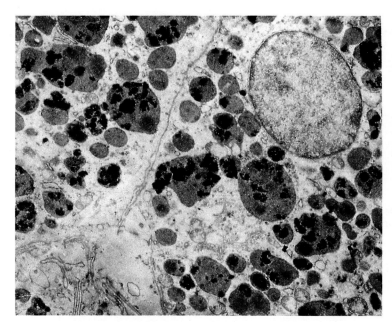

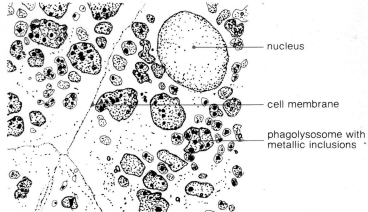

FIGURE 13.41 Electron photomicrograph of synovial cells from a patient with a total hip replacement shows an accumulation of electron-dense material in phagolysosomes in the cytoplasm. These dense particles are metallic.

nucleus

cell membrane

phagolysosome with metallic inclusions

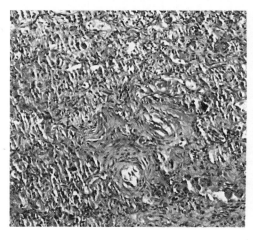

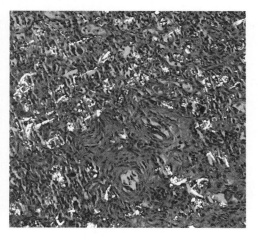

FIGURE 13.42 Photomicrograph of a histologic section taken from the synovium of a patient with a hip prosthesis in which the acetabular component was made of polyethylene. In the transmission light photograph shown here, the subsynovium is infiltrated by large numbers of histiocytes and some chronic inflammatory cells (H&E, x 10 obj.).

FIGURE 13.43 On polarized light microscopy the cells from the section in Figure 13.42 are seen to be filled with threadlike particles of refractile material, which are derived from wear of the polyethylene surface.

rial, can easily be overlooked in transmitted light. However, examination under polarized light will readily, and sometimes dramatically, demonstrate their presence (Figs. 13.42 and 13.43). The largest pieces are surrounded by a layer of fibrous tissue; the smaller pieces are surrounded or engulfed by giant cells and large mononuclear macrophages (Fig. 13.44). On occa-

sion, many of the giant cells are seen to contain "asteroid bodies" (Fig. 13.45).

Debris from a polyethylene component is usually concentrated in the immediate vicinity of the component, in the synovial and pseudocapsular structures of the joint (Fig. 13.46). However, it may also be seen in small amounts deep within the bone and bone marrow away

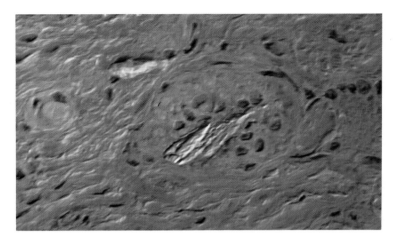

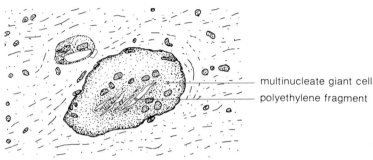

FIGURE 13.44 Photomicrograph of a giant cell reveals fine threadlike particles of polyethylene within the cytoplasm (H&E, Nomarski, x 25 obj.).

multinucleate giant cell
polyethylene fragment

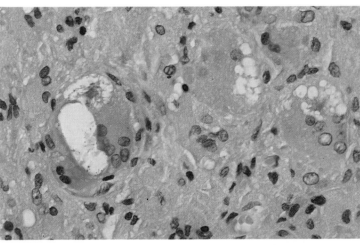

FIGURE 13.45 Photomicrograph of a histiocytic and giant-cell reaction to cement and polyethylene, showing the presence of asteroid bodies in many of the giant cells (H&E, x 40 obj.).

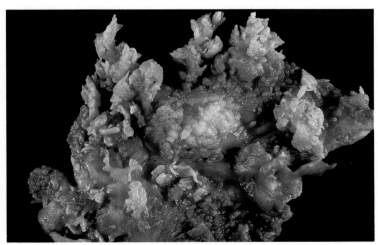

FIGURE 13.46 Photograph of synovium removed from a failed prosthesis showing marked papillary proliferation of the synovium with focal hemosiderin staining. Microscopic examination of this tissue revealed a foreign body reaction to polyethylene and cement debris.

from the polyethylene implant, where it has the appearance of granulomatous infiltrates (Figs. 13.47 to 13.49).

On occasion, the polyethylene component may be a composite of carbon filaments. In this case it is possible to find fragmented carbon filaments in the tissues. Inflammation is usually not apparent, and in the absence of polyethylene debris there is no discernible foreign body giant cell reaction to the carbon particles (Fig. 13.50).

METHYLMETHACRYLATE IN TISSUES

In histologic sections, methylmethacrylate is not seen because it dissolves in the solvents used to process tissues for paraffin embedding. In unstained frozen tissue sections however, the particles are glassy and granular but are not birefringent in polarized light (Fig. 13.51). In paraffin sections the particles of methylmethacrylate

instead appear as cleared-out spaces of widely variable size. The largest spaces are lined with giant cells and are partially filled with granular material, which can be shown to contain barium sulfate that was mixed with the methylmethacrylate to provide radiodensity (Fig. 13.52).

SILICONE RUBBER IN TISSUES

The tissue response to silicone debris is moderate to intense, and consists of an inflammatory infiltrate which includes lymphocytes, plasma cells, eosinophils, macrophages, and foreign body giant cells. The debris is pale yellow and faintly refractile but not birefringent in polarized light, and the particles range in size from 6 to 100 micrometers. The particles are usually intracellular but may also be free in the extracellular connective tissues (Fig. 13.53).

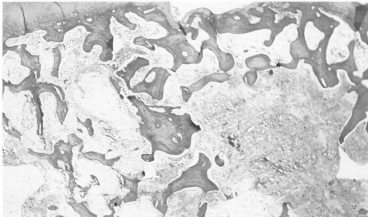

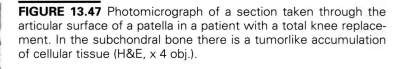

FIGURE 13.47 Photomicrograph of a section taken through the articular surface of a patella in a patient with a total knee replacement. In the subchondral bone there is a tumorlike accumulation of cellular tissue (H&E, x 4 obj.).

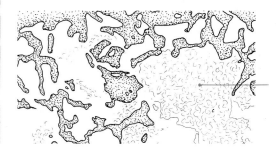

bone erosion following tissue reaction to foreign body

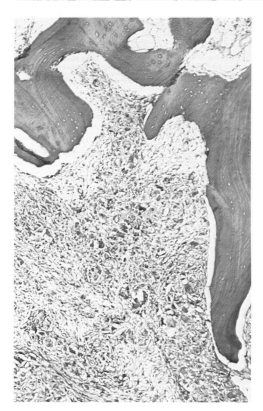

FIGURE 13.48
High-power view of the tissue seen in Figure 13.47 Note histiocytic replacement of the bone and bone marrow (H&E, x 25 obj.).

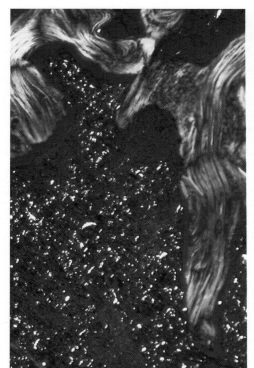

FIGURE 13.49
Polarized light microscopy of tissue shown in Figures 13.47 and 13.48 reveals highly refractile particles of polyethylene debris within the histiocytes and giant cells of the tissue.

CERAMIC IN TISSUES

The major feature of the reaction around a failed ceramic implant is the generation of a thickened membrane with necrosis, fibrosis, and macrophages similar to that seen in failure of the other types of implant. Small particles of debris, less than 5 μ in size, are numerous within the membrane and have a gray-black appearance. These particles are generally found within macrophages. Foreign body giant cells are not usually seen.

CONCLUSION

There are at least three consequences of the shedding of wear particles from articulating implants. First, the total surface area of contact between implant material and the biologic environment is enormously increased by fragmentation, thus facilitating the exchange of potentially toxic elements at the interface for greater systemic dissemination. Second, wear particles of suitable sizes can be phagocytosed and become exposed to intracellular processes, which they might then alter. Third, particles that have been ingested may be transported to sites remote from the implant, such as regional lymph nodes, lungs, and spleen, and may interfere with the functions of these systems.

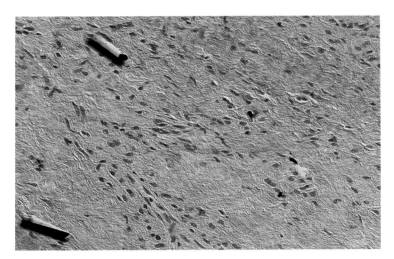

FIGURE 13.50 Photomicrograph demonstrating cylindrical fragments of carbon fiber in the tissue from a patient who had a carbon fiber-reinforced implant. The section also shows a fibroblastic and histiocytic response, which with polarized light reveals extensive polyethylene debris (H&E, x 25 obj.).

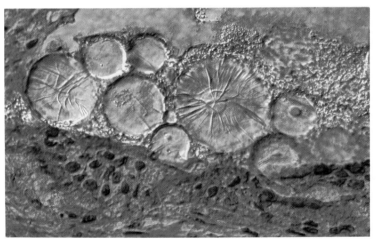

FIGURE 13.51 Photomicrograph of a specimen of synovium cut by frozen section without the use of solvents demonstrates cement in situ. Polymer balls are evident, and between these spheres a finely granular yellow material is seen. This appearance results from the barium sulfate that is mixed with the cement to render it radiopaque (H&E, Normarski, x 25 obj.).

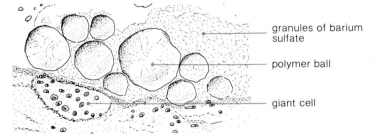

granules of barium sulfate

polymer ball

giant cell

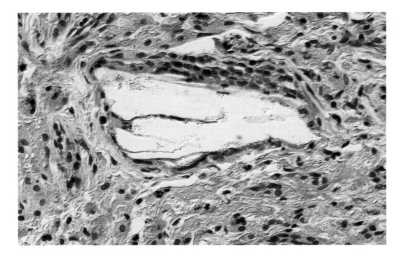

FIGURE 13.52 Photomicrograph demonstrating a giant-cell reaction around a large piece of cement, which appears as an irregular space in the center of the photograph because the cement itself has been dissolved by routine processing methods (H&E, x 40 obj.).

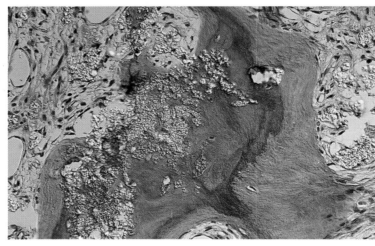

FIGURE 13.53 Photomicrograph showing irregular fragments of silastic within the bone marrow in a patient with a failed silastic implant. The fragments appear as bosselated, glistening irregular particles (H&E, x 10 obj.).

SECTION V

TUMORS

Tumors are uncommon in the clinical practice of orthopedics. However, as is often the case in the teaching of medicine, the weight given to any topic is inversely proportional to how frequently that condition will be encountered. In the case of tumors of the skeleton, the time allocated in the curriculum is perhaps justified by their diversity and by the difficulties encountered in diagnosis.

By far, the most common tumor encountered in orthopedic practice is metastatic carcinoma; in most cases, but by no means in all, the diagnosis is obvious. Among the primary malignant lesions of bone, myeloma is the most common, followed by osteosarcoma, chondrosarcoma, and small-cell or round-cell sarcoma (eg, Ewing's tumor).

Benign bone tumors are perhaps numerically more frequent than primary malignant lesions of bone, but because their nature is usually evident on radiologic examination, they are often not surgically resected. The most common benign lesions are nonossifying fibroma and osteochondroma. Less common are giant-cell tumor, osteoid osteoma, and enchondroma.

The diagnosis of these various lesions can be difficult, requiring a careful correlation of the clinical information with the radiologic and histologic presentation. Discussion of these findings before biopsy or other surgery is in the best interest of the patient and enables the radiologist and pathologist to recommend or plan further studies that might not be possible if immediate surgery is performed.

**Benign tumors -
bony and cartilaginous**

his chapter deals with those benign non-neoplastic processes where either a bony or cartilaginous extracellular matrix is formed by the affected cells. In either case, a fibrous component may also be present.

FIBROUS DYSPLASIA (FIBRO-OSSEOUS DYSPLASIA; FIBRO-OSSEOUS LESION)

Fibrous dysplasia is a relatively common, usually solitary (monostotic), slow-growing hamartomatous lesion composed mainly of bone and fibrous tissue, but occasionally containing foci of cartilage. Rarely, an associated soft-tissue tumor may be present, usually an intramuscular myxoma. The condition is usually manifested in children and adolescents. The clinical course of fibrous dysplasia is most consistent with that of a developmental abnormality, and no familial association is known.

Fibrous dysplasia is usually asymptomatic, and in most instances the lesion is discovered incidentally at radiographic examination. Occasionally a patient with fibrous dysplasia will exhibit symptoms, such as a pathologic fracture or impingement. The femur, tibia, skull, or ribs are most commonly affected, but almost

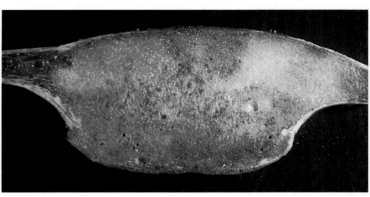

FIGURE 14.2 This gross photograph of fibrous dysplasia in a rib reveals a well-circumscribed expansile lesion with a solid white and tan appearance. Note the normal cancellous and cortical bone of the rib on both sides of the lesion. In such a lesion, the cut surface has a gritty consistency owing to the presence of fine bone spicules, which are responsible for the ground-glass appearance on radiography.

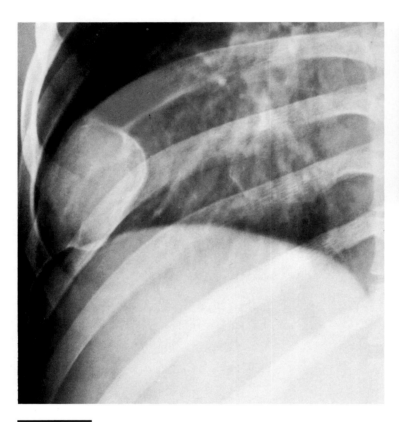

FIGURE 14.1 Radiograph of the chest in a 20-year-old man who complained of a swollen area on the seventh right rib. Note the uniform density of the expanded tumor, which is often referred to as a "ground-glass" appearance.

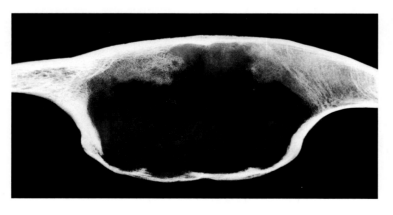

FIGURE 14.3 Radiograph of the specimen shown in Figure 14.2 reveals a relatively lucent expanded zone with marked thinning of the cortex. Throughout the lesion there is a ground-glass appearance due to diffusely distributed fine spicules of bone.

any bone can be involved. Involvement of the craniofacial bones may result in marked asymmetry (unilateral cranial hyperostosis).

The classic appearance of fibrous dysplasia may be seen in a rib as fusiform expansion, with thinning of the cortex and replacement of bone tissue by a firm, whitish tissue of gritty consistency, often containing cysts (Figs. 14.1 to 14.3). The lesion is usually well defined on radiographic examination, although the rim is not usually sclerotic, and the tissue often has a "ground-glass" appearance. Scintigraphy reveals increased isotope uptake in these lesions.

Histologic examination reveals irregular foci of woven (nonlamellar) bone trabeculae in a cellular but otherwise unremarkable fibrous stroma (Figs. 14.4 to 14.6). The bony spicules in fibrous dysplasia are often described as resembling the letters C and Y or Chinese characters. Microscopic evidence of osteoclastic resorption (Fig. 14.7) is frequently associated with these configurations. Osteoblastic rimming of bone, if present, is minimal, which distinguishes this lesion from a so-called ossifying fibroma. (In the latter, the bone spicules are lined with a thin layer of lamellar bone, with prominent osteoblastic rimming.) In a few cases,

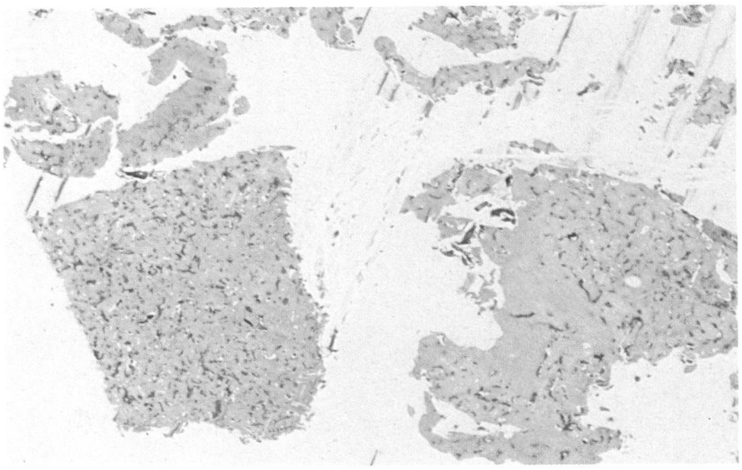

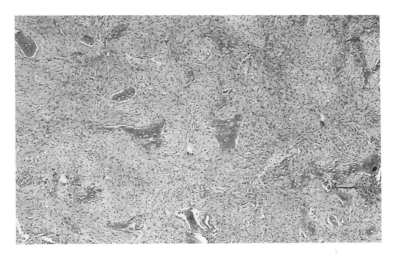

FIGURE 14.4 Low-power view of curetted fragments from a patient with fibrous dysplasia shows a fibrous tissue stroma with islands of bony tissue throughout (H & E, x 1.0 obj.).

FIGURE 14.5 Photomicrograph of fibrous dysplasia shows a background of collagenized fibrous tissue, within which are irregularly shaped spicules of immature bone. Although bone production is readily evident, there are relatively few osteoblasts rimming the bone spicules. This finding suggests a direct metaplasia of bone from the underlying fibrous tissue (H & E, x 10 obj.).

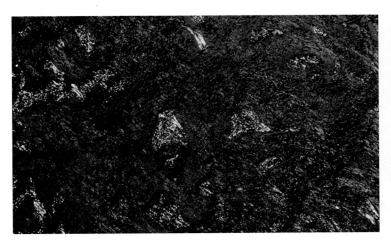

FIGURE 14.6 The same tissue seen in Figure 14.5 viewed with polarized light demonstrates the woven appearance of the collagen within the bone matrix. (This photograph should be compared with the appearance of an ossifying fibroma in Figure 14.16.)

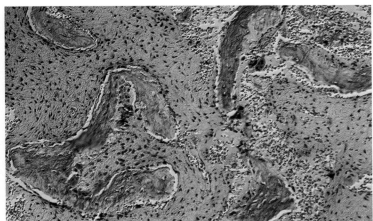

FIGURE 14.7 Photomicrograph demonstrating a feature of fibrous dysplasia not usually illustrated but nevertheless common, ie, osteoclastic resorption of the bone spicules in the fibrous stroma (H & E, x 10 obj.).

we have observed areas which, instead of bone, consisted of dense blue nodules, or "cementicle"-like structures, in the fibrous stroma (Fig 14.8). Occasionally the fibrous stroma exhibits a storiform pattern similar to that seen in a benign fibrous histiocytoma (Fig. 14.9).

Cartilage in lesions of fibrous dysplasia may be intrinsic to the lesion secondary to fracture or may result from disruption of an affected growth plate during development. In either event, the amount of cartilage present in the lesion may lead to confusion in diag-

nosis and the lesion may be mistaken for a chondrosarcoma (Fig. 14.10).

Patients with fibrous dysplasia may exhibit secondary reactive changes caused by a pathologic fracture. These changes include areas of multinucleated giant cells, foamy histiocytes, and fracture callus (Fig. 14.11). If these reactive areas are the only tissues biopsied, the lesion may be mistaken on histologic examination for a primary neoplasm or even a metastatic carcinoma.

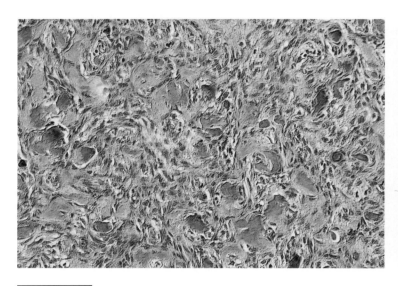

FIGURE 14.8 Photomicrograph showing small, discrete foci of calcified matrix within fibrous dysplasia, which resemble the cementicles occasionally seen in fibromas of the jaw (H & E, x 10 obj.).

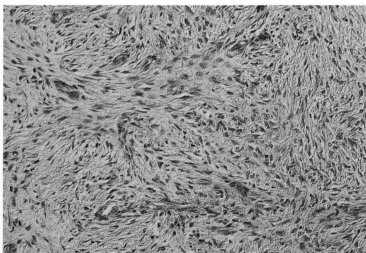

FIGURE 14.9 Photomicrograph of a purely fibrous area within a lesion of fibrous dysplasia demonstrates the "whirling pinwheel" storiform pattern of benign fibrous histiocytoma (H & E, x 10 obj.).

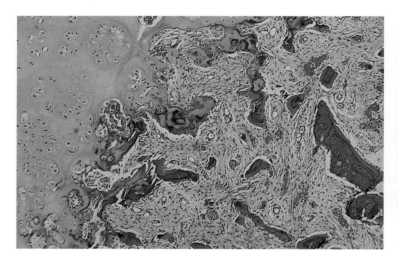

FIGURE 14.10 Photomicrograph demonstrating focus of cellular cartilage within fibrous dysplasia. Occasionally, the cartilaginous areas occupy a considerable portion of the lesion and therefore can be diagnostically confused with chondrosarcoma (H & E, x 10 obj.).

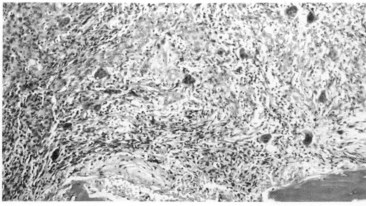

FIGURE 14.11 Photomicrograph taken through an area of fracture in a patient with fibrous dysplasia demonstrates a spindle-cell stroma with many giant cells and a sprinkling of chronic inflammatory cells. A biopsy taken through such an area may be confusing in differential diagnosis (H & E, x 10 obj.).

The classic "shepherd's crook" deformity of the upper end of the femur is the result of multiple sequential fractures, each of which is followed by some residual deformity (Fig. 14.12).

Polyostotic involvement by fibrous dysplasia is decidedly rare. Usually but not always, the multiple lesions affect predominantly one side of the body or a single limb (Fig. 14.13). The histologic features of polyostotic lesions are identical to those of monostotic lesions. The condition may cause severe deformities, and it is sometimes associated with patchy skin pigmentation and various endocrinopathies which are usually associated with precocious puberty, mostly in females (Albright's syndrome).

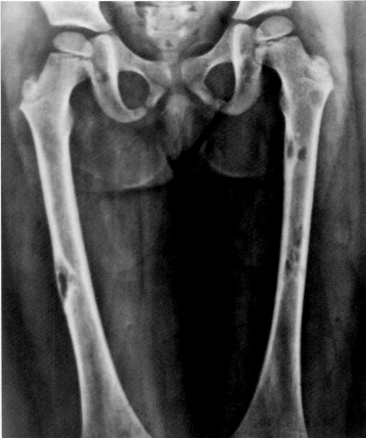

FIGURE 14.13 Radiograph of a 4-year-old girl with multiple bilateral cystic lesions in the femur and pelvis that proved, on histologic examination, to be fibrous dysplasia.

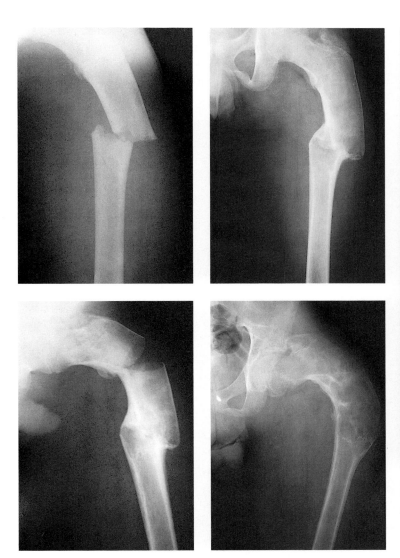

FIGURE 14.12 Radiographs of the upper end of the femur in a patient with fibrous dysplasia shows marked varus ("Shepherd's crook") deformity. This typical deformity in patients with polyostotic fibrous dysplasia results from repeated fractures through the involved section of the proximal femur, with residual deformity after each fracture.

OSSIFYING FIBROMA
(OSTEOFIBROUS DYSPLASIA)

Ossifying fibroma is a fibro-osseous lesion which has been described characteristically in the jaw, and only rarely in the long bones. Although considered by many to be a variant of fibrous dysplasia, others believe that this lesion is a true neoplasm, with aggressive local behavior. In long bones the lesion has a predilection for the tibia; it is most often seen in young children, who present with tibial masses that may be rapidly enlarging but are usually painless. The deformity of the involved leg may be quite dramatic, and the lesion initially behaves in an aggressive fashion. The natural history of this lesion is the subject of much debate, but it appears that ossifying fibroma behaves less aggressively as the affected child gets older. Metastases do not occur.

On radiologic films, the lesion is extensive and involves either the diaphysis or the metaphysis of the tibia; the epiphysis is usually not affected. Characteristic eccentric intracortical osteolysis, with distortion and thinning of the cortex, is evident (Fig. 14.14). The cortical bone may actually be absent in places. Anterior bowing of the tibia is common, as is a multiloculated appearance. The periosteum is usually well preserved.

The histologic appearance of the affected tissue is

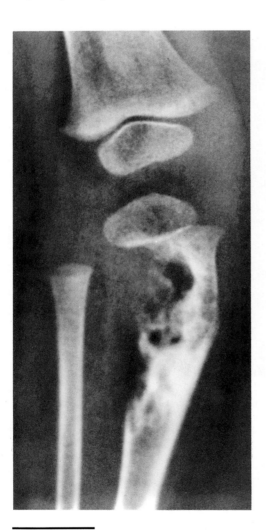 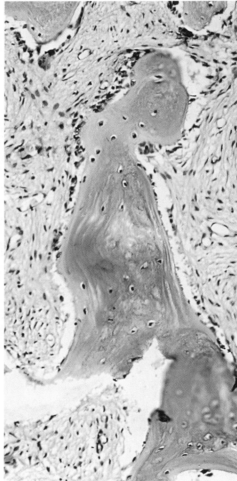 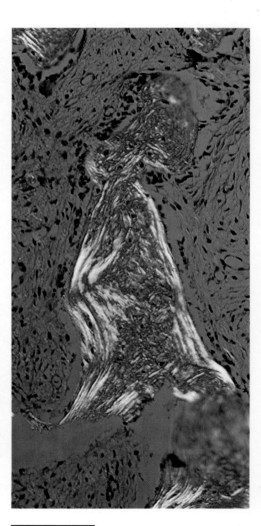

FIGURE 14.14 Radiograph of a 15-month-old boy with a large, lytic, eccentric defect in the upper end of the tibia, which proved on histologic examination to be an ossifying fibroma.

FIGURE 14.15 Photomicrograph of tissue obtained from a patient with ossifying fibroma reveals a cellular spindle cell stroma, with spicules of bone rimmed by plump osteoblasts (H & E, x 25 obj.).

FIGURE 14.16 The field shown in Figure 14.15 viewed under polarized light shows lamellar bone on the bone spicule surface, with a core of woven bone. This finding of peripheral maturation to lamellar bone is characteristic of an ossifying fibroma.

similar to that seen in fibrous dysplasia, with irregular spicules of trabecular bone and unremarkable spindle-cells that produce a collagenous stroma. However, in contrast to fibrous dysplasia, the bone spicules are characteristically lined with osteoblasts that produce a rim of lamellar bone, even though the center of these spicules of bone may have a woven appearance (Figs. 14.15 and 14.16). The finding of woven bone with juxtaposed lamellar bone laid down by prominent, plump osteoblasts is said to be characteristic of ossifying fibroma, and distinguishes it from fibrous dysplasia. Foci of hemorrhage and foamy histiocytes, as well as an occasional area of cartilage (usually in the vicinity of a fracture), may be observed.

ENCHONDROMATOSIS (OLLIER'S DISEASE)

Ollier's disease is a rare developmental abnormality which appears to have no familial association. Characteristically, multiple cartilaginous tumors, ranging from microscopic foci to bulky masses, appear throughout the epiphyses, metaphyses, and diaphyses of the skeleton (Fig. 14.17). The disease usually presents in early childhood. The lesions may be either central or subperiosteal in location. Their distribution is most often unilateral and confined to one limb. Radiographic examination reveals multiple lucent lesions, often within deformed or shortened bone (Fig. 14.18). A short

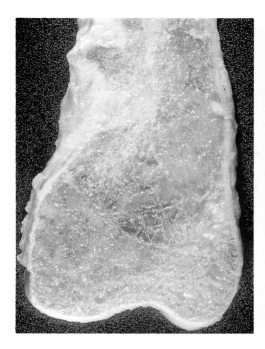
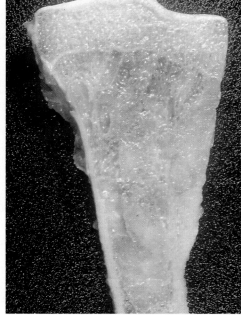
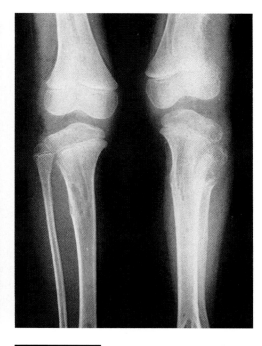

FIGURE 14.17 In the coronal section of a femur *(left)* and tibia *(right)* involved by enchondromatosis, note replacement of the cancellous portion of the bone with circumscribed grayish-blue nodules. In addition to the metaphysis and diaphysis, the epiphysis and periosteal surface are also affected by the disease.

FIGURE 14.18 Radiograph of the lower limbs in a patient with multiple enchondromas. Typically, the lytic lesions are most prominent in the metaphysis and have a striated appearance. However, the lesions also affect the epiphysis and the periosteal surfaces, and may result in bone shortening as well as deformity of the articular ends.

ulna, as is also seen in association with multiple exostoses, is not uncommon. Stippled calcification is common, and the affected bone may have a striated appearance. The histologic features of these lesions resemble those of solitary enchondromas (see Chapter 16), but in enchondromatosis the tumors are more cellular, frequently myxoid and, in general, have a more ominous appearance (Figs. 14.19 to 14.21). Malignant transformation (rare in solitary enchondromas) is reported to occur in approximately one third of cases.

Maffucci's syndrome is a condition characterized by the occurrence of multiple enchondromatosis in association with soft-tissue hemangiomas, including visceral hemangiomas (Fig. 14.22).

OSTEOCHONDROMA (OSTEOCARTILAGINOUS EXOSTOSIS)

Osteochondroma is a common nonfamilial developmental aberration, with the majority of cases presenting in the first two decades. It is approximately one-and-one-half times more common in boys than in girls. The lesion is thought to result from the herniation and separation of a fragment of epiphyseal growth plate cartilage through the periosteal bone cuff that normally surrounds the growth plate (Fig. 14.23). Persistent growth of the herniated cartilage fragment and its subsequent endochondral ossification result in a cartilage-capped subperiosteal bony projection from the bone surface.

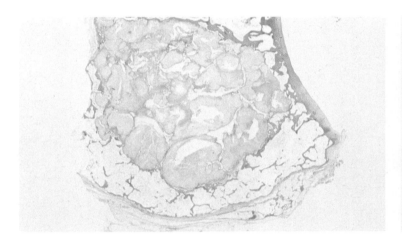

FIGURE 14.19 Low-power photomicrograph of the articular end of a bone demonstrates a cartilaginous nodule extending up to the articular surface. Note the lobular arrangement of the cartilage and the lesion's bony rim (H & E, x 1 obj.).

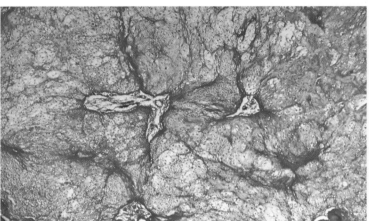

FIGURE 14.20 Photomicrograph of a portion of the lesion shown in Figure 14.19 demonstrates the lobular and cellular appearance of the cartilaginous nodules in enchondromatosis. These lesions usually exhibit more cellularity than is seen in solitary enchondromas (H & E, x 10 obj.).

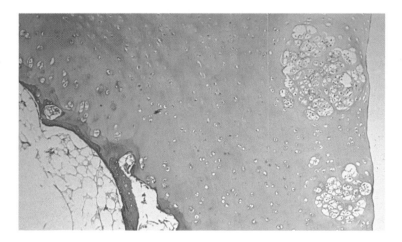

FIGURE 14.21 Histologic section of the cartilaginous end of a bone in a young child with enchondromatosis. Proliferating clones of markedly atypical chondrocytes are seen within the

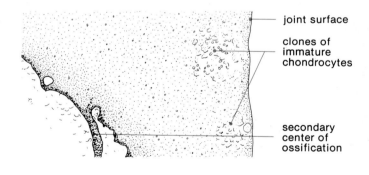

joint surface

clones of immature chondrocytes

secondary center of ossification

cartilaginous epiphysis, thus demonstrating that this condition arises from abnormal clones of chondrocytes within the cartilage anlage of the affected limb (H & E, x 10 obj.).

Rarely, osteochondromas in children may arise after radiation therapy. The most common sites of occurrence are long bones, usually the lower end of the femur and upper end of the tibia (Fig. 14.24). However, involvement of the flat bones, ilium, and scapulae occurs in about 5 percent of cases. Osteochondromas of the spine are rare but may occasionally be encountered. The lesion generally manifests clinically before the third decade, with the patient complaining of pain or a mass. On radiographs, these lesions appear as either a flattened (sessile) or a stalk-like protuberance (exostosis) from the bone shaft in a juxta-epiphyseal

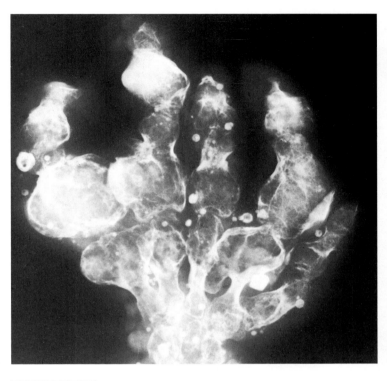

FIGURE 14.22 Radiograph of a hand in a patient with multiple enchondromas reveals many calcified phleboliths in association with soft-tissue hemangiomas. This combination of soft-tissue hemangiomatosis and enchondromatosis is known as Maffucci's syndrome.

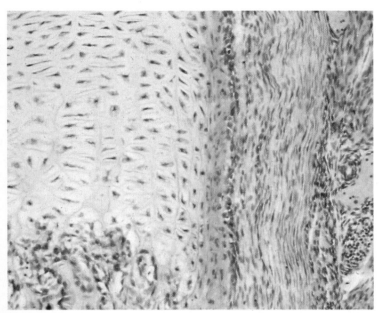

FIGURE 14.23 Histologic section taken from a normal 12-week-old fetus. One can see the cartilage on the left, and the underlying bone metaphysis. To the right of the epiphysis is a thin layer of periosteal bone which forms a cuff around the cartilaginous epiphysis. The perichondral bone cuff is important to the mechanical integrity of the epiphyseal growth plate cartilage (H & E, x 40 obj.).

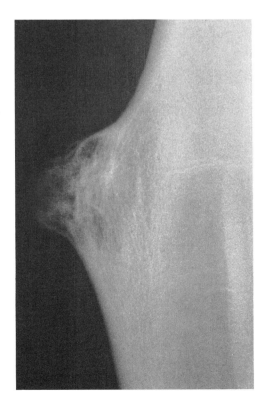

FIGURE 14.24 Radiograph of the metaphyseal end of a femur shows an eccentric irregularity on the cortex, with a lucent cap. The margins of the lesion are contiguous with the surrounding cortex.

location (Figs. 14.25 to 14.29). This bony protuberance is contiguous with the adjacent cortical bone.

The pathologist usually receives an irregular bony protuberance with a bluish-gray cartilaginous cap resembling a cauliflower; the base of the lesion consists of cortical bone contiguous with the normal shaft. Histologic examination reveals a somewhat disorganized cartilaginous cap covered with a thin layer of fibrous periosteum (Figs. 14.30 and 14.31). The older the patient, the thinner the cartilaginous component becomes. After adolescence and closure of the growth plates there is usually no further growth of the osteochondroma. The lesion may recur if it is inadequately excised, and this is particularly a problem with sessile lesions. In very rare cases, a malignant tumor (usually a chondrosarcoma) may be engrafted onto the lesion.

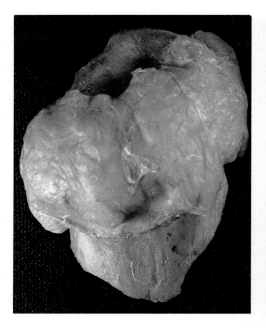

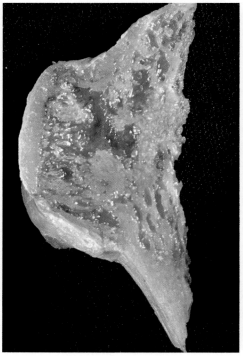

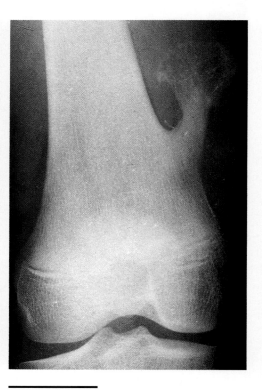

FIGURE 14.25 Photograph of the specimen removed from the femur seen in Figure 14.24. An irregular, cauliflower-like, bluish-gray cartilage mass overlies the cortical bone.

FIGURE 14.26 Cross-section of the specimen shown in Figure 14.25 demonstrates that the lesion seen radiologically is contiguous with the surrounding cortex, but is capped by a thin layer of bluish-gray cartilage.

FIGURE 14.27 Clinical radiograph of a pedunculated osteochondroma in the distal femur. Characteristically, the stalk points away from the adjacent joint surface, and the cortex of the osteochondroma is contiguous with the femoral cortex.

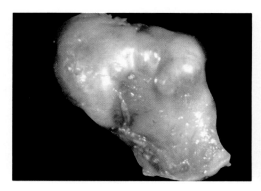

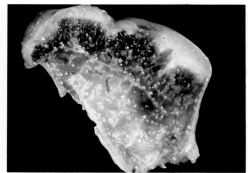

FIGURE 14.28 Surface and cross-section of the osteochondroma removed from the patient seen in Figure 14.27. The cartilage cap varies considerably in thickness.

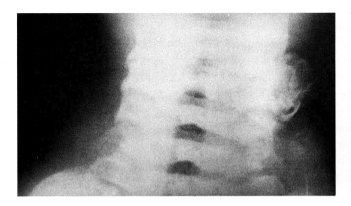

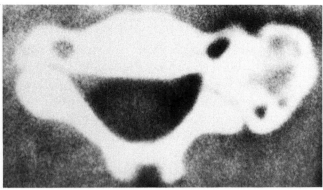

FIGURE 14.29 AP radiograph *(left)* of the lower cervical spine shows a well-corticated bubbly expansile lesion lateral to the lateral masses of C-4 and C-5. A CT section *(right)* through C-4 shows an expansile lesion extending from the left lateral mass. The cortex is thick and is contiguous with that of the pedicle. The neural foramina and spinal canal are uninvolved. The matrix is similar to that of a medullary cavity with coarse trabeculations. There is no evidence of calcified cartilage within the matrix and no associated surrounding soft-tissue component. (From Novick GS, Pavlov H, Bullough PG: Osteochondroma of the cervical spine: Report of two cases in preadolescent males. Skeletal Radiol 8:13-15, 1982)

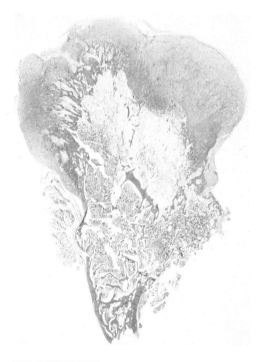

FIGURE 14.30 A histologic preparation of a pedunculated osteochondroma shows a thick proliferating cartilage cap overlying poorly organized cancellous bone. Irregular endochondral ossification is evident at the base of the cartilage cap (H & E, x 1 obj.).

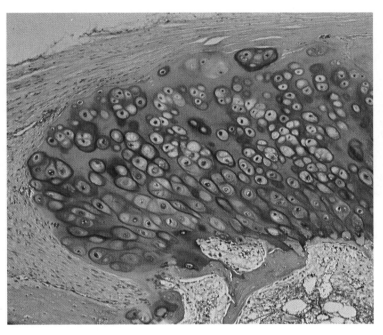

FIGURE 14.31 Photomicrograph of the cartilage cap at a higher power demonstrates the reflected layer of the periosteum over the exostosis, and the irregularity of the chondrocytes within the cartilage cap. Endochondral ossification is apparent at the base of the cap (H & E, x 25 obj.).

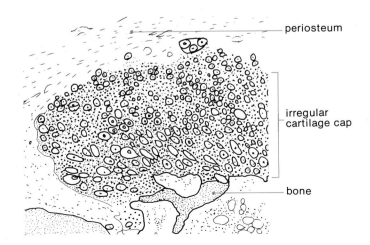

periosteum

irregular cartilage cap

bone

MULTIPLE OSTEOCHONDROMA (HEREDITARY MULTIPLE OSTEOCARTILAGINOUS EXOSTOSES)

The occurrence of multiple osteocartilaginous exostoses is rare. Inherited as an autosomal dominant trait, this condition is usually associated with short stature and other bone deformities (Figs. 14.32 and 14.33). The patients present with disfigurement or with pain induced by pressure on surrounding soft-tissue structures. Individual lesions are radiographically, grossly, and microscopically similar to solitary osteochondromas, although frequently the multiple lesions are more disorganized in structure and tend to have bosselated cartilage caps.

The significance of this disorder for the surgeon lies in the management of the multiple lesions; however, the pathologist must consider that the incidence of malignant transformation, compared with that in solitary osteochondromas, is much higher (about 10 percent). A lesion with suspected malignant transformation is shown in Figs 14.34 to 14.37.

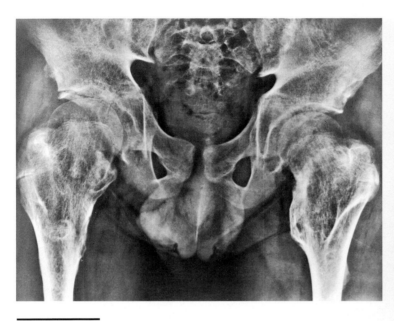

FIGURE 14.32 Radiograph of an adolescent boy with hereditary multiple exostoses. Note the short, wide, deformed femoral neck, on which can be seen several exostoses.

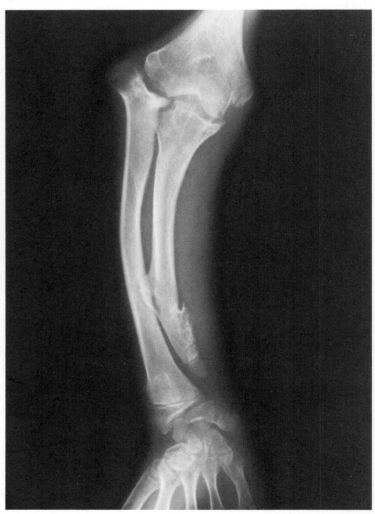

FIGURE 14.33 Radiograph of the forearm of the patient shown in Figure 14.32. Note multiple exostoses, with shortening and deformity of the forearm associated with malformation of the distal ulna.

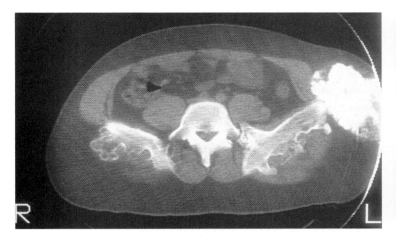

FIGURE 14.34 This CT scan of the pelvis in a 36-year-old man with known multiple exotoses reveals a large mass on the wing of the ilium. The patient's history revealed that this mass had been increasing in size.

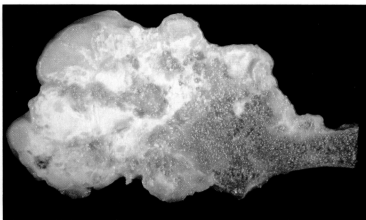

FIGURE 14.35 Transected specimen removed from the patient shown in Figure 14.34. Note the thick cartilage cap on the surface and the extensive calcification (calcified cartilage) within the irregular bosselated lesion.

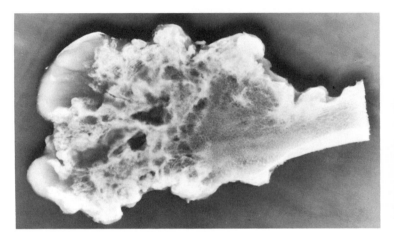

FIGURE 14.36 Radiograph of the specimen shown in Figure 14.35 again reveals the thick cartilage cap and extensive calcification of the cartilage matrix.

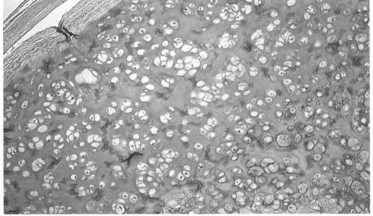

FIGURE 14.37 Photomicrograph of the cartilage cap in the specimen shown in the previous three figures. The cartilage cap is covered with a dense fibrous capsule, and the cartilage matrix is filled with crowded viable chondrocytes. The finding of a thick, active cartilage cap on an exotosis in a skeletally mature individual (especially if the lesion has a history of recent growth) must alert the clinician and the pathologist to the possibility of malignant transformation (H & E, x 10 obj.).

DYSPLASIA EPIPHYSEALIS HEMIMELICA (OSTEOCHONDROMA OF THE EPIPHYSIS; TREVOR'S DISEASE)

Dysplasia epiphysealis hemimelica is a nonfamilial developmental disorder of the skeleton, usually manifested in young children who present with unilateral irregular enlargement of the epiphysis (Figs. 14.38 to 14.40). The disorder most commonly involves the lower femur, the upper tibia, or the talus. Although it is a benign condition, varus or valgus deformities of the limb may ensue. Surgical excision is the treatment of choice.

When excised and examined microscopically, the lesion somewhat resembles an osteochondroma, with a cartilage cap, an underlying zone of endochondral ossification, and normal progression of cancellous bone formation (Figs. 14.41 and 14.42).

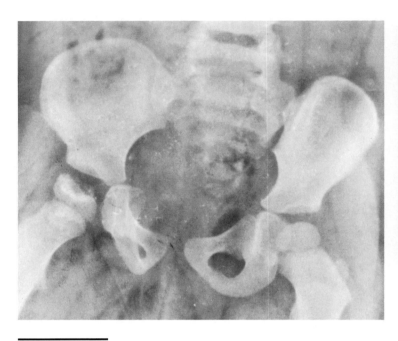

FIGURE 14.38 Radiograph of a child with an eccentrically enlarged, irregular, capital femoral epiphysis due to an epiphyseal osteochondroma (Trevor's disease). It is important not to confuse this condition with Legg–Calvé–Perthes disease.

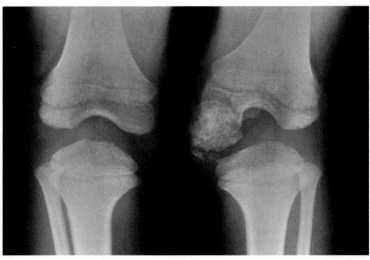

FIGURE 14.39 Radiograph showing a large ossifying protuberance arising in the medial femoral condyle of a patient with Trevor's disease.

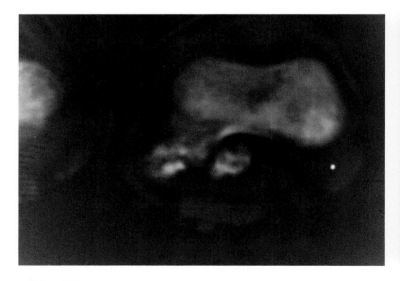

FIGURE 14.40 A computerized axial tomogram through the left medial femoral condyle shown in Figure 14.39 demonstrates the origin of the lesion from the underlying bone.

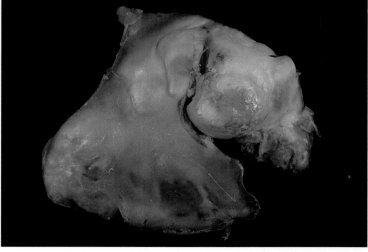

FIGURE 14.41 A gross photograph of the resected specimen of the lesion shown in Figure 14.40. Note the cartilaginous appearance of the lesion, which has focal ossification at its periphery and is partially covered by a fibrous membrane.

BONE ISLAND (SOLITARY ENOSTOSIS)

A solitary fleck of increased density in cancellous bone is not an uncommon incidental finding on radiographs. Scintigraphy may reveal increased uptake of isotope in some of these lesions. Usually these lesions are only 1 or 2 mm in diameter, but occasionally they may measure as much as a centimeter or more (Figs. 14.43 to 14.45).

The lesions are called bone islands or enostoses, and they are probably developmental in origin. They are significant only in differential diagnosis (eg, of osteoid osteoma when they are small or of sclerosing osteosarcoma if they are large).

On gross examination, these foci are found in the intramedullary spongy bone and are composed of compact bone which merges with the surrounding trabecular bone to give a spoke-like pattern at the periphery

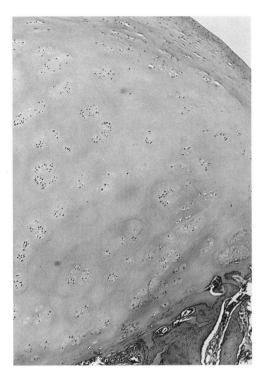

FIGURE 14.42 Photomicrograph of a portion of the cartilage cap on the articular surface demonstrated in Figure 14.41, showing the increased irregular cellularity of the lesional cartilage (H & E, x 10 obj.).

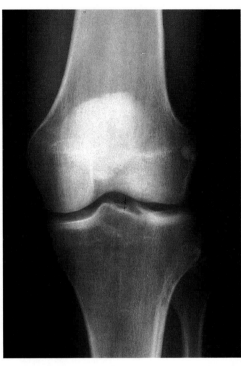

FIGURE 14.43 Anteroposterior radiograph of a knee, showing in the lateral femoral condyle a peripheral island of dense bone delineated by a fine osteolytic rim. (Courtesy of Dr. Leon Sokoloff)

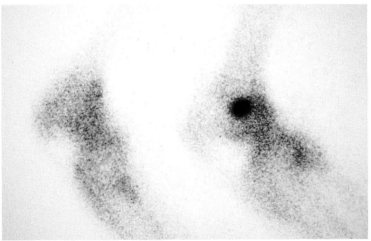

FIGURE 14.44 Scintigram showing increased uptake of ^{99}Tc diphosphonate in the lesion demonstrated in Figure 14.43.

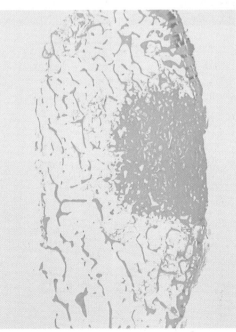

FIGURE 14.45 Photomicrograph of a section through the lesion demonstrated in Figure 14.43 reveals dense cortical bone which merges imperceptibly with the surrounding cancellous bone (H & E, x 1 obj.).(Courtesy of Dr. Leon Sokoloff)

(Figs. 14.46 to 14.48). Microscopic examination of this tissue reveals mature lamellar bone with well-developed haversian and interstitial lamellar systems (Fig. 14.49). No endochondral ossification or calcified cartilage is observed.

OSTEOPOIKILOSIS

Osteopoikilosis is a rare, symptomless, and clinically benign condition. It is inherited as an autosomal dominant trait. On radiographs, the bones show multiple discrete or clustered foci of radiopacity with uniform density, giving the bone a spotted appearance. The disorder is usually symmetrical, affecting both the epiphyseal and metaphyseal zones. It most commonly involves the small bones of the hands and feet, and the ends of the long bones of the extremities (Fig. 14.50). The microscopic features of the lesions are similar to those of solitary bone islands (Fig. 14.51).

Osteopoikilosis has also been reported to occur in association with cutaneous nodules, which usually prove on microscopic examination to be fibrous tissue (eg, fibromatosis, scleroderma-like lesions, or keloids). This finding suggests a general mesenchymal defect in these patients.

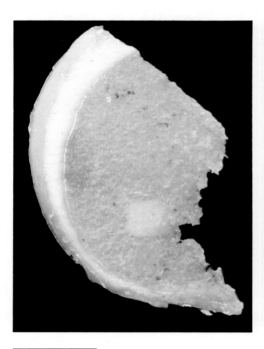

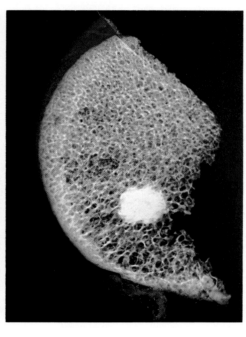

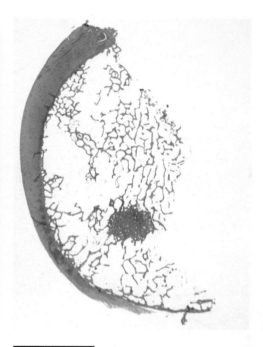

FIGURE 14.46 Coronal section through a femoral head reveals a whitish, circumscribed piece of bone, clearly demarcated from the surrounding cancellous bone.

FIGURE 14.47 Radiograph of the specimen illustrated in Figure 14.46 demonstrates the marked density of the solitary bone island.

FIGURE 14.48 The bone island consists of normal bone distinctly separated from the surrounding cancellous bone spicules, but note that the spicules merge with the nodule in a radial fashion. This bone is found to be lamellar when viewed under polarized light.

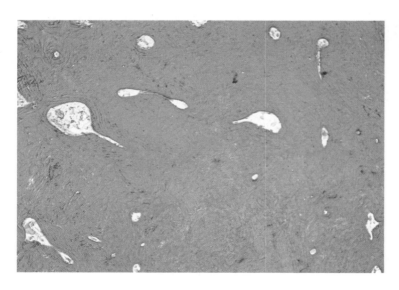

FIGURE 14.49 High-power view of the bone island illustrated in Figure 14.48 shows the mature, dense appearance of the bone.

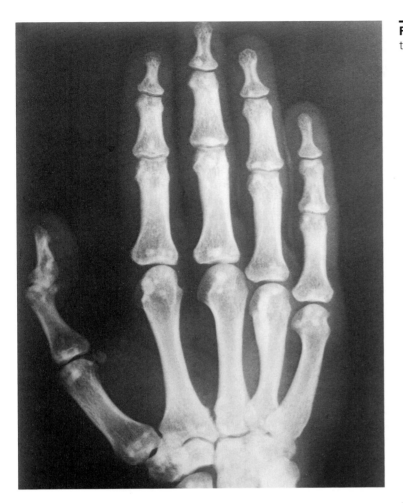

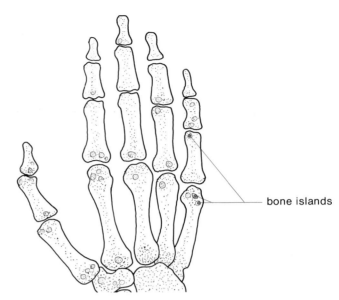

FIGURE 14.50 Radiograph reveals circumscribed dense foci distributed throughout the hand of a patient with osteopoikilosis.

bone islands

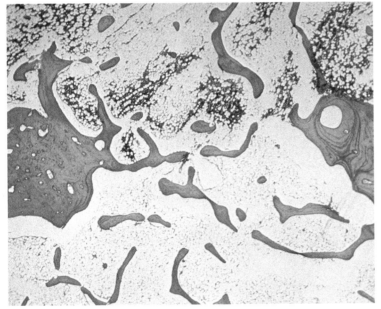

FIGURE 14.51 Nodules of bone with connected spicules of cancellous bone are evident in this specimen from a patient with osteopoikilosis (H & E, x 4 obj.).

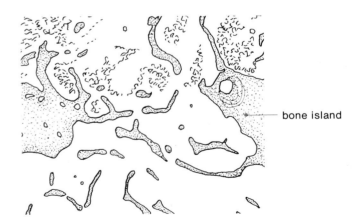

bone island

MELORHEOSTOSIS

Melorheostosis is a rare, nonfamilial, usually unilateral lesion of long bones in which the affected bones display a peculiar irregular cortical hyperostosis, similar in appearance to melting wax dripping down the sides of a candle (see Fig. 14.52). The lesions occur on both the periosteum and the endosteum. Associated cutaneous lesions, including vascular malformations and focal subcutaneous and para-articular fibrosis, are common.

In affected children, the skeleton is characterized by hyperostoses of the bones of the extremities and pelvic girdle, by inequality in the length of the extremities, and by joint contractures resulting in deformity. On radiographs, the lesions may be found to involve the epiphysis, and osseous tissue may be seen crossing the growth plate. In children, prominent soft-tissue fibrosis may predate osseous abnormalities. Attempts at surgical management of the contractures have been unrewarding.

In adult melorheostosis, the patients present with pain, deformity, or limitation of joint motion. The lesion may involve one or many bones. Ectopic bone may be present in para-articular locations. The

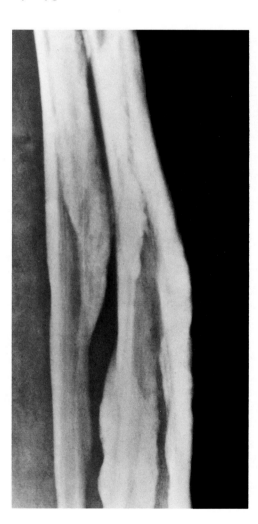

FIGURE 14.52 Radiograph of forearm in a 35-year-old man with generalized bone pain shows the thickened endosteal and periosteal bone "candle-dripping" appearance of melorheostosis.

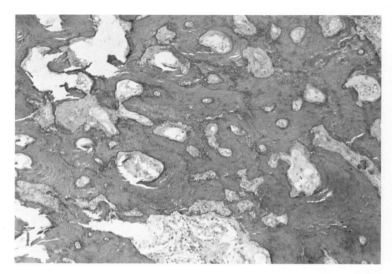

FIGURE 14.53 Biopsy specimen of cortical bone from a patient with melorheostosis reveals markedly irregular bone with relatively little cellular activity on the endosteal surfaces. The marrow may show mild fibrosis (H & E, x 4 obj.).

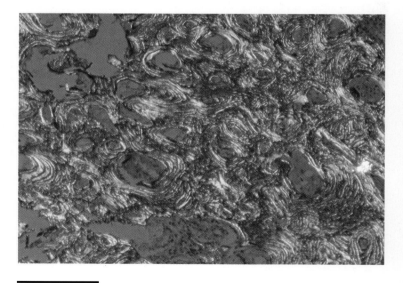

FIGURE 14.54 The same histologic field shown in Figure 14.53, photographed with polarized light. Note the irregular mixture of lamellar and woven bone.

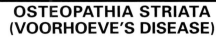

involvement of one side of a bone (or row of bones, in some cases) has suggested a sclerotome distribution.

On gross examination, the periosteal and endosteal surfaces of the affected bones in melorheostosis are irregular, and the bones display thickened trabeculae. The marrow cavity is narrowed. Histologic examination reveals that the new bone is either woven or lamellar (Figs. 14.53 and 14.54). When the new bone tissue is lamellar, it is architecturally irregular. The affected cortical bone in these cases is often quite cellular, and there is a distinct differentiation between the normal and the melorheostotic bone.

OSTEOPATHIA STRIATA (VOORHOEVE'S DISEASE)

Osteopathia striata is a benign, asymptomatic disorder characterized radiographically by usually symmetrical, axially oriented, dense striations. Its presence in association with sclerosis of the base of the skull has been determined to be genetically transmitted as an autosomal dominant condition. When osteopathia striata is seen in association with osteopoikilosis and/or melorheostosis, the condition is referred to as mixed sclerosing bone dystrophy (Figs. 14.55 to 14.56).

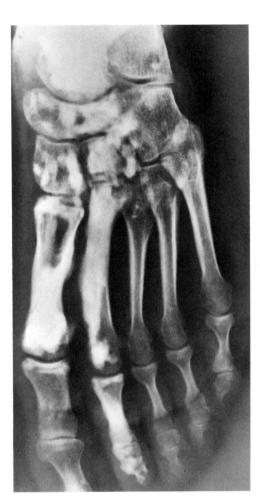

FIGURE 14.55
Many bone islands and evidence of melorheostosis can be seen in the foot of the patient shown in Figure 14.52. This rare pattern of mixed sclerosing bone dystrophy was generalized throughout the skeleton.

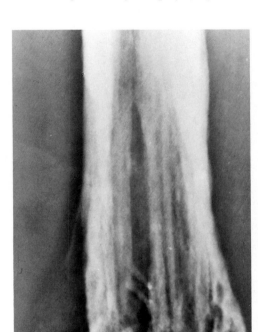

FIGURE 14.56
In this radiograph of the lower femur of the patient shown in Figures 14.52 and 14.55, the striated pattern of Voorhoeve's disease can be clearly seen.

OSTEOID OSTEOMA

Osteoid osteomas are relatively common, small (usually less than a centimeter in diameter), solitary, benign but painful lesions of bone. They are characteristically seen in children and adolescents, with males affected twice as frequently as females. The most commonly involved site is a lower extremity, with lesions tending to occur near the end of the diaphysis. However, almost any bone can be involved.

The characteristic clinical presentation of osteoid osteoma is nocturnal pain which is usually relieved by aspirin. Local swelling may be apparent, and the lesion may be exquisitely tender; mild leukocytosis may also be present. When the lesion is close to or within a joint, the patient may present with joint effusion and symptoms of synovitis; this type of presentation is seen in approximately 20 percent of the cases. Individuals with lesions in the vertebral column may present with scoliosis (Figs. 14.57 and 14.58).

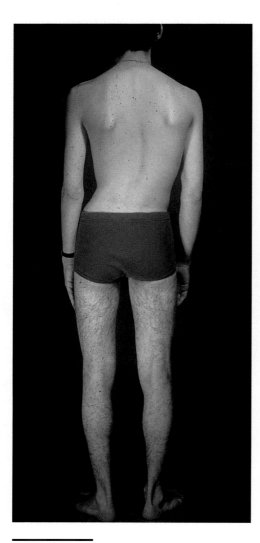

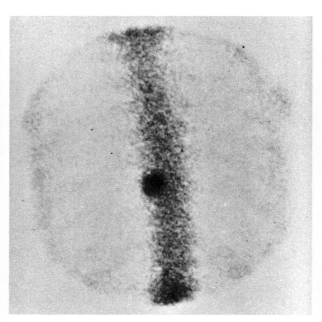

FIGURE 14.58 Technetium scan of the thoracic spine in a patient complaining of severe localized pain, occasionally present at night and relieved by aspirin. The localized area of high uptake, as seen here, is typical of osteoid osteoma.

FIGURE 14.57 Clinical photograph demonstrating mild scoliosis in a teenaged boy with an osteoid osteoma in the lumbar spine. (Courtesy of Dr. David Levine)

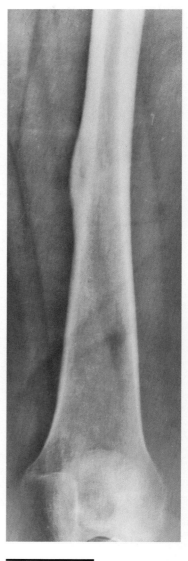

FIGURE 14.59 A 20-year-old man complained of pain in the midshaft of the right femur. Radiograph shows an area of cortical thickening, in the center of which is a lucent defect with an opaque central nidus. An osteoid osteoma in cortical bone produces a considerable amount of reactive bone tissue, as seen in this case. (However, in the cancellous area of the bone it may be difficult to see the lesion because of a lack of reactive bone sclerosis.)

On radiographs, the typical lesion is located within the cortex of a long bone, and exhibits a central lucent zone (or nidus) with density of the surrounding bone (Figs. 14.59 to 14.64). Osteoid osteomas located subperiosteally or in the cancellous portion of the bone show much less surrounding sclerosis. On bone scans these lesions show up as very active foci ("hot spots").

At surgery, the area of involvement is sometimes difficult to ascertain, although there may be a mild pinkish cast to the overlying cortical bone. The lesion itself may appear as a well-demarcated nodule, often cherry red (Figs. 14.65 and 14.66), but occasionally very dense and white.

Osteoid osteomas are characterized microscopically by a maze of small spicules of immature bone, most often lined with prominent osteoblasts and osteo-

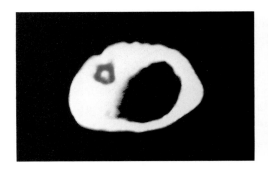

FIGURE 14.60 An osteoid osteoma located in the cortex of the tibia is well demonstrated on this CT scan.

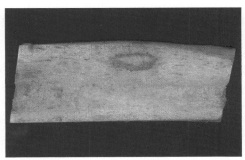

FIGURE 14.61 Gross photograph of a segment of cortical bone containing an osteoid osteoma nidus. Note the dense center in the nidus and the surrounding hyperemia.

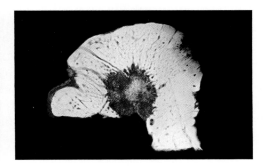

FIGURE 14.62 Radiograph of a slice taken through the nidus shown in Figure 14.61. The nidus is formed of fine bone spicules and, corresponding to the hyperemic zone, a lucent zone lies between the nidus and the surrounding sclerotic cortical bone.

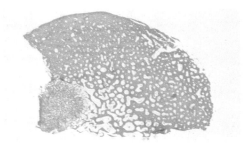

FIGURE 14.63 Photomicrograph of the osteoid osteoma shown in Figures 14.61 and 14.62 shows the central nidus formed of irregular trabeculae of immature woven bone surrounded by a fibrous hyperemic zone and sclerotic cortical bone (H & E, x 1 obj.).

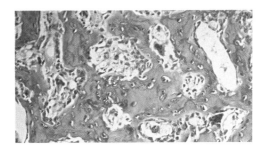

FIGURE 14.64 High-power photomicrograph of the central nidus of an osteoid osteoma shows interconnecting trabeculae of immature woven bone with an extremely vascular stroma. Many osteoclasts and active osteoblasts line the bone trabeculae (H & E, x 10 obj.).

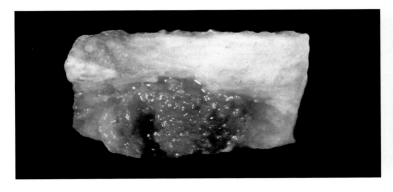

FIGURE 14.65 Gross photograph of an excised osteoid osteoma which appeared on radiographs as a lucent lesion. Note the hyperemic appearance of the tissue.

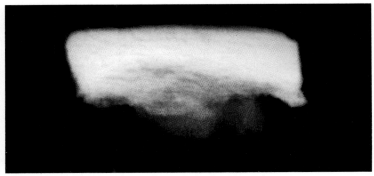

FIGURE 14.66 Radiograph of the specimen shown in Figure 14.65 demonstrates the relative lucency of the nidus. However, there are fine bone trabeculae coursing through the lesion.

clasts. The intervening stroma is sparsely cellular, with readily apparent vascular spaces (Figs. 14.67 to 14.69). Cartilage matrix formation does not occur. Striking amounts of periosteal new bone may appear in the overlying cortex. Very rare cases have been observed in which multiple nidi were present.

The minute size of the lesion often makes it difficult for both the surgeon and the pathologist to locate. A fine-grain radiograph may be helpful in determining the location of the nidus of an osteoid osteoma in tissue submitted for microscopic examination (Fig. 14.70). However, even with this technique and multiple samples, the lesion may be difficult to localize. Preoperative technetium (^{99}Tc) isotope injections with intraoperative localization of radioactivity and postoperative localization by specimen autoimaging on undeveloped film may be of considerable help.

The etiology of this bizarre condition remains obscure. The radiologic differential diagnosis includes a small focus of osteomyelitis or a stress fracture.

OSTEOMAS OF THE CRANIUM AND FACIAL BONES

These lesions are asymptomatic, benign, slow-growing, tumor-like masses that occur in the calvaria and facial bones. The characteristic histologic features of the calvarial lesions differ from the histologic features of the facial lesions.

Osteomas appear on the outer surface of the calvaria as circumscribed, ivory-like excrescences composed of mature lamellar bone (Figs 14.71 and 14.72). Lesions on the facial bones are frequently associated

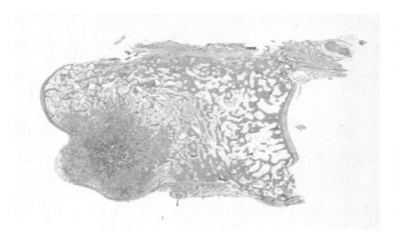

FIGURE 14.67 Low-power photomicrograph of the middle phalanx of a finger. A subperiosteal osteoid osteoma is seen adjacent to the joint margin (H & E, x 1 obj.).

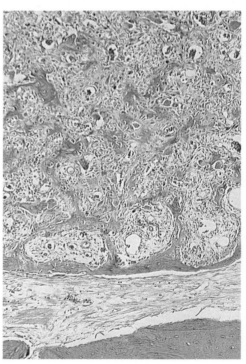

FIGURE 14.68 Photomicrograph showing a portion of an osteoid osteoma nidus and a part of the normal bone at the edge of the lesion. The nidus is composed of vascular fibrous tissue in which there are small, irregular, but connected trabeculae of woven bone, demonstrating both prominent osteoblasts and prominent osteoclasts (H & E, x 1 obj.).

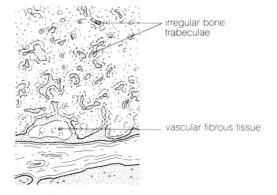

irregular bone trabeculae

vascular fibrous tissue

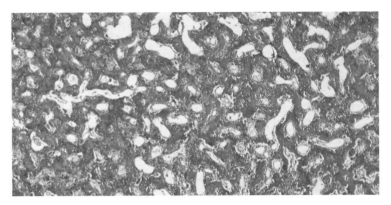

FIGURE 14.69 Photomicrograph of the nidus of a more mature osteoid osteoma, with more dense interconnecting trabeculae of bone and less cellular activity than is seen in Figure 14.68 (H & E, x 4 obj.).

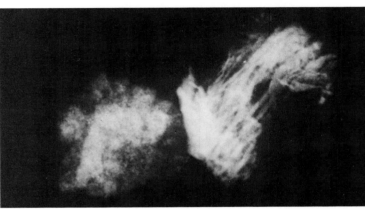

FIGURE 14.70 Radiograph of curetted tissue taken during surgery in a patient with a suspected osteoid osteoma. Radiographs of the specimen were taken immediately, and in this portion of the specimen one can discern a piece of bone with a very fine trabecular pattern typical of an osteoid osteoma (left), and a fragment of more normal cancellous bone (right). When many specimens are received from a patient with an osteoid osteoma, radiographs of the specimens not only help the pathologist to inform the surgeon whether he has removed the lesional tissue, but also enable the pathologist to select the proper pieces for histologic examination.

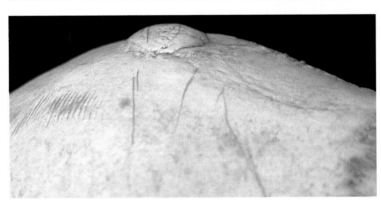

FIGURE 14.71 Gross photograph of an osteoma (or ivory exostosis) of the calvaria shows a well-circumscribed nodular growth distorting the smooth contour of the skull.

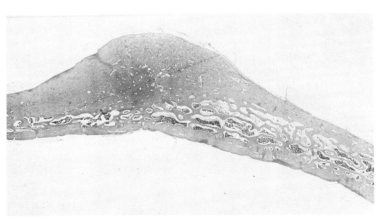

FIGURE 14.72 Photomicrograph of the lesion shown in Figure 14.71 demonstrates that the lesion is composed of mature lamellar bone.

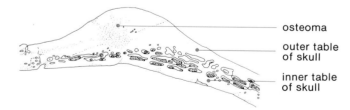

osteoma

outer table of skull

inner table of skull

with the sinuses, and are formed of immature bone, often with active osteoblasts and osteoclasts (Figs. 14.73 to 14.76).

The etiology of facial osteoma is obscure. The lesion does not recur after surgical excision, and it is not associated with malignant change.

It should be remembered that osteomas of the facial bones may be associated with colonic polyps (Gardner's syndrome). Other disorders characteristically grouped with this syndrome are odontomas, supernumerary and unerupted teeth, and soft-tissue tumors including fibromas and epidermal inclusion cysts. Gardner's syndrome is an autosomal dominant genetic disorder, and is of particular importance because of the malignant change that frequently occurs in the adenomatous lesions of the intestine.

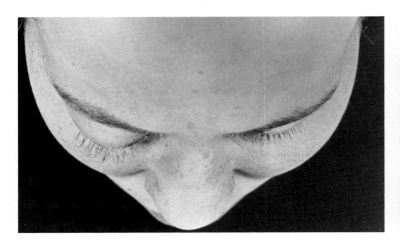

FIGURE 14.73 The protusion of the orbit seen in this patient is caused by an osteoma arising from the bone in the frontal sinus.

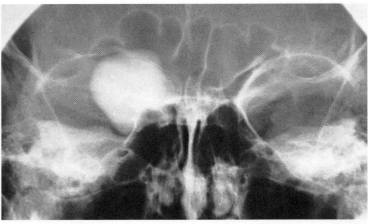

FIGURE 14.74 Radiograph of the patient shown in Figure 14.73 demonstrates a well-circumscribed dense lesion which is distorting the frontal sinus (the cause of the orbital protrusion in the clinical photograph).

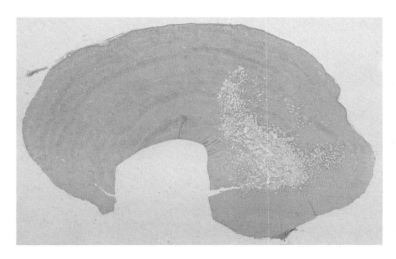

FIGURE 14.75 Histologic section through the lesion excised from the frontal sinus of the patient shown in Figures 14.73 and 14.74. The lesion consists of dense immature bone with a small focal area of fibrous modeling (H & E, x 1 obj.)

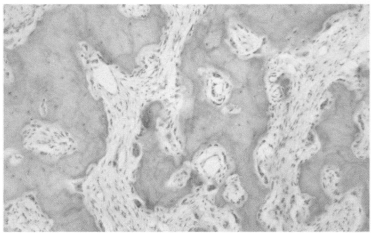

FIGURE 14.76 Close-up of the area of fibrous modeling shown in Figure 14.75 shows irregular bone trabeculae with fibrous marrow and osteoclastic resorption of the bone (H & E, x 25 obj.).

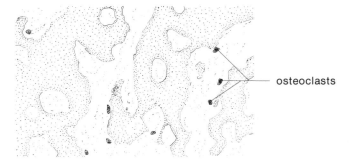

osteoclasts

**Benign tumors-
cystic, fibrous and others**

This chapter will consider both benign cellular non-neoplastic lesions as well as those non-neoplastic lesions in which there is an extracellular matrix of simple fibrous character.

EPIDERMOID INCLUSION CYST

Epidermoid inclusion cysts are cysts bounded by a wall of stratified squamous epithelium and filled with keratin debris (Fig. 15.1). Although these lesions rarely occur in bone, when they are present they usually appear radiologically as sharply outlined, intraosseous lytic areas, most commonly found in the distal terminal phalanx (Fig. 15.2) or the calvaria.

The radiologic differential diagnosis of an epidermoid inclusion cyst in the finger includes enchondroma (which occurs only in the proximal portion of the distal phalanx), giant-cell reparative granuloma, and intraosseous extension of a glomus tumor (Figs. 15.3 and 15.4).

GANGLION CYST OF BONE

Radiographically, intraosseous ganglion cysts are rare uniloculated or multiloculated, well-demarcated lytic defects with a rim of sclerotic bone. Patients with this disorder are usually middle-aged and present with mild localized pain that is increased by weight bearing. The

FIGURE 15.1 Photomicrograph of an epidermoid inclusion cyst. The central space is lined with stratified squamous epithelium and is filled with keratin debris (H & E, x 4 obj.).

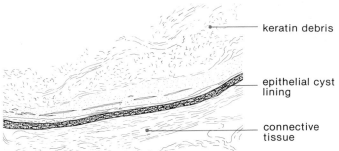

- keratin debris
- epithelial cyst lining
- connective tissue

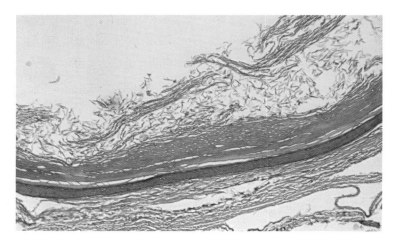

FIGURE 15.2 Anteroposterior *(left)* and lateral *(right)* radiographs showing an epidermoid inclusion cyst. A well-circumscribed lucent defect with a thinned cortical rim is present in the distal

portion of the terminal phalanx. No calcification is evident, and this, together with the location, helps to differentiate this lesion from an enchondroma.

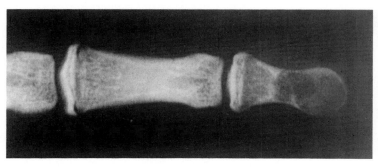

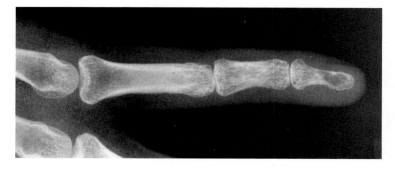

FIGURE 15.3 Radiograph shows a lytic defect in the terminal phalanx of the little finger, caused by the intraosseous extension of a soft-tissue glomus tumor. (Courtesy of Dr. Isao Sugiura)

lesion may be discovered as an incidental finding. Clinically, these defects are most frequently seen at the epiphyseal end of long bones, commonly in the medial malleolus of the ankle (Fig 15.5). Despite its proximity to a joint, a ganglion cyst rarely involves the joint. Occasionally an overlying soft-tissue ganglion is present on clinical examination, and it may communicate with the intraosseous ganglion.

At surgery, the lesion is a unilocular or multilocular cyst lined with a thick, fibrous membrane and filled with a whitish or yellowish gelatinous material. On microscopic examination, the wall of a ganglion cyst is composed of a dense, fibrous connective tissue layer with focal mucoid degeneration, flattened membrane-lining cells, and occasional mononuclear inflammatory cells (Fig. 15.6).

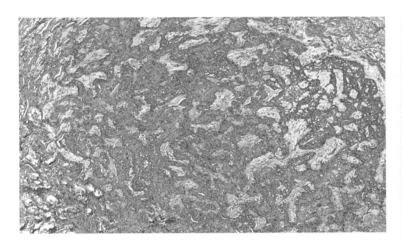

FIGURE 15.4 Photomicrograph of a glomus tumor shows connecting cords of round to oval homogeneous cells with pinkish cytoplasm. The intervening stroma is a vascular fibrous connective tissue that may have a mucinous appearance (H & E, x 10 obj.).

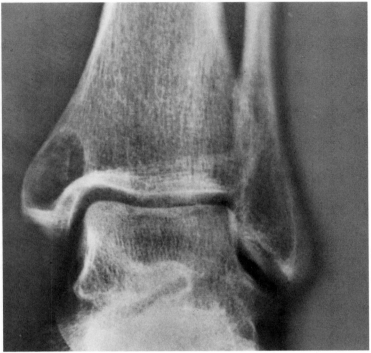

FIGURE 15.5 Ganglionic cyst of bone. In this radiograph of the lower end of the tibia, a well-demarcated, roundish lucent area is evident. Although this lesion is close to the joint space, the joint space is not narrowed, which finding differentiates a ganglionic cyst from an osteoarthritic cyst.

FIGURE 15.6 Microscopic examination of a ganglionic cyst of bone reveals the walls of the lesion to consist of fibrous connective tissue, with focal areas of mucoid degeneration and patchy dense collagen. The membrane may be lined with flattened lining cells (H & E, x 10 obj.).

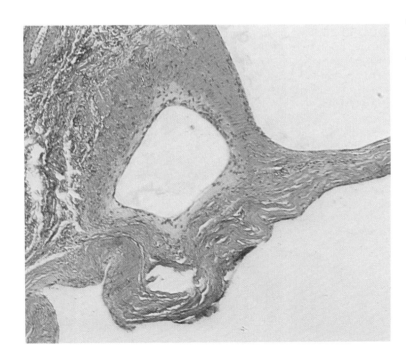

The lack of communication between the cystic bone defect and the articular cavity and the absence of arthritic change distinguish this disorder from marginal cysts and subchondral bone cysts associated with degenerative joint disease (Fig. 15.7).

Treatment by currettage or excision has been curative. Recurrences are rare.

UNICAMERAL BONE CYST (SOLITARY CYST; SIMPLE BONE CYST)

A simple bone cyst is a benign, solitary cystic defect in the metaphyseal region of long bones, usually presenting clinically in children or young adolescents (Fig. 15.8). The classic location for such a lesion is the proxi-

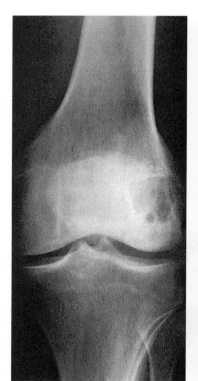

FIGURE 15.7 Anteroposterior radiograph of the knee, showing a well-defined peripheral trabeculated lytic lesion of the lateral femoral condyle, secondary to an intraosseous ganglion.

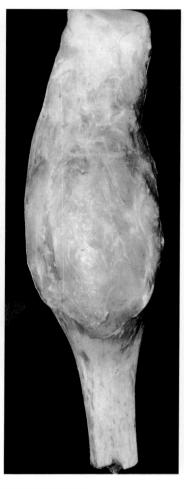

FIGURE 15.8 Gross photograph of fibula with a central bulblike expansion caused by a simple bone cyst. Note the pink color at the margin of the cyst, owing to periosteal bone formation.

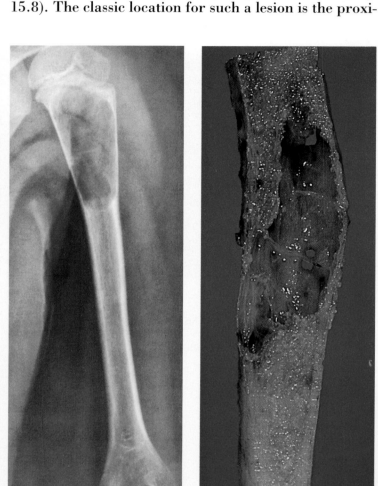

FIGURE 15.9 Radiograph of a simple bone cyst in the proximal humerus of an 8-year-old boy reveals a well-circumscribed lucent area in the metaphysis, extending to the diaphysis. Although the lesion extends up to the epiphysis, the epiphysis is not involved. Thinning of the cortex is evident. (Because these lesions typically present after a fracture, the radiologic appearance may be complicated by callus formation.)

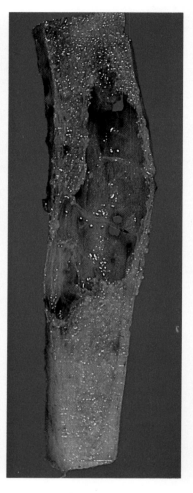

FIGURE 15.10 Longitudinal section of a segment of resected humerus reveals a well-demarcated cystic cavitation in the medullary portion of the bone, with cortical thinning and periosteal elevation leading to a bulging cortex. Note also the glistening cystic lining. (These lesions usually contain a clear, serous-like fluid.)

mal humerus (Figs. 15.9 and 15.10), and the most common clinical presentation is a pathologic fracture through the area of weakened bone. On radiographic studies, the lesion appears as a well-defined lucent area with a thin sclerotic margin. A pseudo-loculated appearance may result from irregular thinning of the cortex by the expanding cyst.

On gross inspection, an unaltered lesion appears as a clear, fluid-filled cyst lined with a thin fibrous membrane (Figs. 15.11 and 15.12). However, because frac-

tures are common complications, "secondary" changes such as hemorrhage and hemosiderin deposits, granulation tissue, cholesterol clefts, fibrin, calcification, and reactive bone (Fig. 15.13) may be observed. In such instances, the lesion may mimic the histologic features of an aneurysmal bone cyst or even a giant-cell tumor. A rarely observed histologic feature is the accumulation of calcified amorphous material which superficially resembles the contents of a cementoma of the jaw (Fig 15.14). This material probably represents calcified fibrin.

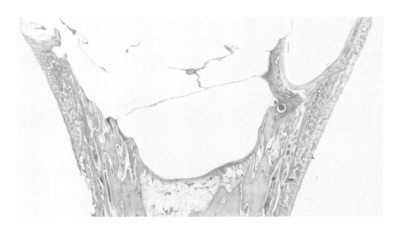

FIGURE 15.11 Low-power photomicrograph of a simple bone cyst reveals a fibrous membrane. Erosion of the cortex is evident, as is periosteal bone formation (H & E, x 1 obj.).

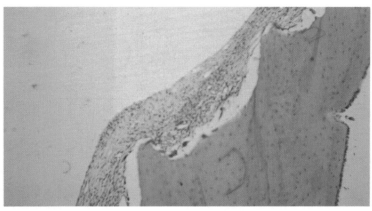

FIGURE 15.12 High-power view of the fibrous lining of a simple bone cyst (H & E, x 4 obj.).

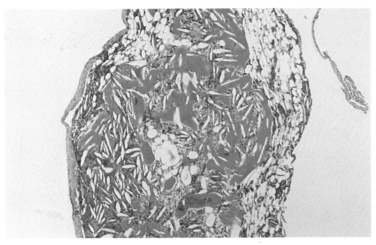

FIGURE 15.13 Photomicrograph of tissue curetted from a simple bone cyst after fracture. Local hemosiderin deposits, chronic inflammation with many cholesterol clefts, and a rapidly forming callus are evident (H & E, x 4 obj.).

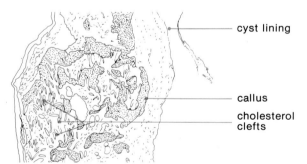

FIGURE 15.14 The membranous wall of this simple bone cyst reveals a peculiar, irregularly arranged calcific matrix which morphologically resembles the tissue present in a cementoma of the jaw (H & E, x 10 obj.).

The lesion, when observed in serial radiographs, appears to migrate from the epiphyseal plate, although in reality the growth plate grows away from the cyst (Fig. 15.15). Because of the difficulty of complete surgical removal of the lesion, there is a high rate of recurrence after surgical curettage, particularly in children under 10 years of age in whom the lesion is characteristically juxta-epiphyseal. Nonsurgical treatment by injection with corticosteroids has met with some success.

ANEURYSMAL BONE CYST

An aneurysmal bone cyst is a solitary, generally eccentric, expansile lesion of unknown etiology. Aneurysmal bone cysts are most commonly seen in individuals under 20 years of age. Swelling, pain, and/or tenderness may be observed in these patients.

Although the lesion usually involves long bones or the spine, any bone can be involved, including flat bones. When a long bone is affected, the lesion appears

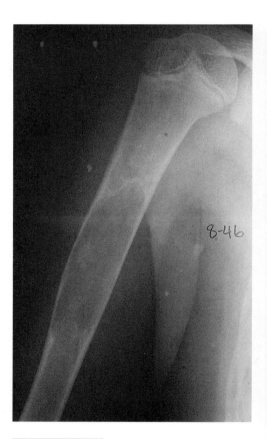

FIGURE 15.15 Radiograph showing a large simple cyst in the humeral diaphysis.

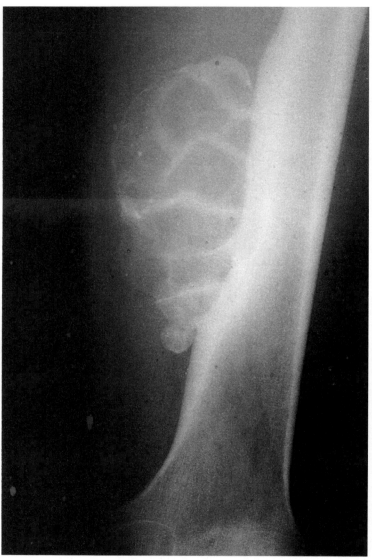

FIGURE 15.16 Radiograph of an aneurysmal bone cyst shows a septated, subperiosteal blowout lesion. Note the irregular cortical margins at the lesion's interface with the shaft of the bone.

on serial radiographic films as a rapidly expansile, eccentric, lucent lesion in the shaft of the bone (Fig. 15.16). The periphery of the lesion is often indistinct, and the tumor itself has a trabeculated appearance. Approximately 15 percent of all aneurysmal bone cysts arise in the spine, where they may occur at any level with the exception of the coccyx. Occasionally multiple vertebrae are affected. Although these tumors mainly involve the vertebral arches, they sometimes extend into the vertebral bodies (Fig. 15.17). Extradural cord compression is fairly common and may cause neurologic complications.

On external gross examination, the wall of an aneurysmal bone cyst is usually soft and fibrous. However, when the cyst is opened, separated spaces containing friable, brownish blood clot usually become apparent (Fig. 15.18). On histologic examination, the lesion is found to contain cystic spaces of different sizes which are filled with blood but are not lined with vascular endothelium. Between the blood-filled spaces are

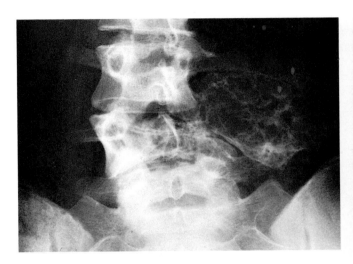

FIGURE 15.17 AP radiograph of the lumbar spine of a woman in her mid-twenties with complaints of low back pain. Examination revealed a scoliotic deformity and slight local tenderness. This film shows collapse of the L-4 body, with a huge expansion of the transverse process. The cortex is intact and the bone has a honeycombed trabeculated appearance; the pedicle is not seen on the affected side. The mild scoliotic deformity has developed as a result of the lesion.

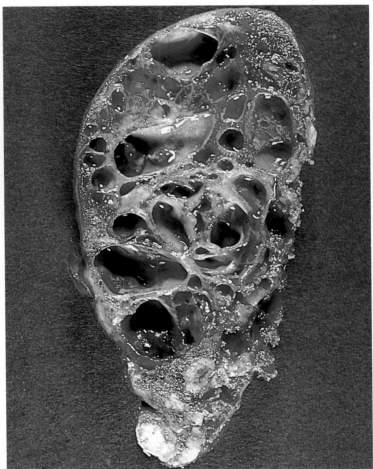

FIGURE 15.18 Viewed grossly, the lesion resected from the patient shown in Figure 15.16 is a spongy, honeycombed, blood-filled mass with cystic spaces of various sizes, some containing osseous tissue within the septated walls.

fibrous septa containing giant cells and foci of immature bone or osteoid (Figs. 15.19 and 15.20). Focal or diffuse collections of hemosiderin or reactive foam cells and chronic inflammatory cells may be seen in the septal zone. Characteristically, the cell morphology appears innocuous. In some instances it is clear from histologic examination that the lesion coexists with another benign tumor, such as an osteoblastoma or chondroblastoma (Figs. 15.21 and 15.22). In about 50 percent of patients the lesion recurs once or several times after curettage.

It is important to differentiate this lesion microscopically from a telangiectatic osteosarcoma, a differential diagnosis that may on occasion be difficult.

GIANT-CELL REPARATIVE GRANULOMA (SOLID ANEURYSMAL BONE CYST)

A giant-cell reparative granuloma is a benign, non-neoplastic, intra-osseous lesion most commonly seen in the mandible or maxilla, but also reported in the small bones of the hands and feet (Fig. 15.23) as well as in other bones. Although these lesions may present at any age, most patients are in the second or third decade. The clinical signs of this lesion are localized pain and swelling of variable duration. Radiographic examination reveals a lucent defect expanding the bone. The cortex is thinned, and there is little evidence of bone destruction and no surrounding sclerosis.

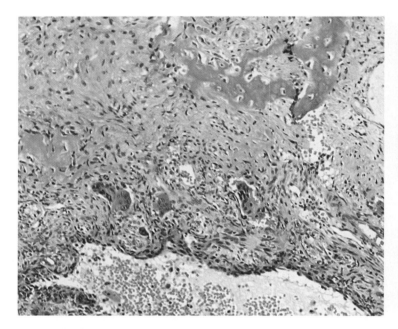

FIGURE 15.19 Low-power photomicrograph reveals that the lining tissue of an aneurysmal bone cyst contains a cellular stroma, often with many giant cells and bone formation (H & E, x 4 obj.).

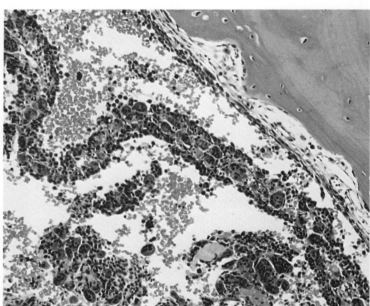

FIGURE 15.20 Higher-power photomicrograph demonstrates the many giant cells lining the septa. This feature distinguishes an aneurysmal bone cyst lining from the fibrous lining space of a simple bone cyst (H & E, x 10 obj.).

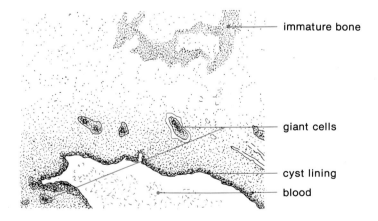

immature bone

giant cells

cyst lining

blood

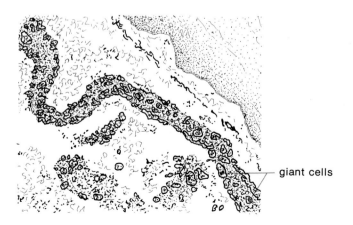

giant cells

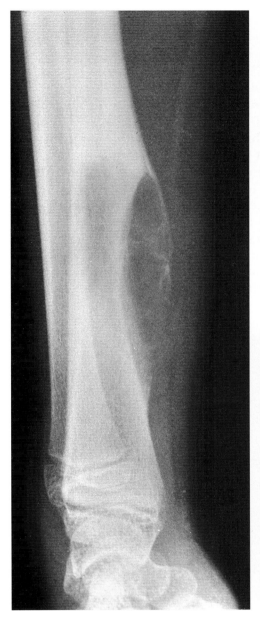

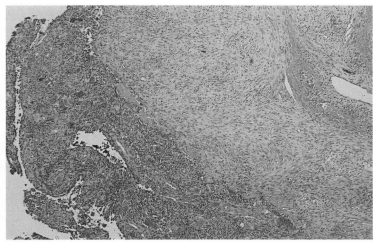

FIGURE 15.22 Photomicrograph demonstrating the juxtaposition of an aneurysmal bone cyst and a focus of coexisting fibrous dysplasia (H & E, x 10 obj.).

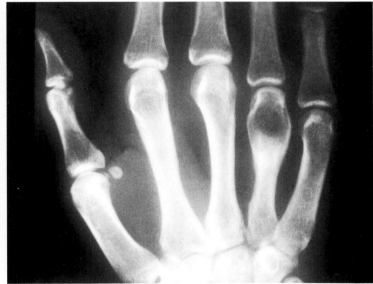

FIGURE 15.21 Radiograph of the lower arm, showing an eccentric and expanded cystic lesion of the lower diaphysis of the distal radius. An intact shell of periosteal bone is seen over most of the lesion. In the shaft of the radius there is a poorly defined central lucency. In this case of aneurysmal bone cyst, there is microscopic evidence of an underlying focus of fibrous dysplasia (see Figure 15.22).

FIGURE 15.23 Radiograph of a giant-cell reparative granuloma of the fourth metacarpal. A lucent lesion expands the bone and there is thinning and expansion of the cortex. No calcification has occurred. The shaft of the bone protudes into the expansile lesion, resembling a finger inside a balloon. This radiologic finding is also common in aneurysmal bone cysts when they affect small tubular bones and is evidence of rapid growth.

On gross examination, tissue obtained from a giant-cell reparative granuloma appears grayish-brown and is often friable. Microscopic observation of the tissue, may reveal varying degrees of cellularity, with predominantly unremarkable fibroblast-like spindle cells (Figs. 15.24 and 15.25). Histiocytes are also present. Characteristically, giant cells clustered in areas of recent and old hemorrhage are scattered throughout the tissue of the lesion. Mitotic activity is rare. New bone formation and osteoid may be seen, again usually at sites of hemorrhage. Focal or scattered lymphocytic infiltration has been noted.

The differential diagnosis of giant-cell reparative granuloma includes "brown" tumor of hyperparathyroidism, giant-cell tumor, and aneurysmal bone cyst. The following considerations may prove helpful in sorting through the differential diagnosis of a suspected giant-cell reparative granuloma. The clinical presentation of a solitary lesion, as well as laboratory findings of normocalcemia and normophosphatemia, militate against a "brown" tumor of hyperparathyroidism. A giant-cell tumor has a more homogeneous morphology, with diffuse but uniform distribution of the giant cells; the stromal cells of a giant-cell tumor are more rounded and less spindle-shaped, and little or no inflammation is evident. A giant-cell reparative granuloma lacks the large blood-filled channels seen in aneurysmal bone cysts. As with all bone tumors, it is important to note that the typical locations and clinical presentations of the various lesions are different.

Treatment of a giant-cell reparative granuloma consists of curettage or excision of the involved bone; however, recurrences are common in curetted lesions of the small bones of the hands and feet.

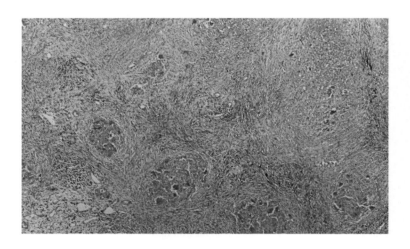

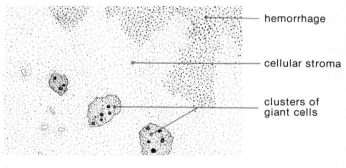

hemorrhage

cellular stroma

clusters of giant cells

FIGURE 15.24 Low-power photomicrograph of a giant-cell reparative granuloma. Spindle-shaped fibroblasts constitute the bulk of the lesion. Foci of giant cells can be seen, particularly in areas of extravasated blood (often accompanied by iron deposits) (H & E, x 4 obj.).

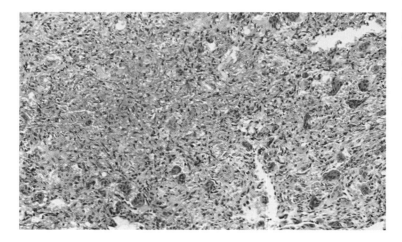

FIGURE 15.25 High-power photomicrograph of a giant-cell reparative granuloma. The cellularity varies, but hypervascularity is usually evident. Changes typical of reactive tissue include focal chronic inflammation. The histologic differential diagnosis includes giant-cell tumors and aneurysmal bone cysts (H & E, x 10 obj.).

HEMANGIOMA OF BONE

Intra-osseous hemangiomas are vascular hamartomas which are usually asymptomatic and solitary. These lesions typically affect the vertebral bodies or the skull, and clinical presentation, when seen, is usually in patients in the middle years of life. There is no familial tendency of these lesions.

Hemangiomas are among the most frequently occurring spinal tumors, although they are usually identified only incidentally on a radiographic survey or after a careful autopsy study. Clinically, they constitute only about 2 to 3 percent of spinal tumors. The most common presentation is that of neurologic symptoms caused by extension of the angiomatous tissue into the epidural space. These lesions occur most commonly in the lower thoracic vertebrae, somewhat less frequently in the lumbar spine, and infrequently in the cervical spine and the sacrum. Erosion of the horizontal trabeculae of the vertebral bodies leads to the typical radiographic appearance of accentuated, somewhat thickened vertical trabeculae (Fig. 15.26). In children, the affected bone may have a stippled or mottled appearance on radiographic examination. Cortical expansion may be seen in flat bones such as ribs and skull (Fig. 15.27).

Gross examination of a sectioned hemangioma reveals a cystic, dark-red cavity (Fig. 15.28). The microscopic structure of this cavity consists of thin-

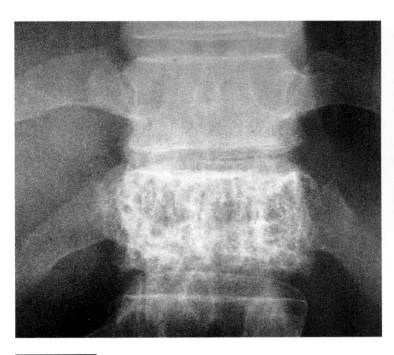

FIGURE 15.26 Radiograph of a hemangioma of a vertebral body demonstrates the characteristic, accentuated coarse trabecular pattern of the lesion.

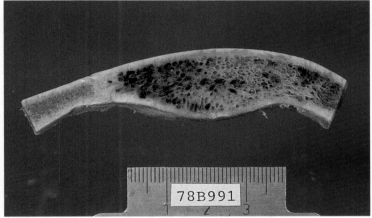

FIGURE 15.27 Gross photograph of a section through a segment of rib which contains an expanding hemangioma. (Courtesy of Dr. Miguel Calvo)

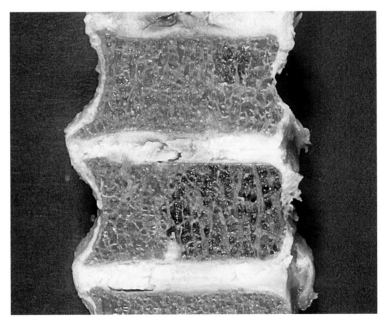

FIGURE 15.28 Gross photograph of hemangiomas of the vertebral bodies shows a well-demarcated, coarsely trabeculated red lesion, clearly from normal cancellous bone.

walled cavernous blood vessels or proliferating capillaries lined with thin, flattened epithelium (Fig. 15.29).

Hemangiomas usually follow an indolent course, but they may be complicated by a fracture or by extraosseous extension.

HEMANGIOMATOSIS/LYMPHANGIOMATOSIS (CYSTIC ANGIOMATOSIS OF BONE, LYMPHANGIECTASIS OF BONE)

Systemic hemangiomatosis/lymphangiomatosis is a hamartomatous malformation involving the skeleton and often the visceral organs. The condition is usually diagnosed incidentally on radiologic examination, or as the result of complications such as pathologic fractures, soft-tissue masses (rarely), or chylous or hemorrhagic effusions. The patients are usually in the first three decades of life at the time of diagnosis. Hemangiomas or lymphangiomas in the skeleton are often seen in association with visceral hemangiomas and lymphangiomas, most commonly involving the spleen, pleura, and skin.

There is no known familial tendency.

The radiographic features of skeletal hemangiomatosis/lymphangiomatosis are similar to those of solitary hemangiomas. The lesions usually have a fine peripheral rim of increased density (Fig. 15.30). Rare cases of diffuse blastic skeletal lesions may mimic metastatic cancer; however, in these cases closer scrutiny reveals central lytic and hemorrhagic areas surrounded by dense sclerotic bone (Figs. 15.31 to 15.33).

Laboratory findings in patients with this condition are usually unremarkable, although increases in alkaline phosphatase activity have been noted.

On gross examination the lesions are cystic, with a reddish fluid indicative of blood or a clear yellow fluid indicating a lymphatic origin. Combinations of hemangiomas and lymphangiomas may be observed. On microscopic examination, the lesions consist of thinwalled vascular spaces lined with flattened endothelial cells and separated by collagen septa (Fig. 15.34).

The prognosis for patients with this disorder is variable, depending on the degree and sites of involvement. The condition is usually self limiting.

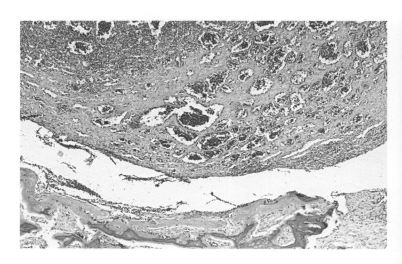

FIGURE 15.29 Photomicrograph of a hemangioma of bone reveals characteristic increased vascular channels of various sizes. Note in the lower part of the photograph reactive bone formation at the rim of the lesion (H & E, x 4 obj.).

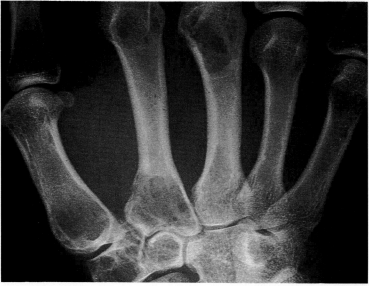

FIGURE 15.30 Radiograph of a hand with multiple hemangiomas. Lucent zones well demarcated from surrounding bone are evident.

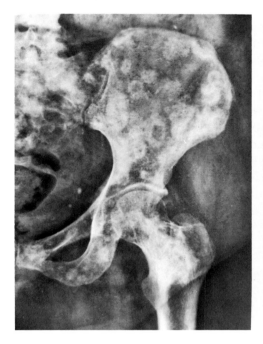 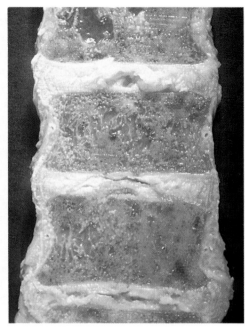 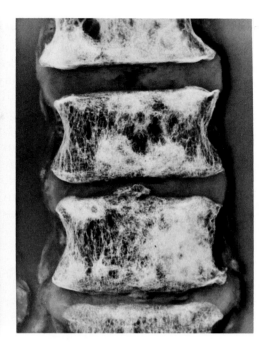

FIGURE 15.31 Hemangiomas are characteristically lucent lesions, although the surrounding bone reaction may be sufficiently sclerotic to give the appearance of density. Sometimes this appearance is the dominant pattern, as seen in this clinical radiograph, with multiple densities throughout the skeleton mimicking a malignant bone-forming metastatic tumor.

FIGURE 15.32 Cross-section of the spine removed at autopsy from the patient with hemangiomatosis shown in Figure 15.31. Note the disruption of the normal cancellous architecture of the vertebral bone. Multiple areas of dense bone, often with dark reddish centers, can be seen adjoining areas of osteopenia, in which the underlying yellow fat is readily evident.

FIGURE 15.33 Radiograph of the specimen shown in Figure 15.32. Within the areas of density there are relatively lucent foci which represent the hemangioma.

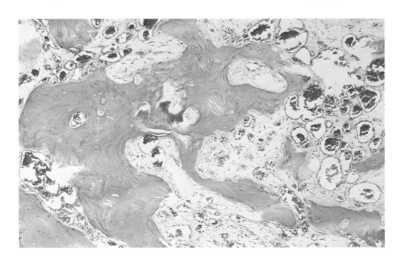

FIGURE 15.34 Photomicrograph of one of the dense lesions illustrated in Figures 15.32 and 15.33. Vascular channels of various sizes and shapes can be seen. The thickened bone appears immature, with increased cellularity and irregular architecture (H & E, x 4 obj.).

SYNOVIAL HEMANGIOMA

A synovial hemangioma is usually a solitary, benign lesion, most commonly seen in the knee joints of children and adolescents. The patient may be asymptomatic, or may have a swollen knee and may experience mild pain or limitation of movement. Patients sometimes report a history of recurrent episodes of joint swelling and pain of several years' duration.

A soft-tissue mass may be evident on radiographic examination, although arthrography may be necessary to show it clearly (Fig. 15.35). In severe cases, a periosteal reaction or lucent zones in the adjacent bones may also be present.

Gross examination of the knee joint in synovial hemangioma reveals a soft, brown, doughy mass with overlying villous synovium which is frequently stained mahogany brown by hemosiderin (Fig. 15.36). When the mass is viewed microscopically, arborizing vascular channels of different sizes are apparent (Fig. 15.37). The overlying synovium is hyperplastic, and in chronic cases with repeated hemarthrosis, copious iron deposition can be observed.

Complete surgical excision (that is, total synovectomy) may be difficult to perform, and this fact probably accounts for the occasionally reported cases of local recurrence.

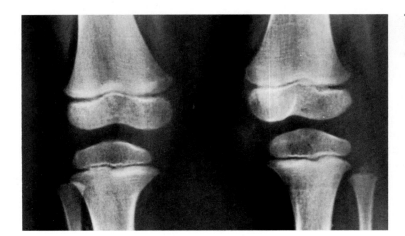

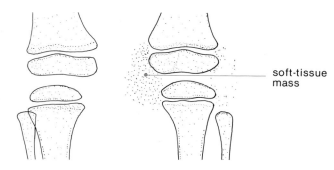

FIGURE 15.35 Radiograph of the knee in a 3-year-old girl with a history of repeated joint effusions. Note the soft-tissue swelling on the medial side of the joint.

soft-tissue mass

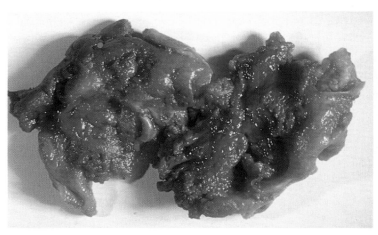

FIGURE 15.36 Gross specimen removed from the knee of a patient with a history of recurrent hemorrhages into the joint. Marked hemosiderin staining of the tissues has occurred, but the synovium does not show either the villous appearance seen in association with hemophilia or the papillary appearance usually seen in patients with pigmented villonodular synovitis.

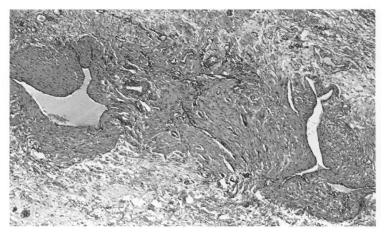

FIGURE 15.37 Photomicrograph of part of the synovial tissue shown in Figure 15.36 demonstrates the vascular malformation in this patient's synovium. At the synovial surface, copius hemosiderin deposits and hyperplastic reactive tissue were evident (H & E, x 10 obj.).

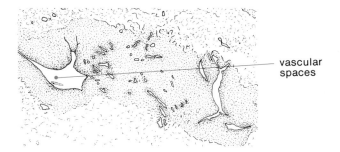

vascular spaces

NONOSSIFYING FIBROMA
(FIBROUS CORTICAL DEFECT;
BENIGN FIBROUS HISTIOCYTOMA)

A nonossifying fibroma is a benign, eccentric, solitary (or, rarely, multiple), well-circumscribed lesion in the metaphyses of the long bones of children. Most commonly the femur or tibia is involved. These lesions usually regress spontaneously. Most cases are detected as incidental findings on radiographic examination, although occasionally a pathologic fracture through a large lesion causes the patient to seek medical attention (Fig. 15.38).

Gross inspection reveals the lesions to be formed of soft, somewhat friable yellow or brown tissue (Figs. 15.39 through 15.41). The microscopic findings include a cellular tissue of unremarkable spindle cells arranged in an interlacing, whorled pattern and interspersed

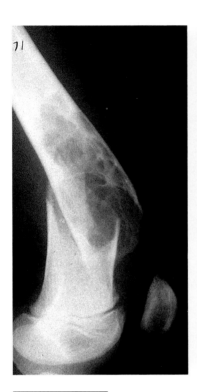 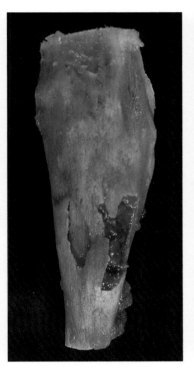 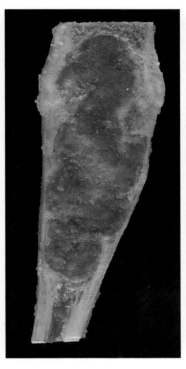 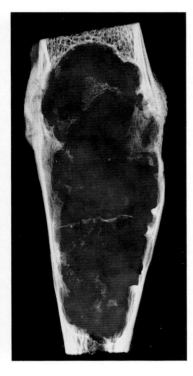

FIGURE 15.38 Radiograph showing a pathologic fracture through a large trabeculated lytic lesion of the lower femoral diaphysis, which proved on biopsy to be a nonossifying fibroma.

FIGURE 15.39 Gross photograph of a resected segment of fibula which contains a nonossifying fibroma. Note the irregular thinning of the cortical bone, which focally reveals underlying mahogany brown tumor tissue.

FIGURE 15.40 Section through the specimen demonstrated in Figure 15.39 shows the scalloped margin of the lesion and the cortical thinning. The reddish-brown color is typical. The focal areas of gray probably represent fibrous tissue, and the areas of yellow discoloration, lipid accumulation.

FIGURE 15.41 Specimen radiograph of the lesion illustrated in Figure 15.40. The radiograph shows cortical erosion, with a thin layer of periosteal bone covering the expanded tumor.

with multinucleated giant cells and foamy, pale histiocytes (Figs. 15.42 through 15.44). The microscopic features may cause diagnostic confusion of a nonossifying fibroma with other giant-cell containing lesions. However, the clinical and radiographic presentation of nonossifying fibroma is so typical that it should rarely be confused with anything else.

Radiologic surveys have shown a 35 percent incidence of fibrous cortical defects in normal children. The lesions range in size from a few millimeters to several centimeters and are characterized on radiographs by their cortical, eccentric position, as well as by their well-demarcated central lucent zones surrounded by scalloped sclerotic margins (Figs. 15.45 to 15.48). Often a nonossifying fibroma is elongated in the longitudinal axis of the bone. Serial radiographs have demonstrated the migration of the defect away from the epiphyseal plate.

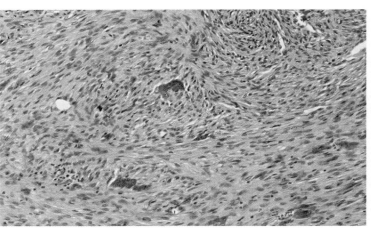

FIGURE 15.43 Low-power photomicrograph of a nonossifying fibroma shows the spindle-cell stroma with occasional giant cells and mitoses. Note that the stromal cells are crowded, with little collagen formation (H & E, x 10 obj.).

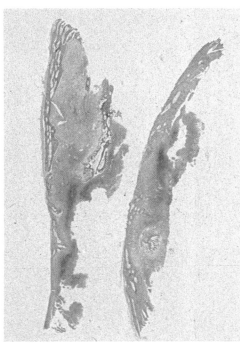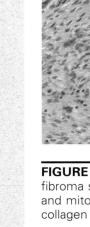

FIGURE 15.42 Low-power photomicrograph of a histologic section demonstrates the variegated appearance of a nonossifying fibroma. In some areas, the lesion is more cellular; in others, it has a pink collagenous stroma (H & E, x 1 obj.).

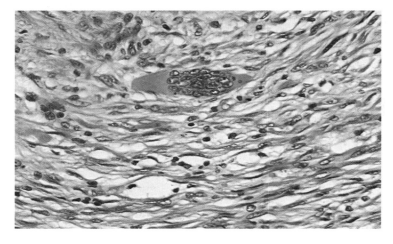

FIGURE 15.44 High-power photomicrograph of the stromal cells shows foamy cytoplasm in some of the cells and one multinucleated giant cell (H & E, x 10 obj.).

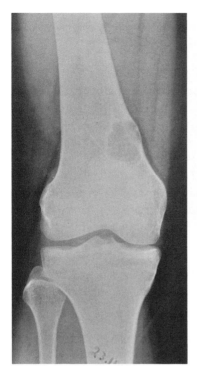

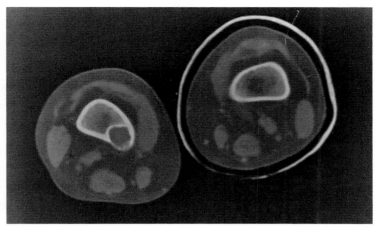

FIGURE 15.46 Computerized axial tomogram through the lesion demonstrated in Figure 15.45 emphasizes the sclerotic margin.

FIGURE 15.45 Radiograph showing a typical nonossifying fibroma eccentrically located in the lower femoral metaphysis.

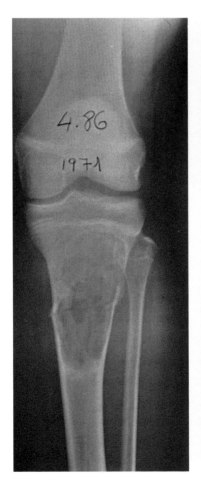

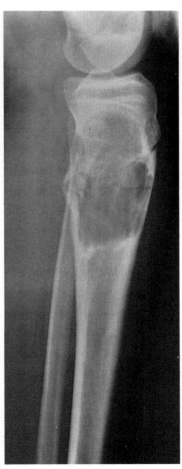

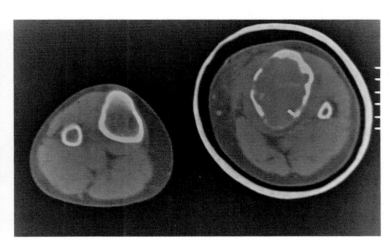

FIGURE 15.48 Computerized axial tomogram of the lesion shown in Figure 15.47.

FIGURE 15.47 Radiograph of the leg shows a large lytic defect due to a nonossitying fibroma involving the upper end of the tibia. A pathological fracture through the lesion has occurred.

Very rarely, lesions that are histologically indistinguishable from nonossifying fibroma may be seen in adults. Radiographically, the lesions may either be lucent or more sclerotic, and their locations are likely to be different from those seen in children (Figs. 15.49 to 15.51). Patients may experience mild pain or they may be asymptomatic. On histologic examination, the spindle-cell stroma has a whorled or "storiform" pattern (Fig. 15.52). The predominant underlying cell, a fibroblast, is mixed with polygonal histiocytic cells which have a more vacuolated cytoplasm. Iron deposits, multinucleated giant cells, sparse chronic inflammatory cells, or lipid-laden cells may be evident.

In adults, such a lesion is often reported as a benign fibrous histiocytoma or a fibroxanthoma.

PERIOSTEAL "DESMOID"

Periosteal desmoid is a common periosteal fibrous lesion that most commonly affects boys in the first two decades of life. It arises on the posteromedial aspect of the lower metaphysis of the femur. Radiographic examination reveals erosion of the cortex, with a sclerotic base (Fig. 15.53). Periosteal desmoids are composed microscopically of dense collagenized tissue with uni-

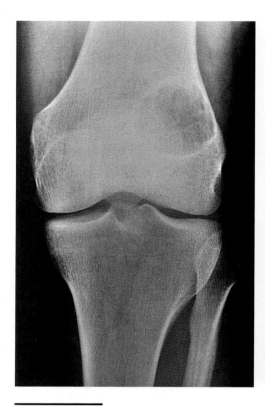

FIGURE 15.49 Radiograph of the right knee of a 30-year-old female complaining of "dull pain" around the knee joint. There is an eccentric, well-defined radiolucency in the metaphysis abutting the peripheral region, which proved on biopsy to be a benign fibrous hystiocytoma.

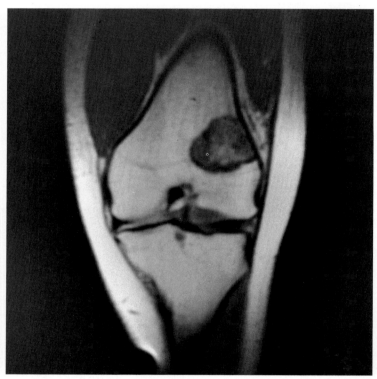

FIGURE 15.50 Magnetic resonance image of the lesion shown in Figure 15.49.

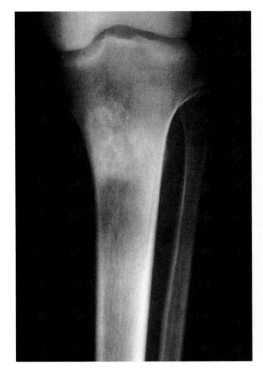

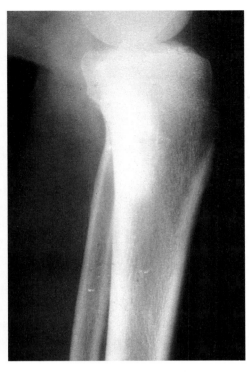

FIGURE 15.51 Anteroposterior *(left)* and lateral *(right)* radiographs of the tibia in a 64-year-old man who had had a bone scan for suspected metastatic disease. The lesion in the tibia was discovered incidentally, and the radiographs show a dense lesion in the metaphysis which is well defined and shows no periosteal reaction.

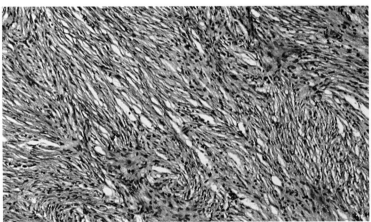

FIGURE 15.52 Photomicrograph of tissue removed from the patient shown in Figure 15.51. The lesion was composed of a benign but cellular spindle-cell stroma, with scattered chronic inflammatory cells and giant cells and a matted storiform pattern. This histologic appearance is similar to that seen in the typical nonossifying fibroma in children; in an adult, this lesion is sometimes referred to as a fibroxanthoma or a benign fibrous histiocytoma (H & E, x 10 obj.).

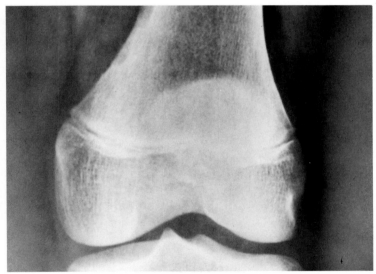

FIGURE 15.53 A scalloped periosteal defect with a sclerotic base in the medial metaphysis of the femur is the characteristic radiographic appearance of a periosteal desmoid tumor.

form, unremarkable fibroblasts and reactive bone formation (Fig. 15.54).

The lesion probably occurs as the result of previous trauma. It is characteristic in location and does not warrant a biopsy.

LIPOMA OF BONE

Benign fatty tumors of bone are among the rarest skeletal tumors. They have been described in patients of all ages, especially in the long bones. They may present as either subperiosteal or intramedullary lesions. In either case they are lytic, although occasionally calcification within necrotic fat may give rise to confusion with a bone infarct (Fig. 15.55). The intramedullary lesions have well-defined borders and occasionally a bubbly appearance. The periosteal lesions are also lytic and usually erode the cortex; sometimes spicules of periosteal new bone are associated with the lesion. Magnetic resonance imaging is particularly useful for localization of such lesions, because fat gives a characteristic signal (Fig. 15.56).

On gross examination, the tumor is characteristically a lobulated soft yellow mass. Microscopic examination reveals mature fat, usually containing thin, residual cancellous bone trabeculae (Figs. 15.57 and 15.58).

HOFFA'S DISEASE (SYNOVIAL LIPOMATOSIS)

Hoffa's disease is a condition clinically characterized by enlargement of the infrapatellar fat pad on either side of the patellar tendon, with resulting pain or deep aching in the anterior compartment of the knee. The pain is aggravated by physical activity or extension of the knee. Swelling or recurrent effusion is a consequence of synovial injury. The treatment of Hoffa's disease is surgical reduction in the volume of extrasynovial fat.

When the lesion is examined macroscopically (Fig. 15.59), the synovium has a marked papillary appearance; microscopically, there is mild hyperplasia of the synovial lining cells overlying abundant unremarkable fat (Fig. 15.60).

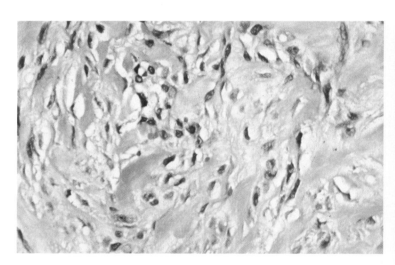

FIGURE 15.54 Photomicrograph of the dense fibrous tissue removed from the lesion illustrated in Figure 15.53. Abundant collagen production by poorly organized but unremarkable fibroblasts has occurred (H & E, x 25 obj.).

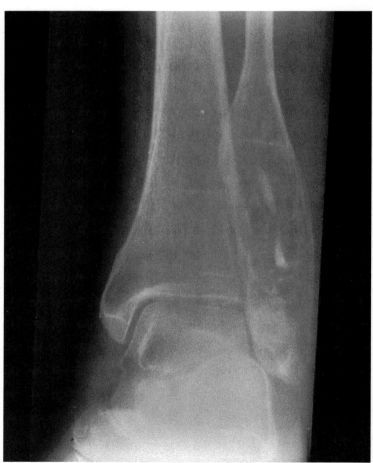

FIGURE 15.55 Radiograph of an ankle shows fusiform swelling of the lower end of the fibula due to a lytic trabeculated intraosseous mass. In the center of the lesion there is focal dense calcification. (Courtesy of Dr. Leonard Kahn)

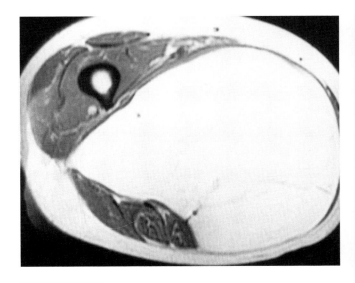

FIGURE 15.56 Lipoma. An MRI showing section through the thigh. There is a large mass in the posterior compartment of the thigh, producing compression of the adjacent muscles. (From *MRI: Musculoskeletal System* by Dr. Javier Beltran, Gower Medical Publishing, 1990).

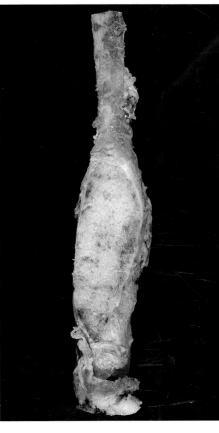

FIGURE 15.57 Photograph of a section through the dissected distal fibula shown in Figure 15.55. The lesion is composed of an admixture of fat and fine cancellous bone. (Courtesy of Dr. Leonard Kahn)

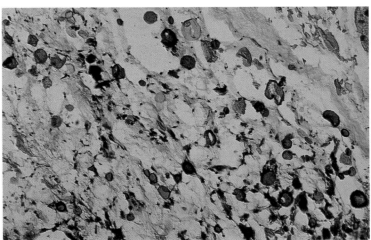

FIGURE 15.58 Photomicrograph of the lesional tissue through the specimen shown in Figure 15.57, demonstrating punctate calcification within an area of fat necrosis (H & E, x 25 obj.).

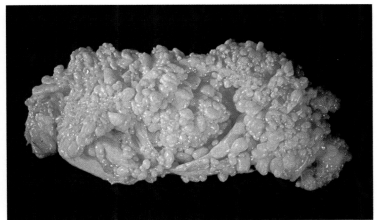

FIGURE 15.59 Gross photograph of the synovium resected from a patient with Hoffa's disease. Note the fatty appearance of the tissue and the papillomatous folds arising on the surface.

FIGURE 15.60 Photomicrograph of a section through the synovium shown in Figure 15.59, showing fatty infiltration of the sub-synovial tissue (H & E, x 10 obj.).

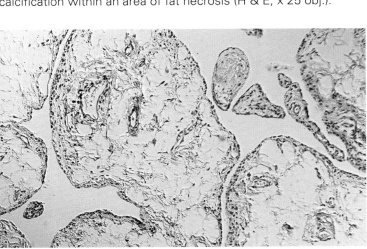

Neoplasms: benign and malignant; bony and cartilaginous

eoplastic lesions in bone usually represent metastases (often carcinomatous) from another site. It is important to realize that a solitary bone metastasis may be the initial clinical presentation for some patients with occult cancer.

Primary neoplasms of bone are rare, with the exception of myelomas, and they range from benign to highly malignant. They will be described in essential detail in this and the following chapter.

OSTEOBLASTOMA

Osteoblastoma is a solitary, benign, osteoid- and bone-forming neoplasm which contains many well-differenti-ated osteoblasts and osteoclasts and usually has a vascular stroma. Osteoblastomas are usually painful lesions which predominantly affect young adults; swelling and tenderness may prompt the patient to seek medical attention. In most cases, the long bones or vertebrae are the sites of involvement. In long bones, the lesion may arise in either the metaphysis or the diaphysis. Approximately 30 percent of osteoblastomas originate in the spine. The lesions affect the vertebral arch, involving the spinous and transverse processes as well as the laminae and pedicles. In only a few cases does the lesion appear to originate within the vertebral bodies. The clinical presentation may include myelopathic and/or radicular symptoms, and thus may suggest

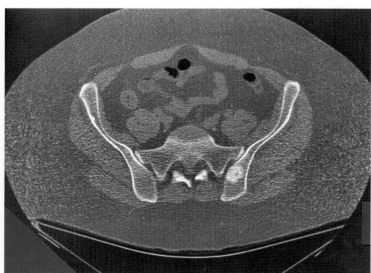

FIGURE 16.2 Computerized axial tomogram shows a circumscribed sclerotic lesion in the ilium adjacent to the sacroiliac joint, which proved to be an osteoblastoma.

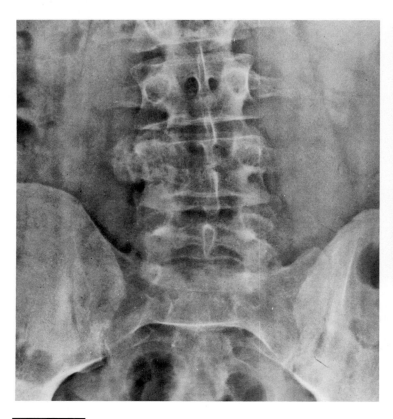

FIGURE 16.1 A 20-year-old man complained of low back pain and was admitted to the hospital with an expanding, destructive lesion affecting the pedicle and transverse process on the right side of L4. On radiographic examination, the margin of the lesion is well defined and there is a patchy increase in density. An excisional biopsy of the lesion proved it to be a benign osteoblastoma.

either an intraspinal tumor or a herniated disc. Progressive scoliosis may also appear. If the cervical spine is affected reversal of the lordotic curve may occur and torticollis may be prominent. Benign osteoblastomas arise with about equal frequency in the cervical and lumbar regions, with the thoracic region being less frequently involved (Fig. 16.1). Occasionally they may involve the sacrum.

On radiographic examination, the lesion character-istically appears as a lucent defect with various degrees of central density; it is usually well circumscribed, without extensive surrounding bone sclerosis and with no periosteal reaction. CT scanning may be particular-ly helpful in delineating these lesions (Fig. 16.2) and isotope scanning will show increased uptake (Fig. 16.3).

At surgery, an osteoblastoma is found to be com-posed of hemorrhagic, granular, friable, and calcified tissue (Fig. 16.4). On microscopic examination, the

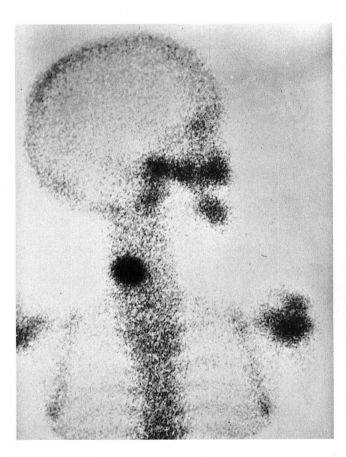

FIGURE 16.3 Radioisotope scan of an osteoblastoma in the transverse process and pedicle of C5. The intense uptake is typical of that seen in association with both osteoblastomas and osteoid osteomas. In this case, the size of the lesion indicates that this is an osteoblastoma.

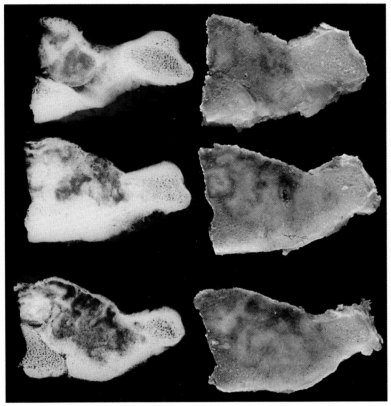

FIGURE 16.4 A series of slices through an osteoblastoma are matched with fine-grain radiographs, to demonstrate the mixed lytic and sclerotic areas seen in osteoblastoma. (Courtesy of Dr. Alberto G. Ayala)

lesion consists of a vascular spindle-cell stroma with abundant irregular spicules of mineralized bone and osteoid (Figs. 16.5 and 16.6). Osteoblasts and multinucleated osteoclasts are readily evident on the bone surfaces, but no cartilage can be seen in the lesion. Treatment consists of curettage or en bloc excision.

Microscopically, it is sometimes difficult to differentiate an osteoblastoma from an osteoid osteoma. However, the tissue pattern appears less regular in an osteoblastoma than in an osteoid osteoma. Furthermore, osteoid osteomas rarely exceed 1 cm in diameter, whereas osteoblastomas may be several centimeters in diameter and have a tendency to enlarge. Nevertheless, the lesions are similar enough that osteoblastomas are occasionally referred to in the literature as giant osteoid osteomas.

On rare occasions, osteoblastomas have been noted to act aggressively, with significant bone destruction and extension into adjacent soft tissues. Retrospective analyses of these lesions have revealed more cellular atypia with large, plump osteoblasts (Fig. 16.7). These lesions do not metastasize, and therefore should be considered aggressive variants of osteoblastoma; however, on occasion it may be difficult to differentiate an aggressive osteoblastoma from osteosarcoma. Changes characteristic of an aneurysmal bone cyst may be present within these lesions, adding to the problem of differential diagnosis.

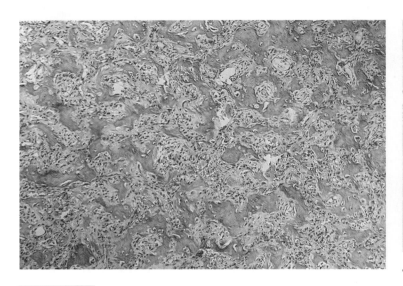

FIGURE 16.5 Photomicrograph of an osteoblastoma shows the usual pattern of disorganized trabeculae of immature bone set in a cellular vascular stroma (H & E, x 4 obj.).

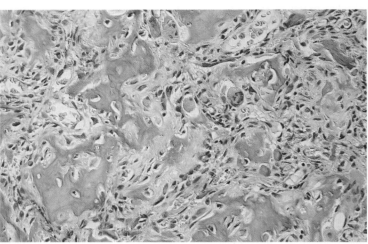

FIGURE 16.6 Photomicrograph of an osteoblastoma at a higher magnification shows marked osteoblastic and osteoclastic activity at the bone surfaces (H & E, x 25 obj.).

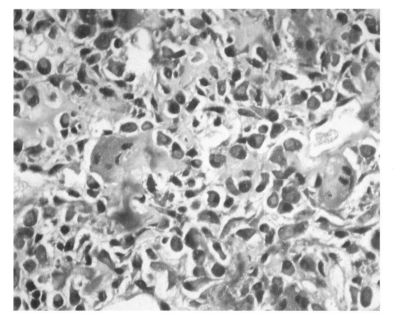

FIGURE 16.7 Photomicrograph of an atypical osteoblastoma with crowded, large epithelioid stromal cells; small irregular foci of woven bone are present. It is important for the pathologist to recognize that an osteoblastoma may be cellular, and to distinguish this pattern from osteosarcoma, a histologic differentiation that can at times be very difficult (H & E, x 40 obj.).

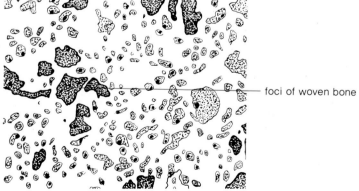

foci of woven bone

OSTEOSARCOMA (OSTEOGENIC SARCOMA)

After myeloma, osteosarcoma is the most common primary neoplasm of bone, accounting for approximately 20 percent of all primary malignant bone tumors. Osteosarcoma is defined as a malignant bone-producing neoplasm in which the bone matrix is formed by the malignant cells (Fig. 16.8). However, the pluripotential nature of the neoplasm is evident in the abundant fibrosarcomatous or chondrosarcomatous tissue matrix present in many of these lesions. Roughly 50 percent of all osteosarcomas are osteoblastic; the rest are chondroblastic or fibroblastic. Recently, a small-cell variant

has also been described (Fig. 16.9). Heterogeneity may lead to confusion of this lesion with a number of entities, including fracture callus (especially following a stress fracture without clinical history of injury), aneurysmal bone cyst, chondrosarcoma, and even giant-cell tumor. This diagnostic dilemma is aggravated if a pathologic fracture through the lesion is also present.

Most osteosarcomas are high-grade lesions, although less common low-grade osteosarcoma may also be encountered, usually as a surface lesion. The discussion that follows will consider high-grade central lesions (the most common), low-grade central lesions, low-grade surface lesions (so-called parosteal or juxtacorti-

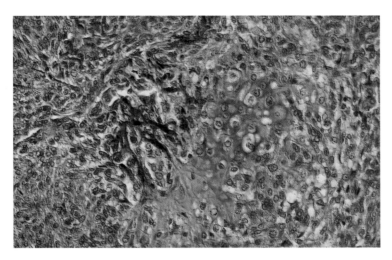

FIGURE 16.8 Photomicrograph of a cellular osteosarcoma showing foci of both bone and cartilage matrix differentiation (H & E, x 25 obj.).

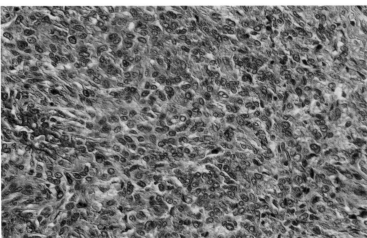

FIGURE 16.9 Photomicrograph of an intraosseous tumor principally characterized by packed small, round spindled cells. As can be appreciated in this photograph, fine spicules of bone matrix are being formed by the tumor cells (H & E, x 25 obj.).

cal osteosarcoma), high-grade surface lesions, periosteal osteosarcoma, intracortical osteosarcoma, soft-tissue osteosarcoma and, finally, lesions that complicate Paget's disease or those seen after radiation therapy.

In very rare cases, an osteosarcoma may present with more than one focus of tumor. In such a case it may be difficult to determine whether one is dealing with a multifocal origin or whether the other lesions are metastatic. However there are some points that characteristically suggest a multifocal origin and these include symmetrical and simultaneous involvement with distal metaphyseal lesions in long bones, and sparing of the visceral organs, particularly the lungs (Figs. 16.10 to 16.15).

CENTRAL OSTEOSARCOMA, HIGH GRADE

Central high-grade osteosarcoma, the most common variant, usually affects children (before the closure of the growth plates) and occurs more often in boys than in girls. More than 90 percent of the lesions occur at the ends of long bones, especially around the knee joint. Localized swelling, often accompanied by pain (and sometimes by a fracture), develops in children who are otherwise in good health. Alkaline phosphatase levels in these patients are two to three times that found in normal individuals.

Radiographic examination may reveal a sclerotic (in about 35 percent) (Fig. 16.16), lytic (in about 25 percent) (Fig. 16.17), or mixed destructive lesion in the

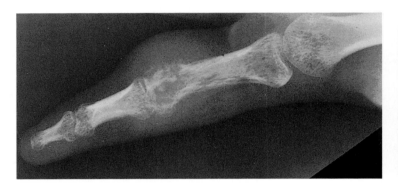

FIGURE 16.10 A radiograph shows a destructive lesion of the distal end of the proximal phalanx, with soft tissue invasion which on biopsy proved to be an osteosarcoma.

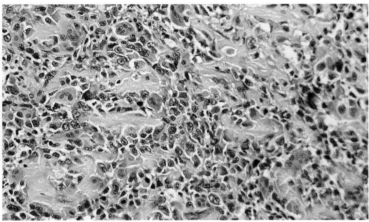

FIGURE 16.11 Photomicrograph of the lesional tissues obtained from the tumor demonstrated in Figure 16.10. There are foci of immature bone formation and the cellular components show pleomorphic nuclei (H & E, x 25 obj.).

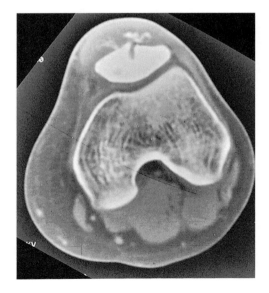

FIGURE 16.12 Computerized axial tomogram through the right knee of the patient shown in Figure 16.10. The patella is extremely dense and an osseous mass is seen in the prepatellar region. The linear defects in the anterior part of the patella represent the area of the biopsy.

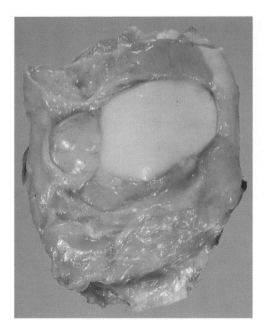

FIGURE 16.13 Gross photograph of the articular surface of the resected patella with surrounding soft tissue. Adjacent to the patella is a pink/gray nodule which represents part of the soft-tissue extension of the patellar tumor.

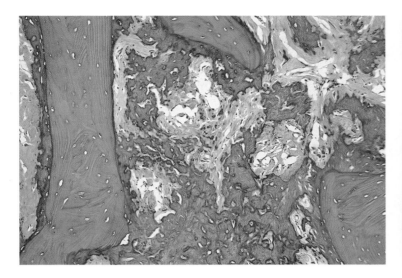

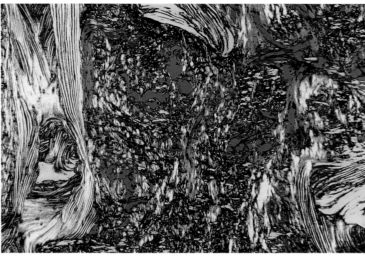

FIGURE 16.14 Photomicrograph of the patellar lesion shown in Figure 16.13 showing sclerosing osteosarcoma of poor cellularity, which is invading the marrow space and plastered onto the surface of residual trabecular bone within the medular cavity (H & E, x 10 obj.).

FIGURE 16.15 Photomicrograph of the same field shown in Figure 16.14, photographed in polarized light, demonstrates the "irregular" woven appearance of the collagen matrix produced by the tumor bone. The lamellar pattern of the residual bone is clearly seen.

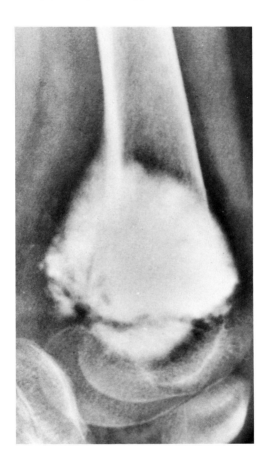

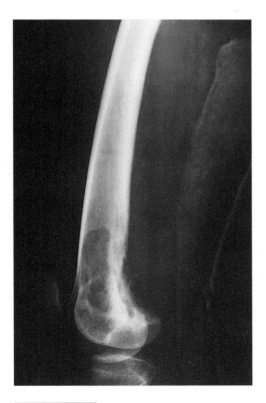

FIGURE 16.16 A 10-year-old boy presented with complaints of pain around the knee joint. On physical examination, some fullness was felt in the lower femur, which was noted to be warmer than the surrounding tissue. Radiograph shows a radiodense tumor involving the metaphyseal end of the femur, with extension of the tumor both anteriorly and posteriorly into the soft tissue. It is difficult to determine whether or not the epiphyseal end of the bone is involved because of the two-dimensional radiologic image of the three-dimensional bone. (This radiograph should be compared with Figure 16.23, a gross photograph of the specimen resected from this patient.)

FIGURE 16.17 Lateral radiograph shows a lytic osteosarcoma of the lower femur. Posterior extension of the tumor into the soft tissue is evident.

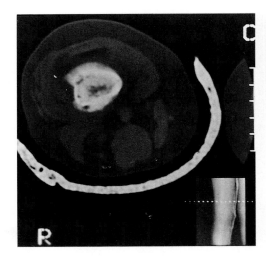

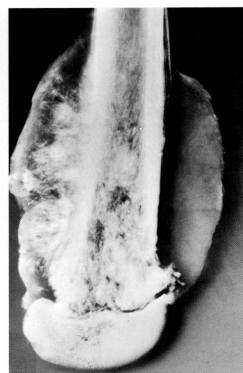

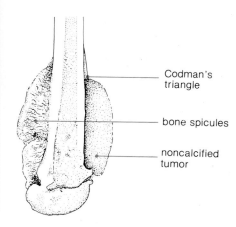

FIGURE 16.18 Computerized axial tomogram demonstrates bone matrix formation in an intramedullary osteosarcoma.

FIGURE 16.19 Specimen radiograph of an osteosarcoma demonstrates that in the anterior part of the tumor the lesion is purely lytic, without bone formation. Posteriorly, bone formation has occurred, and the newly formed bone spicules are oriented at right angles to the surface of the bone, producing a sunburst pattern. A well-defined Codman's triangle is apparent at the upper end of the lesion.

Codman's triangle

bone spicules

noncalcified tumor

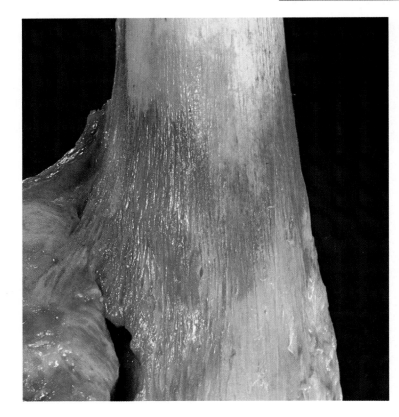

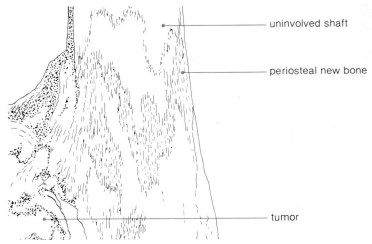

FIGURE 16.20 Gross photograph of part of an osteosarcoma of the lower end of the femur. At the upper end of the photograph a portion of the uninvolved femoral shaft can be seen, and at the lower end of the photograph the tumor is seen to break through the cortex of the bone. Between the tumor and the normal cortex is a hyperemic zone which has an irregular margin with the cortical bone. This hyperemic zone is composed of reactive bone formed by the periosteum, and would appear on a radiograph as Codman's triangle.

uninvolved shaft

periosteal new bone

tumor

metaphysis. The tumor has often invaded the cortex and extended into the soft tissues at the time of presentation, and in many cases there is abundant periosteal new bone formation (which sometimes shows a "sunburst" pattern) (Fig. 16.18). At the edge of the tumor, elevation of the periosteum may result in a triangle of bone visible on radiologic films; this is referred to as Codman's triangle. The sides of the triangle are formed by the periosteum, the underlying cortex, and the narrow margin of the tumor mass. However, the triangle itself is made up of benign reactive bone, and this tissue may cause diagnostic problems if biopsy specimens are obtained only from this area (Figs. 16.19 to 16.22).

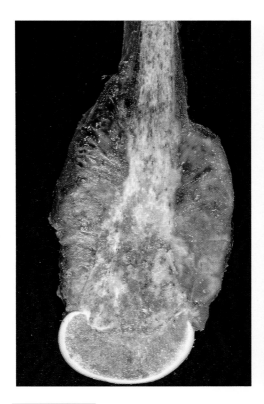

FIGURE 16.21 Gross photograph of the lesion shown in Figure 16.19 shows a bulky and more vascular osteosarcoma. Again, extensive soft-tissue extension and involvement of the epiphysis may be observed.

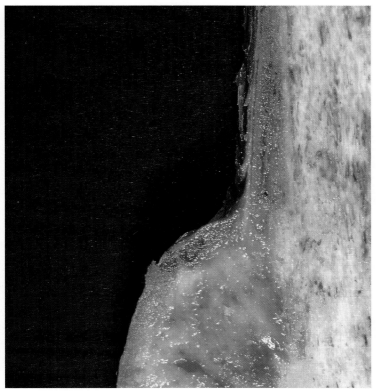

FIGURE 16.22 A slice taken through the specimen shown in Figure 16.20 demonstrates the reactive periosteal bone above and the tumor below. If this reactive periosteal bone is the site of biopsy, it will fail to produce any histological evidence of malignant tumor.

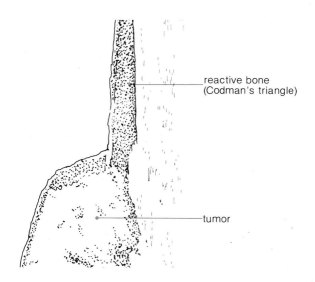

reactive bone
(Codman's triangle)

tumor

The gross appearance of osteosarcoma varies according to the type of matrix (bony, fibrous, or cartilaginous) produced by the lesion (Figs. 16.23 and 16.24). Penetration of the cortex is common and of the epiphysis less common, but the joint space is rarely involved.

Most osteosarcomas have in common a pleomorphic and anaplastic cell population that produces bone matrix and, as previously stated, may form cartilage matrix or may be mainly fibroblastic (Fig. 16.25). However, the histologic diagnosis rests on the finding of malignant bone matrix formation (Figs. 16.26 and 16.27).

Osteosarcomas metastasize, primarily hematogenously and most commonly to the lungs. Favorable prognostic factors include small and distal lesions.

Telangiectatic osteosarcoma is a variant of central high-grade osteosarcoma which is characterized radiographically by a large lytic defect, grossly by its blood-filled cavity (Fig. 16.28), and microscopically by dilated vascular channels lined with multinucleated giant cells and an anaplastic sarcomatous stroma with evident bone formation (Figs. 16.29 and 16.30). Occasionally this lesion is difficult to distinguish from an aneurysmal bone cyst.

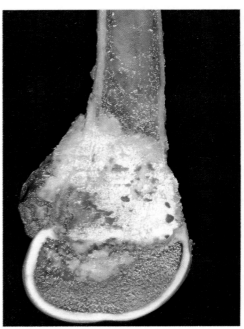

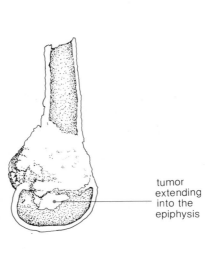

tumor extending into the epiphysis

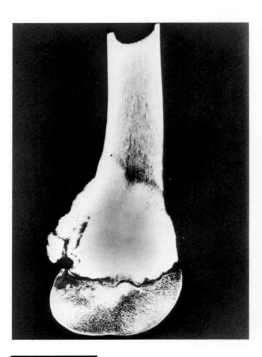

FIGURE 16.23 Gross photograph shows a dense osteoblastic osteosarcoma in the lower end of the femur. It has extended through the cortex into the soft tissue, and is also present in the epiphysis.

Although epiphyseal extension is rarely seen on clinical radiographs, it is commonly present when the resected specimen is examined grossly (compare with Figure 16.16).

FIGURE 16.24 Specimen radiograph of the lesion shown in Figure 16.23 reveals extensive bone formation by the tumor (an osteoblastic osteosarcoma).

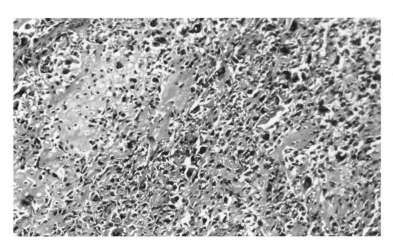

FIGURE 16.25 Low-power photomicrograph of tissue from an osteosarcoma shows a cellular pleomorphic tumor which is producing a collagenous matrix; focally, this matrix has the appearance of primitive bone (H & E, x 10 obj.). (An osteosarcoma may exhibit primitive bone or cartilage matrix formation, together with areas of malignant spindle-cell tumor and giant-cell tumor.)

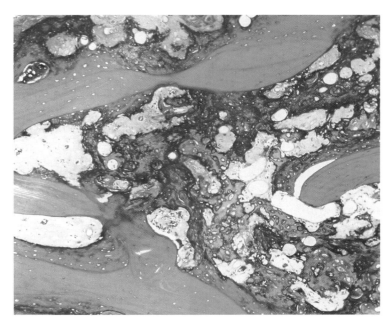

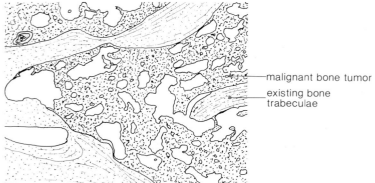

FIGURE 16.26 A characteristic feature of osteosarcoma is the observation of a malignant tumor which forms an abundant mineralized matrix and infiltrates through the marrow spaces between the existing trabeculae of the bone. The malignant tumor tissue becomes firmly attached to the surface of the existing bone, as seen in this photomicrograph (H & E, x 4 obj.).

malignant bone tumor

existing bone trabeculae

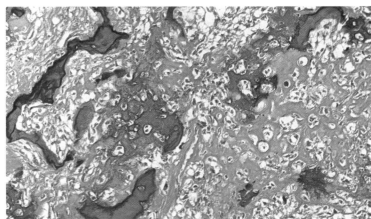

FIGURE 16.27 Photomicrograph of a sclerotic osteoblastic osteosarcoma shows extensive primitive bone matrix formation which is focally calcified. Sometimes, as seen here, it is difficult to distinguish cartilage matrix formation from bone matrix formation, since the primitive matrix being formed has features of both (H & E, x 25 obj.).

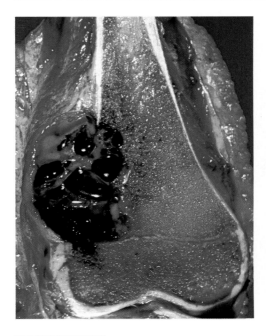

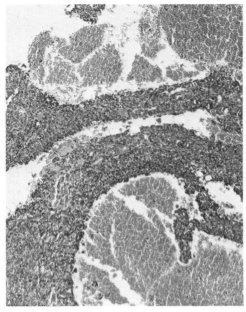

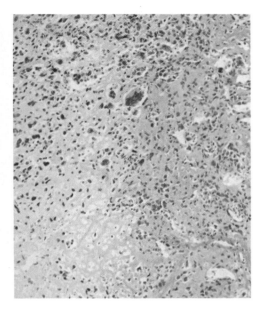

FIGURE 16.28 Gross photograph of a telangiectatic osteosarcoma at the lower end of the femur. Note the extremely hemorrhagic appearance of this tumor, which on radiographic examination appeared completely lytic.

FIGURE 16.29 Low-power photomicrograph of a telangiectatic osteosarcoma. Septa of cellular tissue are separated by large blood-filled spaces. At this magnification the lesion can easily be confused with an aneurysmal bone cyst (H & E, x 4 obj.).

FIGURE 16.30 Higher-power view of one portion of the tumor illustrated in Figure 16.29 demonstrates the anaplastic malignant quality of the tumor tissue. Such tissue may be difficult to find in a telangiectatic osteosarcoma and must be carefully looked for in this type of hemorrhagic tumor (H & E, x 10 obj.).

CENTRAL OSTEOSARCOMA, LOW GRADE

Rarely, an intramedullary bone-forming tumor of low-grade malignancy may be encountered. This tumor is usually seen in somewhat older individuals, although a wide age range may be affected. Males and females are affected with equal frequency.

Radiographically, these lesions are usually sclerotic and may mimic large bone islands (Fig. 16.31), osteoblastoma, or foci of solitary fibrous dysplasia (Figs. 16.32 and 16.33). On microscopic examination, they commonly have a fibrous stroma with rather bland-looking foci of bone formation similar to the appearance of a conventional surface or parosteal lesion. In other cases, dense sclerotic bone formation is observed. The key to the microscopic diagnosis of these lesions is identification of the invasive character of the lesion, which is typified by the presence of islands of residual lamellar bone within the lesion and evidence of malignant tumor bone plastered on and surrounding these islands of residual bone (Fig. 16.34). In such a case, the prognosis is much better than it is in the case of the classic high-grade intramedullary osteosarcoma.

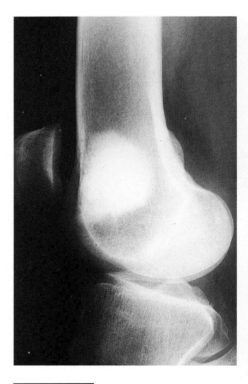

FIGURE 16.31 Lateral radiograph of the knee shows a large intramedullary sclerotic lesion which has a spiculated periphery suggestive of a large bone island. On biopsy, this lesion proved to be a low grade osteosarcoma. (Courtesy of Dr. Lauren Ackerman)

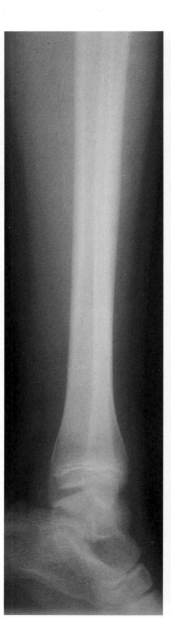
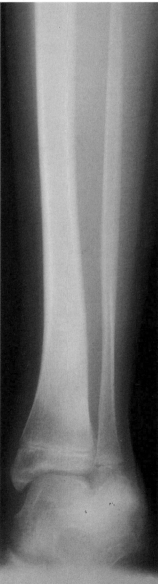
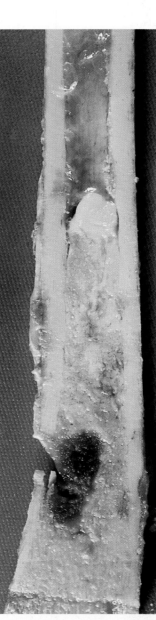
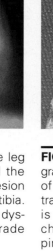

FIGURE 16.32 Anteroposterior and lateral views of the leg in a young patient complaining of vague pain around the ankle. The radiograph shows an ill-defined sclerotic lesion involving the distal diaphysis and metaphysis of the tibia. The initial impression was that this represented fibrous dysplasia. However, a biopsy proved it to be a low-grade osteosarcoma.

FIGURE 16.33 Gross photograph of a longitudinal section of the tibia in the case illustrated in Figure 16.32. There is an intramedullary mass characterized by firm pink/gray tissue, the upper margin of which is well delineated from the bone marrow.

PAROSTEAL OSTEOSARCOMA, LOW GRADE (JUXTACORTICAL OSTEOGENIC SARCOMA)

Parosteal osteosarcoma is usually a histologically low-grade, slow-growing osteosarcoma that occurs on the external surface of a bone, most commonly on the back of the lower end of the femur (the popliteal region) in patients over 20 years of age. In general, this lesion has a much better prognosis than the classic high-grade intramedullary osteosarcoma. However, it is important to recognize that some fully malignant osteosarcomas may present as juxtacortical lesions.

On radiographic films, the lesion appears as a large, well-circumscribed, generally dense juxtacortical mass, although lytic areas may be present (Figs. 16.35 and 16.36). The mass may be separated

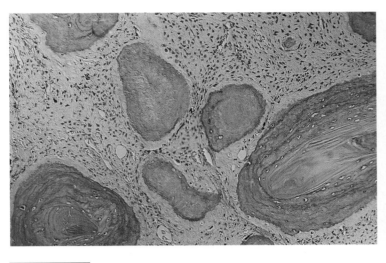

FIGURE 16.34 Photomicrograph of the lesion illustrated in Figure 16.33. The fibrous stroma, although somewhat cellular, has a relatively bland appearance. However, islands of bone are being formed by the tumor and, significantly, this bone is seen surrounding residual trabecular bone. This was a feature of the case and is not seen with fibrous dysplasia. The diagnosis in this case was a low-grade osteosarcoma (H & E, x 25 obj.).

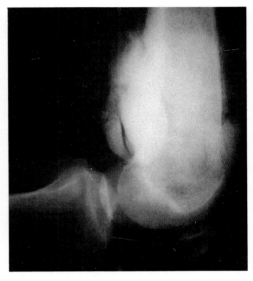

FIGURE 16.35 Lateral radiograph of the knee demonstrates a sclerotic bone tumor involving the lower end of the femur. In this view it is not possible to determine the precise involvement of the bone.

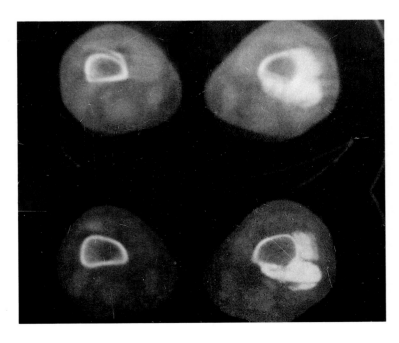

FIGURE 16.36 Computerized axial tomograms of the lesion shown in Figure 16.35 demonstrate that the tumor is entirely confined to the periphery of the bone, with no involvement of the intramedullary bone. (Figures 16.35 and 16.36 courtesy of Dr. Leonard Kahn)

from the cortical bone by a fine, relatively lucent line (Fig. 16.37).

Grossly, the tumor is firmly adherent to the bone and on cut section may exhibit bony, cartilaginous, and fibrous areas (Figs. 16.38 to 16.40). Microscopically, the lesion consists of a well-defined lobulated mass, with extensive bone and (occasionally) cartilage formation. Most tumors contain a bland, well-differentiated fibrosarcomatous stroma (Figs. 16.41 and 16.42).

The treatment of choice is surgical removal of the mass. However, in some cases intramedullary extension of the lesion may have occurred, so that excision of the lesion and the attached cortex may not be adequate treatment. Computerized axial tomography should be performed on these lesions to gauge the extent of intramedullary extension.

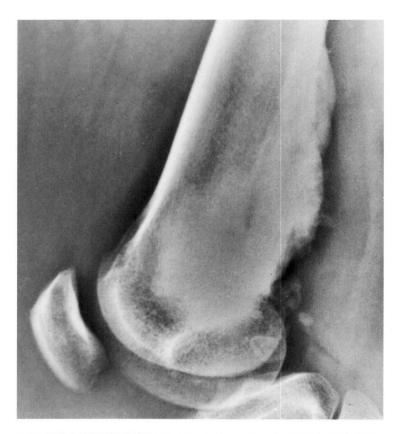

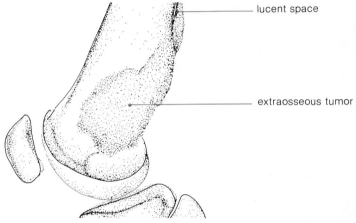

FIGURE 16.37 Radiograph of a 35-year-old woman who complained of pain in the lower end of the femur above the knee. An irregular radiodense tumor can be seen on the surface of the bone, particularly posteriorly but also to some extent laterally at the lower end of the femur. The margins of the tumor are well defined, and between the tumor and the underlying cortex a fine radiolucent line is focally apparent. In a case of juxtacortical osteosarcoma such as this, it is difficult to determine radiographically whether or not the medullary cavity is involved. For this reason, a CT scan can be extremely useful in determining the extent of the tumor.

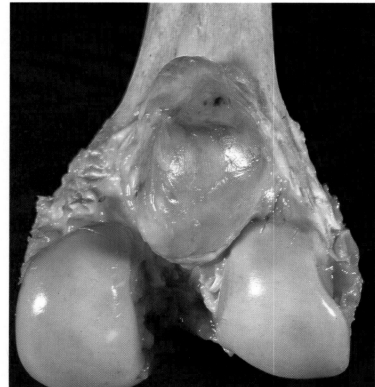

FIGURE 16.38 Gross photograph of the lower end of the femur resected from a patient with a juxtacortical osteosarcoma. A large mass is present on the cortex of the bone just above and between the two femoral condyles. This location is typical for juxtacortical osteosarcoma.

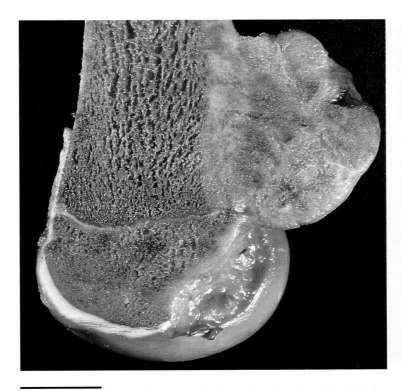

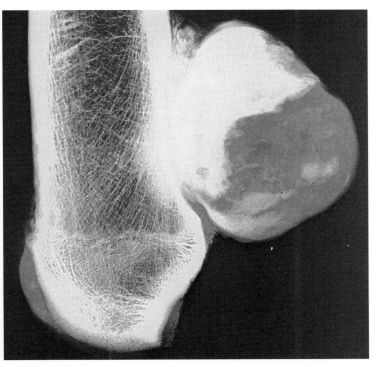

FIGURE 16.39 Gross photograph of a sagittal section through the lesion shown in Figure 16.38 demonstrates that the lesion is well encapsulated and formed of bone-producing tissue. As in the case shown here, the lesion frequently extends for a short distance through the cortex into the medullary cavity. For this reason, when surgical treatment of a juxtacortical osteosarcoma is planned, medullary extension should be carefully sought and taken into account if local recurrence is to be prevented.

FIGURE 16.40 Radiograph of the specimen in Figure 16.39. A juxtacortical osteosarcoma, as shown here, may contain a large area of tumor which is either purely fibrous or purely cartilaginous, and therefore radiolucent.

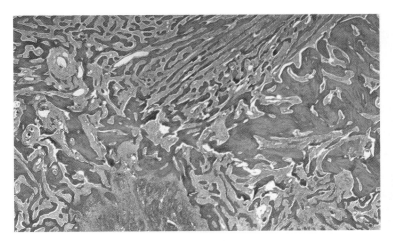

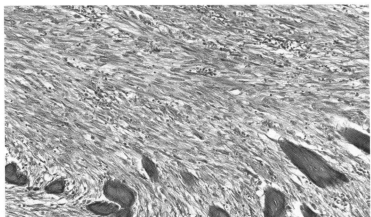

FIGURE 16.41 Low-power photomicrograph of a juxtacortical osteosarcoma shows the typical appearance of a heavily collagenized fibrous matrix with irregular trabeculae of bone (H & E, x 4 obj.).

FIGURE 16.42 Higher-power photomicrograph shows the cellular, though unremarkable, fibrous stroma of a juxtacortical osteosarcoma with islands of bone tissue (H & E, x 25 obj.).

PAROSTEAL OSTEOSARCOMA, HIGH GRADE

On occasion, a juxtacortical lesion may be identified as being a fully malignant tumor when examined microscopically; therefore, it should not be assumed that because the lesion has a juxtacortical location it necessarily has a better prognosis. Fully malignant parosteal lesions may account for as many as 25 percent of all parosteal lesions. On microscopic examination, the features of a malignant parosteal osteosarcoma are those of a high-grade central lesion.

Because the lesion may have an intramedullary component, it can sometimes be difficult to decide whether a particular case is a surface lesion or a central lesion with a large soft-tissue component. However, in either case the prognosis is similar (ie, poor).

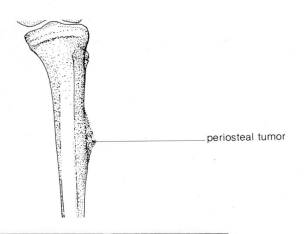

FIGURE 16.43 Radiograph of a 14-year-old boy who complained of pain in the upper part of the leg. In the upper part of the diaphysis is a peripheral lesion apparently confined to the surface of the bone. It is composed of an irregular bone-forming lesion, and there is reactive periosteal new bone both superiorly and inferiorly. Histologic examination proved this to be a cartilage-rich periosteal osteosarcoma.

periosteal tumor

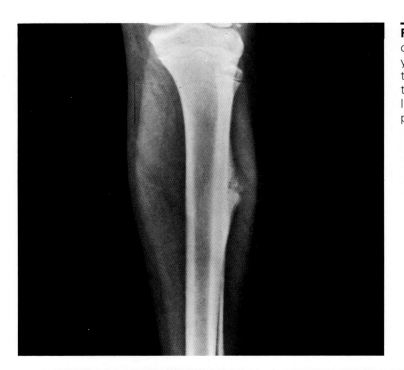

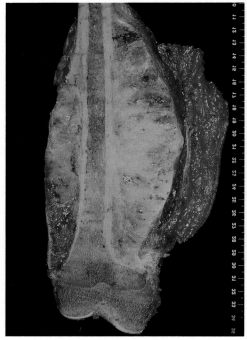

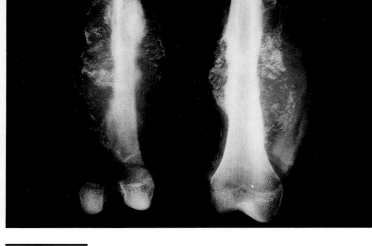

FIGURE 16.45 Radiograph of the dissected specimen shown in Figure 16.44 confirms the osseous component of the tumor. (Figures 16.44 and 16.45 courtesy of Dr. Leonard Kahn)

FIGURE 16.44 Gross photograph of a longitudinal section through the lower end of the femur demonstrates a large surface tumor composed of gray/white glistening tissues and admixed bone.

PERIOSTEAL OSTEOSARCOMA

Periosteal (peripheral) osteosarcoma is a rare, predominantly cartilage-forming osteosarcoma, characterized on radiographs by ill-defined swelling and formation of periosteal new bone, which often has a "sunburst" appearance (Fig. 16.43). The lesion usually occurs at the midshaft of the femur or tibia in children. It is usually small at the time of presentation, although larger lesions may be encountered (Figs. 16.44 and 16.45). The microscopic appearance is typical, with abundant

cartilage formation and a cellular stroma (Fig. 16.46). However, malignant bone matrix formation is present and distinguishes the lesion from a juxtacortical chondroma or chondrosarcoma.

INTRACORTICAL OSTEOSARCOMA

Cases of osteosarcoma that have an intracortical origin have been only rarely described. One such case of intracortical osteosarcoma is illustrated in figures 16.47 to 16.49.

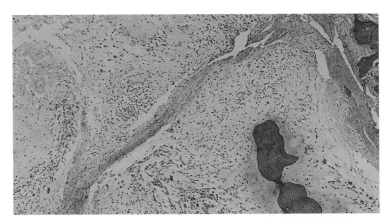

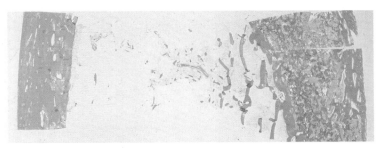

FIGURE 16.46 Photomicrograph demonstrating the features of a periosteal osteosarcoma. These lesions tend to be fairly cellular and for the most part to form, as here, a cartilaginous extracellular matrix; however, foci of bone formation can be found if searched for (H & E, x 10 obj.).

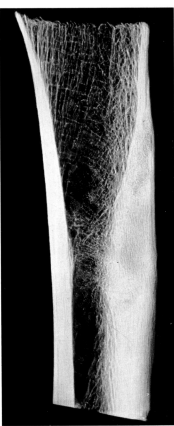

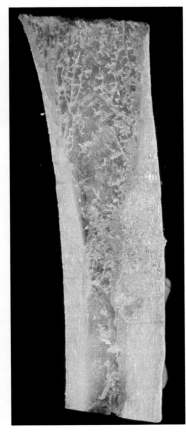

FIGURE 16.49 Histologic section through the shaft of the tibia shown in Figure 16.48 shows an osteosarcoma confined to the cortex of the bone (H & E, x 1 obj.).

FIGURE 16.47 A teenage boy complained of pain in the shin. Radiograph shows marked cortical thickening with a dense intracortical lesion, and a biopsy of this lesion revealed evidence of an osteosarcoma.

FIGURE 16.48 The resected specimen from the patient in Figure 16.47 demonstrates tumor confined to the cortical area of the bone.

SOFT-TISSUE OSTEOSARCOMA

Rare cases of bone-forming mesenchymal tumor have been described in the soft tissues, usually intramuscularly. These are usually small, round to ovoid lesions which exhibit finely trabeculated bone formation throughout. They occur in older individuals and have a better prognosis than conventional high-grade central lesions (Figs. 16.50 to 16.52).

PAGET'S SARCOMA

Rarely, patients with Paget's disease also develop sarcoma. These patients usually have advanced polyostotic Paget's disease (Fig. 16.53). However, on rare occasions sarcoma may occur in patients with monostotic disease (for example, in a single vertebral body).

The tumor most frequently associated with Paget's disease is osteosarcoma (Figs. 16.54 and 16.55),

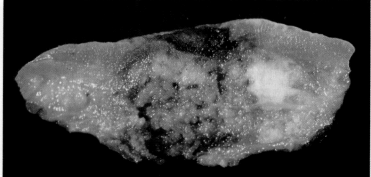

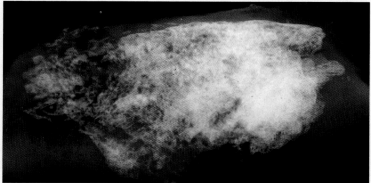

FIGURE 16.51 Gross lesion resected from the patient in Figure 16.50 *(upper)* and radiograph of the specimen *(lower)*. The radiograph shows the formation of mineralized tissue throughout the lesion. There is no evidence of maturation of the bone toward the periphery, a finding in contrast to those in myositis ossificans, a lesion that can be mistaken for a soft-tissue osteosarcoma.

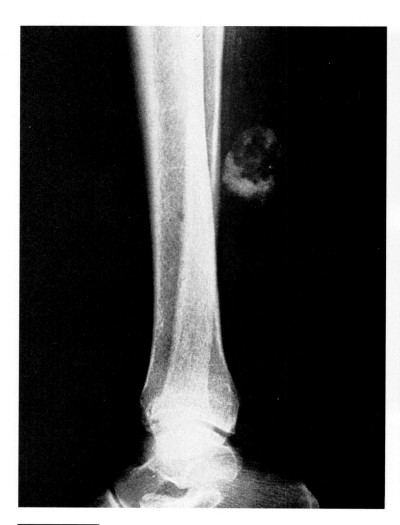

FIGURE 16.50 Radiograph of a 50-year-old man who presented with a small painful mass in the calf region. A well-defined ossified lesion is evident in the soft tissue.

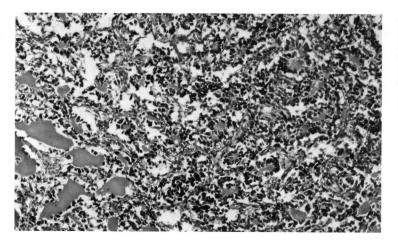

FIGURE 16.52 Photomicrograph of a portion of the tumor shown in Figures 16.50 and 16.51 demonstrates the hypercellular anaplastic nature of the lesion and the microscopic foci of osteoid that are being formed by the tumor cells. This is in marked contrast to the histologic picture found in cases of myositis ossificans circumscripta (see Figures 14.42 to 14.45) (H & E, x 10 obj.).

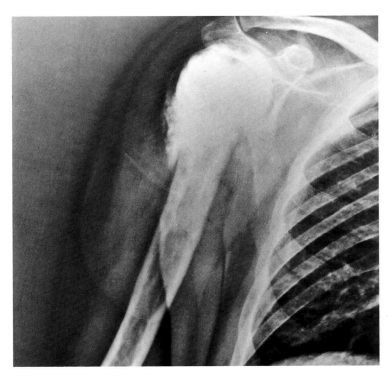

FIGURE 16.53 Radiograph of a 65-year-old man, who presented with severe pain in the upper end of the right humerus, shows a large destructive and sclerotic tumor in the upper end of the humerus extending into the soft tissue. Note that the cortex of the bone below the tumor is thickened and indistinct, characteristic of Paget's disease.

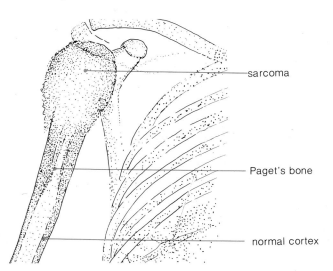

sarcoma

Paget's bone

normal cortex

FIGURE 16.54 Sagittal section through the humerus of the patient shown in Figure 16.53 shows a large destructive tumor at the upper end. The tumor has extended through the cortex into the soft tissue. (Often, sarcoma in Paget's disease occurs in the mid-shaft of the bone, and this finding contrasts with that of primary osteosarcoma, which is more often seen in the metaphysis.) Note the thickened hyperemic cortical bone involved by Paget's disease.

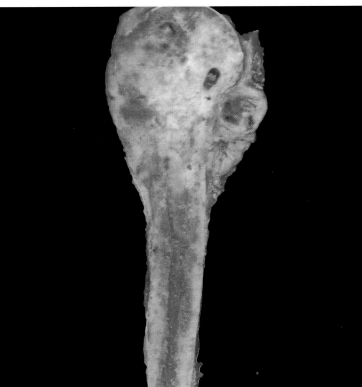

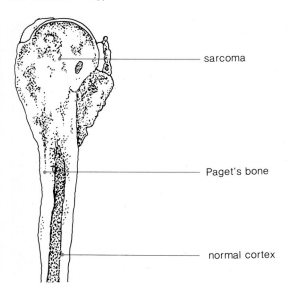

sarcoma

Paget's bone

normal cortex

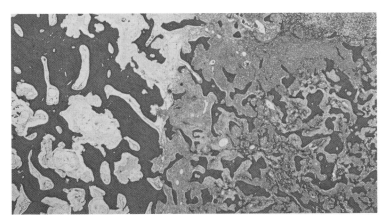

FIGURE 16.55 Photomicrograph of tissue removed from the patient in Figure 16.54. On the left, is pagetoid bone; on the right, a cellular bone-forming tumor (H & E, x 4 obj.).

although occasionally other patterns of sarcoma (eg, chondrosarcoma, malignant fibrous histiocytoma) may be encountered and, rarely, a benign giant-cell tumor occurs. The prognosis for sarcomas arising in patients with Paget's disease is very poor.

RADIATION SARCOMA

Osteosarcoma and fibrosarcoma are the most commonly encountered radiation-induced sarcomas, although chondrosarcoma, malignant fibrous histiocytoma, or undifferentiated sarcoma may be seen. The time interval between radiation and the diagnosis of postirradiation sarcoma may be as much as 40 years, but the average is around 10 to 12 years. If the interval between radiation and tumor diagnosis is less than 2 years, a causal relationship should be seriously doubted. The vast majority of cases have received a radiation dose of more than 3000 rads. The incidence of sarcomatous degeneration appears to be related to the dose given. In general, radiation sarcomas behave in a highly malignant way.

The tumors present in the radiation field, and the most commonly treated lesions that give rise to postirradiation sarcomas are gynecologic cancer and breast cancer (Fig. 16.56). Among primary bone lesions, giant-cell tumors treated by radiation therapy seem to be particularly associated with postirradiation sarcoma.

ENCHONDROMA

Enchondroma is a common, usually asymptomatic (especially in long bones), benign intramedullary cartilaginous neoplasm. Enchondromas commonly arise in the short tubular bones of the hands and feet of adults, but may also occur in the long bones. Enlarging lesions may fracture, and this complication is the usual reason for clinical presentation. In rare cases, an eccentric chondroma may cause bulging of the cortex. This appearance has been referred to as enchondroma protuberans.

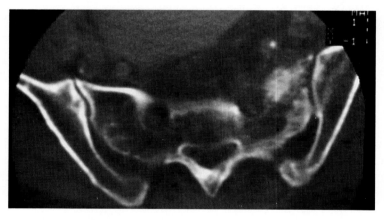

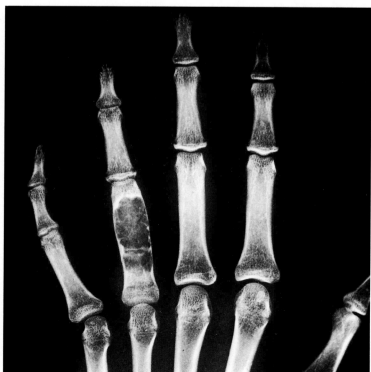

FIGURE 16.56 Computerized axial tomogram through the sacroiliac joint of a 52-year-old woman shows an expanding and destructive bone-forming tumor involving the left ala of the sacrum. Biopsy confirmed the diagnosis of sarcoma secondary to previous irradiation of a cervical carcinoma.

FIGURE 16.57 Radiograph of a hand shows a well-defined lytic lesion with small punctate calcifications in the proximal phalanx of the ring finger. At the proximal end of the lesion is a line of density suggesting a fracture through the tumor. This appearance is characteristic of enchondroma.

Radiographically, enchondroma usually appears as a well-delineated, solitary lucent defect in the metaphyseal region of the bone, although in the small tubular bones the entire shaft is usually involved. The cortex is usually intact unless a fracture through the weakened bone has occurred. Calcification is usually present in the lesion, appearing as fine, punctate stippling or small broken rings of radiodensity (Fig. 16.57). When calcification is pronounced, the lesion may be suggestive of a bone infarct (Fig. 16.58).

Gross inspection of the lesion reveals bluish-gray lobules of firm, translucent tissue. On microscopic examination these lobules are found to be proliferating nests of cartilage cells without obvious atypia. Foci of calcification are usually present (Fig. 16.59), and a thin layer of lamellar bone rimming the cartilage nodules is sometimes observed (Fig. 16.60). Occasionally, evidence of endochondral ossification is seen. However, invasive infiltration of the bone marrow spaces is not characteristic of benign enchondromas,

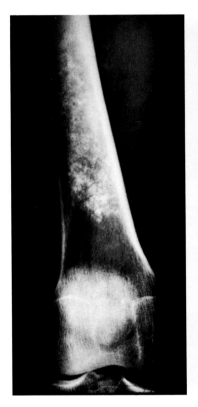
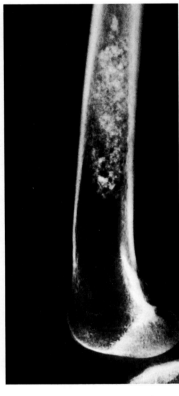

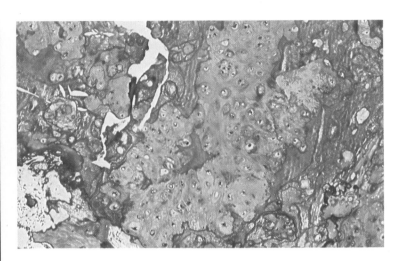

FIGURE 16.59 Photomicrograph of the lesion shown in Figure 16.58 reveals a calcified cartilaginous lesion. The cartilage cells are uncrowded and unremarkable (H & E, x 10 obj.).

FIGURE 16.58 Anteroposterior *(left)* and lateral *(right)* radiographs of a 52-year-old man with pain in the knee joint show a heavily calcified intramedullary lesion in the lower end of the femur. There were no apparent symptoms related to this lesion. Histologic examination revealed a heavily calcified cartilage tumor, interpreted as an enchondroma.

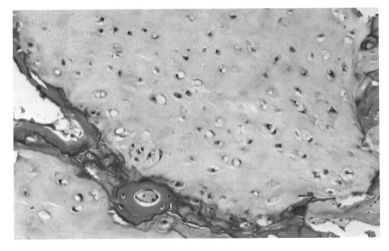

FIGURE 16.60 Frequently, in an enchondroma, the cartilage lobules are surrounded by a narrow rim of bone, as shown in this photomicrograph (H & E, x 25 obj.).

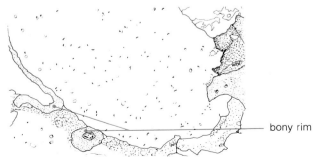

bony rim

and this finding helps to distinguish the lesion from a chondrosarcoma. Rarely, a chondrosarcoma develops in a preexisting enchondroma, usually in long tubular bones (Fig. 16.61).

Although it may be difficult on histologic examination to differentiate an enchondroma from a low-grade chondrosarcoma, small peripheral cartilage tumors usually tend to be benign, whereas large axial tumors tend to be malignant.

Sometimes examination of cross-sections of a femoral head reveals small nodules of cartilage within the bone, which are usually less than a centimeter in diameter. Such nodules are perhaps best regarded as benign cartilage rests (Fig. 16.62).

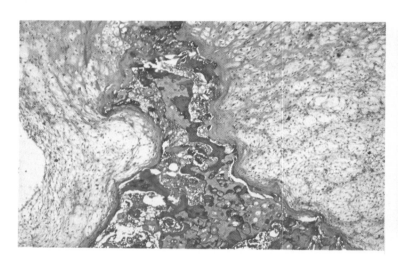

FIGURE 16.61 Photomicrograph demonstrates the development of a chondrosarcoma in a patient with preexisting enchondroma. In the lower center part of the photomicrograph a heavily calcified enchondroma is apparent. In the upper left and right parts a cellular myxoid chondrosarcoma is present (H & E, x 4 obj.).

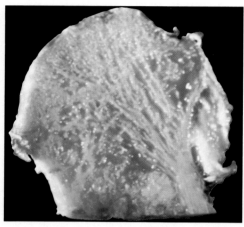

FIGURE 16.62 Gross photograph of a femoral head resected for osteoarthritis. A small cartilage rest is present in the neck of the femur. Note the glistening, lobulated, bluish-white appearance of the cartilaginous tissue.

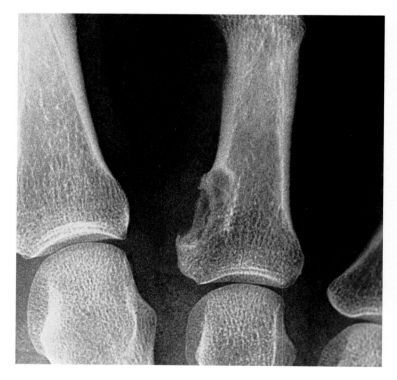

FIGURE 16.63 Radiograph of a hand shows a well-defined saucer-like depression of the cortex at the proximal end of one phalanx. This radiographic picture is typical of a juxtacortical chondroma.

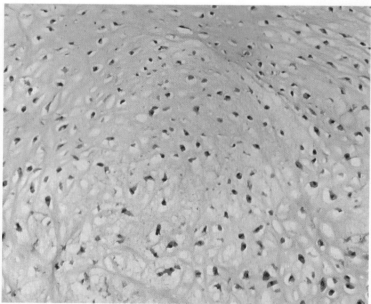

FIGURE 16.64 Photomicrograph of the lesion illustrated in Figure 16.63 shows a cellular but benign cartilaginous lesion (H & E, x 10 obj.).

JUXTACORTICAL CHONDROMA (PERIOSTEAL CHONDROMA)

Juxtacortical chondroma is a benign cartilaginous lesion characterized by its location in the metaphyseal cortex of both long and short tubular bones. A cup-shaped or scalloped cortical defect with a sclerotic margin is evident on radiographs, and the lesion, which is rarely more than 3 to 4 cm in diameter, typically has overhanging edges (Fig. 16.63). Calcified material and, in some instances, a soft-tissue mass may be seen. On gross inspection, juxtacortical chondroma is a well-circumscribed lesion which is partially embedded in cortical bone and covered by the periosteum. Its cut surface is grayish-white or bluish and lobulated. When examined microscopically, proliferating chondrocytes show minimal pleomorphism and nuclear abnormalities (Fig. 16.64). Focal calcification and ossification may occur within the cartilage.

The treatment of a juxtacortical chondroma is en bloc resection.

SOFT-TISSUE CHONDROMA

Cartilaginous lesions in the soft tissues are rare. Most soft-tissue chondromas have been seen in the hands or feet of patients in the older age group. In general, the lesions measure between 1 and 2 cm in diameter and are densely calcified on radiographic examination (Fig. 16.65).

Grossly, the lesions are usually firmly adherent to adjacent structures and have a hard, gritty consistency. Microscopic examination usually reveals heavy granular calcification and many necrotic chondrocytes. Viable cartilage tissue is often limited to the periphery of the lesion (Fig. 16.66).

CHONDROBLASTOMA

Chondroblastoma is an uncommon, benign cellular neoplasm located in the epiphysis of long bones, and is usually diagnosed in the patient's second decade. On

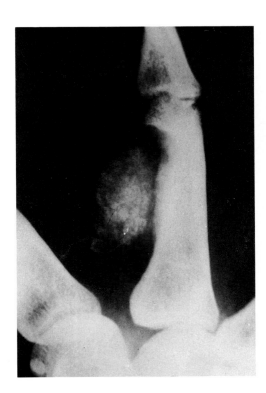

FIGURE 16.65 Radiograph showing a heavily calcified tumor on the volar aspect of a proximal phalanx. Note the punctate appearance of the calcification.

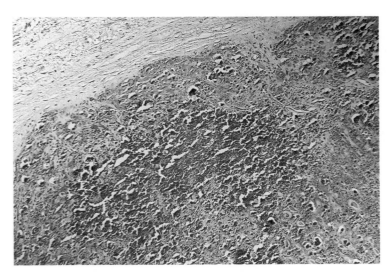

FIGURE 16.66 Photomicrograph of a portion of the periphery of the lesion illustrated in Figure 16.65 shows heavily calcified cartilage with only a few viable chondrocytes at the periphery, consistent with soft tissue chondroma (H & E, x 10 obj.).

rare occasions these lesions occur in older individuals and in odd locations, such as the spine or a flat bone.

The characteristic radiographic signs of chondroblastoma include a well-demarcated lucent defect with mottled calcification, located in the epiphysis and sometimes extending into the metaphysis of long bones (Fig. 16.67). The cortical bone may be intact or expanded. The lesion has a predilection for the upper end of the humerus, the upper and lower ends of the femur, and the upper end of the tibia.

The gritty, grayish-pink tissue of this lesion is characterized microscopically by round and ovoid cells, often mixed with a scattering of giant cells. Focally, an intercellular chondroid matrix is produced in which a lace-like deposit of calcium granules is typically observed (so-called "chicken-wire" calcification) (Figs. 16.68 to 16.70). On occasion the lesions are cystic and hemorrhagic (cystic chondroblastoma), and this finding

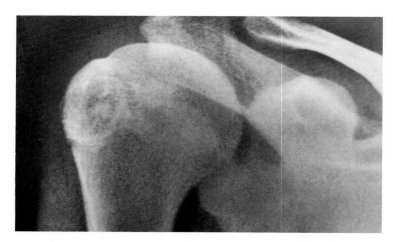

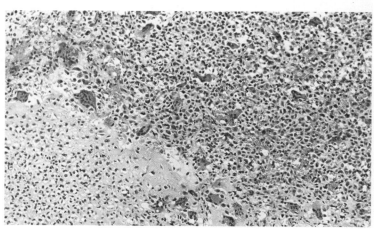

FIGURE 16.67 Radiograph of an 11-year-old boy with complaints of pain and limitation of motion in the right shoulder. An eccentric lytic lesion with patchy calcification involves the apophysis of the humerus laterally. Curettage of this lesion proved it to be a chondroblastoma. The radiographic appearance and location shown here are typical. Occasionally, the lesion may extend into the metaphysis.

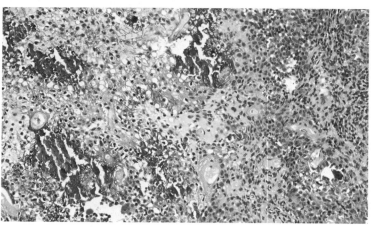

FIGURE 16.68 Photomicrograph of a chondroblastoma demonstrates the varied appearance of this lesion. Cellular areas mixed with areas of cartilage matrix formation and calcification can be seen (H & E, x 10 obj.).

FIGURE 16.69 Photomicrograph reveals the juxtaposition of an area of chondroid matrix on the lower left, with a more cellular area of polyhedral cells and admixed giant cells on the right (H & E, x 10 obj.).

FIGURE 16.70 Fine stippled calcification is characteristic of chondroblastoma and frequently extends around the individual chondroblasts, producing a "chicken-wire" appearance (H & E, x 25 obj.).

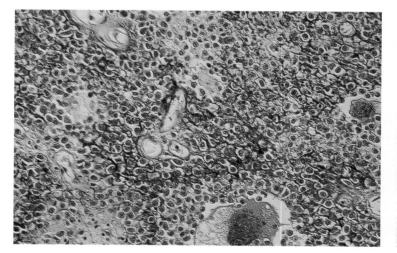

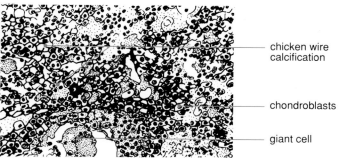

chicken wire calcification

chondroblasts

giant cell

may cause confusion of chondroblastomas with aneurysmal bone cysts. (The presence of cartilage and giant cells in chondroblastomas may also lead to diagnostic confusion of the lesion with either chondrosarcoma or giant-cell tumors of bone.)

Curettage or local excision is the treatment of choice. In very rare cases, lung metastases have occurred; when present, they are usually rimmed with bone. These metastases should be surgically removed.

CHONDROMYXOID FIBROMA

Chondromyxoid fibroma is a rare, benign bone neoplasm most often discovered during the patient's second or third decade. The lesion occurs most commonly in the femur and upper metaphysis of the tibia, but it may occasionally develop in other bones. Patients may experience pain and local swelling. On radiographs, the lesion is usually characterized by an eccentric lucent defect with a thin, well-defined scalloped border of sclerotic bone (Fig. 16.71).

Inspection of intact gross specimens reveals that the lesion is sharply demarcated and covered on its outer surface with a thin rim of bone or periosteum. Examination of the cut surface demonstrates a firm, lobulated, grayish-white mass, sometimes with small cystic foci and areas of hemorrhage (Fig. 16.72).

On microscopic examination, chondromyxoid fibroma has a lobulated pattern, with sparsely cellular lobules alternating with more cellular zones. The sparsely cellular lobules show spindle and stellate cells without distinct cytoplasmic borders in a myxoid or chondroid matrix. Running between the lobules are areas of increased cellularity, with multinucleated giant cells. Some nuclear pleomorphism may be evident but mitotic figures are rare (Fig. 16.73).

Because recurrence of the lesion after curettage is frequent, en bloc excision is the preferred treatment.

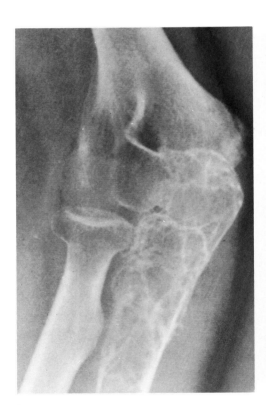

FIGURE 16.71 Radiograph of the elbow joint in a young adult man who complained of pain shows a well-defined, trabeculated lytic lesion, with cortical thinning but no obvious soft-tissue extension. This soap-bubble appearance is rather typical of chondromyxoid fibromas, although these lesions are so rare that the diagnosis is usually not made until after histologic examination.

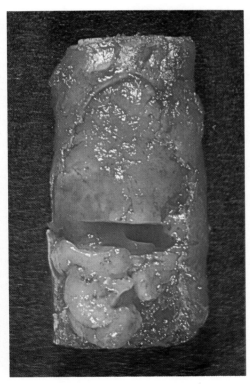

FIGURE 16.72 Gross photograph of a segment of resected fibula with a chondromyxoid fibroma. Note the well-demarcated lesion and the glistening fleshy appearance.

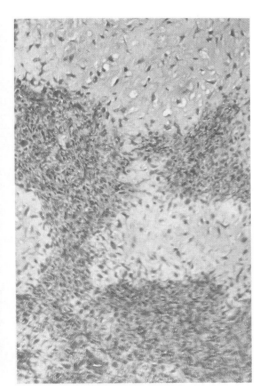

FIGURE 16.73 Photomicrograph of a chondromyxoid fibroma shows the typical lobulated and variegated appearance of this lesion. Lobules of chondromyxoid tissue and septa of cellular fibrous tissue are evident, with occasional multinucleated giant cells running between the lobules (H & E, x 10 obj.).

FIBROMYXOMA

Fibromyxoma is microscopically superficially similar to a chondromyxoid fibroma, but it is rarer and occurs in older individuals. In addition, fibromyxoma lacks both the lobular pattern and the chondroid matrix that typify a chondromyxoid fibroma.

This lesion is so rare that no radiographic characteristics have been substantiated. The radiograph in Fig. 16.74 was thought to show a giant-cell tumor. However, histologic examination (Fig. 16.75) showed it to be a fibromyxoma. Follow-up of the few cases described in the literature has revealed no instances of local recurrence or metastases.

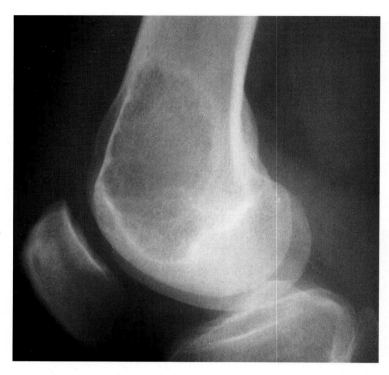

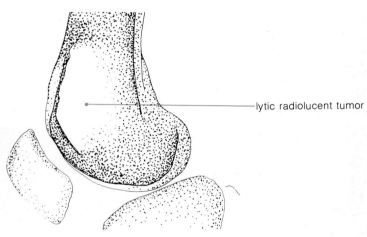

FIGURE 16.74 Radiograph of the lower end of the femur in a 38-year-old man who complained of pain in the knee joint. A lytic destructive lesion involves both the epiphysis and the metaphysis of the femur; on radiographs, this lesion resembles a giant-cell tumor.

lytic radiolucent tumor

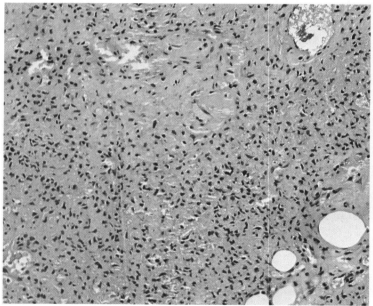

FIGURE 16.75 Photomicrograph of the lesion shown in 16.74 shows loose fibromyxomatous tissue without lobulation and without obvious chondroid areas. A few such cases have been reported, usually in older people, and these lesions have been designated as fibromyxomas (H & E, x 10 obj.).

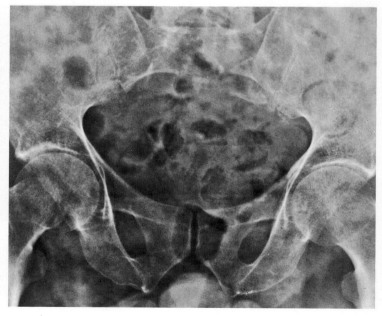

FIGURE 16.76 Radiograph of a 60-year-old man, who complained of pain in the coccygeal region, reveals destruction of the sacrum and the coccyx by a large, lytic, expansile lesion, which on biopsy proved to be a chordoma.

CHORDOMA

Chordoma is a neoplasm that arises from remnants of the notochord, and therefore occurs in the midline of the axial skeleton. About half the cases occur in the sacrococcygeal region (Fig. 16.76), whereas one third are present at the base of the skull. The remaining cases arise at different sites along the vertebral column, most commonly in the cervical region. Chordoma is a slow-growing neoplasm whose clinical symptoms depend on its location. Cranial lesions usually are smaller than sacrococcygeal lesions at the time of initial presentation. Males are more frequently affected than females, and the average age at diagnosis is approximately 55 years.

Bone destruction is the radiographic hallmark of chordoma; however, about half of the patients exhibit focal calcifications within the lesion. Localization of the lesion is greatly aided by the use of newer imaging techniques, particularly in cases of intracranial chordoma (Fig. 16.77). When chordomas affect areas of the spine other than the two common sites (ie, sacrococcygeal and cervical), the lesions are likely to be lytic, located centrally within the vertebral body, and slowly expansile. When the cervical vertebrae are affected, extension anteriorly into the soft tissues may result in dysphagia (Fig. 16.78), whereas posterior extension may lead to neurologic complications. Systemic metastases to the regional lymph nodes, lung, liver, and bone have been reported in about half the cases.

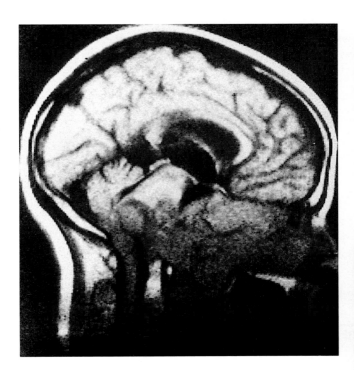

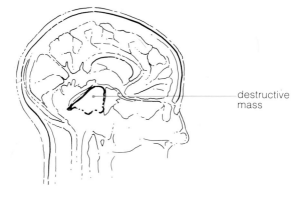

FIGURE 16.77 A sagittal spin–echo MRI shows an enormous mass filling the nasal cavity and ethmoid sinus anteriorly. It has obliterated the nasopharynx, extending inferiorly into the hypopharynx. Rostral to the odontoid process, it extends into the cranial cavity, completely destroying the clivus. It has invaded or displaced the brain-stem, extending directly to the anterior aspect of the fourth ventricle.

destructive mass

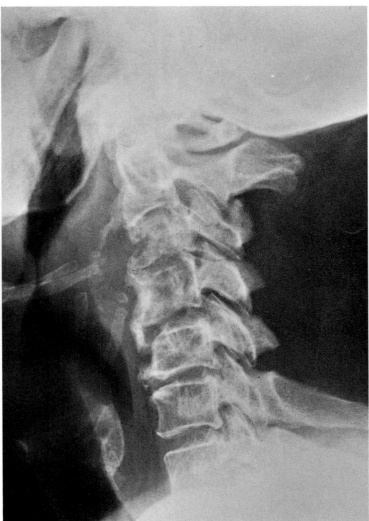

FIGURE 16.78 Lateral radiograph of a 40-year-old male who presented with dysphagia and myelopathy. There is a destructive lesion involving C3 and C4, with an anterior soft-tissue extension that partially occludes the airway.

On gross examination, chordomas are generally soft and appear well encapsulated. Lobulations are apparent on cut section, and the tumor usually has a bluish-gray color with extensive gelatinous translucent areas which are focally cystic and hemorrhagic (Fig. 16.79). Grossly, the tissue may suggest a chondrosarcoma or even a mucinous carcinoma. Histologic examination, however, reveals a characteristic arrangement of tumor cells separated into lobules by fibrous septa of different thicknesses. The tumor cells are of various sizes and shapes, arranged in both cords and sheets, with an eosinophilic cytoplasm associated with both extracellular and intracellular mucin that may be minimal or abundant (Fig. 16.80). The vacuoles may be very prominent and thus may displace the nucleus to one edge, producing the so-called physaliphorous cell (Fig. 16.81); pools of mucin also are seen in the extracellular space.

Approximately one third of spheno-occipital chordomas contain a significant chondroid component, and these lesions can easily be confused with chondrosarcomas, especially with chondrosarcomas having a predominantly myxoid structure (Fig. 16.82). Rarely, there is an associated malignant mesenchymal tumor in a chordoma, either a malignant fibrous histiocytoma or another poorly differentiated sarcoma; at least some of these cases are associated with a history of radiation therapy.

PRIMARY SYNOVIAL CHONDROMATOSIS (PRIMARY SYNOVIAL CHONDROMETAPLASIA)

Primary synovial chondromatosis is a rare condition characterized by the proliferation of islands of irregularly cellular cartilage in the synovium of a joint (or tendon sheath) without any underlying arthritis. This

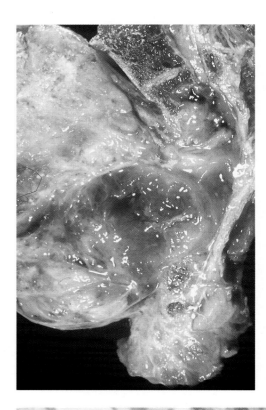

FIGURE 16.79 Photograph of a sagittal section obtained at autopsy through the lower lumbar spine and sacrum of a patient with chordoma. The tumor has largely destroyed the sacrum and is involving L5. A large anterior component is present. The tumor tissue shows a characteristic lobulated, firm blue-gray tissue mass, with focal hemorrhage and cystification. (Courtesy of Dr. Mario Campanacci)

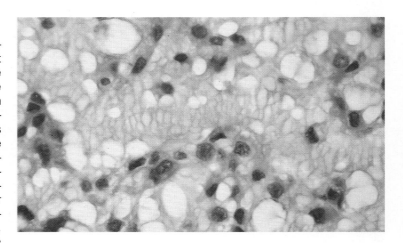

FIGURE 16.80 In some areas of chordoma, large mucoid foci are present; in these mucoid areas, cords of eosinophilic cells may be present (as in this photomicrograph) (H & E, x 40 obj.).

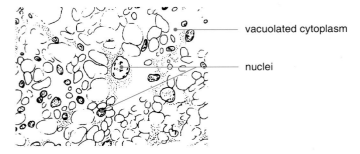

FIGURE 16.81 Photomicrograph shows the large variegated and vacuolated cells characteristic of chordoma (physaliphorous cells) (H & E, x 40 obj.).

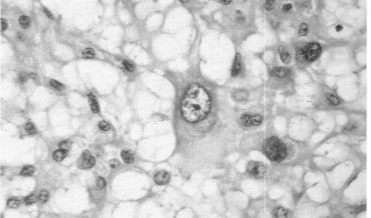

vacuolated cytoplasm

nuclei

finding distinguishes primary synovial chondromatosis from the much more commonly observed occurrence of articular cartilage fragments, often with associated reactive metaplastic cartilage, in the synovial tissues of patients with various types of arthritis. Patients with primary synovial chondromatosis have been observed in their second through seventh decades of life, and they usually report the gradual onset of pain, stiffness, or an enlarged mass around the affected joint. Pain and limitation of motion are characteristic findings on clinical examination. About half the cases involve the hip or the knee, while most of the remaining cases occur in the tendon sheaths of the hands or feet.

The radiologic signs of this disorder include multiple loose bodies of variable size, which may or may not be radiopaque (Fig. 16.83). Contrast arthrography may be necessary to demonstrate these lesions (Figs. 16.84 and 16.85). In some cases of synovial chondromatosis affecting the hip joint, erosion of the bone has been observed.

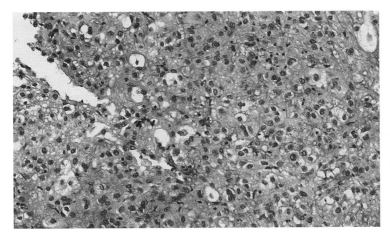

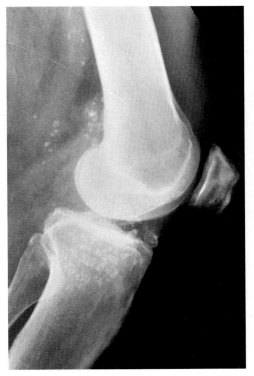

FIGURE 16.82 In some patients with chordomas arising in the area of the clivus, the tumor has a distinctly chondroid appearance (as in this photomicrograph). This chondroid pattern is important to recognize, since the prognosis for patients with chondroid chordomas in the base of the skull is much better than for patients with a conventional pattern of chordoma in that area (H & E, x 10 obj.).

FIGURE 16.83 Lateral radiograph of the knee joint of a middle-aged man complaining of vague knee pain and swelling. Multiple small opacifications both in and around the joint are particularly prominent in the popliteal space. On biopsy, this proved to be due to primary synovial chondromatosis.

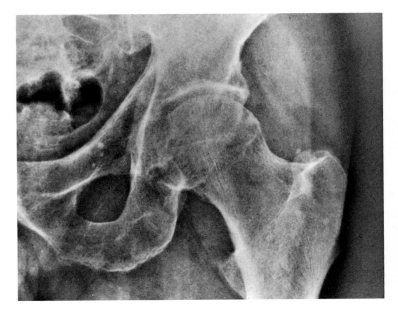

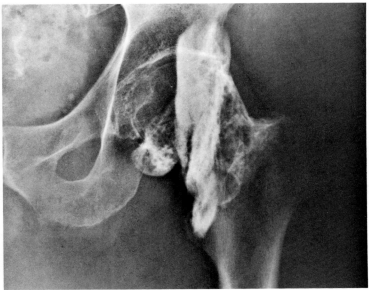

FIGURE 16.84 Radiograph of a 65-year-old man, who presented with an intermittent 20-year history of mild pain in the right hip, shows no obvious lesion in the joint. (Courtesy of Dr. Alex Norman)

FIGURE 16.85 Arthrogram of the patient shown in Figure 16.84 demonstrates many small, round filling defects in the synovium, consistent with synovial chondromatosis. The individual nodules of cartilage were neither calcified nor ossified, and therefore failed to show up on plain radiographs. (Courtesy of Dr. Alex Norman)

At surgery, there are usually multiple cartilaginous loose bodies, both free in the joint and attached to the synovium (Figs. 16.86 and 16.87). Microscopic examination reveals discrete nodules of cartilaginous tissue in the synovium, characterized by markedly disorganized cartilage cloning with cytologic atypia (Figs. 16.88 and 16.89). This disordered appearance helps to differentiate primary synovial chondromatosis from the much more common secondary chondromatosis, which occurs in association with traumatic loose bodies and osteochondritis dissecans, for example (see Chapter 18). Although calcification and endochondral ossification of the cartilage nodules may occur, they are usually irregular and patchily distributed.

These lesions frequently recur after excision.

CHONDROSARCOMA

Chondrosarcoma is a malignant neoplasm whose cells produce cartilage matrix. Bone matrix made by the malignant cells is not present in chondrosarcoma, although on occasion there may be foci of benign reactive bone. Chondrosarcoma is characteristically seen in adults, most frequently occurring in the medullary cavity of the femur and humerus (central chondrosarcoma) and on the surface of the pelvis and spine (peripheral chondrosarcoma) (Figs. 16.90 to 16.93). Patients initially complain of mild pain and local swelling.

On radiography, chondrosarcomas in the long bones are located in the metaphysis and often extend into the diaphysis to produce a fusiform, lucent defect

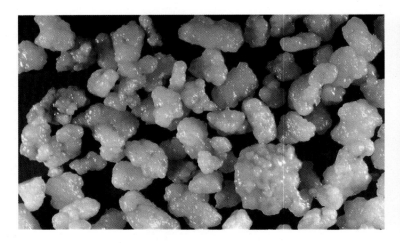

FIGURE 16.86 Gross photograph of multiple loose bodies removed from a patient with synovial chondromatosis.

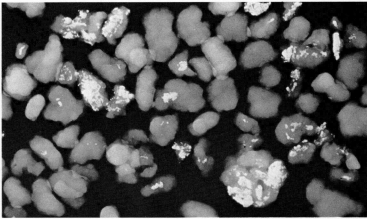

FIGURE 16.87 Radiograph of the tissue shown in Figure 16.86 demonstrates that only a few of the loose bodies contain calcium.

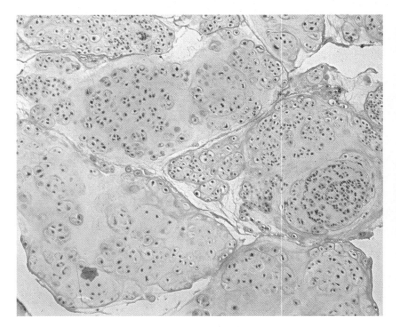

FIGURE 16.88 Photomicrograph of the synovium removed from a patient with primary synovial chondromatosis shows nodules of irregular cellular cartilage within the synovium (H & E, x 10 obj.).

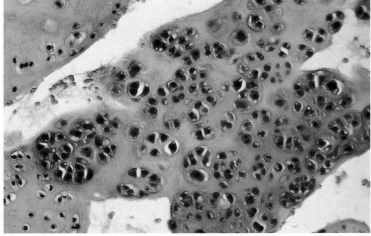

FIGURE 16.89 Higher-power view of primary synovial chondromatosis lesion shows atypical cells which are crowded and clumped. This histologic picture helps to distinguish primary synovial chondromatosis from the secondary chondromatosis that is frequently seen in association with osteoarthritis and trauma (H & E, x 25 obj.).

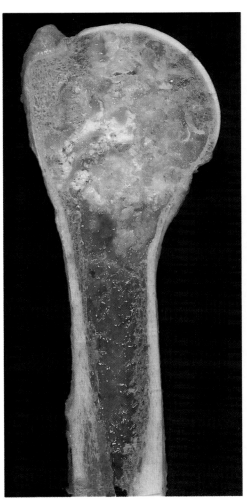

FIGURE 16.90
Gross photograph of a central chondrosarcoma arising from the medullary cavity of the humerus.

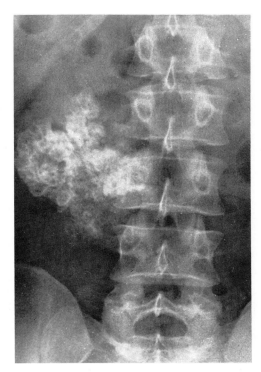

FIGURE 16.91
In this radiograph a large calcified mass is present adjacent to the lumbar spine. This lesion proved to be a chondrosarcoma.

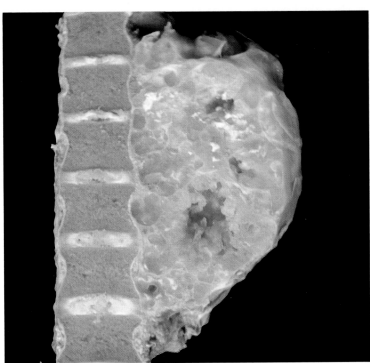

FIGURE 16.92 Gross photograph of a chondrosarcoma arising from the vertebral column.

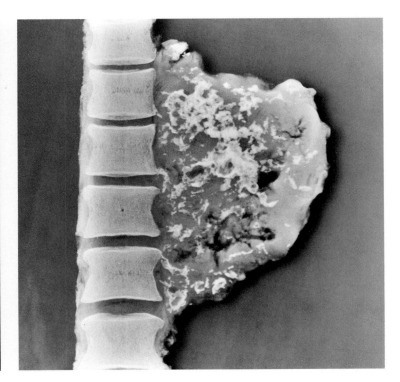

FIGURE 16.93 Radiograph of the specimen shown in Figure 16.92 demonstrates irregular areas of calcification within the lesion.

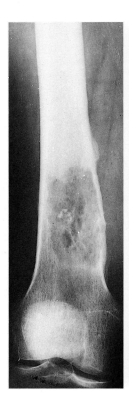
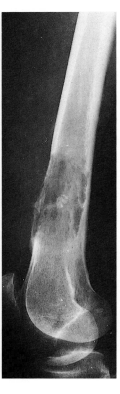

FIGURE 16.94
Anteroposterior and lateral radiographs of the lower femur in a 50-year-old man complaining of acute onset of pain. The margin of the lesion is fairly well defined, and thinning of the cortex gives rise to a trabeculated appearance. Soft-tissue extension of the tumor is evident anteriorly and medially. In the center of the lesion, small foci of punctate calcifications are apparent consistent with a diagnosis of chondrosarcoma.

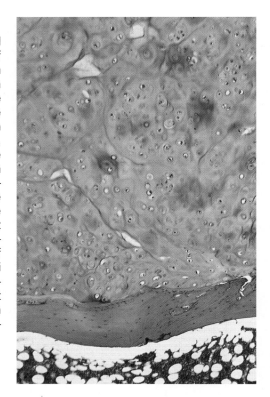

FIGURE 16.95 Photomicrograph of a low grade chondrosarcoma. The chondrocytes though somewhat crowded, are not particularly atypical. Although this tumor is frequently edged by bone, as seen here, it does not particularly invade through the spaces (H & E, x 4 obj.).

FIGURE 16.96 In a fully malignant high-grade chondrosarcoma, the hallmark of the lesion is that the tumor invades between the bone spicules, as illustrated here. In addition, when compared with the low-grade lesion, there is much more crowding and atypicality of the chondrocytes (H & E, x 10 obj.).

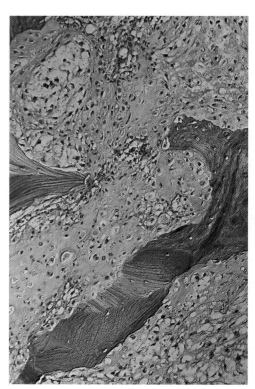

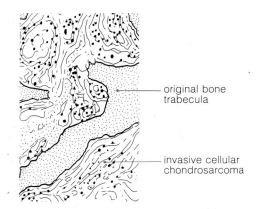

— original bone trabecula

— invasive cellular chondrosarcoma

with a scalloped inner cortex. Frequent punctate or stippled calcifications are characteristic Fig. 16.94). Occasionally, extensive calcification may give rise to the radiologic confusion of chondrosarcoma with a bone infarct.

Grossly, chondrosarcomas are lobulated, grayish-white or blue, focally calcified masses, often with areas of mucoid degeneration or necrosis. The lesions can be distinguished microscopically from benign cartilage tumors by their increased cellularity and pleomorphism (Figs. 16.95 to 16.98). Attempts have been made to grade chondrosarcomas on the basis of their degree of differentiation, variation in nuclear size, the presence of double nuclei and multinucleated giant cells, and the frequency of mitoses, although mitoses are usually rare. (Adequate sampling of cartilage tumors is

necessary to discern these features.) It is usually convenient to classify these lesions as either low grade or high grade. Low-grade chondrosarcomas are difficult to differentiate from benign enchondromas on microscopic examination. It is generally true that lesions in the axial skeleton and the proximal portions of the appendicular skeleton are more likely to pursue a malignant course than tumors in the distal skeleton. [However, it is important to recognize that on rare occasions chondrosarcomas may arise in the digits (Fig. 16.99).] Furthermore, infiltration of the marrow spaces occurs in chondrosarcomas, so that trabeculae of normal bone may be found embedded in the tumor. In assessment of low-grade chondrosarcomas, this finding can be a useful way of distinguishing the lesion from an enchondroma (Fig. 16.100).

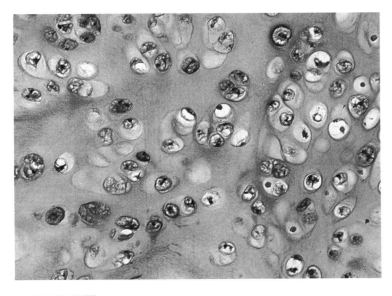

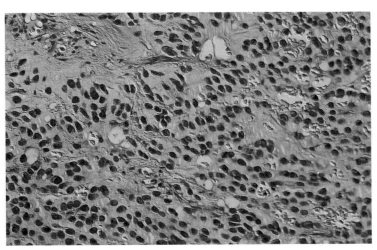

FIGURE 16.98 Photomicrograph from an area within a chondrosarcoma that exhibits crowded round cells lying in a myxoid matrix (H & E, x 10 obj.).

FIGURE 16.97 Photomicrograph of a fully malignant, anaplastic chondrosarcoma shows marked cellular atypia and crowding (H & E, x 40 obj.).

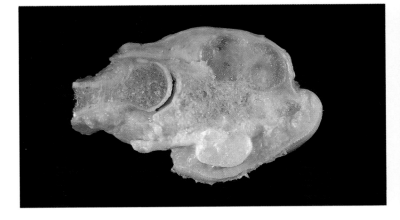

FIGURE 16.99 Sagittal section through a great toe in which a chondrosarcoma of the distal phalanx has extensively grown out into the surrounding soft tissues. Microscopically, this proved to be a high-grade malignant chondrosarcoma.

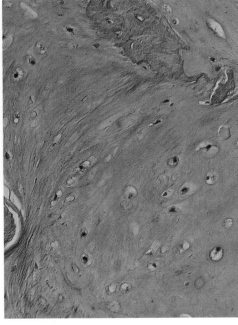

FIGURE 16.100
Photomicrograph taken from a low-grade chondrosarcoma illustrating the invasive quality of the lesion, with islands of mature lamellar bone embedded within the cartilaginous tumor tissue. From its cellularity, the lesion shows no evidence of malignancy in this field (H & E, x 40 obj.).

The clinical course of chondrosarcoma depends on several factors. In general, well-differentiated tumors rarely metastasize, but they recur locally after incomplete excision. Anaplastic, fully malignant tumors metastasize early, primarily to the lung. Complete surgical excision of the tumor is the treatment of choice. (Cartilage lesions do not usually respond to chemotherapy or radiation therapy.)

About 10 percent of all chondrosarcomas undergo dedifferentiation in one area or another and become highly malignant sarcomas with spindle cells and bizarre giant cells (features of fibrosarcoma or malignant fibrous histiocytoma) (Figs. 16.101 to 16.103). These dedifferentiated tumors carry a poor prognosis and often metastasize widely, the metastases frequently showing only the fibrosarcomatous component of the tumor. Radiographs may reveal a poorly defined and destructive lucent zone in an otherwise typical chondrosarcoma with stippled calcification.

MESENCHYMAL CHONDROSARCOMA

Mesenchymal chondrosarcoma is a rare, malignant bone tumor which has been seen most commonly in individuals in the second and third decades of life. Almost any bone may be affected, although there is a reported predilection for the ribs and jaw. Approximately one third of the lesions have been found in soft tissue. Patients may experience pain and/or swelling.

An ill-defined osteolytic lesion with irregular calcifications may be noted on radiographs, and this radiologic appearance corresponds to the grayish-white or yellow tumor mass with evident foci of cartilage and calcification found on gross examination (Figs. 16.104 to 16.106). On microscopic examination, the tumor is composed of sheets of small, uniform, round- to spindle-shaped cells that resemble those of Ewing's tumor. The perivascular arrangement of the cells results in a

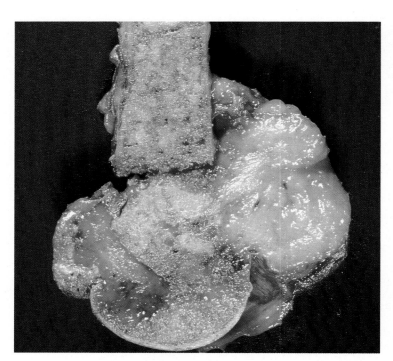

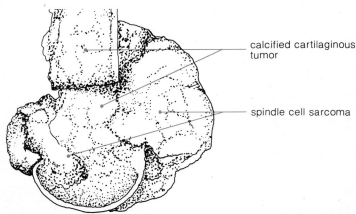

FIGURE 16.101 Gross photograph of the lower end of a femur removed from a patient with a long-standing cartilaginous tumor that had begun to grow rapidly. The transected specimen exhibits a lobulated bluish-gray tissue filling the medullary cavity of the bone. However, at the lower end of the femur, filling the medulla and extending to the soft tissue, a fleshy yellow-tan tumor can be seen. This area proved to be a malignant spindle-cell tumor.

calcified cartilaginous tumor

spindle cell sarcoma

FIGURE 16.102 Specimen radiograph of the malignant spindle-cell tumor shown in Figure 16.101. Although the cartilaginous portion of the tumor is heavily calcified, the dedifferentiated spindle-cell component is entirely radiolucent.

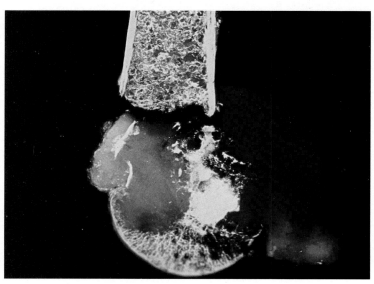

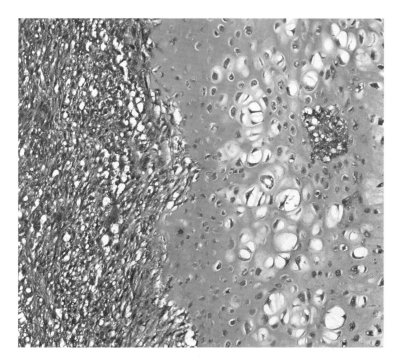

FIGURE 16.103 Photomicrograph of the dedifferentiated spindle-cell tumor that developed in the chondrosarcoma illustrated in Figures 16.101 and 16.102. The spindle-cell tumor has the pattern of a malignant fibrous histiocytoma and is seen here abutting the chondrosarcoma (H & E, x 10 obj.).

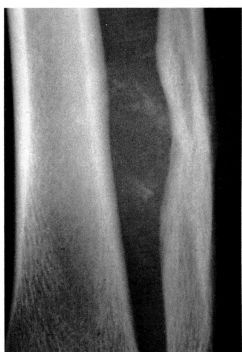

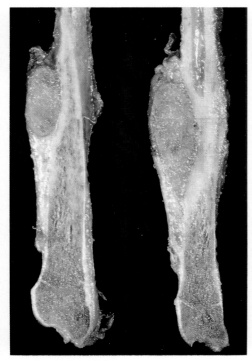

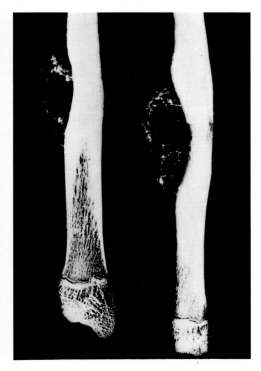

FIGURE 16.104 Clinical radiograph of a young man who presented with leg pain and swelling. A soft-tissue mass is eroding the adjacent bone between the fibula and the tibia. Focal calcification is evident within the tumor mass. In this case, the differential diagnosis would include synovial sarcoma.

FIGURE 16.105 Gross photograph of the resected specimen from the patient in Figure 16.104 shows a soft-tissue tumor eroding the cortex of the adjacent fibula.

FIGURE 16.106 Specimen radiograph of the lesion shown in Figure 16.105. Focal calcification is seen, particularly at the periphery of the lesion.

hemangiopericytoma pattern of the cellular component. The characteristic feature of these lesions is the biphasic pattern, and a mesenchymal chondrosarcoma has focal admixed areas of cartilaginous or chondroid matrix arranged in a lobular pattern (Figs. 16.107 and 16.108)

Mesenchymal chondrosarcoma metastasizes primarily to the lungs, but osseous and soft-tissue metastases have been documented.

CLEAR-CELL CHONDROSARCOMA

Clear-cell chondrosarcoma, considered by some to represent an aggressive variant of chondroblastoma, is a very rare, destructive low-grade malignant tumor which presents in adults. It affects the epiphyseal ends of long bones, most often the upper femur. On radiographs, these tumors are well-circumscribed mixed lucent and sclerotic defects, often with a thin sclerotic

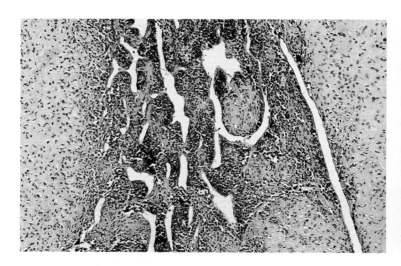

FIGURE 16.107 Photomicrograph of a portion of a mesenchymal chondrosarcoma showing nodules of cellular chondroid tissue on either side and between a vascular cellular tumor (H & E, x 4 obj.).

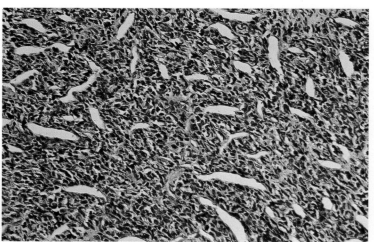

FIGURE 16.108 Higher-power photomicrograph of the cellular vascular component shown in Figure 16.107. Note the small closely packed spindle cells surrounding the vascular spaces and resembling the pattern of a hemangiopericytoma (H & E, x 40 obj.).

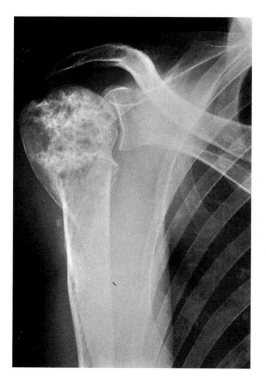

FIGURE 16.109 Radiograph of a 35-year-old man with a 7-year history of pain in the right shoulder. The patient was seen because of acute pain secondary to a pathologic fracture. There is extensive replacement of the cancellous bone by a calcified tumor which is extending to the articular surface. (Courtesy of Dr. Takeo Matsuno)

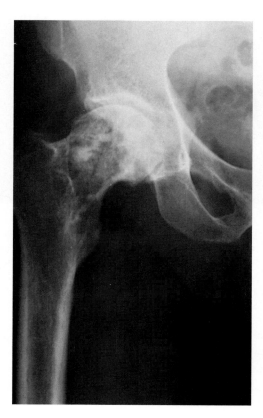

FIGURE 16.110 Radiograph of the right hip in a middle-aged man with a long-term history of pain in the hip, who recently developed acute pain due to pathologic fracture. A heavily calcified tumor involves a good deal of the femoral head and neck. No soft-tissue extension is evident.

border (Figs. 16.109 to 16.112) and scattered calcification. They are most likely to be diagnosed radiologically as chondroblastoma.

On histologic examination, a clear-cell chondrosarcoma contains many cells with abundant clear, vacuolated cytoplasm, which often lie between heavily calcified trabeculae of cartilage matrix that may superficially resemble bone. Frequently, scattered giant cells are seen and, between the cells, a scant chondroid matrix (Figs. 16.113 and 16.114). The vacuolated clear cells may suggest the presence of a renal-cell carcinoma, but the scattered giant cells and the scant chondroid matrix should help to differentiate that lesion from a clear-cell chondrosarcoma.

Clear-cell chondrosarcomas are locally aggressive, and metastases have been reported.

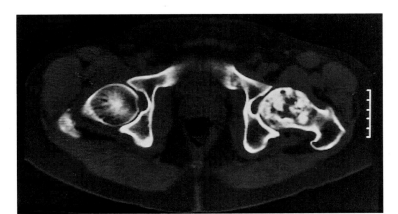

FIGURE 16.111 Computerized axial tomogram through the body of the lesion illustrated in Figure 16.110 demonstrates the focal character of the calcification within the lesion.

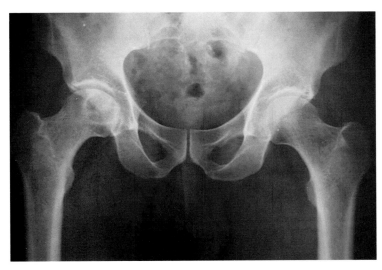

FIGURE 16.112 Radiograph of the pelvis of the patient shown in Figures 16.110 and 16.111, taken 13 years previously, shows a clearly defined lytic lesion which is mostly confined to the right capital femoral epiphysis.

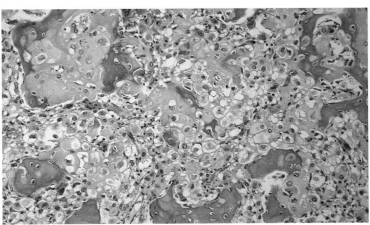

FIGURE 16.113 Photomicrograph demonstrating the typical histology of a clear-cell chondrosarcoma. Note the crowded vacuolated cells, with minimal cartilage matrix between them and scattered foci of bone embedded within the lesional tissue (H & E, x 10 obj.).

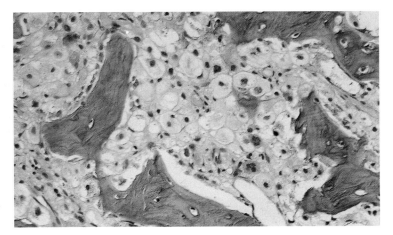

FIGURE 16.114 Higher-power photomicrograph from a clear-cell chondrosarcoma shows the clear vacuolated cytoplasm of the tumor cells typical of the lesion, together with occasional giant cells (H & E, x 40 obj.).

**Neoplasms: benign and
malignant; fibrous,
small cell and others**

I n this chapter, both cellular neoplasms and neoplasms in which there is an extracellular matrix of a simple fibrous character are considered.

DESMOPLASTIC FIBROMA

Desmoplastic fibroma is a rare, intraosseous, collagen-producing fibrous tumor which is well differentiated and is characterized clinically by pain. The tumor usually arises in patients during the first three decades of life, and most commonly develops towards the end of a long bone or in the pelvis. Most radiographs reveal a lucent defect which may expand the cortex and on occasion has a trabeculated appearance (Fig. 17.1). In some cases there may be cortical destruction simulating malignant tumor. Microscopically, the most prominent features are interlacing bundles of dense collagen. The cells are usually sparse and exhibit no cytologic atypia (Fig. 17.2). The histologic similarity of desmoplastic fibroma to certain fibrous lesions elsewhere (such as palmar fibromatosis and desmoid tumors) suggests that it is an intraosseous counterpart of those lesions (Fig. 17.3). The tumor has a tendency to recur locally but does not metastasize. The lack of bone production in this lesion characteristically distinguishes it from fibro-osseous lesions of bone, including fibrous dysplasia and ossifying fibroma.

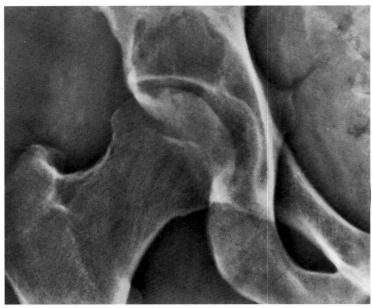

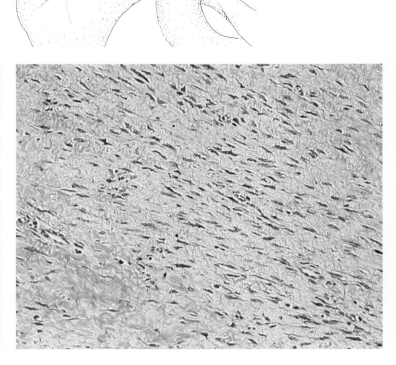

FIGURE 17.1 Radiograph of a young adult patient who complained of pain in the hip joint reveals a large lytic defect in the ilium, just above the acetabulum. The margins of the lesion are fairly well defined, without obvious sclerosis. On curettage, this lesion proved to be a densely fibrous tumor, characterized microscopically as a desmoplastic fibroma.

lytic lesion

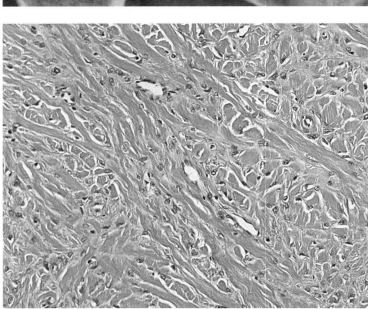

FIGURE 17.2 Low-power photomicrograph of a desmoplastic fibroma shows the dense, collagenized matrix of this lesion (H & E, x 10 obj.).

FIGURE 17.3 Photomicrograph of another area of desmoplastic fibroma which is somewhat more cellular than that seen in Figure 17.2. Note the innocuous appearance of the fibroblasts and the extensive collagen production (H & E, x 10 obj.).

FIBROSARCOMA

Fibrosarcoma is a rare, malignant spindle-cell neoplasm which produces a sparse collagen matrix and has no other matrix differentiation. The lesion usually occurs in the metaphyseal ends of the long bones, especially around the knees, in adults who are usually between 20 and 60 years of age. Pain or swelling in the affected area is frequently exacerbated by a pathologic fracture. About a quarter of the reported cases are associated with a preexisting condition such as Paget's disease, fibrous dysplasia, or an irradiated giant-cell tumor.

On radiographic examination, fibrosarcomas appear as lucent lesions, often with cortical destruction and, at the time of presentation, extension into soft tissue. The involved bone often has a mottled or motheaten pattern. Bone margins are irregular (Fig. 17.4). On gross examination the tumor is usually discrete, grayish-white, and rubbery (Fig. 17.5). On microscopic examination, fibrosarcomas are found to be either well or poorly differentiated. The well-differentiated lesions contain homogeneous spindle-shaped fibroblasts with ovoid nuclei, relatively little pleomorphism, and infrequent mitoses (Fig. 17.6). The tumor matrix usually has

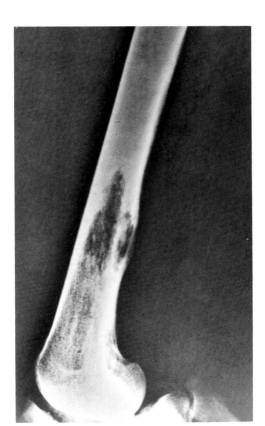

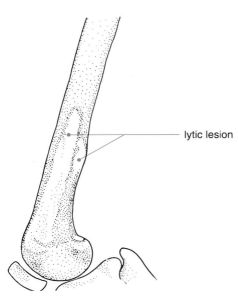

lytic lesion

FIGURE 17.4 Radiograph of the lateral aspect of the femur in a 40-year-old man who complained of pain in the lower thigh shows an intramedullary lytic area extending into the posterior cortex. The margin is ill-defined, and the lesion has at its periphery a permeative appearance. On biopsy, this lesion proved to be a fibrosarcoma.

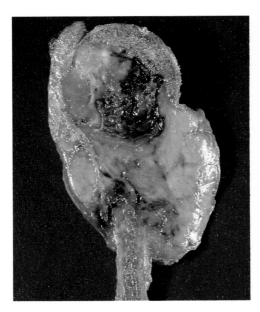

FIGURE 17.5 Photograph of a transected humerus shows a solid tumor at the upper end of the humerus, extending into the soft tissue. Focal hemorrhage is evident. When examined histologically, this tumor proved to be a fibrosarcoma.

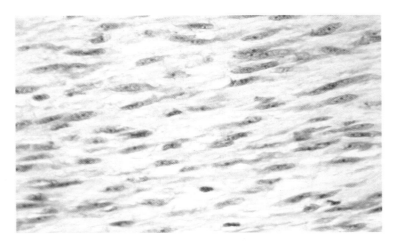

FIGURE 17.6 Most fibrosarcomas of bone are well differentiated, as seen in this high-power view. On low power, this type of lesion shows a characteristic herringbone pattern (H & E, x 25 obj.).

a characteristic "herringbone" pattern (Fig. 17.7). Poorly differentiated tumors are considerably more crowded with pleomorphic cells, abundant mitotic activity, and bizarre hyperchromatic nuclei (Fig. 17.8). Whereas well-differentiated tumors grow slowly, a poorly differentiated fibrosarcoma metastasizes to the lung early in its course. The treatment of choice is radical surgical excision with adjuvant radiation therapy.

The differential diagnosis of primary fibrosarcoma should include metastatic carcinoma, which may demonstrate a spindle-cell pattern (eg, carcinoma of the kidney), and metastatic melanoma.

It should be noted that sarcomas arising in patients with chronic, long-standing osteomyelitis, Paget's disease, irradiated bone, bone infarcts, or giant-cell tumors following radiation may also have a predominantly malignant spindle-cell appearance. However, the pattern is more likely to be that of a malignant fibrous histiocytoma.

MALIGNANT FIBROUS HISTIOCYTOMA

Malignant fibrous histiocytoma is a malignant sarcoma characterized by a heterogeneous population of pleomorphic spindle cells organized in a characteristic storiform or "starry-night" pattern, which was first described about 30 years ago. In the older literature, cases of this type were usually classified as undifferentiated sarcoma, malignant giant-cell tumor, liposarcoma, or osteosarcoma. When it occurs in bone, this tumor primarily affects adults, who may be of any age, and usually involves the lower femur or upper tibia.

On radiographs, malignant fibrous histiocytoma appears as a poorly delineated lucent defect, often with cortical destruction. Minimal periosteal new bone formation may be evident (Fig. 17.9). In some cases this tumor has been found in association with a preexisting bone infarct (Figs. 17.10 to 17.13).

The characteristic microscopic features of malignant fibrous histiocytoma are bundles and whorls of

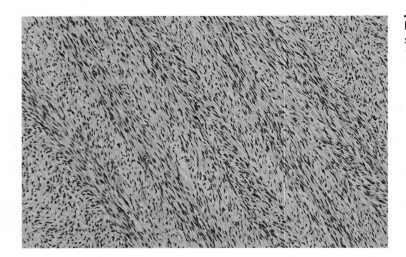

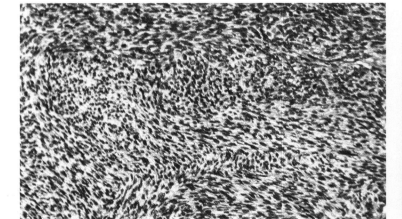

FIGURE 17.8 Photomicrograph of a poorly differentiated fibrosarcoma shows the cell crowding and pleomorphism typically associated with this lesion (H & E, x 10 obj.).

FIGURE 17.7 Photomicrograph of a fibrosarcoma clearly demonstrates the typical herringbone pattern of these lesions (H & E, x 10 obj.).

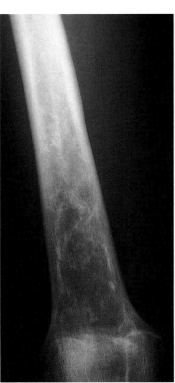

FIGURE 17.9 Radiograph of the lower femur in a man with a long history of pain recently increasing in intensity. This extensive lytic and sclerotic lesion proved on biopsy to be a malignant fibrous histiocytoma.

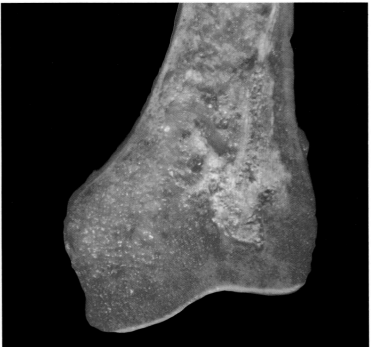

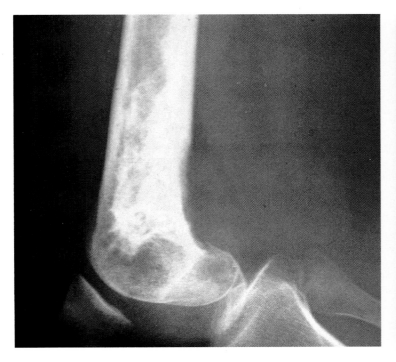

FIGURE 17.10 Radiograph of the femur in a patient with a long-standing history of bone infarction resulting from his being a caisson worker. Recently, the patient had experienced severe pain in the lower end of the femur, and on the radiograph a lytic area can be discerned at the lower end of the infarcted zone.

FIGURE 17.11 Photograph of the transected specimen of the femur removed from the patient in Figure 17.10. The infarcted bone, seen as an area of opaque yellow tissue, is clearly delineated from the surrounding normal bone. The lower end of the femur exhibits admixed, fleshy gray tissue which, on microscopic examination, proved to be a malignant tumor.

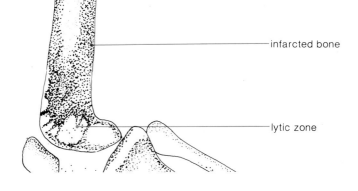

— infarcted bone

— lytic zone

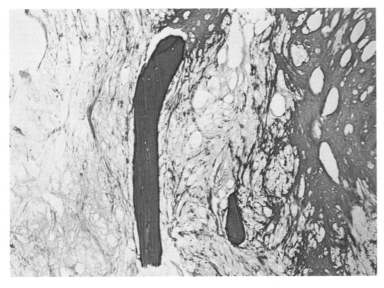

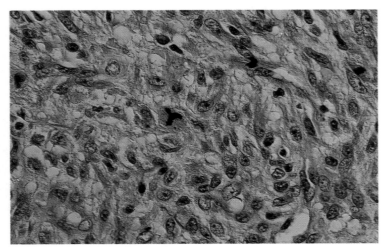

FIGURE 17.12 Photomicrograph of the infarcted area of the lesion illustrated in Figures 17.10 and 17.11 (H & E, x 4 obj.).

FIGURE 17.13 Photomicrograph of a portion of the fleshy tumor shown in Figure 17.11 demonstrates the pleomorphic cellular pattern of the tumor, with vacuolated cytoplasm and, in the center, a tripolar mitosis (H & E, x 40 obj.).

pleomorphic spindle-shaped cells with patchy or extensive reticulin fiber production. The cells and fibers often meet at right angles, and sometimes take on a pinwheel (storiform) pattern (Fig. 17.14). Foci of rounded cells with foamy or vacuolated cytoplasm may be observed, as well as giant-cells and multiple, often atypical, mitotic figures. There is often evidence of phagocytosed intracytoplasmic material, including hemosiderin, hematin, and lipofuchsin pigments. An infiltration of chronic inflammatory cells is characteristically present. The complicated microscopic appearance of the tumor is best understood in light of evidence supporting a pluripotential cell that has features of both a macrophage (hence "histiocyte") and a collagen-producing cell (hence "fibroblast").

Although malignant fibrous histiocytoma is not as aggressive as osteosarcoma, it is a fully malignant and metastasizing tumor, and radical treatment is recommended.

Rare instances of multicentricity have been reported.

GIANT-CELL TUMOR

Giant-cell tumor of bone is a locally aggressive neoplasm most commonly seen in the epiphyseal ends of long bones (usually the lower end of the femur, the upper end of the tibia, or the lower end of the radius). In rare cases the jaw or the spine may be involved, and in such cases evidence of preexisting Paget's disease should be sought. This tumor most often occurs in the third and fourth decades of life, and is rare in skeletally immature subjects. Females are affected about one and a half times more frequently than males. Affected individuals may complain of pain, show signs of local swelling, or have a pathologic fracture through the lesion.

Radiographs reveal a well-defined defect in the metaphysis and epiphysis which is usually eccentrically located and extends to the subchondral bone end plate of the articular surface. There is usually no evidence of sclerosis around the lesion (Figs. 17.15 and 17.16).

The unaltered lesional tissue appears rather homogeneous, with a tan color and a moderately firm consistency (Fig. 17.17). However, foci of hemorrhage and/or necrosis may be observed in many tumors.

The microscopic features of the tumor include a background of proliferating, homogeneous mononuclear cells. These have a round to ovoid shape, relatively large nuclei with inconspicuous nucleoli, and display multinucleated giant cells dispersed evenly throughout the tissue (Figs. 17.18 and 17.19). In some cases, foci of reactive bone are also present, particularly at the periphery of the tumor (Fig. 17.20). In other areas,

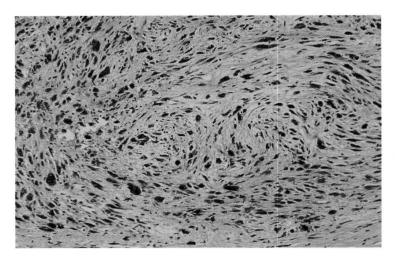

FIGURE 17.14 Photomicrograph of a malignant fibrous histiocytoma demonstrating the marked nuclear pleomorphism, with giant-cell forms and the typical storiform or "starry-night" pattern (H & E, x 25 obj.).

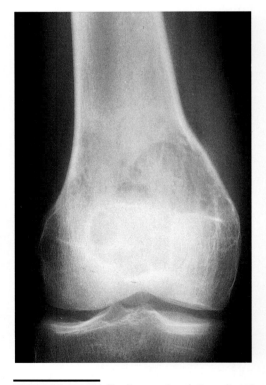

FIGURE 17.15 Radiograph of the distal femur and knee joint of a 30-year-old woman with complaints of pain shows a sharply demarcated lytic and eccentric lesion involving the epiphysis and metaphysis in a manner characteristic of a giant-cell tumor.

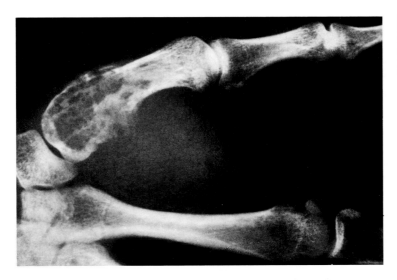

FIGURE 17.16 Radiograph of a lytic lesion in the proximal end of the first metacarpal bone, through which there has been a pathologic fracture. On biopsy, this lesion proved to be a conventional giant-cell tumor.

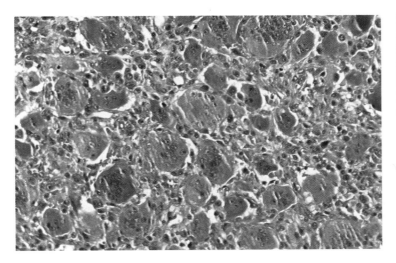

FIGURE 17.17 Photograph of the transected specimen removed from the patient in Figure 17.16. The pinkish-tan soft tissue seen here is typical of a giant-cell tumor.

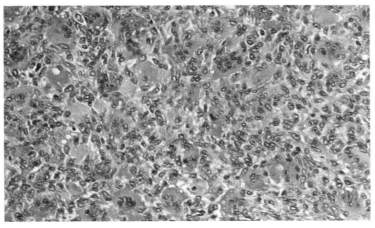

FIGURE 17.18 Photomicrograph of a conventional giant-cell tumor reveals the cellular nature of the lesion and the giant cells that are evenly distributed throughout (H & E, x 10 obj.).

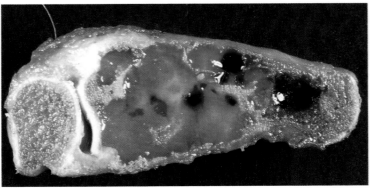

FIGURE 17.19 Photomicrograph demonstrates the homogeneous, mononuclear stromal cells and the evenly distributed multinucleated giant-cells. However, compared with the previous photomicrograph the giant cells here are much larger. (The presence of giant cells alone does not confirm the diagnosis of giant-cell tumor. Many lesions contain giant cells; it is the combination of mononuclear stromal cells and giant cells that is diagnostic of giant-cell tumor.) (H & E, x 10 obj.)

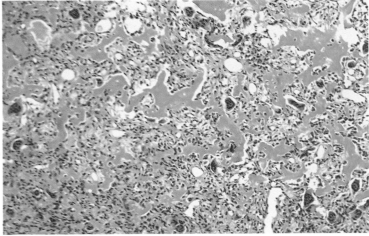

FIGURE 17.20 Photomicrograph demonstrating irregular and extensive bone formation in the periphery of an otherwise typical conventional giant-cell tumor (H & E, x 10 obj.).

involutional changes with lipid-filled histiocytes may be observed (Fig. 17.21).

Multicentric lesions have been reported but are very rare. Although malignant degeneration is also rare, it occurs in about 10 percent of irradiated lesions after five to eight years. The histologic features of malignant degeneration include crowding of the cell stroma, marked atypia, and increased mitotic activity, usually with atypical forms (Fig. 17.22). Many cases that in the past were diagnosed as malignant giant-cell tumor would probably now be classified as malignant fibrous histiocytoma. In order to confidently diagnose a lesion as malignant giant-cell, tumor foci of conventional giant-cell tumors should be identified. After curettage, giant-cell tumors have a high local recurrence rate (50 percent). Surgical excision is the treatment of choice.

In conventional giant-cell tumors, lung metastases only rarely appear, and can be successfully treated by surgical excision. However, metastases are common in the rare, fully malignant giant-cell tumor.

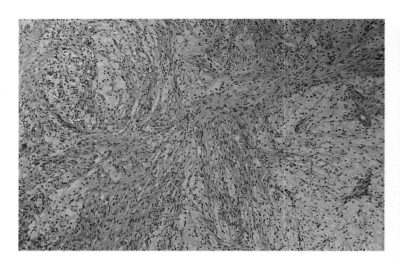

FIGURE 17.21 Photomicrograph of tissue obtained from a giant-cell tumor of long standing shows foci of lipid-laden macrophages, fibrosis, and chronic inflammation. In some cases, especially following fractures, such involutional areas may be widespread (H & E, x 10 obj.).

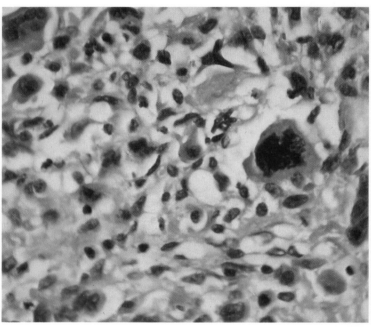

FIGURE 17.22 Photomicrograph of a malignant giant-cell tumor of bone shows marked pleomorphism and nuclear atypia, with sparse atypical giant cells scattered throughout the lesion (H & E, x 40 obj.).

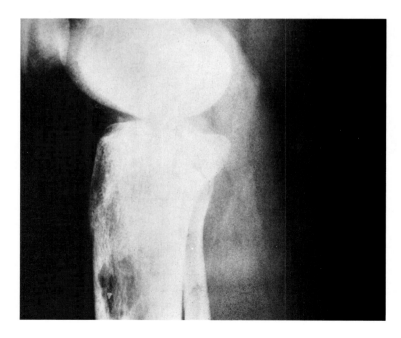

FIGURE 17.23 A 50-year-old man was admitted to the hospital complaining of pain in the upper part of the leg. Lateral radiograph reveals a lytic and permeative lesion in the upper tibia, which on biopsy proved to be a well-differentiated vascular neoplasm.

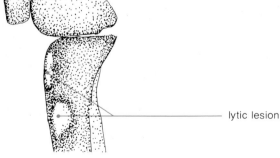

lytic lesion

VASCULAR NEOPLASMS

Vascular neoplasms of bone are rare. They include tumors arising from the endothelium (hemangioendothelioma or angiosarcoma) and tumors arising from the pericytes (hemangiopericytoma). Endothelial tumors vary from differentiated and locally aggressive lesions (hemangioendothelioma) to highly anaplastic, poorly differentiated metastasizing neoplasms (angiosarcoma). The presence of multiple intraosseous lesions at the time of initial diagnosis is common in both well-differentiated and poorly differentiated tumors.

WELL-DIFFERENTIATED ENDOTHELIAL TUMORS

Hemangioendothelioma is a locally aggressive tumor which predominantly affects the long bones in adults. Complaints of pain or swelling are common. These tumors are osteolytic and may be poorly demarcated on radiographs (Fig. 17.23). Periosteal new bone formation is unusual in hemangioendotheliomas. Macroscopically, a multiloculate hemorrhagic tumor mass is typically found (Figs. 17.24 and 17.25).

The tumor is characterized microscopically by anastomosing cords of vascular channels lined with plump endothelial cells which lack pleomorphism or significant mitotic activity. Solid foci of polygonal cells may also be seen (Fig. 17.26).

Wide resection is the treatment of choice. Although these tumors may recur they rarely metastasize.

POORLY DIFFERENTIATED ENDOTHELIAL TUMORS

Angiosarcoma is a fully malignant, metastasizing neoplasm. These tumors are characterized by rapid growth and extensive bone destruction, with erosion of the cortices and extension into soft tissues. Metastases to the lungs and other organs are common. The lesion consists

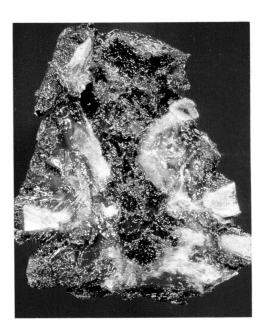

FIGURE 17.24 Gross photograph of the sternum of a patient with a well-differentiated vascular tumor. The tumor has extensively involved the sternum and extends into the adjacent soft tissue.

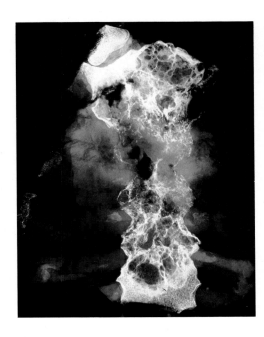

FIGURE 17.25 Specimen radiograph of the tumor shown in Figure 17.24. Note the lytic, destructive character of the tumor.

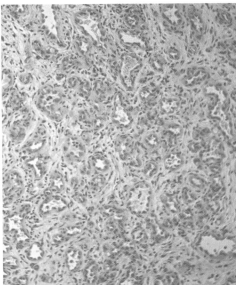

FIGURE 17.26 Photomicrograph of the tumor illustrated in Figures 17.24 and 17.25 shows a fibrous stroma filled with proliferating vascular channels, lined with plump endothelial cells which lack obvious pleomorphism or significant mitotic activity (H & E, x 4 obj.).

of irregular, anastomosing vascular channels lined with malignant cells which exhibit prominent intravascular budding and striking cellular anaplasia with frequent mitoses (Fig. 17.27). Solid undifferentiated areas are often present and may suggest a poorly differentiated carcinoma or an anaplastic lymphoma. As with other sarcomas, foci of necrosis are common. Immunoperoxidase staining for factor VIII may be helpful in some cases.

Radical surgery is the treatment of choice.

HEMANGIOPERICYTOMA

Hemangiopericytoma is a rare, low-grade vascular tumor which occasionally occurs as a primary intraosseous lesion. Patients may present with localized pain. Radiographs are nonspecific and may reveal either lysis or focal sclerosis. Gross examination is likely to show a solid tumor (Figs. 17.28 and 17.29).

The intervascular stroma contains typical spindle-shaped mononuclear cells believed to arise from a perivascular precursor cell (the pericyte) with the characteristics of smooth muscle. The key to the diagnosis of hemangiopericytoma is recognition that the neoplastic cells surround the vascular spaces and are not formed from the endothelial lining cells (Fig. 17.30). This finding can be confirmed by immunoperoxidase or reticulin staining (Fig. 17.31). Because in some cases of mesenchymal chondrosarcoma the predominant pattern may be that of a hemangiopericytoma, it is important to look for evidence of cartilage formation when the diagnosis of hemangiopericytoma is being considered. Since microscopic foci of cartilage have been described in some cases of hemangiopericytoma, the differential diagnosis is sometimes difficult.

Surgery is the treatment of choice; the prognosis is guarded, as metastases may occur.

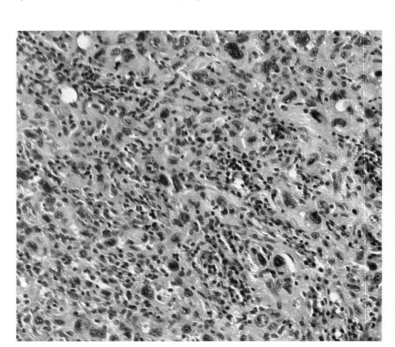

FIGURE 17.27 Photomicrograph of a malignant angiosarcoma of the bone shows the striking pleomorphism of the lesion, with many malignant giant cells. In such a case the true nature of the lesion may be difficult to determine, and the differential diagnosis would include poorly differentiated metastatic carcinoma as well as malignant lymphoma. Reticulin staining would assist in demonstrating the intraluminal position of the malignant cells (H & E, x 10 obj.).

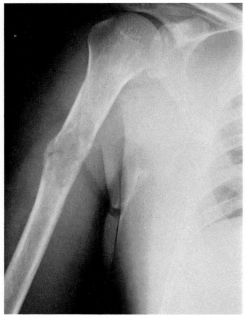

FIGURE 17.28 Radiograph of a 30-year-old male with a one-year history of vague pain in the left arm. A recent acute injury necessitated admission. A well-demarcated lytic lesion of the upper diaphysis is apparent.

EWING'S SARCOMA

Ewing's sarcoma is a small-cell malignant neoplasm of bone which develops in the diaphysis or metaphysis of long bones, most often the femur, tibia, and humerus, as well as in the pelvis, scapulae, ribs, and other bones. It is essentially a tumor of childhood, with most patients being under 20 years of age. Males and females are about equally affected. Ewing's tumors may very rarely arise in soft tissues.

Patients usually complain of pain or tenderness in the affected bone of several weeks' or months' duration. Physical examination may reveal swelling and tenderness. Fever, anemia, leukocytosis, and elevated erythrocyte sedimentation rates often suggest a diagnosis of osteomyelitis and, because of the histologic appearance of the tumor, osteomyelitis is the most important differential diagnosis of Ewing's tumor, not only clinically, but also radiologically as well as histologically.

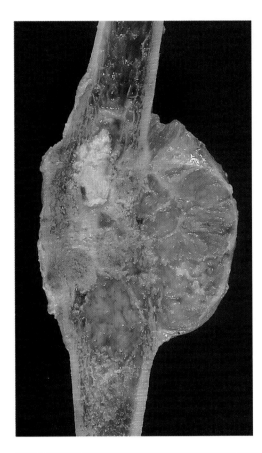

FIGURE 17.29 Section through the resected segment of humerus from the patient in Figure 17.28 shows a fleshy tumor extending into the soft tissue from the intramedullary space. The opaque yellow infarcted area may be related to a past fracture in this area.

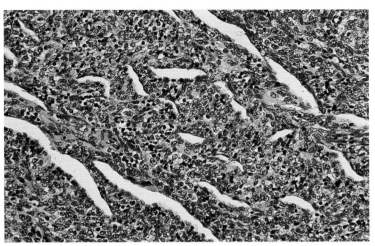

FIGURE 17.30 Photomicrograph of tissue obtained from the case shown in Figures 17.28 and 17.29 shows crowded, uniform round cells surrounding vascular spaces in a pattern characteristic of hemangiopericytoma (H & E, x 25 obj.).

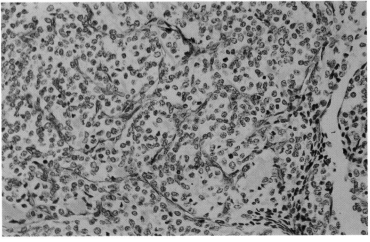

FIGURE 17.31 Photomicrograph of a portion of a hemangiopericytoma stained with Ulex europaeus agglutinin demonstrates the fine capillary network running between the nests of tumor cells (x 40 obj.).

Radiographic examination reveals a lytic, moth-eaten, mottled appearance (Fig. 17.32), or sometimes even sclerosis; classically, laminated periosteal reactive bone is present, likened by some to an onion peel (Fig. 17.33). (However, this onion-peel appearance should not be considered diagnostic of Ewing's tumor.) Bone formation mays in some cases, suggest the radiologic diagnosis of osteosarcoma.

Gross examination of intact specimens reveals poorly demarcated, grayish-white tumor tissue with areas of hemorrhage, cystic degeneration, and necrosis. The actual extent of bone destruction is usually greater than that evident on radiographs, and extension of the tumor into adjacent soft tissue is common.

Ewing's sarcoma consists of a homogeneous population of densely packed small cells. Nuclei are regular and lack prominent nucleoli (Figs. 17.34 and 17.35). The cell wall is indistinct but may be visible on tissue-touch imprints (Fig. 17.36). Mitoses are infrequent. Reticulin fibers are sparse, but glycogen is evident after

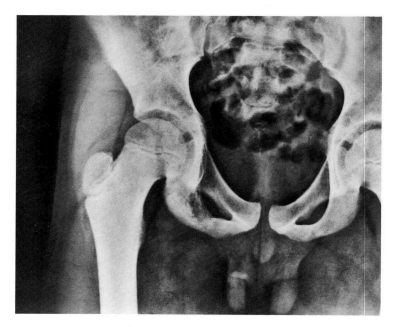

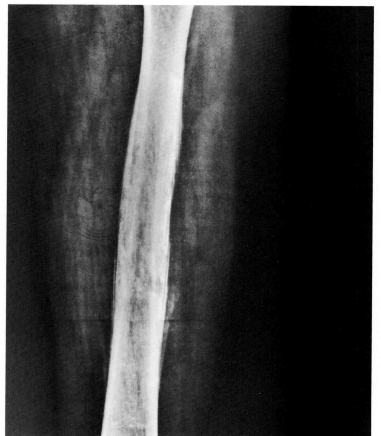

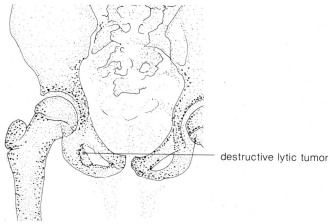

FIGURE 17.32 Radiograph of a 9-year-old child complaining of the pain in the left hip joint shows a permeative destructive lesion of the ischium. Biopsy of this area showed a malignant round-cell tumor consistent with Ewing's sarcoma.

destructive lytic tumor

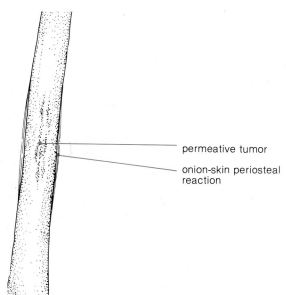

FIGURE 17.33 Radiograph of the femur in a 13-year-old child complaining of pain in the thigh shows an extensive permeative lesion in the midshaft of the femur, with elevation of the overlying periosteum, and periosteal new bone formation which is present in several layers, giving an onion-skin appearance. Ewing's tumors are frequently located in the diaphysis, and in this respect are to be distinguished from osteosarcoma, the other common malignant primary tumor of bone in childhood, which usually occurs in the metaphysis.

permeative tumor

onion-skin periosteal reaction

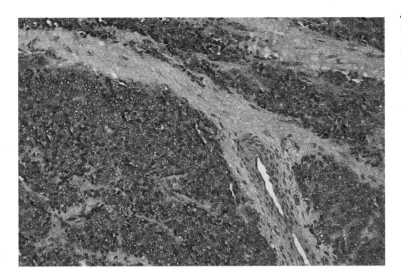

FIGURE 17.34 Photomicrograph of a portion of a Ewing's tumor shows the monotonous, homogeneous cell population with focal, pyknotic nuclei. It is common for the lesion to show extensive necrosis or hemorrhage (H & E, x 10 obj.).

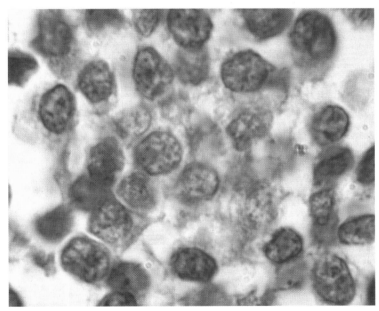

FIGURE 17.35 High-power view of a portion of a Ewing's tumor shows the small round cells and the indistinct lacy appearance of the cytoplasm. Note the lack of prominent nucleoli in these cells (H & E, x 100 obj.).

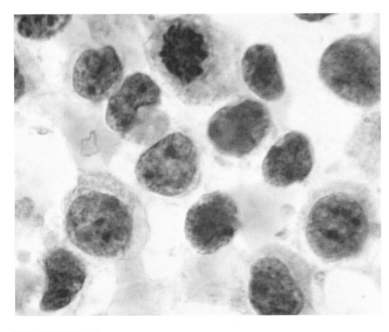

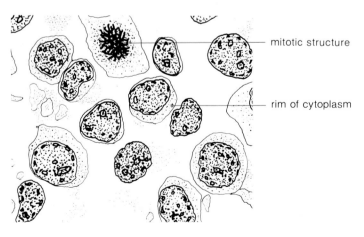

mitotic structure

rim of cytoplasm

FIGURE 17.36 Photomicrograph of a direct imprint of fresh tumor tissue on a glass slide, subsequently stained with hematoxylin and eosin. By this technique, the cytologic detail of the cells is clearly demonstrated. A thin rim of delicate cytoplasm is seen around the vesicular nuclei, which lack any obvious nucleoli. A mitotic structure is noted in the upper part of the field (x 100 obj.).

PAS staining and is usually found to be abundant on ultrastructural examination (Figs. 17.37 and 17.38). Areas of hemorrhage and necrosis are typically present. Although commonly referred to as a "small-cell" tumor, Ewing's cells are actually two to three times larger than lymphocytes.

The microscopic differential diagnosis of Ewing's sarcoma includes osteomyelitis, eosinophilic granuloma, and the group of small-cell tumors that includes lymphoma, leukemia, and metastatic neuroblastoma (and, in the case of soft-tissue Ewing's sarcoma, embryonal rhabdomyosarcoma).

Ewing's sarcoma unfortunately has a high incidence of early metastatic spread, usually to the lungs or to other bones. However, the recent use of adjuvant chemotherapy with radiation and surgical resection has considerably improved the outlook for patients with this tumor.

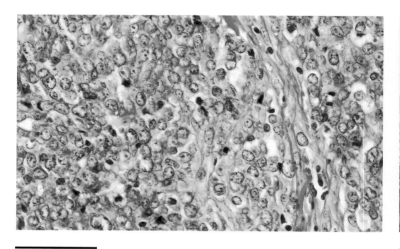

FIGURE 17.37 Photomicrograph of a portion of a Ewing's tumor stained by the PAS method demonstrates glycogen in the cytoplasm of most of the tumor cells (x 40 obj.).

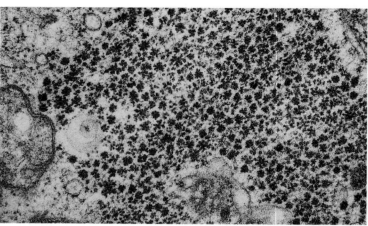

FIGURE 17.38 Electron photomicrograph of a Ewing's sarcoma cell shows the packing of cytoplasm with glycogen granules (x 30,000).

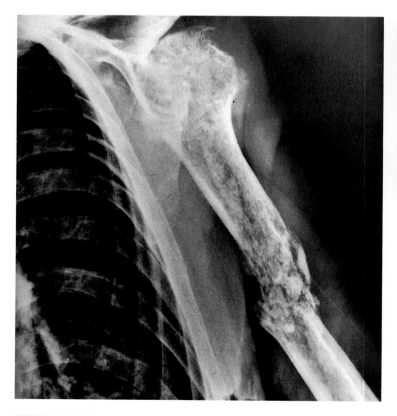

FIGURE 17.39 A 45-year-old man complained of sudden onset of pain in the left arm. Radiograph shows a pathologic fracture through an area of permeative destruction of cortical and medullary bone, which proved to be due to lymphoma. The fracture is recent, and there is little or no periosteal reaction either to the tumor or to the complicating fracture.

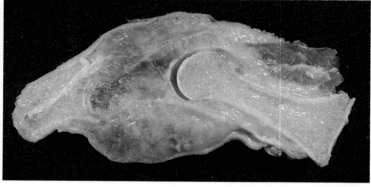

FIGURE 17.40 An amputated toe from a patient with a primary non-Hodgkin's lymphoma of the bone. The middle phalanx has been completely destroyed by a fleshy pink tumor which has extended both dorsally and ventrally into the soft tissue.

LYMPHOMA

In clinical cases of lymphoma, secondary involvement of the bone is present in approximately 20 percent of all patients. Primary intraosseous lymphomas are uncommon, but it is important to recognize that patients with primary bone lymphomas and no systemic involvement have a substantially better prognosis than those with disseminated disease.

The tumor can occur at any age but is rare in patients during the first decade of life (cf, Ewing's sarcoma). Although local pain is usually present at the time of initial evaluation, the overall general health of the patient is good. Early changes on radiographs include vague, mottled lucent areas. Considerable bone destruction may result from long-standing lesions.

PRIMARY NON-HODGKIN'S LYMPHOMA

Primary non-Hodgkin's lymphomas of bone are usually large-cell lymphomas of B-cell origin. At one time, these tumors were generally referred to as reticulum-cell sarcomas. They usually involve the bones of the extremities, and occur mostly in patients over 20 years of age. The characteristic clinical picture is that of a patient in generally good health but with complaints of localized pain, swelling, or tenderness. No fever or marked weight loss is noted in the typical case.

On radiographs, osteolysis is the predominant change observed, with the resulting appearance of a moth-eaten destructive lesion with no periosteal reaction (Fig. 17.39). Gross examination reveals grayish-white tissue infiltrating the bone (Fig. 17.40).

Histologically, the tumor consists of sheets of lymphoid cells with variable nuclear characteristics that depend on the type of lymphoma (Figs. 17.41 to 17.43). Most commonly, primary lesions are composed of a mixture of large cells with irregular cleaved nuclei, large cells with oval nuclei containing prominent nucleoli, and small cells with cleaved, hyperchromatic nuclei. Some lesions have a decidedly spindled appearance and may be difficult to recognize as lymphoma. Secondary lesions usually have a predominance of small cells, regardless of the nodal pattern. The lack of

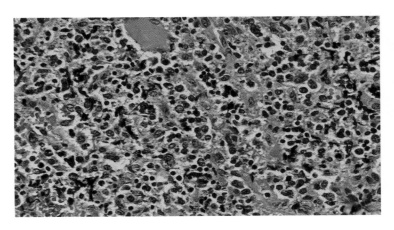

FIGURE 17.41 Low-power photomicrograph of an area of non-Hodgkin's lymphoma shows the crowded irregular cells. At high power these cells frequently show nuclear indentation and clefts. Compared with the cells of Ewing's tumor, these cells are larger and the cytoplasmic borders are more distinct. The cells in a non-Hodgkin's lymphoma usually lack glycogen (H & E, x 10 obj.).

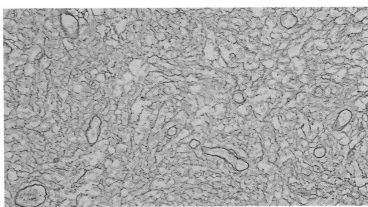

FIGURE 17.42 Reticulin staining of the tumor shown in Figure 17.41 reveals a fine network of reticulum separating small groups of cells as well as individual cells (x 10 obj.).

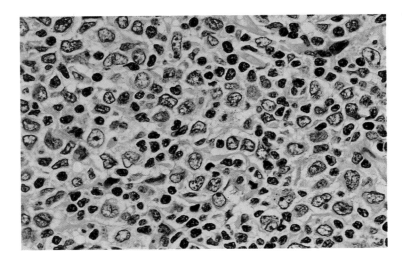

FIGURE 17.43 Photomicrograph of a primary non-Hodgkin's lymphoma in the bone. The crowded cells are larger and more irregular in outline than those seen in Ewing's sarcoma. Note the mixed cell population and the large irregular cleaved cells with prominent nucleoli (H & E, x 50 obj.).

glycogen (indicated by negative PAS staining) and the abundance of reticulin fibers separating each cell help to differentiate most lymphomas from Ewing's sarcoma. In addition to Ewing's tumor, the differential diagnosis includes poorly differentiated metastatic carcinoma, melanoma and, if the tissue is poorly preserved, osteomyelitis.

The treatment of choice is local radiation, with or without chemotherapy depending on the stage.

Rare cases of solitary granulocytic tumors (chloroma) have been described. These are likely to be initially diagnosed as some other form of small-cell sarcoma. Diagnosis depends on demonstration of the typical intracytoplasmic granules by Wright–Giemsa staining and chloracetate esterase staining.

HODGKIN'S DISEASE

Hodgkin's disease is characterized by pain and tenderness, sometimes with a palpable mass. Unlike non-Hodgkin's lymphoma, which is more common in the long bones, Hodgkin's disease may appear anywhere in the skeleton. However, primary osseous involvement is rare. Lesions in the ribs and sternum may result in significant swelling and extension into soft tissues. Vertebral involvement may cause neurologic disorders.

The radiographic features of Hodgkin's disease are variable; lesions may be lytic, blastic, or mixed. The radiologic finding of a solitary, dense "ivory" vertebra is a classic presentation (Fig. 17.44).

Microscopically, a characteristic mixed cell popula-

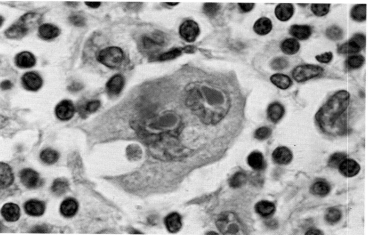

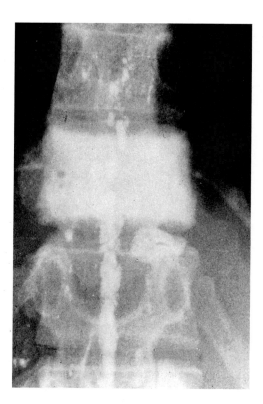

FIGURE 17.44 AP radiograph of a 35-year-old male who presented with vague back pain. A single dense sclerotic vertebra is seen in the lower thoracic spine which, on biopsy, proved to be Hodgkin's disease. In the bone, Hodgkin's disease frequently exhibits considerable marrow fibrosis and reactive bone formation, which may be so severe as to obscure the lymphomatous tissue.

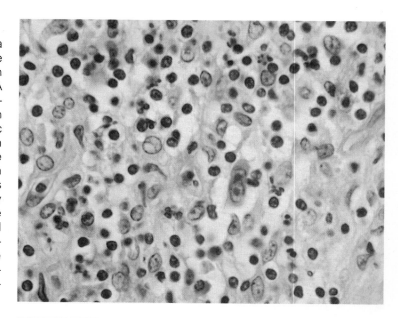

FIGURE 17.45 Photomicrograph of an area of Hodgkin's disease in bone shows a fibrous stroma with mixed cellular infiltrate of small round cells and larger histiocytes (H & E, × 40 obj.).

FIGURE 17.46 High-power photomicrograph demonstrates a binucleate Sternberg–Reed cell with prominent eosinophilic nucleoli (H & E, × 100 obj.).

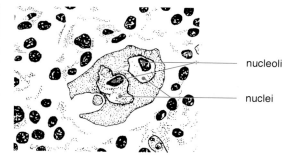

nucleoli

nuclei

tion can be observed, including plasma cells, lymphocytes, histiocytes, and eosinophils (Fig. 17.45). A large amount of fibrous stroma may complicate the diagnostic process, but the pathognomonic finding is the Sternberg–Reed cell. The Sternberg–Reed cell is large, with sharply delineated, abundant cytoplasm and a mirror-image double nucleus with a large, prominent, central eosinophilic nucleolus (Fig. 17.46). Large, irregular mononuclear cells are also present, with similar nuclear pleomorphism and prominent eosinophilic nucleoli. These cells are referred to as "Hodgkin's cells."

LEUKEMIA

Acute lymphocytic leukemia in young patients is often accompanied by bone changes. A characteristic finding in children is a radiolucent band in the metaphysis of the long bones; similar bands may be found in the vertebral bodies just beneath the end plates (Fig. 17.47). However, the most common radiographic finding is dif-

fuse demineralization of the spine with compression fractures, usually seen as anterior wedging. Epidural extension of the tumor is not uncommon in leukemia, and sometimes constitutes the presenting symptom. In addition, replacement of bone marrow by leukemic tissue may lead to ischemic necrosis of the affected bone and bone marrow (Fig. 17.48).

MULTIPLE MYELOMA

Multiple myeloma is the most common primary tumor of bone. The tumor has a predilection for marrow-containing bones and the spine is almost always involved, although the primary presentation may be in the skull, ribs, sternum, or pelvis. This tumor usually affects individuals over the age of 50 but is occasionally seen at a younger age. The usual clinical picture is one in which pain predominates. Anemia is common, the ESR is usually elevated, and occasionally, especially in association with bed rest and concomitant osteoporosis, hypercalcemia is present. The most important diagnos-

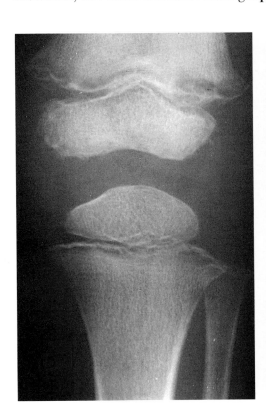

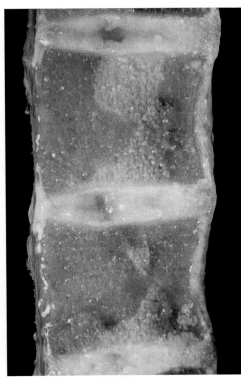

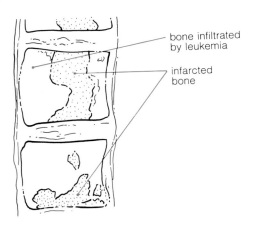

FIGURE 17.48 Photograph of a segment of the spine from a child who died of leukemia. Within the vertebral bodies are geographic areas of necrosis identified as yellow opacification of the bone and marrow. These are surrounded by a thin rim of hyperemic tissue. Note that the viable bone marrow has a fleshy tan color, reflecting the leukemic infiltrate.

bone infiltrated by leukemia

infarcted bone

FIGURE 17.47 Anteroposterior radiograph of the knee in an infant with recent onset of fever, showing a radiolucent zone in the metaphysis adjacent to the growth plate, which is a classic radiologic sign of acute leukemia.

tic test involves the identification of a monoclonal protein by serum electrophoresis (see Fig. 17.49). Light-chain subunits of immunoglobulins (Bence–Jones proteins) are usually found in the urine.

Multiple myeloma is characterized radiographically by the presence of round lytic defects in the bone, with no significant sclerotic reaction surrounding them (Fig. 17.50). Occasionally, however, lytic defects may not be apparent and the radiographic picture suggests a diffuse osteopenia. In such cases, the differential diagnosis from osteoporosis must be made by laboratory examination. Very rarely, multiple myeloma produces sclerotic lesions, such that the correct diagnosis may not at first be considered. In more than half of patients, pathologic fractures lead to an overall loss of vertebral body height, with swelling of the adjacent interverte-bral discs into the affected bodies and a resulting "fish-mouth" appearance (Fig. 17.51).

Gross examination of the affected bones reveals either a diffuse gelatinous red infiltration of the marrow or tan tumor nodules (Figs. 17.52 and 17.53). Microscopic examination reveals sheets of plasma cells, which may exhibit various degrees of differentiation; however, the atypicality of the cells (Fig. 17.54) has no prognostic significance. In approximately 10 percent of patients with myeloma, amyloidosis occurs as a complication and amyloid deposits can be found within the bone (Fig. 17.55).

Multiple myeloma is a strikingly aggressive tumor, usually leading to early death. However, in a few cases palliative chemotherapy and bone marrow transplantation have been effective in prolonging the survival time.

Serum Protein Electrophoresis

	%	NORMAL RANGE
ALBUMIN	32.3	56.4–71.6
ALPHA 1	3.6	1.9–4.5
ALPHA 2	5.3	7.3–15.0
BETA	6.8	6.2–11.5
GAMMA	52.0	7.8–18.2

Quantitative Immunoglobulin

	mg/dL	NORMAL RANGE
IgG	275	600–1450
IgA	2964	60–340
IgM	10.4	25–200

Immunofixation Electrophoresis Gel

SPE   IgG   IgA   IgM   κ   λ

INCREASED IgA LAMBDA PRESENT

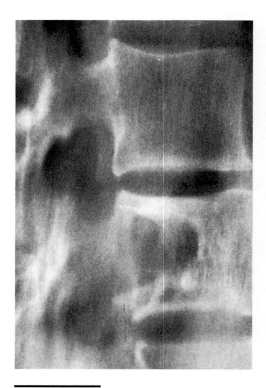

FIGURE 17.49 Immunoelectro-pherogram of the serum from a patient with myeloma. Note that there is an excess of gammaglobulin, which is overwhelmingly IgA (L).

FIGURE 17.50 Lateral tomogram of L2, with parts of L1 and L3, in a 55-year-old male with multple myeloma, demonstrating the well-defined lytic lesions, devoid of significant sclerosis, which are characteristic of this disease.

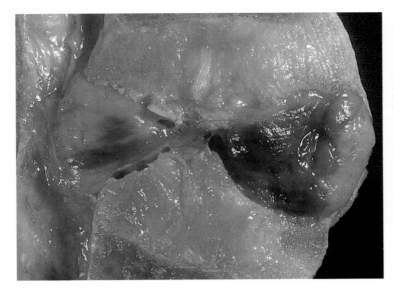

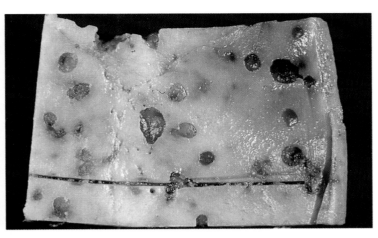

FIGURE 17.52 A portion of the skull removed from a patient with multiple myeloma shows many round defects filled with pinkish-gray tissue.

FIGURE 17.51 Collapse of the fifth lumbar vertebra and replacement by a gelatinous, pinkish-gray tissue is seen in this gross photograph of the lower spine removed at autopsy from a patient with multiple myeloma.

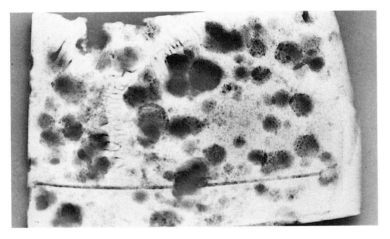

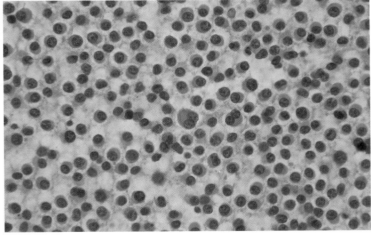

FIGURE 17.53 Radiograph of the portion of skull shown in Figure 17.52 demonstrates the clearly demarcated, lytic, punch-out lesions.

FIGURE 17.54 Photomicrograph of multiple myeloma shows closely packed plasma cells with some variation in shape and size, and an occasional double nucleus (H & E, x 40 obj.).

FIGURE 17.55 In some cases of multiple myeloma, foci of smooth, homogeneous pink material (amyloid) may be found, as shown in this photomicrograph (H & E, x 40 obj.).

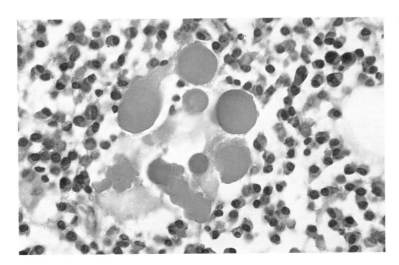

SOLITARY (LOCALIZED) MYELOMA (PLASMACYTOMA)

The occurrence of a large solitary focus of plasma cell proliferation associated with radiologic evidence of bone destruction can be considered a distinct entity from multiple myeloma if the following criteria are met: there are no other radiographically evident lesions; a bone marrow biopsy from a site other than the solitary focus reveals no malignant cells; and no significant protein or immunoglobulin abnormality is discernible in serum and urine analyses (or, if a monoclonal spike is present on serum electrophoresis, this disappears after treatment of the solitary lesion).

Patients who meet these criteria tend to be younger than those with multiple myeloma and have a much better prognosis. The site of involvement is usually a long bone or a vertebral body (or, in exceptional cases is confined to soft tissue). Long-bone lesions may be expansile, and often present with a pathologic fracture (Figs. 17.56 and 17.57).

In the spine, solitary myelomas are quite likely to present with rapidly developing paraplegia and gibbous deformity as a result of vertebral collapse (Fig. 17.58). In fact, paraplegia is much more frequently associated with solitary myeloma than with multiple myeloma, probably because patients with multiple myeloma die before paraplegia can develop. About 70 percent of

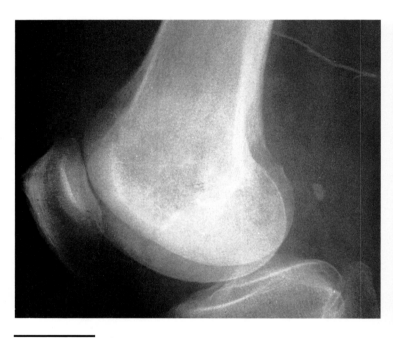

FIGURE 17.56 Radiograph of a 54-year-old man who complained of severe pain in the knee shows a well-demarcated lytic lesion on the femur which, when biopsied, was found to contain only plasma cells.

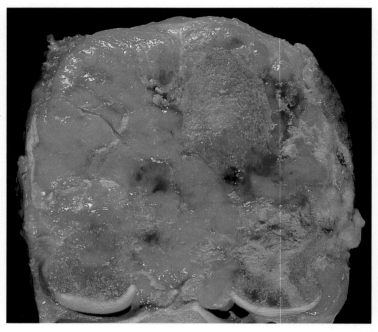

FIGURE 17.57 Gross photograph of the specimen obtained from the patient shown in Figure 17.56. At the time of resection no other evidence of myeloma was present in this patient.

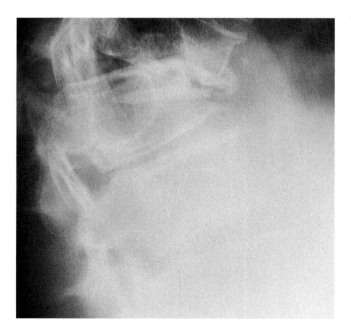

FIGURE 17.58 Lateral radiograph of a 45-year-old male who presented with severe thoracolumbar pain following a fall. A fracture-dislocation of T10 and T12 is demonstrated, with virtual absence of T11. Biopsy of the area showed myeloma. No other sites of myeloma were demonstrated on radiographic survey. The patient received local radiation therapy and a 10-year follow-up showed no evidence of local or generalized disease.

patients who present with an apparently solitary focus of myeloma will develop multiple myelomatosis and will usually die within five years. The remaining patients may be cured after radiation therapy or surgical en bloc resection. A few cases may develop generalized disease only after many years.

ADAMANTINOMA OF LONG BONES

Adamantinoma is a slow-growing neoplasm which usually affects the jaw bones but sometimes occurs in long bones, most often the diaphysis of the tibia. Patients with long bone lesions are usually between 15 and 30 years of age. Males are somewhat more frequently affected than females. The principal clinical sign of adamantinoma is the insidious onset of pain, sometimes developing over many years. The characteristic radiographic finding is a multicystic ("soap-bubble") osteolytic lesion with surrounding sclerosis, cortical thinning, and expansion (Fig. 17.59).

The tumor is generally well circumscribed and rubbery in texture; however, focal areas of hemorrhage or necrosis may be evident on gross inspection. The microscopic finding of a biphasic appearance of spindle-shaped, collagen-producing cells, alternating with sinewy cords or nests of epithelioid cells, is characteristic (Figs. 17.60 and 17.61).

The histogenesis of this tumor is disputed. Epithelial, vascular, and synovial origins have been

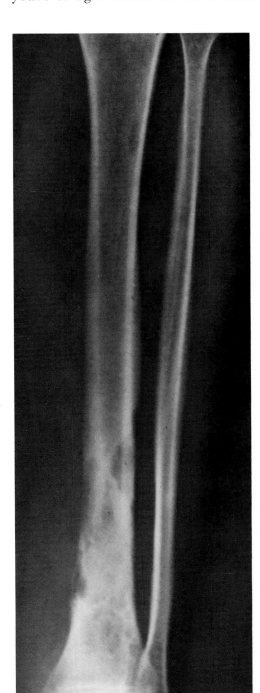

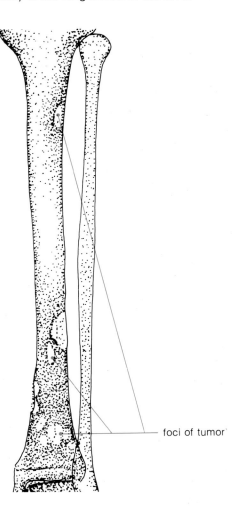

foci of tumor

FIGURE 17.59 Radiograph of the left leg in a young adult patient who complained of an aching leg pain shows multiple lytic lesions in the bone, particularly in the lower third of the diaphysis. The lytic, bubbly appearance of the tumor, together with the presence of satellite lesions, is characteristic of adamantinoma in the tibia. Occasionally, adamantinomas may also be seen in the fibula, and even more rarely in the long bones of the forearm.

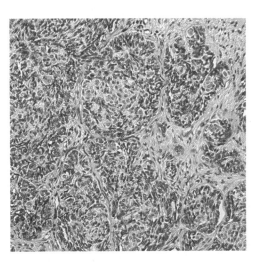

FIGURE 17.60 Photomicrograph of an adamantinoma of the tibia shows a fibrous stroma with islands of basophilic epithelioid cells which may be focally sparse and show cleft-like spaces (as shown in Figure 17.61) (H & E, x 10 obj.).

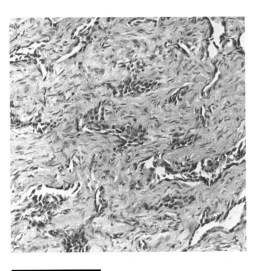

FIGURE 17.61 Photomicrograph of an adamantinoma with a dense fibrous stroma and cleft-like spaces lined with epithelioid cells (H & E, x 25 obj.).

hypothesized, but on the basis of immunoperoxidase studies an epithelial origin is favored. In rare cases adamantinoma has been described in association with foci of fibrous dysplasia elsewhere. Adamantinoma is a neoplasm of low-grade malignancy. It is locally invasive and may metastasize late in its course in about 20 percent of cases.

Treatment of adamantinoma consists of adequate surgical excision; the margins of resection should be carefully planned if recurrence is to be avoided, because satellite lesions may occur at some distance from the major tumor mass (Fig. 17.62).

SYNOVIAL SARCOMA (MALIGNANT SYNOVIOMA)

Synovial sarcomas are rare malignant neoplasms of unknown histogenesis which involve soft tissue around the joints (Fig. 17.63). Although usually sharply circumscribed, these tumors may extend along fascial planes and invade bone. Only a very small percentage of the lesions directly involve the synovium.

Patients with synovial sarcoma present with pain or with a slow-growing mass. Most tumors are located in the lower extremity; the major sites of involvement are

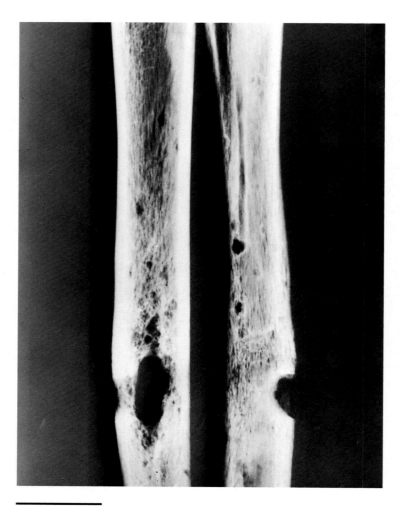

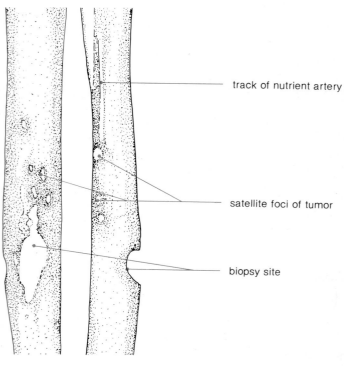

track of nutrient artery

satellite foci of tumor

biopsy site

FIGURE 17.62 Anteroposterior *(left)* and lateral *(right)* radiographs of a portion of the tibial diaphysis removed from a 9-year-old boy with adamantinoma of the tibia. Small punch-out lesions not connected with the main tumor mass are clearly evident; on histologic examination, each of these lesions contained tumor. When such satellite lesions are found, radical resection is necessary if recurrence is to be avoided.

the knee joint, the foot, and the thigh. Affected individuals are usually in their third or fourth decade of life; this tumor is decidedly rare in children. A lobulated soft-tissue shadow may be seen on radiographs, and irregular spotty calcification is often evident (Fig. 17.64). Although the lesion may grossly appear to be encapsulated, on microscopic examination it usually exhibits diffuse infiltration of the surrounding tissues.

The tumor has a rubbery consistency and may contain evidence of hemorrhage and cysts. Calcifications are usually visible on gross examination.

On histologic examination, synovial sarcoma displays a biphasic pattern of pleomorphic spindle cells and well-differentiated cuboidal to columnar cells forming gland-like spaces (Fig. 17.65). The glandular zone contains mucus-like material which stains posi-

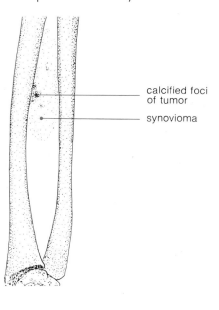

FIGURE 17.64 Radiograph of a young adult patient who complained of pain and swelling in the right arm reveals a soft-tissue mass lying between the radius and the ulna; focal areas of calcification are apparent within this mass. On biopsy, this lesion proved to be a synovioma.

calcified foci of tumor

synovioma

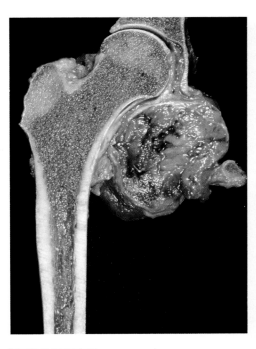

FIGURE 17.63 Transected gross specimen of the upper end of the femur and acetabulum shows a soft-tissue solid tumor abutting against the neck of the femur. Histologically, this tumor proved to be a synovioma. (Typically, synoviomas do not involve the joint space.)

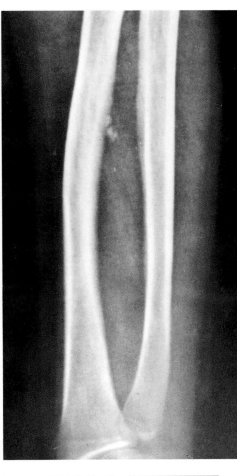

FIGURE 17.65 Photomicrograph of a malignant synovioma demonstrates the biphasic appearance of such lesions. Glandlike spaces lined with tall columnar cells are seen, as well as a fibrosarcomatous stroma. The ratio of these two components may vary considerably (H & E, x 25 obj.).

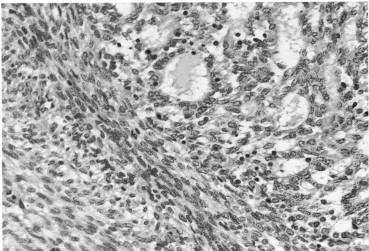

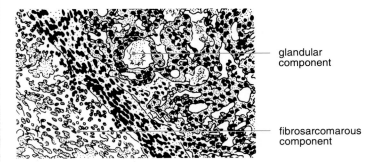

glandular component

fibrosarcomarous component

tively with PAS. Microscopic calcifications are usually found. Synovial sarcoma has a high rate of local recurrence, as well as metastasis.

Recently, attention has been given to malignant soft-tissue tumors with a monophasic pattern (Fig. 17.66). These tumors are characterized by a malignant spindle-cell population but they lack the gland-forming components typically seen in classic synovial sarcoma.

Some clinicians report a poorer prognosis for patients with the so-called monophasic variant of synovial sarcoma.

The histogenesis of synovial sarcoma remains obscure, and although the name implies origin from synovial lining cells, true intra-articular synovial sarcomas are decidedly rare.

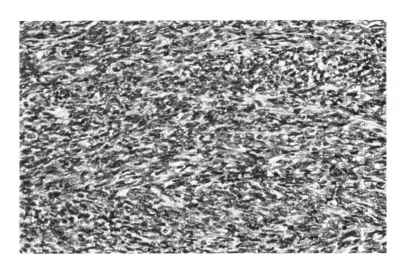

FIGURE 17.66 Occasionally, soft-tissue lesions with the clinical presentation of a malignant synovioma have a histologic appearance similar to that demonstrated in this photomicrograph. A cellular spindle-cell tumor is evident, without any of the biphasic glandular pattern seen in conventional synoviomas, leading some authors to designate these lesions as monophasic synoviomas (They may also be considered poorly differentiated spindle-cell tumors.) (H & E, x 10 obj.)

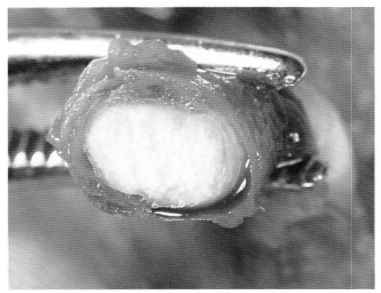

FIGURE 17.67 In this patient with an epithelioid sarcoma, the tumor initially arose in the distal portion of the tendon sheath of the extensor policis longus. At amputation, as demonstrated in this photograph, the tumor was found to be in the subsynovial space, wrapping around tendon.

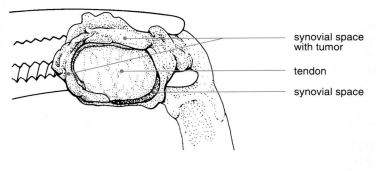

synovial space with tumor

tendon

synovial space

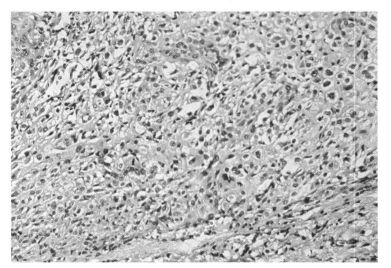

FIGURE 17.68 Photomicrograph of an epithelioid sarcoma shows plump, oval to polyhedral cells which have a dense eosinophilic cytoplasm. The predominant pattern here is epithelial, but in other areas a spindle fibrosarcomatous appearance can be expected (H & E, x 25 obj.).

EPITHELIOID SARCOMA

Epithelioid sarcoma is a fully malignant, painless soft-tissue sarcoma. These lesions occur in the superficial or deep tendon sheaths (Fig. 17.67) of the hand, wrist, or fingers, but may also extend to involve the skin. The histogenesis of this neoplasm remains obscure, but a synovial origin has been suggested.

On microscopic examination, epithelioid sarcoma is a nodular growth composed of a densely eosinophilic polyhedral cell population with prominent nucleoli and an epithelial appearance (Fig. 17.68). Pleomorphism is variable, and central necrosis may be evident. These tumors have a tendency to recur and may disseminate via the lymphatic and vascular systems, eventually leading to lung metastases.

Because of the histologic appearance of epithelioid sarcoma, the differential diagnosis includes a benign reactive granuloma. The treatment of choice is wide excision.

PIGMENTED VILLONODULAR SYNOVITIS (GIANT-CELL TUMOR OF TENDON SHEATH; BENIGN SYNOVIOMA)

Pigmented villonodular synovitis (PVNS) is a locally aggressive synovial tumor which affects both large joints and tendon sheaths. The most common sites involved are the knee or fingers, but this tumor sometimes occurs in the hip, ankle, toe, or wrist. The lesion is usually painless or only mildly painful; the pain appears to be more severe when the lesion is clinically diffuse throughout a major joint. In general, the condition is confined to a single joint or tendon sheath. (These nodules may also be discovered as an incidental finding at surgery, but this presentation is rare.)

The radiologic signs of PVNS depend on the site of occurrence. In the finger, only soft-tissue swelling may be evident, although cortical bone erosion may occur (Figs. 17.69 to 17.72). In the knee, the only consistent radiographic change is soft-tissue swelling in and

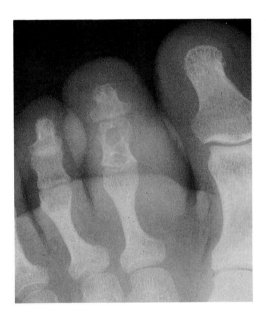

FIGURE 17.69 Radiograph of the foot in a middle-aged male with a swelling of the second toe shows, in addition to a soft-tissue mass, several intraosseous lytic areas in the middle phalanx.

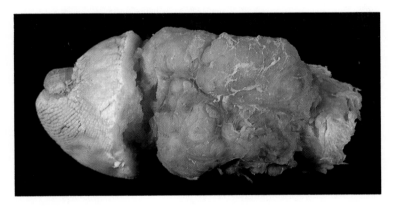

FIGURE 17.70 Lateral view of the amputated second toe in the patient shown in Figure 17.69 shows a tan tumor enveloping the bone.

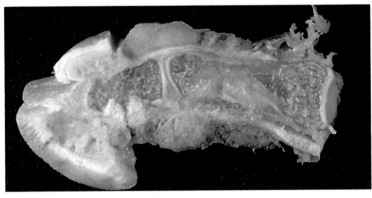

FIGURE 17.71 Gross photograph of a section through the specimen shown in Figure 17.70. A soft-tissue tumor can be seen extending around and involving the distal interphalangeal joint. The lesion is also invading the medullary cavity of the phalanx. Focally, the tumor has a tan color. Histologically, this lesion proved to be PVNS.

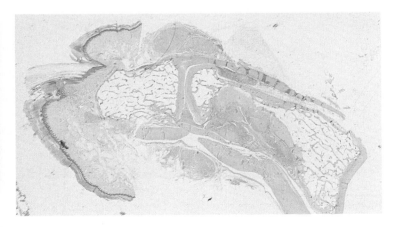

FIGURE 17.72 Photomicrograph of a sagittal section through the toe shown in Figure 17.71. Tumor tissue is seen both in the soft tissue and invading the bone and joint space. The pinker areas within the tumor tissue represent areas of collagenization (phloxine and tartrazine, x 1 obj.).

around the joint, which may be massive. In the hip, joint narrowing and lytic defects in the bone may be present on both sides of the joint (Figs. 17.73 and 17.74). Local juxta-articular bone destruction may also be prominent in joints such as the wrist and ankle.

On gross examination, the lesion is usually solitary and well circumscribed when it occurs in the tendon sheath of a finger (Fig. 17.75). In the knee joint it may consist of multiple nodules, often with dramatic associated hyperplastic villous changes in the synovium and extensive hemosiderin deposition (Fig. 17.76). The lesions tend to have a tan color, which is often more

prominent at the periphery.

On microscopic examination, the lesion is composed of proliferating, collagen-producing polyhedral cells, often with scattered, multinucleated giant cells (Figs. 17.77 and 17.78). Iron deposits and aggregates of foam cells may be present, but these are usually seen in the periphery of the lesion and are most consistent with secondary changes following hemorrhage into the lesion (Fig. 17.79). Abundant production of collagen may be evident in patients with long-standing disease (Fig. 17.80). Occasionally, the cellularity of the lesion, associated with a trabecular pattern, may give a pseudosar-

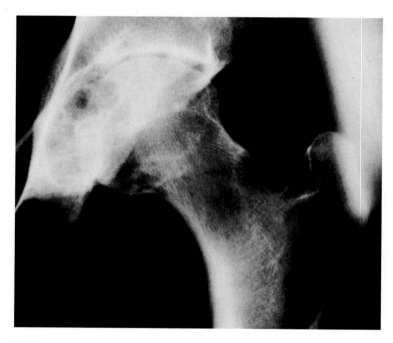

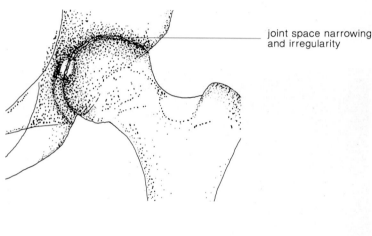

joint space narrowing and irregularity

FIGURE 17.73 Radiograph of a young woman with a history of rapid deterioration of function in the hip shows destructive changes on both sides of the joint, with marked narrowing of the joint space. Because of these radiographic findings, a diagnosis of tuberculosis was considered; however, at surgery abundant hemosiderotic synovium containing nodular fleshy areas was found.

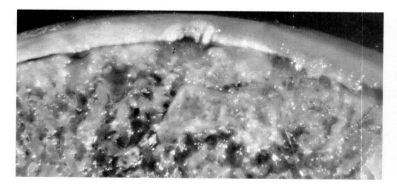

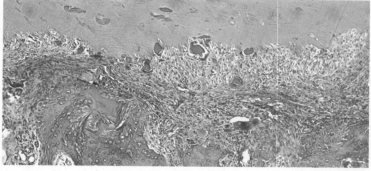

FIGURE 17.74 Gross section of the femoral head *(left)* reveals dissection of the articular cartilage, with proliferation of soft tissue between the bone and cartilage. Histologic section of this tissue *(right)* reveals proliferating mononuclear cells and giant cells in the subchondral bone. A diagnosis of PVNS was confirmed in this patient (H & E, x 10 obj.).

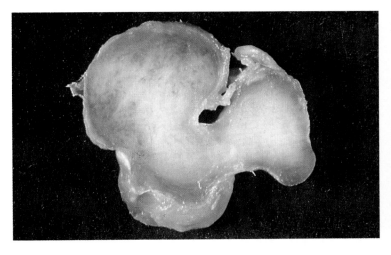

FIGURE 17.75 Photograph of a transected nodule removed from a finger. The nodule is firm to palpation, its center has a white-yellow appearance, and pigmentation seems to be confined to the periphery of the lesion. This appearance is often found in lesions of PVNS and probably occurs as a result of secondary hemorrhage into the lesion following trauma.

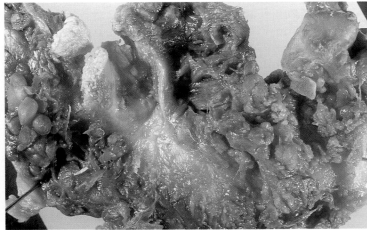

FIGURE 17.76 Gross photograph of synovium resected from the knee of a patient with PVNS. Note the reddish-brown staining due to hemosiderin deposition, as well as the plump papillary projections which result from cell proliferation. This appearance often causes diagnostic confusion with hemosiderotic synovitis.

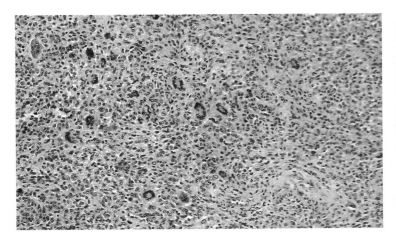

FIGURE 17.77 Photomicrograph of an area of pigmented villonodular synovitis shows the subsynovial nodular accumulation of mononuclear cells with interspersed giant cells, which have frequently peripherally arrayed nuclei, characteristic of PVNS (H & E, x 4 obj.).

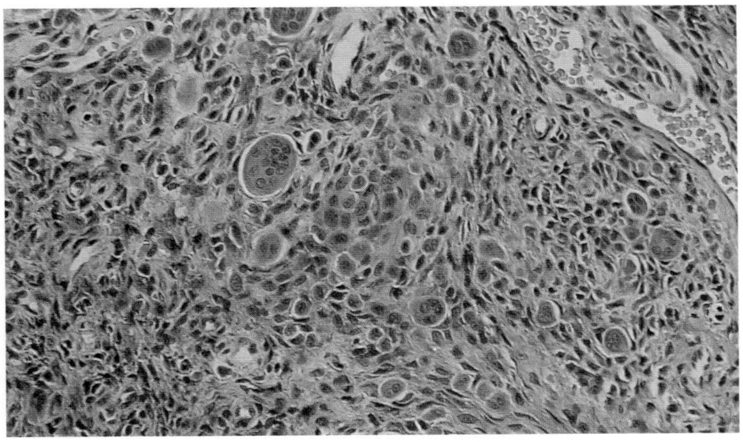

FIGURE 17.78 Photomicrograph of a cellular area of PVNS shows large histiocytic cells with some spindled-out fibroblasts, scattered giant cells, and interstitial hemorrhage (H & E, x 25 obj.).

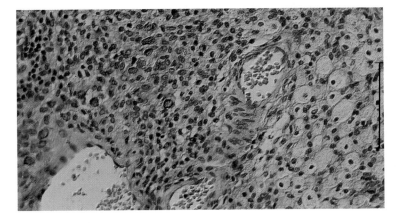

FIGURE 17.79 Photomicrograph showing areas of lipid-laden macrophages and scattered hemosiderin-containing macrophages in PVNS (H & E, x 40 obj.).

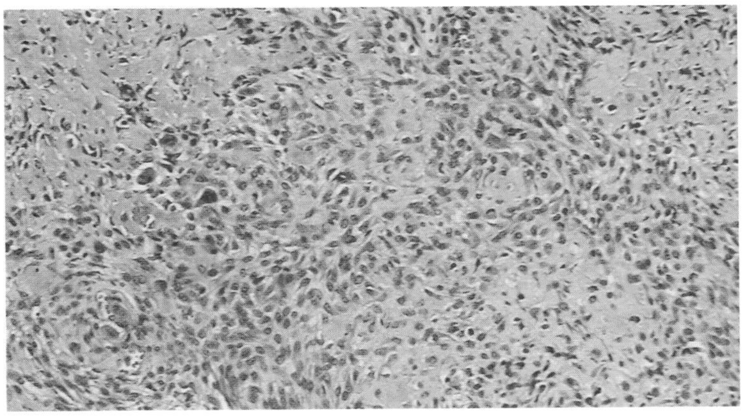

FIGURE 17.80 Photomicrograph of an area of PVNS showing a collagenous extracellular condensation focally resembling primitive bone matrix. The stromal cells in this area are somewhat spindled and have a storiform pattern (H & E, x 25 obj.).

comatous appearance (Fig. 17.81).

The lesion appears to be localized below the synovial membrane lining cells, suggesting that it arises from a submembrane cell such as a fibrohistiocyte, and it is usually noninflammatory or contains only a scattering of mononuclear cells, lymphocytes, and plasma cells. The differential diagnosis of PVNS includes hemosiderotic synovitis, which is seen in patients with chronic intra-articular bleeding (eg, hemophilia). Although a hemosiderotic synovitis lesion contains significant pigmentation, it lacks the distinct submembranous mononuclear and giant-cell nodular cell proliferation that characterizes PVNS. The treatment of PVNS is excision; however, because complete surgical removal is very difficult, clinical recurrence is fairly frequent. Very rare cases of malignant change in PVNS have been described.

METASTATIC CANCER

Metastatic cancer is the most frequent malignant tumor of bone. It is considerably more common than primary bone tumor, and it usually causes pain. Reflecting the general prevalence of cancer in the population, most bone lesions are metastases from primary lesions in the breast, prostate, lung, kidney, thyroid, or colon. A diagnosis of neuroblastoma, rhabdomyosarcoma, or retinoblastoma should be considered in young children.

On radiographs, metastatic tumors may appear as sclerotic or lytic, solitary or multiple. In general, whereas purely blastic or sclerotic lesions are seen with prostate and breast carcinoma, kidney and thyroid metastases are destructive and frequently "expansile." It is not unusual for patients with an undiagnosed primary tumor (eg, in the kidney) to present initially with

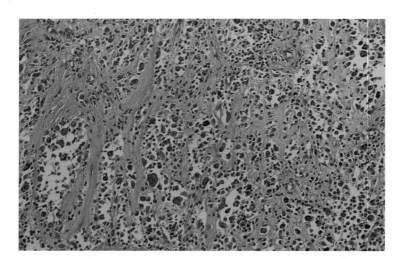

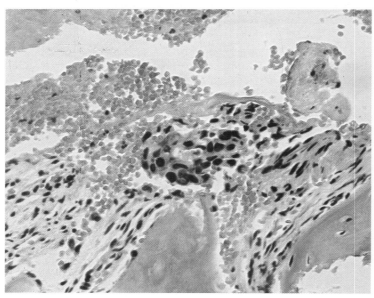

FIGURE 17.82 Photomicrograph of a needle biopsy taken from a vertebral body with a sclerotic lesion suspected of arising from metastatic cancer. There is obviously active new bone formation as well as fibrous scarring, and a clump of atypical cells is strongly suggestive of tumor. Definitive diagnosis may be difficult on this type of tissue; however, the aspirated clot seen in Figure 17.83 is frequently diagnostic (H & E, x 40 obj.).

FIGURE 17.81 Photomicrograph of a case of PVNS in which the collagen is seen in a trabeculated pattern with loose pseudoalveolar spaces between. This pattern, together with the heterogeneity of the cells, gives a pseudosarcomatous appearance to the tissue (H & E, x 10 obj.).

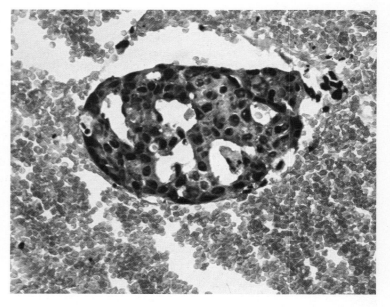

FIGURE 17.83 Within the aspirated clot is evidence of adenocarcinoma. Often, in needle biopsies of bone, severe crushing artifacts preclude interpretation of the tissue sample. For this reason, aspirated blood should always be submitted for examination, and will frequently give positive results where the tissue is negative or equivocal (H & E, x 40 obj.).

a lytic lesion in the bone. Scintigraphy has greatly facilitated the identification of bone metastases.

The diagnosis of metastatic disease is often aided by fine-needle aspiration biopsy. In these circumstances, smears should be made to facilitate the interpretation of fine cytologic detail, and both core bone and blood (clot) should be processed and examined. The blood clot may exhibit evidence of cancer in many cases in which crushed tumor tissue precludes interpretation of the bone sample (Figs. 17.82 and 17.83).

Microscopic identification of the primary site from which the metastasis has originated may be difficult, especially in poorly differentiated neoplasms. Squamous pearls may be seen in association with well-differentiatiated tumors if they are from a squamous carcinoma, and mucin-producing glands if they stem from an adenocarcinoma. (It should be noted that whereas gastrointestinal adenocarcinomas usually produce mucin, those from the lung may not, and those from the kidney rarely do.) The clear cells of renal cancer may create considerable diagnostic confusion, suggesting a clear-cell chondrosarcoma or chordoma.

The preferential deposition of tumor cells in bone marrow may be explained by the latter's rich vascularity and large sinusoidal channels.

In the case of osteoblastic metastases, the bone formed is reactive and is present as fine spicules of woven bone adherent to the residual existing bone (Fig. 17.84).

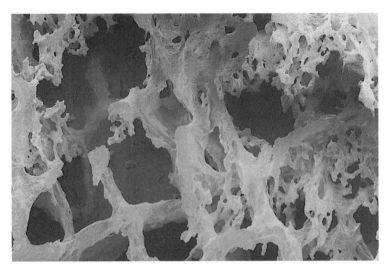

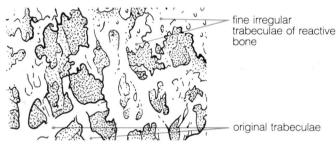

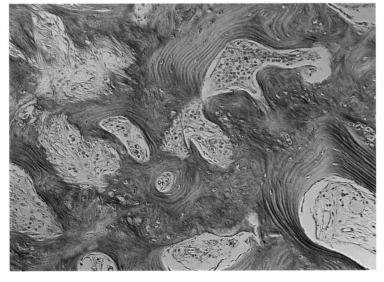

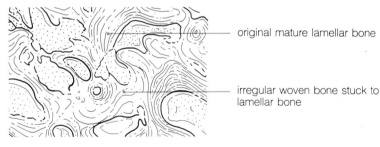

FIGURE 17.84 *(top)* Scanning electronmicrograph of a portion of bone obtained from metastases from an osteoblastic prostatic carcinoma (x 15 magnification). The fine trabeculae of bone produced in response to the tumor are apparent. Photomicrograph *(bottom)* of the same specimen shows the woven character of the new bone, which is firmly adherent to the surface of the lamellar bone of the vertebral body. The spaces in between are filled with fibrous tissue and malignant cells (H & E, x 4 obj.).

COMMON BUT UNEXCITING ORTHOPEDIC CONDITIONS

This section reviews a variety of conditions that are frequently seen and treated by orthopedic surgeons but that have not been dealt with in previous sections of this book. For many of these diseases the etiology is unknown, but for others the causative factor is believe to be mechanical trauma.

C H A P T E R 18

**Miscellaneous orthopedic
bone conditions**

T he term "bony" used in this chapter's title refers both to lesions within the bone and lesions which occur in close proximity to a bone and are themselves ossified, as is the case with myositis ossificans.

BONE INFARCTION

The relatively frequent occurrence of bone infarcts in caisson workers who have had decompression sickness and in patients with sickle-cell anemia, Gaucher's disease, and other hematologic disease, as well as in association with cortisone therapy, is generally recognized.

Most cases involve the femoral head or other convex articular surfaces, as already described in Chapter 11. However, on rare occasions, infarction may affect other sites, usually the metaphysis of a long bone or even, on occasion, a flat bone. The lesions may be multiple and symmetrical. Most of the patients are middle-aged or older, and some may complain of pain. In other cases the lesion is discovered as an incidental radiologic finding.

The early stage of a bone infarct can be observed only at autopsy, where it appears grossly as an elongated pale area with a hyperemic border which is rather sharply demarcated from the surrounding bones

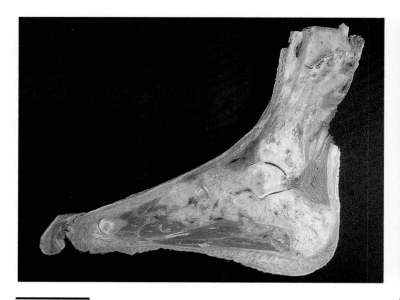

FIGURE 18.1 Photograph of a sagittal section through the lower leg and foot of a 68-year-old male with multiple sclerotic lesions radiographically and a non-union of a fracture of the tibia. The multiple areas of chalky white, opaque tissue in the tibia and in the bones of the foot proved microscopically to be the result of infarction.

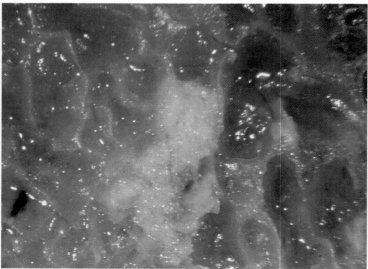

FIGURE 18.2 Close-up photograph of cancellous bone to demonstrate a small focus of marrow and bone necrosis recognized by its opacity, yellowish-white color, and failure to retract like the surrounding viable tissue.

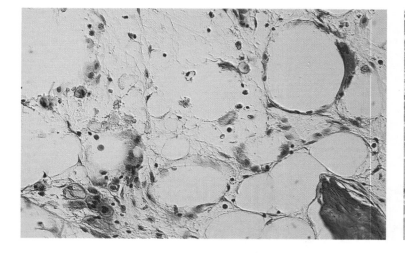

FIGURE 18.3 Photomicrograph to demonstrate early fat necrosis. There is breakdown of the walls of the fat cells resulting in large irregular cystic spaces which are surrounded by foamy histiocytes and giant cells (H & E, x 10 obj.).

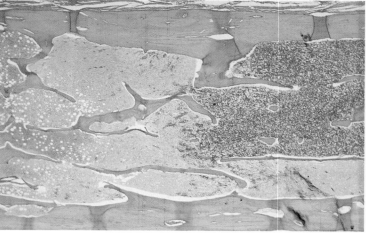

FIGURE 18.4 Photomicrograph to demonstrate necrosis of the hematopoietic marrow (viable blue-staining marrow, for comparison, is seen in the upper right). Necrosis of the marrow is the most obvious microscopic finding associated with bone necrosis (H & E, x 4 obj.).

(Figs. 18.1 and 18.2). At this stage, there has not been enough time for changes in the architecture of the bone trabeculae to develop, and therefore little if any change is seen on the radiograph.

Microscopically, large spaces are seen in the marrow, which result from breakdown of the walls of fat cells and local hemorrhage (Fig. 18.3). The bone trabeculae are nonviable, as evidenced by lacunae that do not contain stainable osteocytes. However, the most obvious evidence of early infarction is seen in bone that contains hematopoietic tissue, since this tissue is extremely vulnerable to ischemia (Fig. 18.4).

With the passage of time, ingrowth of granulation tissue takes place at the periphery of the lesion, and "creeping substitution" of the nonviable cancellous bone by layering of new viable bone on the trabecular surfaces is also seen at the periphery. In most cases the healing process is aborted and a rim of highly collagenized connective tissue forms about the periphery of the lesion. This connective tissue wall becomes infiltrated with calcium salts (Fig. 18.5). Subsequently, the central part of the lesion may undergo liquefaction necrosis and eventually cysts may form.

Radiographs of the lesion in the later stages of development have a typical appearance (Fig. 18.6). A moderately thick, radiopaque serpentine border can be observed, often outlining an elongated area of central radiolucency. This appearance may be likened to a coil of smoke. In some cases, particularly in solitary lesions, radiographs may suggest a calcified enchondroma. Usually, however, the foci of calcified matrix in enchondroma or chondrosarcoma are discrete and scattered diffusely throughout the lesion, and the margin of the lesion is not so clearly outlined as with an infarct.

It has been suggested that some lesions presenting as bone infarcts may in fact represent calcified and cystified lipomas of bone. However, in view of the rarity of intraosseous lipomas, this must be rare.

The occasional development in a bone infarct of a malignant tumor, usually a malignant fibrous histiocytoma, is a well-recognized complication and has been referred to in Chapter 17.

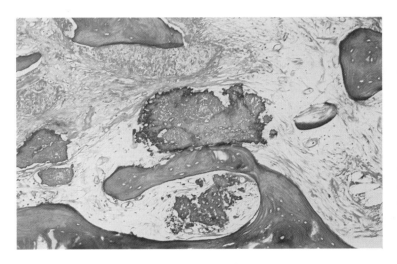

FIGURE 18.5 Photomicrograph to demonstrate calcium deposition in necrotic marrow (H & E, x 10 obj.). (If there is heavy calcium deposition, it may lead to an obvious increase in radiodensity on clinical radiographs.)

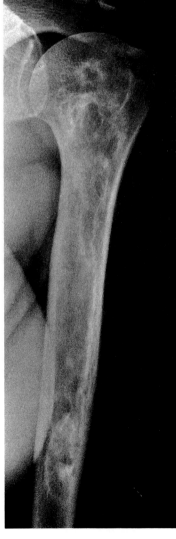

FIGURE 18.6 In a medullary bone infarction, seen here in the proximal humerus of a 36-year-old man with sickle-cell disease, there is no endosteal scalloping of the cortex, and the calcified area is surrounded by a thin, dense sclerotic margin—the hallmark of a bone infarct.

CONGENITAL PSEUDARTHROSES

A pseudarthrosis (false joint) usually occurs as a complication of a fracture. However, it may also manifest at birth or during infancy, commonly in the shaft of the tibia (or rarely the ulna). The lesion is usually observed at the level of the junction of the middle and lower third of the bone shaft. This type of pseudarthrosis is considered congenital and constitutes a distinct orthopedic entity.

Radiographic evaluation of an infant with congenital pseudarthrosis reveals a lucent defect in the diaphysis of the affected bone, associated with a characteristic tapering of the bone ends at the site of the pseudarthrosis (Figs. 18.7 and 18.8). Histologic examination reveals dense, fibrous connective tissue filling the defect (Fig. 18.9).

Neurofibromatosis is present in a high percentage of children with this condition, and as many as 10 percent of patients with neurofibromatosis have the disorder. Nevertheless, neurofibromas are not usually visible on microscopic examination of histologic specimens from the involved site.

These lesions usually prove to be very refractory to treatment.

SLIPPED CAPITAL FEMORAL EPIPHYSIS (ADOLESCENT COXA VARA)

Slipped capital femoral epiphysis is the spontaneous disruption of the epiphyseal plate of the femoral head, usually occurring in overweight adolescent boys at the time of the growth spurt. The condition may be unilateral or bilateral. Early clinical complaints are pain or limping, with eventual limitation of mobility.

On radiographs, early displacement may be evident only on lateral films, where it appears as a backward (or dorsal) displacement (Fig. 18.10). Eventually there is obvious separation of the femoral head and neck, with resultant coxa vara (Figs. 18.11 and 18.12). Valgus presentation is rare.

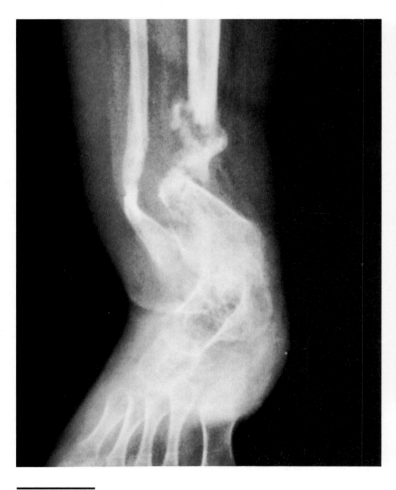

FIGURE 18.7 Anteroposterior radiograph of a young boy with congenital pseudarthrosis of the tibia and fibula. The appearance of the lesion at the junction of the middle and lower third of the bones and the tapering of the bone ends are characteristically found in patients with congenital pseudarthrosis.

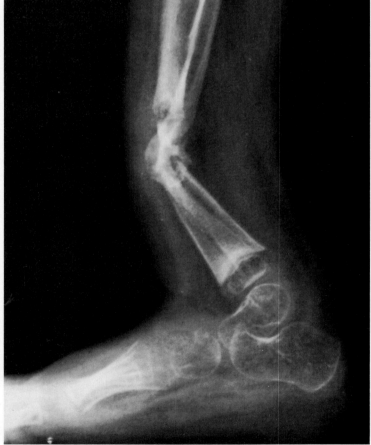

FIGURE 18.8 Lateral radiograph of the case shown in Figure 18.7.

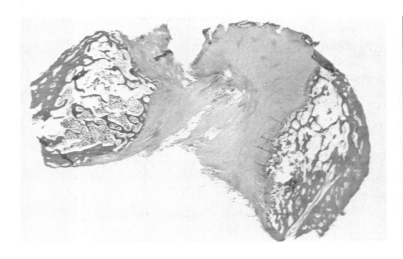

FIGURE 18.9 Histologic section of a congenital pseudarthrosis of the clavicle shows that the gap in the bone is filled with dense, fibrous connective tissue, with no significant new bone formation (H & E, x 1 obj.).

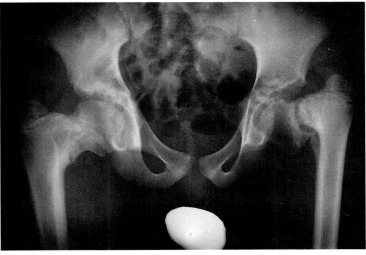

FIGURE 18.11 Radiograph to demonstrate bilateral slip of the capital femoral epiphysis. On the left side, the epiphysis is almost completely dislocated with respect to the metaphysis.

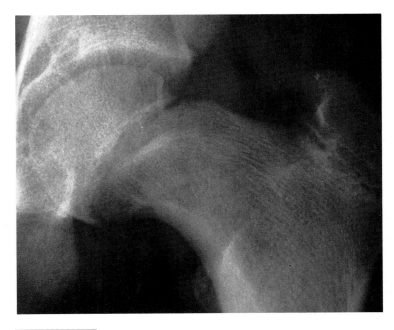

FIGURE 18.10 Clinical radiograph of the hip joint in a patient with a significant slipped epiphysis. The displacement of the capital femoral epiphysis on the neck of the femur can be readily appreciated.

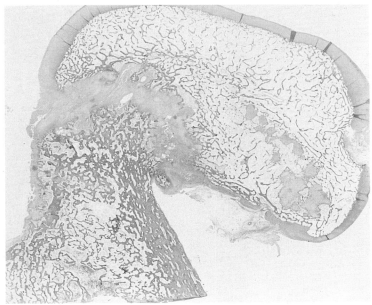

FIGURE 18.12 Photomicrograph of a section through the femoral head and neck of a case of slipped capital femoral epiphysis. The epiphyseal end of the bone has totally separated from the growth plate, a portion of which is seen on the outer surface of the lower left hand side of the photograph (H & E, x 1 obj.).

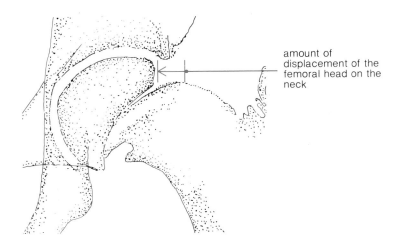

amount of displacement of the femoral head on the neck

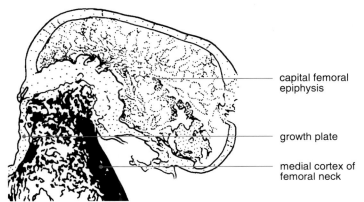

capital femoral epiphysis

growth plate

medial cortex of femoral neck

Microscopically, the epiphyseal growth plate in an affected individual may appear markedly irregular and thicker than normal. Hemorrhage is often present between the growth plate and the primary spongiosa, thus effectively blocking the ingrowth of the metaphyseal capillaries into the growth plate and preventing endochondral ossification (Figs. 18.13 and 18.14).

The condition may result from the widening of the growth plate and the increase in vascularity that accompany the period of accelerated skeletal growth. These circumstances would lead to an increased propensity for shear failure in the angulated growth plate of the femoral neck.

Treatment of a slipped epiphysis is generally by internal fixation of the femoral head.

In blacks, an increased incidence of chondrolysis has been noted in association with a slipped epiphysis. Patients with the combined disorder have elevated levels of immunoglobulins and the C3 component of complement. These findings suggest a localized antigen–antibody-mediated effect as part of a systemic disorder.

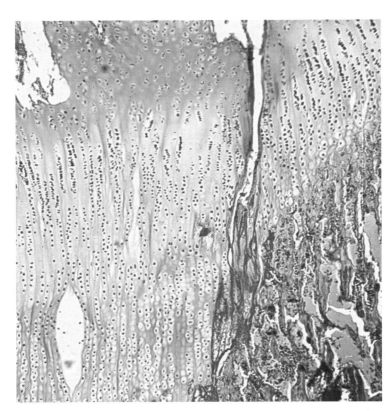

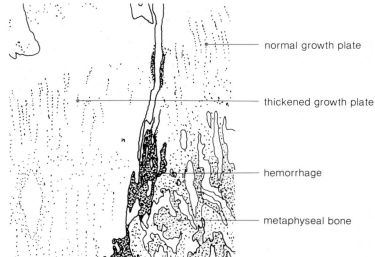

FIGURE 18.13 Low-power photomicrograph taken during an early stage of slipped epiphysis, before extensive displacement has occurred. Focal thickening of the growth plate and separation of the growth plate from the underlying metaphysis by hemorrhagic tissue can be seen (Masson trichrome stain, x 4 obj.).

normal growth plate

thickened growth plate

hemorrhage

metaphyseal bone

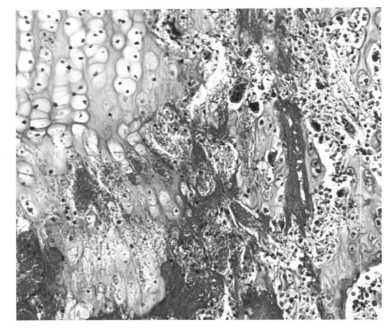

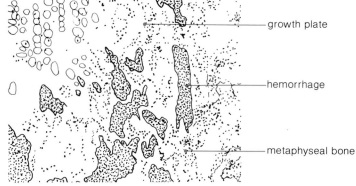

FIGURE 18.14 High-power photomicrograph of the tissue in Figure 18.13 shows focal hemorrhage between the growth plate and the metaphysis. It is postulated that such hemorrhagic tissue serves to block continued endochondral ossification, and consequently the growth plate becomes thicker owing to the lack of endochondral ossification and conversion to bone (Masson trichrome stain, x 25 obj.).

growth plate

hemorrhage

metaphyseal bone

CONGENITAL DISLOCATION OF THE HIP

Congenital dislocation of the hip is a relatively uncommon abnormality in which the femoral head is not properly positioned in the acetabular fossa at the time of birth (Fig. 18.15). Not being a true congenital malformation, it results from either mechanical and/or physical factors that lead to instability of the hip in a newborn. These factors may include tight maternal abdominal and uterine musculature, breech presentation, maternal hormones such as estrogen and relaxin (which affect fetal as well as maternal ligamentous laxity), or forced hip extension following birth. The left hip is more often involved, but bilateral dislocation is present in more than 25 percent of patients.

Treatment consists of early detection and reduction, ie, the return of the femoral head to its normal position as soon as possible after birth. However, in persistent dislocation resulting from delayed diagnosis, the bone and soft tissue adjacent to the joint undergo reactive changes which preclude easy reduction. Both the acetabulum and femoral head become irregularly contoured (Fig. 18.16). Attempts at forcible reduction may compromise the blood supply and lead to avascular necrosis.

In untreated patients, secondary osteoarthritis de-

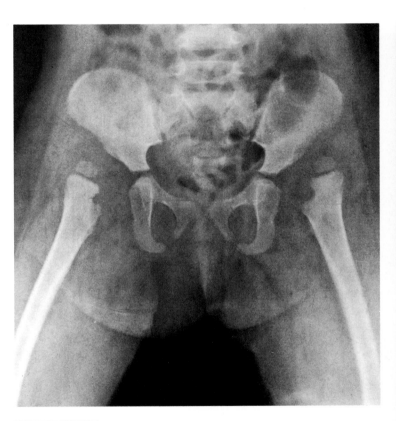

FIGURE 18.15 Radiograph of a young child with untreated congenital dislocation of the hips reveals that both hips are dislocated, and the roof of the acetabulum appears poorly formed. After reduction this patient developed avascular necrosis of the right hip, a common complication.

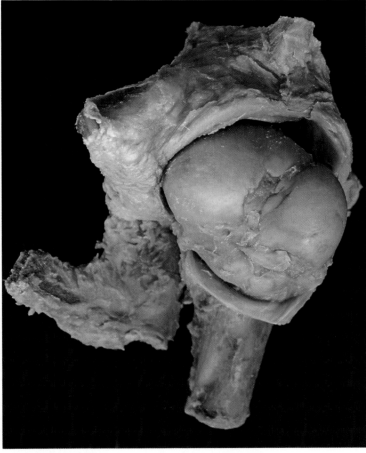

FIGURE 18.16 An anatomic dissection from a young child with congenital dislocation of the hip that was not reduced. Note the deformity of the femoral head, which has developed a saddle-shaped groove across its superior portion. On clinical radiographs this groove may give the appearance of a double head.

velops relatively early in life. Sometimes hip dysplasia (malformation of the joint) occurs without an obvious cause such as congenital dislocation of the hip (Fig. 18.17). This type of congenital malformation also contributes to the early onset of secondary osteoarthritis.

OSTEOCHONDRITIS DISSECANS

Osteochondritis dissecans is a benign noninflammatory condition of diarthrodial joints which affects young adults. The disorder is characterized by a well-demarcated fragment of bone and overlying articular cartilage, which may or may not be separated from the articular surface at the time of presentation. The condition usually involves the lateral aspect of the medial femoral condyle or, less commonly, the posteromedial aspect of the talus and anterolateral aspect of the capitellum. Patients complain of joint pain, often with joint effusions and occasional locking of the joint.

Although osteochondritis dissecans is unilateral in most instances, it may be bilateral and symmetrical. Familial cases of osteochondritis have been reported, and in these the disorder is probably transmitted as an autosomal dominant trait. Affected children are often short in stature and may have an associated endocrine dysfunction. The underlying defect in osteochondritis dissecans may well be an accessory center of ossifica-

tion, although trauma must play an important role in the initiation of clinical disease.

Radiographs reveal a well-demarcated defect in the articular surface of the affected joint (Fig. 18.18). The gross appearance of a resected specimen is usually that of a flat, smooth nodule formed of avascular bone, with overlying viable articular cartilage (Fig. 18.19). A layer of dense, fibrous connective tissue or fibrocartilage usually forms on the bone surface (Fig. 18.20).

Treatment consists of reattachment of the loose body (where feasible) or excision.

HYPERTROPHIC PULMONARY OSTEOARTHROPATHY (MARIE-BAMBERGER SYNDROME)

Hypertrophic pulmonary osteoarthropathy involves the formation of symmetrical periosteal new bone along the diaphyses of the bones of the appendicular skeleton. This condition is seen in association with both neoplastic and non-neoplastic diseases of the lung and, less commonly, of other organs. The classic presentation is an adult with complaints of arthralgia and/or aching bone pain, with or without clubbing of the fingers and toes.

The striking radiographic feature of hypertrophic pulmonary osteoarthropathy is symmetrical "onion-

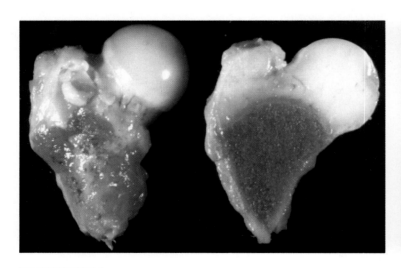
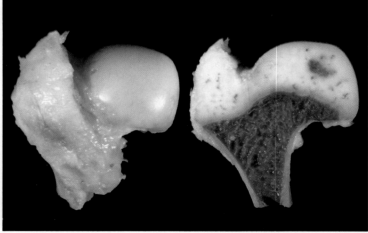

FIGURE 18.17 *(left)* The upper end of the femur, whole and in coronal section, from a normally developed hip in a newborn. *(right)* The upper end of the femur, whole and in coronal section, from an infant with hip dysplasia shows the abnormal configuration of the femoral head and growth plate.

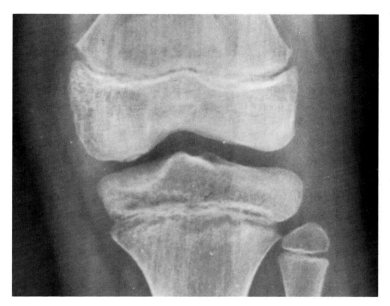

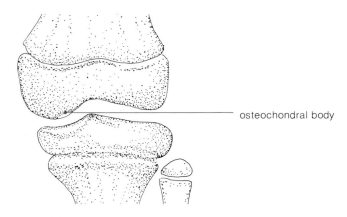

osteochondral body

FIGURE 18.18 Radiograph of the knee in a 12-year-old boy who complained of discomfort in the joint shows a well-demarcated defect on the articular surface of the medial femoral condyle. At this point the osteochondral body has not separated from the condyle and is still in situ.

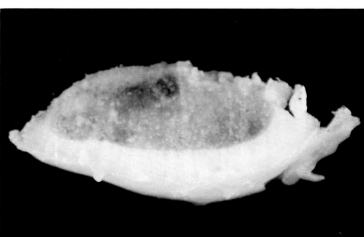

FIGURE 18.19 Photograph of a section through a loose body removed from a patient with osteochondritis dissecans. There is a layer of intact articular cartilage on the lower surface with an overlying disc of attached bone which itself has a fibrous covering on its inferior surface.

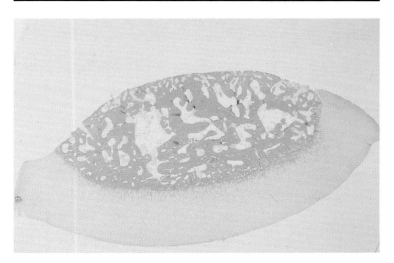

FIGURE 18.20 Photomicrograph of a loose body removed from a patient with osteochondritis dissecans. The bone may or may not be necrotic depending upon whether or not it is still attached to the affected epiphysis (H & E, x 1 obj.).

skin periostitis" of the shafts of long bones, which is confined to the diaphyses but progresses proximally (Fig. 18.21). Densities in the sites of insertions of ligaments and tendons have also been noted. The patient's level of serum alkaline phosphatase may be elevated. Although the joints do not show significant radiographic change, patients may have painful effusions that are characteristically noninflammatory. The arthralgia is usually relieved by aspirin.

On microscopic examination, there is marked periosteal new bone formation. The outer layer of the periosteum may show a mononuclear cell infiltrate. No endosteal bone deposition is seen (Fig. 18.22).

The etiology of pulmonary osteoarthropathy remains obscure. Treatment should be directed at the underlying disease.

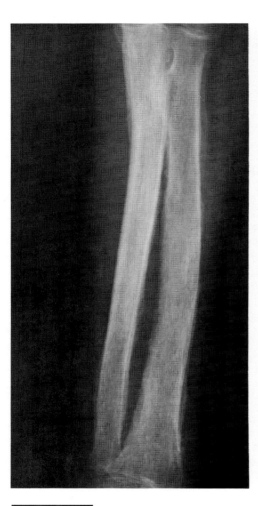

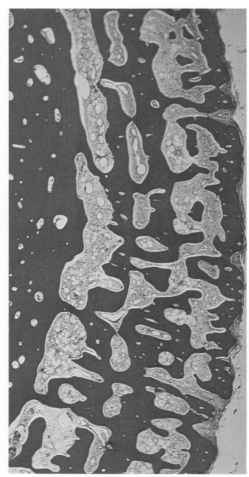

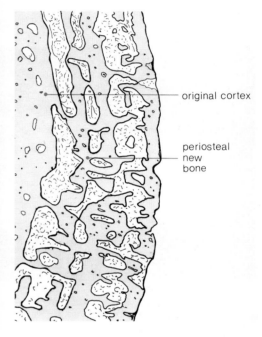

FIGURE 18.22 Photomicrograph of a biopsy of cortical bone from a patient with pulmonary osteoarthropathy. Note the three layers of new periosteal bone (H & E, x 4 obj.).

— original cortex

— periosteal new bone

FIGURE 18.21 Radiograph of the forearm in a patient with carcinoma of the lung shows periosteal bone formation on both the radius and the ulna. In this patient all the long bones demonstrated dramatic periosteal new bone.

INFANTILE CORTICAL HYPEROSTOSIS (CAFFEY'S DISEASE)

Infantile cortical hyperostosis (ICH) is a disease of infants, who present with a classic triad of hyperirritability, soft tissue swelling, and palpable hard masses over multiple and often symmetric bones. Patients may be feverish and acutely ill, and the disease often follows a recent upper respiratory infection. Radiography reveals diffuse, usually symmetric cortical thickening. Many bones are affected, but especially the mandible, clavicle, and ribs (Fig. 18.23). Involvement of the long bones occurs less often, and the vertebral column and tubular bones of the hands and feet are usually spared.

Histologic examination of tissue from affected areas reveals a thickened periosteum, often with marked periosteal new bone formation and mild infiltration by acute chronic inflammatory cells (Fig. 18.24).

Laboratory findings in patients with ICH may include an increased erythrocyte sedimentation rate, anemia, and leukocytosis with a shift to the left. These findings are highly suggestive of an infection; however, in the vast majority of cases no organism has been isolated.

Infantile cortical hyperostosis usually follows a protracted course with several exacerbations and remissions, but spontaneous recovery usually occurs in a few months.

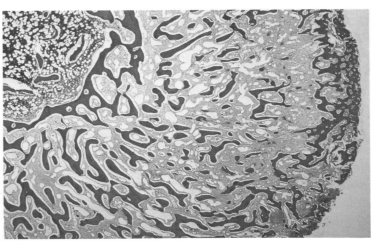

FIGURE 18.24 Histologic section of tissue affected by ICH reveals extensive periosteal new bone formation, with vascularized fibrous tissue lying between the bone spicules. Although not seen here, a scattering of chronic inflammatory cells is commonly found.

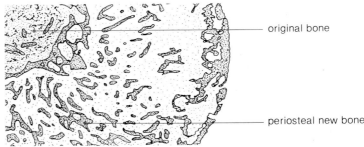

original bone

periosteal new bone

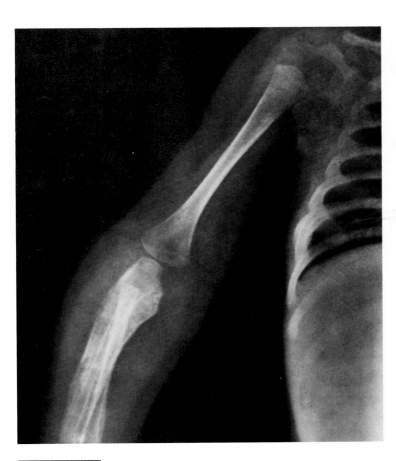

FIGURE 18.23 Radiograph of an infant admitted to the hospital with fever and enlargement of the forearm shows extensive periosteal new bone formation causing enlargement of the ulna. In addition, there is thickening and widening of the seventh rib, as well as bilateral thickening of the mandible (not shown here).

MYOSITIS OSSIFICANS

Two entirely separate conditions are described by the general diagnostic term myositis ossificans: myositis ossificans circumscripta and myositis ossificans progressiva. Two conditions which appear to be related to myositis ossificans circumscripta, subungual exostosis and reactive periostitis, will also be discussed below.

MYOSITIS OSSIFICANS PROGRESSIVA

Myositis ossificans progressiva is a rare progressive disease in which groups of muscles, tendons, and ligaments (usually the muscles of the back and those around major joints) become progressively ossified, thereby producing severe functional disability (Figs. 18.25 and 18.26). Symptoms of the disease usually begin in childhood or adolescence. In some cases the condition is inherited, and several members of a family may be affected.

Microscopic examination reveals poorly organized bone (both lamellar and woven), dense, fibrous scar tissue, and islands of poorly formed cartilage (Figs. 18.27 and 18.28). This disorder is usually fatal because of progressive functional disability, including impairment of pulmonary function.

MYOSITIS OSSIFICANS CIRCUMSCRIPTA

Myositis ossificans circumscripta is a solitary, nonprogressive, benign ossifying lesion of soft tissues. The patient usually presents with a lump in a muscle which has been evident for some weeks and may have been somewhat painful. A history of trauma can usually be elicited, but these traumatic incidents are, more often than not, trivial in nature. A radiograph taken soon after the onset of symptoms may not reveal any calcification (Fig. 18.29), but within a week or two a poorly defined area of opacification will appear. Over succeeding weeks the periphery of this shadow becomes increasingly well delineated from the surrounding soft tissue (Fig. 18.30).

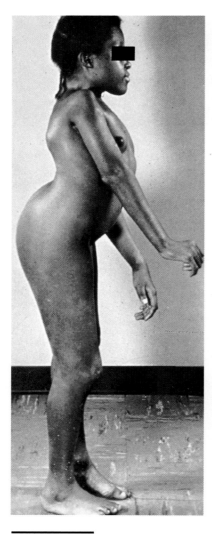
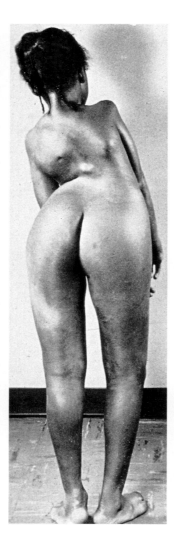
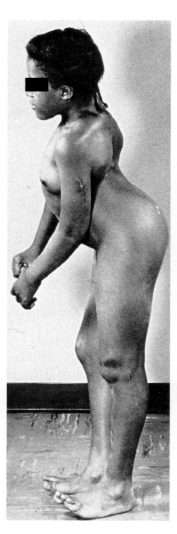
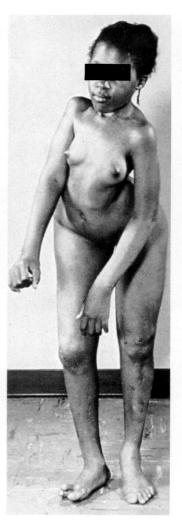

FIGURE 18.25 These photographs demonstrate severe deformities of the limbs, spine, and neck resulting from myositis ossificans progressiva.

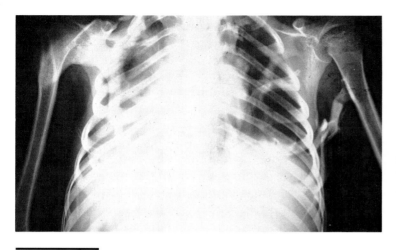

FIGURE 18.26 Clinical radiograph of the patient in Figure 18.25 shows ossification around both shoulder joints as well as in the paravertebral area.

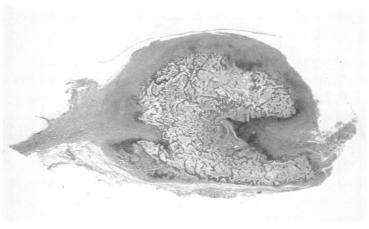

FIGURE 18.27 Photomicrograph of a portion of ossified soft tissue taken from the hip joint of a patient with myositis ossificans progressiva demonstrates both immature bone and cartilage formation, with areas of dense fibrous connective tissue also in evidence (H&E, x 1 obj.).

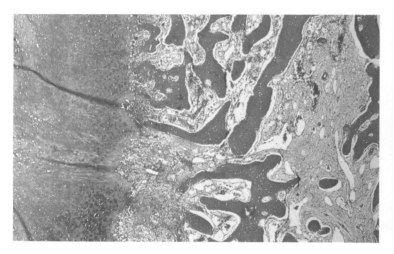

FIGURE 18.28 Higher-power photomicrograph of the tissue in Figure 18.27 shows bone and cartilage formation within the soft tissue (H & E, x 10 obj.).

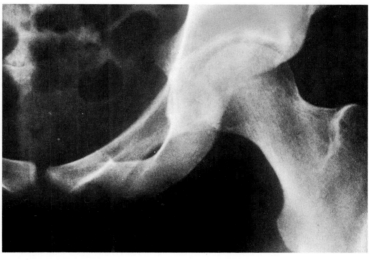

FIGURE 18.29 Clinical radiograph of a young woman who developed pain in the region of the pubis after childbirth reveals no obvious abnormality.

FIGURE 18.30 This radiograph of the patient in Figure 18.29 taken one month later, demonstrates a well-defined ossifying mass in the soft tissue adjacent to the pubis.

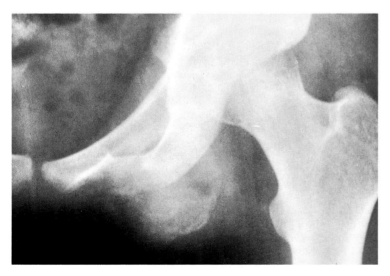

Gross examination of a focus of myositis ossificans circumscripta that has been present for a month or two reveals a shell of bony tissue with a soft reddish-brown central area. The lesion is usually 2 to 5 cm in diameter and is adherent to the surrounding muscle (Fig. 18.31).

Microscopic examination of myositis ossificans circumscripta reveals an irregular mass of active, immature fibroblastic cells in the center of the lesion, with foci of interstitial microhemorrhage that are rarely extensive (Fig. 18.32). At some distance from the center of the lesion, depending on the age of the entity in question, small foci of osteoid production can be seen. The resulting tissue may be disorganized and hypercellular (Fig. 18.33). Near the periphery, more and more clearly defined trabeculae are evident (Fig. 18.34). The bone is usually of the immature woven type, with large, round, and crowded osteocytes; however, in long-standing lesions the bone may be mature and have a lamellar pattern.

It may be difficult to differentiate a focus of myositis, especially in its acute stage, from a sarcoma on the basis of histologic evidence alone. Careful correlation of the clinical and radiologic findings is therefore essential. An important distinction to be emphasized is that whereas myositis ossificans is most mature at its periphery and least mature at its center (Fig. 18.35), the opposite is true of osteosarcoma (see discussion of soft-tissue osteosarcoma in Chapter 16). Treatment of this condition is usually conservative, with excision of the mass an option.

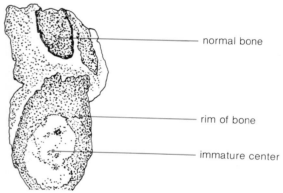

FIGURE 18.31 Gross photograph of the specimen removed from the patient in Figure 18.29. In the upper part can be seen a segment of normal bone, and immediately underlying this segment is a well-circumscribed ossified mass which had been attached to the periosteum but did not arise from the bone tissue.

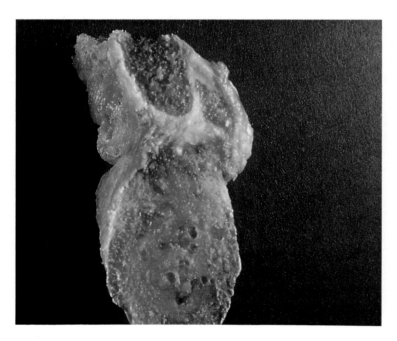

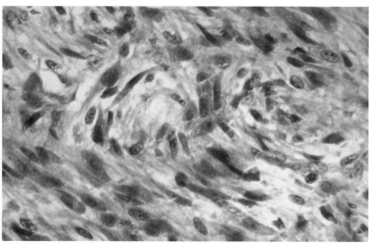

FIGURE 18.32 High-power photomicrograph of tissue taken from the center of the mass shown in Figure 18.31 demonstrates a spindle-cell lesion. The cells have a disorderly arrangement and are producing collagen (H & E, x 40 obj.).

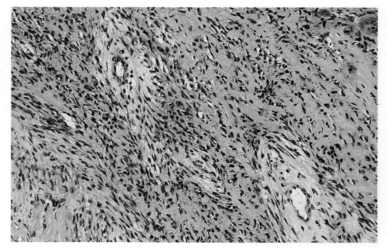

FIGURE 18.33 Photomicrograph of an area adjacent to the tissue seen in Figure 18.32 demonstrates immature bone matrix formation. The cellularity of this tissue might cause concern and lead to an erroneous diagnosis of sarcoma (H & E, x 25 obj.).

SUBUNGUAL EXOSTOSIS

Subungual exostosis is a rare osteocartilaginous lesion arising from a distal phalanx, most commonly that of the big toe. Clinically, the lesion must be differentiated from other lesions that may cause ulceration of the nail bed, including subungual verrucae, glomus tumor, epidermal inclusion cyst, subungual melanoma, carcinoma of the nail bed, and pyogenic granuloma.

Most of the patients are adolescents, but occasionally older individuals are affected. The symptoms are likely to have been present for a few months and growth of the lesion may be rapid, although it is limited. A history of trauma is rarely elicited, although it seems most likely that the lesion is posttraumatic rather than representing a true osteochondral or osteocartilaginous exostosis.

On radiographic examination, the exostosis arises from the dorsal aspect of the tip of the distal phalanx and grows distally. Early in the course of the lesion it appears as a soft-tissue density without attachment to the underlying bone. Later, however, as it calcifies it begins to show a trabecular pattern and eventually connects to the underlying bone (Fig. 18.36).

The microscopic appearance also depends on the stage of maturation. In the early stages the lesion appears as a foci of proliferating fibrous tissue with areas of cartilaginous metaplasia. Later in its development it shows focal calcification and ossification. However, even in a mature lesion there is no distinct layer of peri-

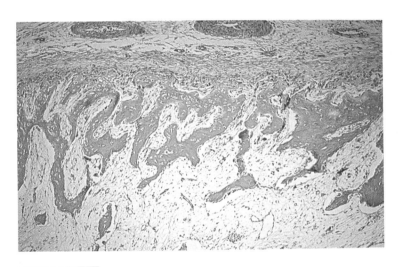

FIGURE 18.34 Histologic section taken from the periphery of the lesion demonstrated in the previous three figures shows mature bone formation, characteristic of myositis ossificans circumscripta (H & E, x 10 obj.).

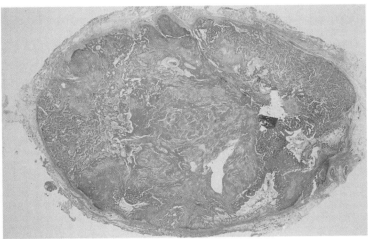

FIGURE 18.35 Photomicrograph of a section through an intact specimen of myositis ossificans circumscripta clearly shows the fibrous cellular center and the limiting outer layer of more mature bone (H & E, x 1 obj.).

FIGURE 18.36 Radiograph of the forefoot to demonstrate subungual exostosis of the big toe. (From Pavlov H, Torg JS, Hirsh A, Freiberger RH: The Roentgen Examination of Runners Injuries. Radiographics 1:17-34, 1981.)

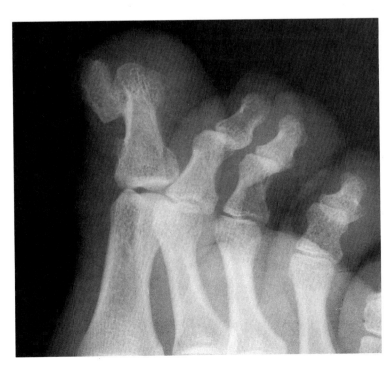

osteum covering the cartilage cap, as is seen with a true osteocartilaginous exostosis (Fig. 18.37); rather, the fibrocartilaginous tissue at the periphery of the lesion blends with the overlying fibrous connective tissue. The microscopic findings are similar to those of reactive periostitis and, like that lesion, may be mistaken for a malignant lesion, especially if biopsy tissue has been obtained only from the periphery of the lesion. The lesion is likely to recur unless it is completely excised, especially if it is removed in the early stages of the disease.

REACTIVE PERIOSTITIS (PARAOSTEAL FASCIITIS)

Reactive periostitis is a rare calcifying and ossifying soft-tissue lesion which occurs most commonly in the hands and less commonly in the feet. The lesion is likely to originate along the margin of a phalanx, and although in the early stages no mineralization may be seen on radiographic examination at the time of clinical presentation, calcification is usually present (Fig. 18.38). A history of trauma may not be given, but it is generally believed that, as in the case myositis ossificans circumscripta and subungual exostosis (lesions to which reactive periostitis is closely related), the lesion is posttraumatic. Microscopically, especially in the early phases, the disordered fibroblastic proliferation, mitotic activity, and immature bone formation may suggest osteosarcoma (Fig. 18.39). However, as with myositis ossificans, there is maturation of the tissue towards the periphery of the lesion, and the edge of the lesion is usually encased in a shell of bone.

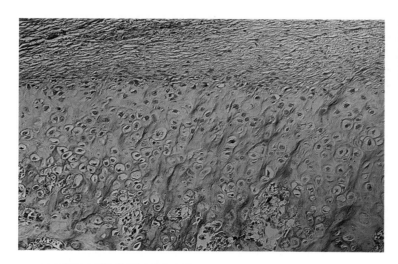

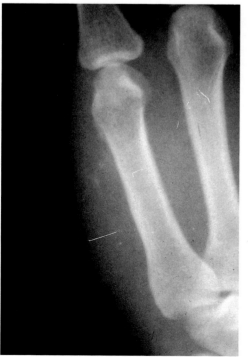

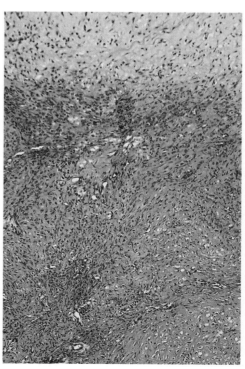

FIGURE 18.37 Photomicrograph of a portion of the periphery of a subungual exostosis showing the merging of the cartilaginous portion with overlying proliferative fibrous tissue and underlying bone formation (H & E, x 25 obj.).

FIGURE 18.38 Radiograph of a 31-year-old drummer who had had a 5 month history of pain in the little finger. In addition to soft tissue swelling along the ulnar side of the proximal phalanx there is poorly defined ossification. In this case, the differential diagnosis would include myositis ossificans or other reactive lesion, synovioma, or a benign or malignant cartilage lesion. (Courtesy of Dr. L. Kahn)

FIGURE 18.39 Photomicrograph of the tissue obtained from a case of reactive periostitis showing the zoning phenomenon seen at the edge of these lesions. A loose myxoid tissue gives way to more dense proliferative fibrous tissue. In the lower part of the picture extracellular matrix is being formed, giving rise to tissue resembling primitive bone or cartilage (H & E, x 10 obj.). (Courtesy of Dr. L. Kahn)

Miscellaneous orthopedic soft-tissue conditions

Some of the soft tissue lesions discussed in this chapter, such as ganglia, carpal tunnel syndrome and Morton's neuroma, are among the most common complaints which bring a patient to consult with an orthopedist.

GANGLION

A ganglion is a fibrous-walled cyst filled with clear mucinous fluid and usually lacking a recognizable lining of differentiated cells (Figs. 19.1 to 19.3). Ganglia occur in the soft tissues, usually dissecting between tendon planes. They are often seen in the hands and feet, particularly on the extensor surfaces near joints. (The most common location is around the wrist joint.)

Ganglia may arise either as herniations of the synovium or from cystification of foci of myxoid degenera-

tion within dense fibrous connective tissue, possibly secondary to trauma. Rarely, a communication with the joint cavity can be demonstrated. On occasion, these lesions may erode the adjacent bone and subsequently become totally intraosseous. The most common site for such an intraosseous ganglion is the medial malleolus of the tibia (see Chapter 14). Similar cystic lesions are seen in the parameniscal tissue of the knee joint, usually in proximity to the lateral meniscus (Figs. 19.4 and 19.5).

On microscopic examination, the wall of a ganglion cyst is formed of dense, collagenized fibrous tissue, often with foci of myxoid tissue (Fig. 19.6). Chronic inflammatory cells may be observed, especially if the cyst has been previously ruptured.

If clinically troublesome, surgical excision of the cyst is the treatment of choice.

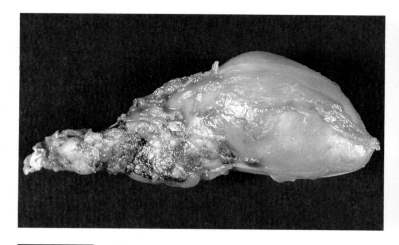

FIGURE 19.1 Gross photograph of an intact, excised ganglion cyst. Note the smooth fibrous wall and the translucent appearance.

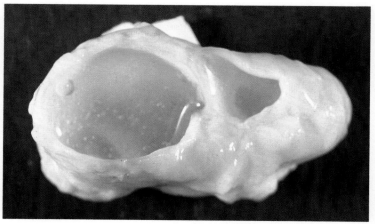

FIGURE 19.2 Gross photograph of a bisected ganglion shows a multiloculated cyst filled with clear glairy fluid.

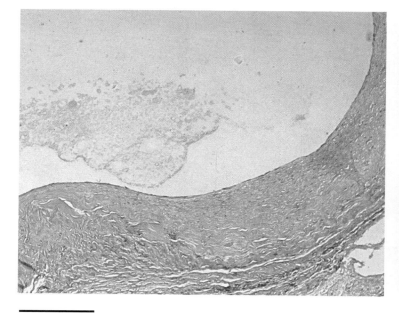

FIGURE 19.3 Photomicrograph of a ganglion shows the dense fibrous connective tissue wall, with a thin layer of flattened cells lining the cyst (H & E, x 10 obj.).

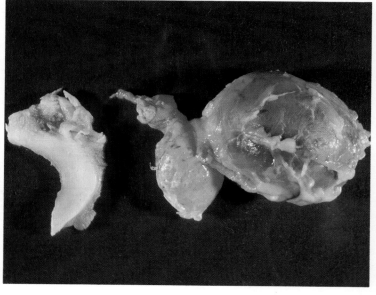

FIGURE 19.4 Gross photograph of the lateral meniscus (left) and a parameniscal cyst (right). As is apparent here, cysts of the lateral meniscus may occasionally grow to a very large size.

BURSITIS

Acute or chronic bursitis is clinically characterized by pain, redness, and/or swelling of one of the many synovium-lined bursae that lie between muscles, tendons, and bone prominences, especially around the joints. Bursitis is usually caused by chronic trauma. It often occurs in the shoulders of professional athletes and in the prepatellar and infrapatellar bursae of those who frequently kneel (eg, housewives and the religiously inclined). Bursitis is sometimes observed as a complication of rheumatoid arthritis or infection. In cases of rheumatoid arthritis, a cyst may occur particularly in the popliteal area (where it is known as a Baker's cyst) and may extend far into the calf (Fig. 19.7). Bursitis may also result from infection, and in the past this was frequently due to tuberculosis. Sometimes extensive calcification may complicate a chronically inflamed bursa, which renders it visible on radiologic examination. The bursa may also be involved in other conditions that commonly affect the synovial membrane (eg, gout, synovial chondromatosis, or pigmented villonodular synovitis).

On gross examination of an inflamed bursa, the wall

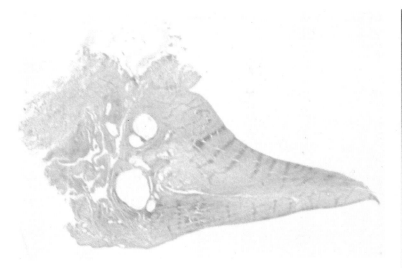

FIGURE 19.5 Photomicrograph of a cross-section of the lateral meniscus shows focal cystic degeneration in the outer third of the meniscus. Microscopic foci of myxoid degeneration and cystification are common findings in histologic sections of the meniscus (H & E, x 4 obj.).

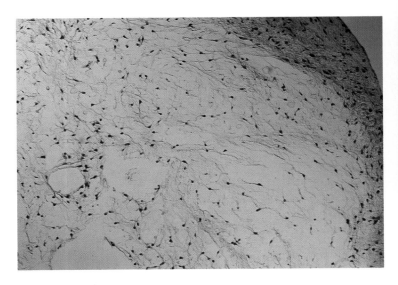

FIGURE 19.6 Photomicrograph of a portion of the wall of a ganglion showing extensive myxoid change (H & E, x 10 obj.).

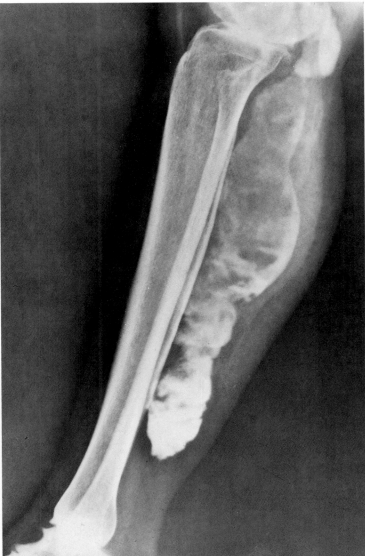

FIGURE 19.7 Radiograph of a leg from a young woman with a history of juvenile rheumatoid arthritis who complained of fullness in the leg. Injection of a radiopaque dye clearly demonstrates the extent of a Baker's cyst in the popliteal region.

of the bursal sac is usually markedly thickened and the lining often appears injected and shaggy owing to fibrinous exudation into the cavity (Fig. 19.8). The microscopic findings depend on the etiology, and the various diseases that might affect the synovium, including infection, should be carefully sought. However, in most cases of posttraumatic origin, scarring and chronic inflammation predominate.

Treatment depends on the etiology and the extent of the lesion.

CARPAL TUNNEL SYNDROME

Carpal tunnel syndrome is an entrapment neuropathy caused by pressure on the median nerve as it passes under the transverse carpal ligament and over the hollow of the carpal bones (Fig. 19.9). Patients usually complain of night pain, often accompanied by paresthesia in the distribution of the median nerve. In advanced cases, wasting of the thenar muscles may occur. The cause of the increased pressure varies, but most often it results from posttraumatic fibrosis or synovitis. Occasionally carpal tunnel syndrome may herald rheumatoid arthritis or other synovial disease and, on rare occasions, it has been found to result from amyloid deposits.

Microscopic examination usually reveals nonspecific fibrosis and occasional fibrocartilaginous metaplasia. This syndrome is treated by surgical division of the transverse carpal ligament. At operation, the nerve is often seen to be congested above the ligament, and constricted and pale where it lies under the ligament (Fig. 19.10).

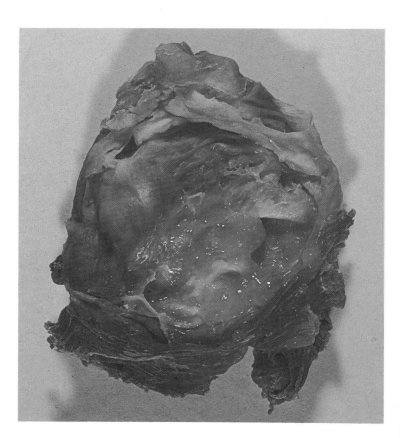

FIGURE 19.8 Gross photograph of an excised popliteal cyst, which was opened to demonstrate a thick fibrous wall with a roughened lining, and a fibrinous exudate.

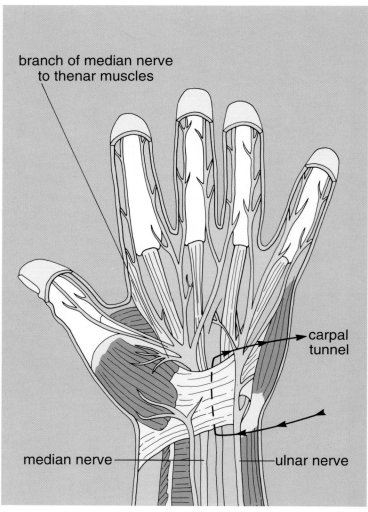

branch of median nerve to thenar muscles

carpal tunnel

median nerve

ulnar nerve

FIGURE 19.9 This diagram of a dissected hand shows the median nerve passing through the carpal tunnel and under the transverse carpal ligament.

Two conditions that may be related to carpal tunnel syndrome are trigger finger and de Quervain's disease (stenosing tenovaginitis of the common tendon sheath of the abductor pollicis longus and the extensor pollicis brevis). In both of these conditions the free movement of the tendon is blocked by a focal thickening of the tendon sheath which results from fibrocartilaginous metaplasia (Fig. 19.11). The treatment is excision.

MORTON'S NEUROMA

Morton's neuroma is a distinct clinicopathologic entity characterized by thickening and degeneration of one of the interdigital nerves of the foot, most commonly that between the third and fourth metatarsal heads. The patient, usually a woman, experiences sharp shooting pains that are worse when standing. These pains characteristically begin in the sole of the foot and radiate to the exterior surface. At surgery, a fusiform swelling proximal to the bifurcation of the plantar interdigital nerve is usually seen. When dissected, the resected specimen usually includes the neurovascular bundle (Fig. 19.12).

Histologic sections generally show three characteristic microscopic features: endarterial thickening of the digital artery, often with thrombosis and occlusion of the lumen; extensive fibrosis both around and within

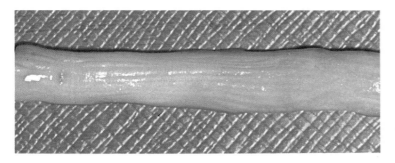

FIGURE 19.10 Gross photograph of a segment of the median nerve, resected at autopsy from the part of the nerve that had entered the carpal tunnel. Note the slight constriction and pale appearance in the area of the nerve that had coursed under the transverse carpal ligament (on the left) as compared with the pink appearance of the nerve proximal to the ligament (on the right).

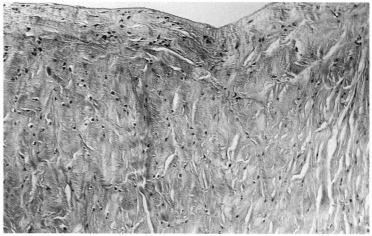

FIGURE 19.11 Photomicrograph of a portion of tissue excised from the thickened tendon sheath in a case of trigger finger. Note the fibrocartilaginous metaplasia of the subsynovial tissue (H & E, with Normarski, x 10 obj.).

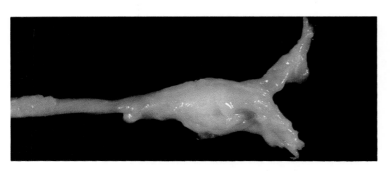

FIGURE 19.12 Gross photograph of a segment of the plantar interdigital nerve resected from the space between the third and fourth metatarsal heads in a patient with Morton's neuroma shows fusiform swelling of the neurovascular bundle just proximal to the bifurcation.

the nerve, giving rise to demyelinization and a marked depletion of axons within the digital nerve; and evidence of Schwann-cell and fibroblast proliferation (Figs. 19.13 to 19.16). These findings are most consistent with recurrent nerve trauma, probably caused by the wearing of poorly fitting shoes.

Morton's neuroma should be differentiated from amputation (traumatic) neuroma which may also occur in the interdigital nerves of the feet, although very much more rarely. Amputation neuroma is caused by transection of a nerve bundle, and a history of lacerating injury is usually given. The lesions are frequently painful, and at operation a bulbous swelling is usually found at the severed nerve ending (Fig. 19.17). On microscopic examination the bulbous swelling shows many proliferating and interdigitating nerve fibers within scar tissue (Fig. 19.18).

COMPARTMENT SYNDROME (VOLKMANN'S ISCHEMIC CONTRACTURE)

Compartment syndrome, ie, swelling and ultimate loss of viability of a muscle group, is caused by compromised circulation within a confined anatomic space. The condition most commonly involves the anterior tibial compartment and the deep posterior tibial compartment of the leg, the volar compartment of the forearm, or the interosseous compartments of the hand.

In general, compartment syndrome results from trauma to an extremity (usually a fracture or crash injury). Recently, the disorder has been noted in patients suffering from drug overdose. Vascular occlusion from either direct injury or increased pressure within the anatomic compartment leads to diminished tissue viability and function. Pain and swelling are prominent

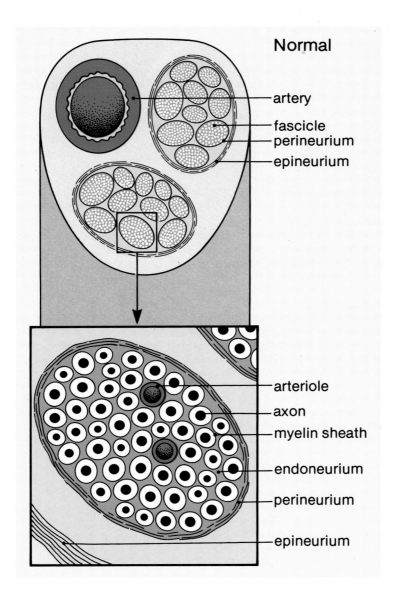

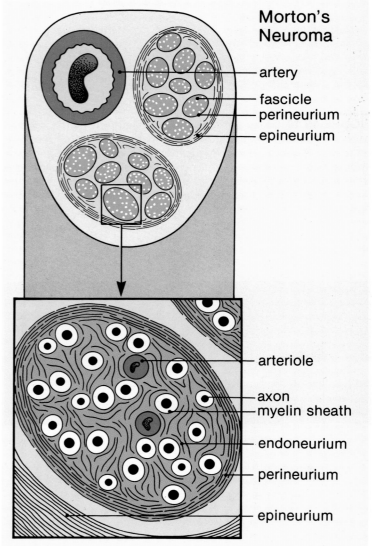

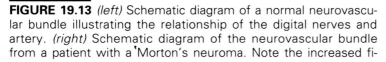

FIGURE 19.13 *(left)* Schematic diagram of a normal neurovascular bundle illustrating the relationship of the digital nerves and artery. *(right)* Schematic diagram of the neurovascular bundle from a patient with a Morton's neuroma. Note the increased fibrosis in the epineurium, perineurium, and endoneurium. In addition, there is marked endothelial thickening of the artery, with narrowing of the lumen.

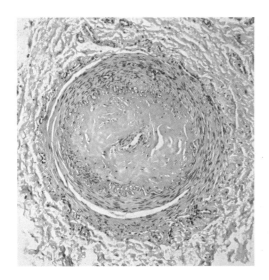

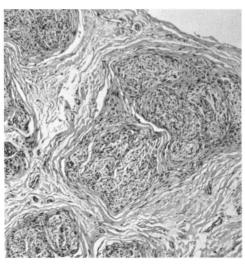

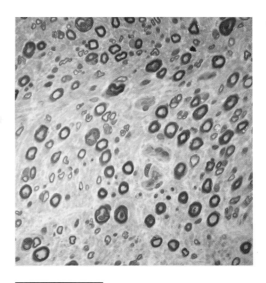

FIGURE 19.14 Histologic section of a narrowed and occluded vessel from a patient with Morton's neuroma (H & E, x 4 obj.).

FIGURE 19.15 Morton's neuroma. The increased fibrosis of the nerve can be appreciated in this histologic section (H & E, x 10 obj.).

FIGURE 19.16 High-power photomicrograph of a single nerve fascicle shows the loss of myelinated nerve fibers together with increased endoneural fibrosis (H & E, x 100 obj.).

FIGURE 19.17 Low-power histologic section of an amputation neuroma stained with Masson trichrome shows the increased fibrous scar tissue. The proximal nerve stump is seen at left (x 1 obj.).

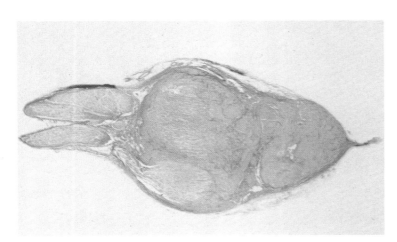

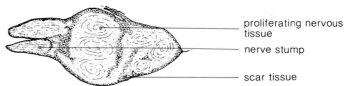

proliferating nervous tissue

nerve stump

scar tissue

FIGURE 19.18 High-power photomicrograph of the section shown in Figure 19.17 demonstrates the proliferating irregular nerve fibers coursing through the scar tissue, characteristic of an amputation neuroma (Masson trichrome, x 25 obj.).

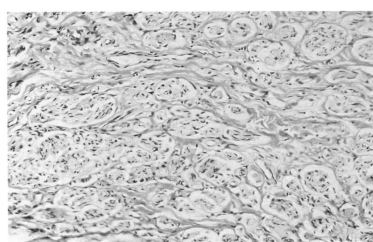

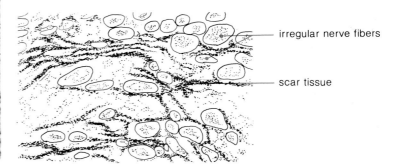

irregular nerve fibers

scar tissue

symptoms. Muscle necrosis ensues, and eventually the original tissue is replaced by dense, fibrous connective tissue, with subsequent deformity and loss of function (Figs. 19.19 to 19.21). Microscopic findings depend on the stage at which the tissue is obtained. Muscle necrosis, granulation tissue, scar tissue, and calcification may all be present.

Treatment of the acute condition is aimed at relieving the pressure by fasciotomy, the removal of tight bandages, or whatever is appropriate to the circumstances.

PALMAR AND PLANTAR FIBROMATOSIS

Under the generic term of the fibromatoses are grouped a number of conditions that are characterized by fibroblastic tissue which, by its cellularity and capacity to infiltrate surrounding tissue, mimics a fibrosarcoma. However, these lesions do not metastasize. They may arise in many parts of the body and are known by a variety of names (eg, desmoid tumor, Peyronie's disease etc.). Of particular interest to the orthopedic surgeon

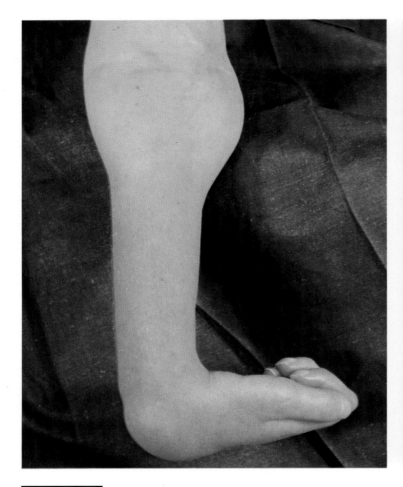

FIGURE 19.19 Clinical photograph of the arm in an untreated patient who had developed compartment syndrome after multiple injuries to the elbow and forearm some months earlier. Note the severe flexion contractures.

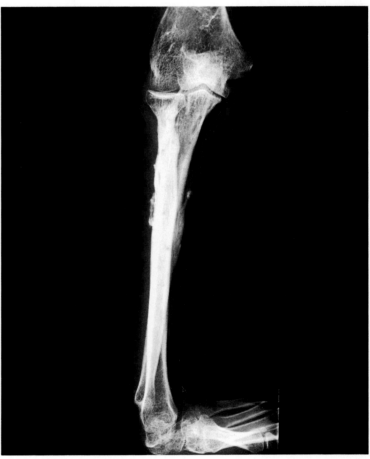

FIGURE 19.20 Radiograph of the arm shown in Figure 19.19. In addition to evidence of traumatic arthritis, there is also some shortening of the ulna and mature bone formation around the ulna and radius in the upper third of the forearm.

FIGURE 19.21 Histologic section through a part of the muscle mass of the anterior tibial compartment involved in compartment syndrome reveals extensive muscle necrosis, with an inflammatory reaction and fibrous replacement at the margin of the infarcted tissue (H & E, x 4 obj.).

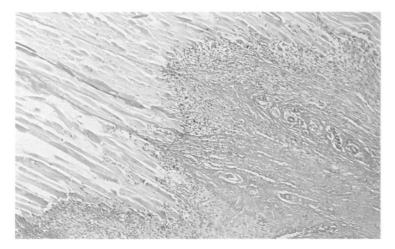

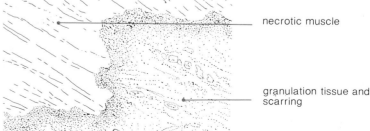

necrotic muscle

granulation tissue and scarring

are palmar fibromatosis (Dupuytren's contracture) and its plantar equivalent.

DUPUYTREN'S CONTRACTURE

Palmar fibromatosis usually occurs in older adults; it is more common in men than in women and is frequently bilateral. In some instances it is associated with alcoholic cirrhosis of the liver. Patients present with nodu-

lar thickening of the palmar fascia (Fig. 19.22) and flexion contracture of the fingers (usually the third, fourth, and fifth). On histologic examination, the lesions vary in cellularity; some are very cellular and others are heavily collagenized (Figs. 19.23 to 19.25). The cellular lesions are in all probability the more recently formed, whereas the collagenized lesions have been present for a longer period of time.

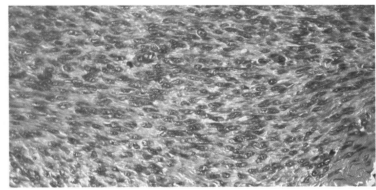

FIGURE 19.22 Cross-section of thickened palmar fascia removed from a patient with Dupuytren's contracture. The aponeurotic tissue has a grayish-white, glistening appearance, and within this tissue can be seen thickened nodular areas having a more opaque, white-orange appearance. These areas represent foci of proliferating fibromatosis. In long-standing Dupuytren's contracture, the entire aponeurosis may be scarred, and the proliferating nodules are no longer evident.

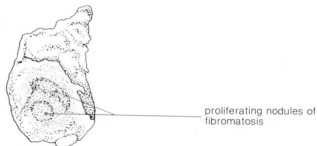

proliferating nodules of fibromatosis

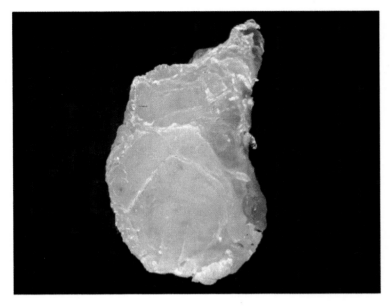

FIGURE 19.23 Low-power photomicrograph of one of the proliferative nodules found in Dupuytren's contracture shows strands of dense collagenized tissue passing through a cellular stroma (H & E, x 4 obj.).

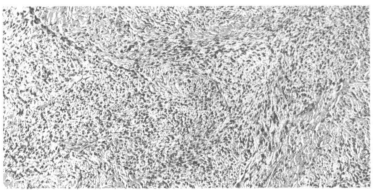

FIGURE 19.24 High-power photograph of Figure 19.23 shows the packed but regular spindle cells characteristically found in Dupuytren's contracture. Mitoses are evident and may be quite numerous; however, atypical mitoses are not seen (H & E, x 25 obj.).

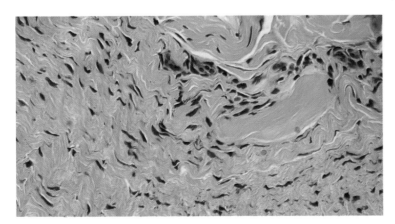

FIGURE 19.25 Photomicrograph of a section through a nodule from a case of long-standing Dupuytren's contracture shows heavily collagenized stroma without the obvious cellular proliferation characteristic of early lesions (H & E, x 25 obj.).

PLANTAR FIBROMATOSIS

Plantar fibromatosis tends to occur in younger patients, is more aggressive, and presents with larger nodules than is usually the case in patients with palmar fibromatosis (Figs. 19.26 to 19.29). However, plantar fibromatosis is not associated with the formation of contractures.

Surgical excision is the treatment of choice; however, because of the infiltrative nature of the lesion local recurrence is common.

CALCIFYING APONEUROTIC FIBROMA (JUVENILE APONEUROTIC FIBROMATOSIS)

Calcifying aponeurotic fibroma usually presents as a slowly growing painless mass commonly in the hands or, less commonly, in the feet of children or young adults. The mass has usually been present for several months or even years at the time of presentation (Fig. 19.30). Radiographically, calcific stippling may be apparent (Fig. 19.31). Grossly, the lesion is usually an ill-defined, firm, white-gray nodular mass less than 3 cms in diame-

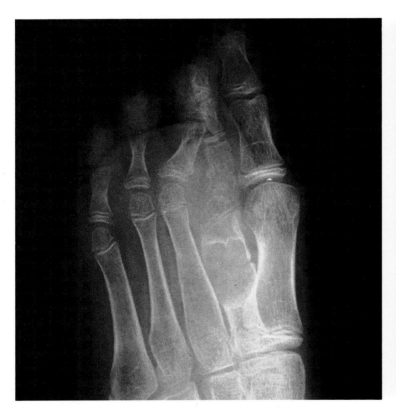

FIGURE 19.26 Radiograph of a 13-year-old girl with a history of two excisions of plantar fibromatosis who was admitted to the hospital because of recurrence with bone involvement. Both soft-tissue swelling and invasion of the second metatarsal bone can be appreciated.

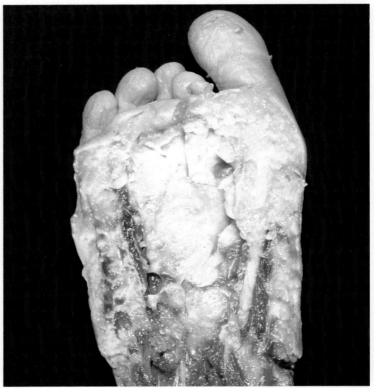

FIGURE 19.27 This amputated specimen from the patient in Figure 19.26 with plantar skin removed, clearly shows the extent of the tumor.

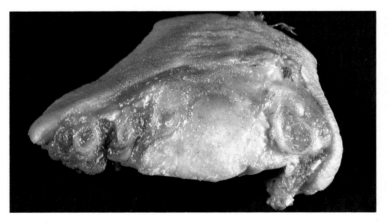

FIGURE 19.28 Cross-section of the foot shown in Figure 19.27 demonstrates the extent of tumor infiltration and involvement of the second metatarsal bone.

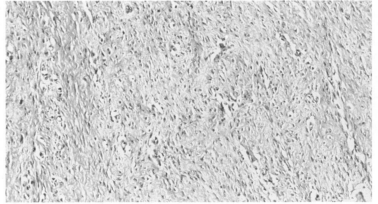

FIGURE 19.29 Low-power photomicrograph of the tumor illustrated in the previous three figures demonstrates the bland appearance of the plantar fibromatous tissue (H & E, x 10 obj.).

ter. Because of calcification it may have a gritty consistency when sectioned. Microscopic examination shows foci of plump cellular fibroblasts separated by more densely collagenized tissue. Mitotic figures are rare. Foci of calcification are generally present within the lesion and are usually associated with areas of cartilaginous metaplasia. However, in very young children calcification may not be evident, making the differentiation from infantile fibromatosis difficult. In such cases, the location in the fingers or the palm of the hand should suggest the diagnosis.

In older patients the lesion may suggest soft-tissue chondroma (Fig. 19.32). However, in calcifying aponeurotic fibroma the calcification is more focal and does not have the diffuse pattern of calcification seen in soft-tissue chondroma. Conservative surgical management is generally recommended.

CRANIAL FASCIITIS

Cranial fasciitis is a rare and only recently described condition which is seen exclusively in the cranium of infants and small children.

Radiologic examination usually reveals a defect in the outer table of the skull, in addition to a soft-tissue mass (Figs. 19.33 and 19.34). Gross examination of the resected tissue reveals a firm, rubbery mass which may

be a few centimeters in diameter and on cut section may have a glistening appearance. Microscopic examination reveals a proliferation of plump fibroblasts in a mucoid matrix. Some mitotic activity is usually present (Figs. 19.35 and 19.36).

Because of its rarity, rapid growth, and pseudosarcomatous appearance, the lesion may be misdiagnosed as fibrosarcoma. However, the lesion is entirely benign and self-limited.

ELASTOFIBROMA

Elastofibroma is an uncommon, self-limited lesion found in older adults which, with rare exceptions, occurs in the soft tissue between the rib fascia and the inferior portion of the scapula. On gross examination the lesion is firm and rubbery in consistency and, although circumscribed, is not encapsulated but rather merges with the surrounding tissue (Fig. 19.37).

On microscopic examination the lesion is formed of dense collagen and fat, interspersed with eosinophilic globules and fibers. Histochemically and ultrastructurally, these fibers and globules consist of elastin (a fibrous protein) and elastin precursors (Figs. 19.38 and 19.39).

It is generally agreed that the lesion occurs posttraumatically. Treatment is usually by surgical excision.

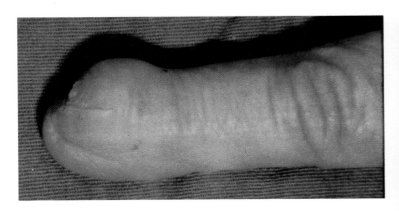

FIGURE 19.30 This elderly woman had had a swelling on the distal end of the index finger for 20 years which had recently got bigger. At operation, there was a poorly defined non-encapsulated mass which merged with the surrounding tissues. Microscopic examination proved this lesion to be an aponeurotic fibroma.

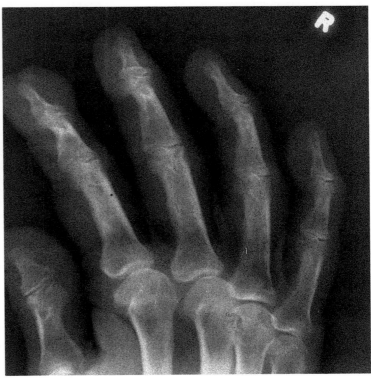

FIGURE 19.31 A radiograph of the case demonstrated in Figure 19.30 shows a soft tissue mass. (Courtesy of Dr. L. Kahn)

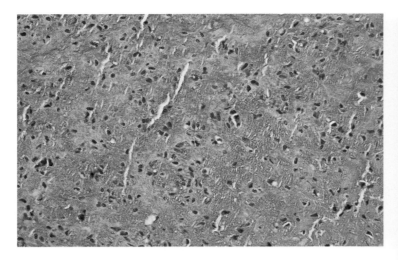

FIGURE 19.32 Photomicrograph of a portion of the lesion shown in Figures 19.30 and 19.31 demonstrates a fibrocartilaginous appearance consistent with the diagnosis of aponeurotic fibroma in an elderly subject (H & E, x 10 obj.). (Courtesy of Dr. L. Kahn)

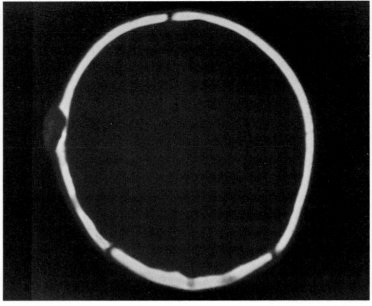

FIGURE 19.34 The CT scan shows that the lesion is extraosseous and involving the bone by secondary erosion.

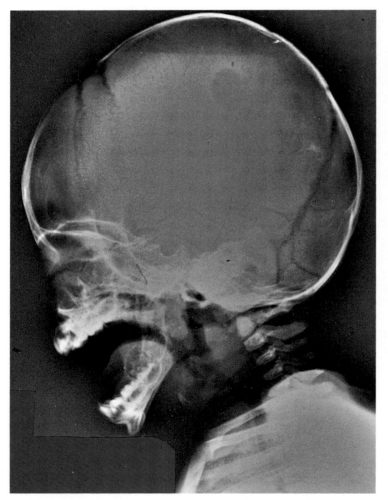

FIGURE 19.33 Radiograph of a 5-month-old infant with a slowly growing mass on the head present since shortly after birth. The radiograph suggests a differential diagnosis including epidermoid inclusion cyst, eosinophilic granuloma, or cranial fasciitis.

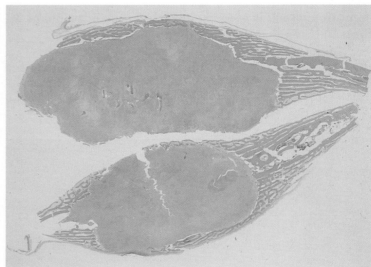

FIGURE 19.35 Photomicrograph of the tissue removed from the case illustrated in Figures 19.33 and 19.34. The lesional tissue has a fibrous appearance (H & E, x 1 obj.).

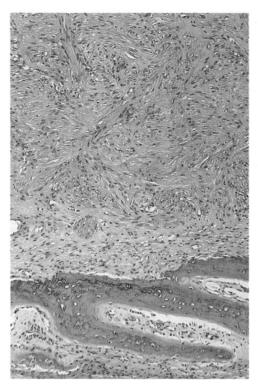

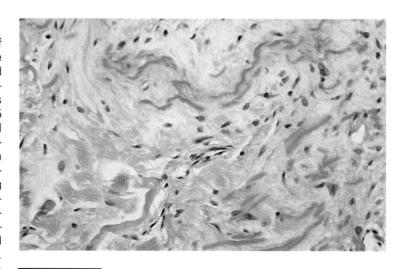

FIGURE 19.36
Photomicrograph of a portion of the tumor removed from the patient illustrated in Figures 19.33 through 19.35 shows the typical loose, swirling pattern of fasciitis, with immature fibroblastic cells producing an extracellular matrix rich in proteoglycan (foci of basophilic staining) and sparse collagen. Scattered chronic inflammatory cells are present (H & E, x 10 obj.).

FIGURE 19.38 Photomicrograph of a portion of the mass illustrated in Figures 19.37 to demonstrate the disorderly collagenous matrix and bland cellular appearance of the lesional tissue (H & E, x 25 obj.).

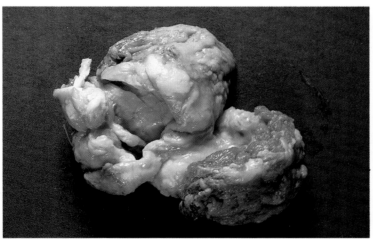

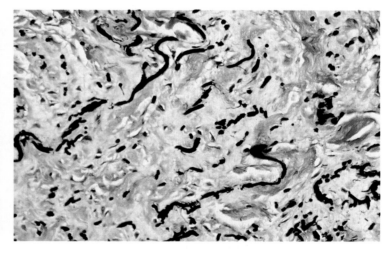

FIGURE 19.37 Photograph of a mass excised from the soft tissues overlying the scapula. The lump had been present clinically for several years.

FIGURE 19.39 The same tissue as shown in Figure 19.38, stained with an elastic tissue stain. Note the abundant fragmented elastic fibers in the tissue typical of an elastofibroma (Verhoeff–van Gieson, x 25 obj.).

BIBLIOGRAPHY

GENERAL READINGS

Bullough PG, Boachie-Adjei O: Atlas of Spinal Diseases. Gower Medical Publishing, New York, 1988.

Dahlin D: Bone Tumors: General Aspects and Data on 6,221 Cases, 4th ed. Charles C Thomas, Springfield, IL, 1986.

Dalinka MK, Zlatkin MB, Chao P, Kricun ME, Kressel HY: The use of magnetic resonance imaging in the evaluation of bone and soft-tissue tumors. Radiol Clin North Am 29:461–470, 1990.

Dobson J: Pioneers of Osteogeny, John Hunter: 1728–1793. J Bone Joint Surg 30-B:361–364, 1948.

Hall BK: Bone (4 vols.). Telford Press, Caldwell, NJ, 1990.

Hirohata K, Morimoto K, Kimura H: Ultrastructure of Bone and Joint Diseases, 2nd ed. Igaku-Shoin, New York, 1981.

Jaffe HL: Metabolic, Degenerative, and Inflammatory Diseases of Bones and Joints. Lea & Febiger, Philadelphia, 1972.

Jaffe HL: Tumors and Tumorous Conditions of the Bones and Joints. Lea & Febiger, Philadelphia, 1958.

Meisel AD, Bullough PG: Atlas of Osteoarthritis. Lea & Febiger, Philadelphia, 1984.

Mirra JM: Bone Tumors: Clinical, Radiologic, and Pathologic Correlations (2 vols.). Lea & Febiger, Philadelphia, 1989.

Ortner D, Putschar W: Identification of pathological conditions in human skeletal remains. Smithsonian Contributions to Anthropology, No. 28. Smithsonian Institution Press, Washington, DC, 1981.

Owen R, Goodfellow J, Bullough P: Scientific Foundations of Orthopaedics and Traumatology. WB Saunders, Philadelphia, 1980.

Rang M: Anthology of Orthopaedics. E & S Livingstone, Edinburgh & London, 1966.

Resnick D, Niwayama G: Diagnosis of Bone and Joint Disorders (3 vols.). 2nd ed. WB Saunders, Philadelphia, 1988.

Schajowicz F: Tumors and Tumorlike Lesions of Bone and Joints. Springer-Verlag, New York, 1981.

Schajowicz F, McGuire MH: Diagnostic difficulties in skeletal pathology. Clin Orthop Relat Res 240:281–310, 1989.

Schmorl G, Junghanns H: The Human Spine in Health and Disease. 2nd Am ed., Grune & Stratton, New York, 1971.

Sissons HA, Murray RO, Kemp HBS: Orthopaedic Diagnosis, Clinical, Radiological and Pathological Coordinates. Springer-Verlag, Berlin, Heidelberg, 1984.

Spjut HJ, Dorfman HD, Fechner·RE, Ackerman LV: Tumors of bone and cartilage. Atlas of Tumor Pathology, 2nd series. Armed Forces Institute of Pathology, Washington, DC, 1971 (and Suppl, 1981).

Thompson D'Arcy: On Growth and Form, abridged ed. by Bonner JT. Cambridge University Press, London, 1961.

Trueta J: Development and Decay of the Human Frame. Heinemann, London, 1968.

SECTION I—NORMAL

Chapter 1 Normal Bone Structure and Development

Gross Structure and Function

Brookes M: The Blood Supply of Bone. Butterworths, London, 1971.

Canalis E, McCarthy T, Centrella M: Growth factors and the regulation of bone remodeling. J Clin Invest 81:277–281, 1988.

Crock HV: The Blood Supply of the Lower Limb Bones in Man. Churchill Livingstone, Edinburgh, 1967.

Crock HV, Yoshizawa H: The Blood Supply of the Vertebral Column and Spinal Cord in Man. Springer-Verlag, New York, 1977.

Murray PDF: Bones: A Study of the Development and Structure of the Vertebrate Skeleton. Cambridge University Press, London, 1936.

Ogden JA: Changing patterns of proximal femoral vascularity. J Bone Joint Surg 56A:941, 1974.

Treharne RW: Review of Wolff's law and its proposed means of operation. Orthop Rev 10:35, 1981.

Wolff J: The Law of Bone Remodelling, translated by Maquet P, Furlong R. Springer-Verlag, New York, 1986.

Wright TM, Burstein AH: Musculoskeletal biomechanics. In Evarts CM (ed.) Surgery of the Musculoskeletal System, 2nd ed. Churchill Livingstone, Edinburgh, 1990.

The Matrix

Anderson HC: Mechanism of mineral formation in bone. Lab Invest 60:320–330, 1989.

Boskey AL: Noncollagenous matrix proteins and their role in mineralization. Bone Miner 6:111–123, 1989.

Burgeson RE: New collagens, new concepts. Annu Rev Cell Biol 4:551–577, 1988.

Carando S, et al.: Orientation of collagen in human tibial and fibular shaft and possible correlation with mechanical properties. Bone 10:139–142, 1989.

Evered D, Harnett S (eds.): Symposium on Cell and Molecular Biology on Vertebrate Hard Tissues, held at the Ciba Foundation, London, 13–15 October 1987. Cell and Molecular Biology of Vertebrate Hard Tissues. Wiley, Chichester, New York, 1988.

Marks SC Jr, et al.: Bone cell biology: The regulation of development, structure and function in the skeleton. Am J Anat 183:1–44, 1988.

Martin TJ, Wah K, Suda T: Bone cell physiology. Endocrinol Metab Clin North Am 18:833–858, 1989.

McDonald JA: Extra-cellular matrix assembly. Annu Rev Cell Biol 4:183–207, 1988.

Ruoslahti E: Structure and biology of proteoglycans. Annu Rev Cell Biol 4:229–255, 1988.

Histology

Cooper RR, Misol S: Tendon and ligament insertion. J Bone Joint Surg 52-A:1, 1970.

Ham AW, Cormack DH: Histology, 9th ed. Lippincott, Philadelphia, 1987.

Hann SL, Fletcher BD, et al: Magnetic resonance imaging of disseminated bone marrow disease in patients treated for malignancy. Skel Radiol 20:79–84, 1991.

Jee WSS: The skeletal tissues. In Weiss L (ed.) Histology, Cell and Tissue Biology. Elsevier Biomedical, New York, 1983.

Martin L, Boyde A, Trine F, Jones S (eds.): Scanning Microscopy of Vertebrate Mineralized Tissues. Scan Microsc Int, AMF O'Hare, IL, 1988.

Mitchell DG, Rao VM, Dalinka M, et al: Hematopoietic and fatty bone marrow distribution in the normal and ischemic hip: New observations with 1.5-T MR imaging. Radiology 161:199–202, 1986.

Tonna EA, Cronkite EP: The periosteum: Autoradiographic studies on cellular proliferation and transformation utilizing tritiated thymidine. Clin Orthop Relat Res 30:218–232, 1963.

The Joints

Bullough PG, Goodfellow JW: The significance of the fine structure of articular cartilage. J Bone Joint Surg 50-B:852–857, 1968.

Bullough PG, Jagannath A: The morphology of the calcification front in articular cartilage. J Bone Joint Surg 65B:72–78, 1983.

Frank CB, Woo SS-Y, Andriacchi T, et al.: Normal ligament: Structure, function and composition. In Woo SS-Y, Buckwalter JA (eds.) Injury and Repair of the Musculoskeletal Soft Tissues, Am Orthop Soc, 45–101, 1987.

Goodfellow JW, O'Connor JJ: The design of synovial joints. In Owen R, Goodfellow J, Bullough P (eds.) Scientific Foundations of Orthopaedics and Traumatology, WB Saunders, Philadelphia, 1980.

Henderson B: The synovial lining cell and synovitis. Scand J Rheumatol (Suppl) 76:33–38, 1988.

MacConaill MA: The movements of bones and joints. J Bone Joint Surg 32B:244, 1950.

Ogston A: On articular cartilage. J Anat Physiol 10:4–73, 1876.

Schenk RK, Eggli PS, Hunziker EB: Articular cartilage morphology. In Kuetnner J (ed.) Articular Cartilage Biochemistry. Raven Press, New York, 1986.

Bone Growth and Development

Enlow DH: Principles of Bone Remodelling. Charles C Thomas, Springfield, IL, 1963.

Hunter SJ, Caplan AI: Control of cartilage differentiation. In Hall BK (ed.) Cartilage. New York, Academic Press, 1983.

Ogden JA: Skeletal Injury in the Child, 2nd ed. WB Saunders, Philadelphia, 1990.

Chapter 2 Methods of Examination

Anderson C: Manual for the Examination of Bone. CRC Press, Boca Raton, FL, 1982.

Bullough PG, Bansal M, DiCarlo EF: The tissue diagnosis of metabolic bone disease—role of histomorphometry. Orthop Clin North Am 21:65–79, 1990.

Clark G (ed.): Staining Procedures Used by the Biological Stain Commission, 4th ed., Williams & Wilkins, Baltimore, 1980.

Cutignola L, Bullough PG: Photographic reproduction of anatomical specimens using ultraviolet illumination. Am J Surg Pathol (in press).

Dickson GR (ed.): Methods of Calcified Tissue Preparation. Elsevier, New York, 1984.

Frost HM: Relation between bone-tissue and cell population dynamics, histology and tetracycline labelling. Clin Orthop 49:65–75, 1966.

Milch R, Rall D, Tobie J: Fluorescence of tetracycline antibiotics in bone. J Bone Joint Surg 40A:897–910, 1958.

Recker RR (ed.): Bone Histomorphometry: Technique and Interpretation. CRC Press, Boca Raton, FL, 1983.

SECTION II—RESPONSE TO EXOGENOUS INJURY

Chapter 3 Injury and Repair

Allbrook DB: Muscle breakdown and repair. In Owen R, Goodfellow J, Bullough P (eds.) Scientific Foundations of Orthopaedics and Traumatology, WB Saunders, Philadelphia, 1980.

Byers PD, Gray JC, Mostafa Agsa, Ali SY: The healing of bone and articular cartilage. In Glynn LE (ed.) Tissue Repair and Regeneration. Handbook of Inflammation. Elsevier North-Holland, Amsterdam, 1981.

Heppenstall RB (ed.): Fracture Treatment and Healing. WB Saunders, Philadelphia, 1980.

Ogden JA: Skeletal Injury in the Child, 2nd ed., WB Saunders, Philadelphia, 1990.

Ordman LJ, Gillman T: Studies in the healing of cutaneous wounds. Arch Surg 93:857,883,911, 1966.

Peacock EE: Wound Repair, 3rd ed. WB Saunders, Philadelphia, 1984.

Sunderland S: The anatomic foundation of peripheral nerve repair techniques. Orthopaed Clin North Am 12:245, 1981.

Ver dan C: Tendon surgery of the hand. Churchill Livingstone, New York, 1979.

Walter JB & Israel M: General Pathology. 6th edition. Churchill Livingstone, Edinburgh, 1987.

Chapter 4 Bone and Joint Infection

Ashby ME: Serratia osteomyelitis in heroin users. J Bone Joint Surg 58A:132, 1976.

Autzen B, Elberg JJ: Bone and joint tuberculosis in Denmark. Acta Orthop Scand 59:50–52, 1988.

Bjarnason DF, Forrester DM, Swezey RL: Destructive arthritis of the large joints. A rare manifestation of sarcoidosis. J Bone Joint Surg 55A:618, 1973.

Fyfe B, et al.: Intraosseous echinococcosis: A rare manifestation of echinococcal disease. Southern Med J 83:66–68, 1990.

Gifford DB, Patzakis M, Ivler D, et al.: Septic arthritis due to Pseudomonas in heroin addicts. J Bone Joint Surg 57A:631, 1975.

Green NE, Edwards K: Bone and joint infections in children.

Orthop Clin North Am 18:555–76, 1987.

Greenspan A, Norman A, Steiner G: Case report 146: Squamous cell carcinoma arising in chronic, draining sinus tract secondary to osteomyelitis of right tibia. Skel Radiol 6:149, 1981.

Gustilo RB, et al. (eds.): Orthopaedic Infection: Diagnosis and Treatment. WB Saunders, Philadelphia, 1989.

Hooper J, McLean I: Hydatid disease of the femur. J Bone Joint Surg 59A:974, 1977.

Lemley DE, Katz P: Granulomatous musculoskeletal disease: Sarcoidosis versus tuberculosis. J Rheumatol 14:1199–1201, 1987.

Lieberman J: Sarcoidosis. Grune & Stratton, Orlando, FL, 1985.

Mascola L, Pelosi R, et al.: Congenital syphilis. Why is it still occurring? JAMA 252:1719–1722, 1984.

Nade S: Infection after joint replacement: What would Lister think? Med J Aust 153:394–397, 1990.

Rasool MN, Govender S: The skeletal manifestations of congenital syphilis: A review of 197 cases. J Bone Joint Surg 71B:752–755, 1989.

Rosenberg ZS, Norman A, Soloman G: Arthritis associated with HIV infection radiographic manifestations. Radiology 173:171–176, 1989.

Shannon FB, Moore M, Houkom JA, Waecker NJ Jr.: Multifocal cystic tuberculosis of bone, report of a case. J Bone Joint Surg 72A:1089–1092, 1990.

Stephens MM, MacAuley P: Brodie's abscess. A long-term review. Clin Orthop 234:211–216, 1988.

Waldvogel FA, Papageorgiou PS: Osteomyelitis: The past decade. N Engl J Med 303:360, 1980.

Walker AN, Fechner RE: Granulomatous inflammation of bones and joints. In Joachim HL (ed.) Pathology of Granulomas. Raven Press, New York, 1983.

SECTION III—METABOLIC DISTURBANCES

Chapter 5 Diseases Resulting from Abnormal Synthesis of Matrix Components

Collagen Disturbances

Bullough PG, Davidson DD, Lorenzo JC: The morbid anatomy of the skeleton in osteogenesis imperfecta. Clin Orthop 159:42–57, 1981.

Cetta G, Ramirez F, Tsipouras P: Third international conference on osteogenesis imperfecta, in Annals of The New York Academy of Sciences, vol. 543. The New York Academy of Sciences, New York, 1988.

Minor RR: Collagen metabolism. A comparison of diseases of collagen and diseases affecting collagen. Am J Pathol 98:225, 1980.

Prockop DJ: Mutations in type I procollagen genes: An explanation for brittle bones and a paradigm for other diseases of connective tissue. Trans Am Clin Climatol Assoc 100:70–80, 1988.

Vitto J, Bauer EA: Diseases associated with collagen abnormalities. In Weiss JB, Jayson MV (eds.) Collagen in Health and Disease. Churchill Livingstone, New York, 1982.

Vitamin A Intoxication

Caffey J: Chronic poisoning due to excess of vitamin A. Am J Roentgenol 65:12, 1951.

Wolke RE, Nielsen SW: Pathogenesis of hypervitaminosis A in growing porcine bone. Lab Invest 16:639, 1967.

Mucopolysaccharidoses

Eggli KD, Dorst JP: The mucopolysaccharidoses and related conditions. Semin Roentgenol 21:275–294, 1986.

Lorincz A: The mucopolysaccharidoses: Advances in understanding and treatment. Pediatr Ann 7:104, 1978.

Alkaline Phosphatase Disturbances

Caffey J: Familial hyperphosphatasemia with ateliosis and hypermetabolism of growing membranous bone: Review of the clinical, radiographic and chemical features. Prog Pediatr Radiol 4:81, 1972.

Horwith M, Nunez EA, Krook L, et al.: Hereditary bone dysplasia with hyperphosphatasaemia: Response to synthetic human calcitonin. Clin Endocrinol 5 (Suppl):341, 1976.

Whyte MP: Hypophosphatasia. In Scriver CR, Beaudet AL, Sly WS, Valle D (eds.) The Metabolic Basis of Inherited Disease, 6th ed. McGraw-Hill, New York, 1989.

Fluoride and Bone

Courvoisier B, Donath A, Baud CA (eds.): Fluoride and bone. Second Symposium CEMO, Nyon, Switzerland, October 9–12, 1977. Hans Huber Publishers, Berne, Switzerland, 1978.

Meunier PJ: Fluoride salts and osteoporosis. In Christiansen C, Overgaard K (eds.) Osteoporosis 1990, from the Third International Symposium on Osteoporosis, Copenhagen, Denmark, 14–20 October, 1990. Osteopress ApS, Copenhagen, Denmark, 1990.

Dwarfism

Dutton RV: A practical radiologic approach to skeletal dysplasias in infancy. Radiol Clin North Am 25:1211–1233, 1987.

Wynne-Davies R, Hall CM, Apley AG: Atlas of skeletal dysplasias, Churchill Livingstone, Edinburgh, 1985.

Chapter 6 Diseases Resulting from Disturbances in Cell Linkage

Favus MJ (ed.): Sclerosing bone dysplasias. In Primer on Metabolic Bone Diseases and Disorders of Mineral Metabolism, 1st ed., American Soc Bone Miner Res, Kelseyville, CA 70:215–227, 1990.

Johnston CC, Melton LJ III, Lindsay R, et al.: Clinical indication for bone mass measurement. J Bone Miner Res 4: (Suppl 2) 1989.

McAfee JG: Radionuclide imaging in metabolic and systemic skeletal diseases. Semin Nucl Med 17:334–349, 1987.

Osteopetrosis

Bevier WC, Wiswell RA, Pyka G, et al.: Relationship of body composition, muscle strength, and aerobic capacity to bone mineral density in older men and women. J Bone Miner Res 4:421–432, 1989.

Bollerslev J, Andersen PE Jr: Radiological, biochemical and hereditary evidence of two types of autosomal dominant osteopetrosis. Bone 9:7–13. 1988.

Marks SC Jr.: Osteopetrosis—multiple pathways for the interception of osteoclast function. Appl Pathol 5:172-183, 1987.

Shapiro F, Glimcher MJ, Holtrop M, et al.: Human osteopetrosis. J Bone Joint Surg 62A:384, 1980.

Paget's Disease

Barry HC: Paget's disease of bone. E & S Livingstone Ltd, Edinburgh, London, 1969.

Basle MF, Mazaud P, et al.: Isolation of osteoclasts from pagetic bone tissue: Morphometry and cytochemistry on isolated cells. Bone 9:1–6, 1988.

Monson DK, Finn HA, et al.: Pseudosarcoma in Paget disease of bone, a case report. J Bone Joint Surg 71A:453–455, 1989.

Paget J: On a form of chronic inflammation of bones. Medchirurg Trans 60:37–63, 1877.

Rebel A, Basle M, Pouplard A, et al.: Bone tissue in Paget's disease of bone. Arthritis Rheum 23:1104, 1980.

Resnick D: Paget disease of bone: Current status and a look back to 1943 and earlier. AJR 150:249–256, 1988.

Osteosclerosis Associated with Increased Osteoblastic Activity

Sparkes RS, Graham CB: Camurati-Engelmann disease. J Med Genet 9:73, 1972.

Van Buchem FSP, Hadders HN, Hansen JF, et al.: Hyperostosis corticalis generalisata. Am J Med 33:387, 1962.

Osteopenic Conditions

Bullough PG: Massive osteolysis. NY State J Med 71:2267, 1971.

Christiansen C, Overgaard K: Osteoporosis 1990, Proc 3rd Int Symposium on Osteoporosis, Copenhagen, Denmark, 1990.

Christiansen C, Rus BJ, Rodbro P: Screening procedures for women at risk of developing postmenopausal osteoporosis. Osteoporosis Int 1:35–40, 1990.

Dickson GR, Hamilton A, et al.: An investigation of vanishing bone disease. Bone 11:205–210, 1990.

Lakharpal S, Ginsburg WW, et al.: Transient osteoporosis. A study of 56 cases and a review of the literature. Ann Intern Med 106:444–450, 1987.

Parfitt AM: Bone remodeling: Relationship to the amount and structure of bone and the pathogenesis and prevention of fractures. In Riggs BL, Melton LJ (eds.) Osteoporosis: Etiology, Diagnosis and Management. Raven Press, New York, 1988.

Whedon GD: Disuse osteoporosis: Physiological aspects. Calcif Tissue Int, 36:S146–150, 1984.

Chapter 7 Diseases Resulting from Disturbances in Mineral Homeostasis

Boyce BF: Focal osteomalacia due to low-dose diphosphonate therapy in Paget's disease. Lancet 821–824, 1984.

Burr DB, Martin RB: Errors in bone remodeling: Toward a unified theory of metabolic bone disease. Am J Anat 186:1–31, 1989.

Burtis WJ, Wu TL, Insogna KL, et al.: Humoral hypercalcemia of malignancy. Ann Intern Med 108:454–456, 1988.

Favus MJ (ed.): A Primer on Metabolic Bone Diseases and Disorders of Mineral Metabolism, 1st ed. Am Soc Bone Miner Res, Kelseyville, CA, 1990.

Genat HK, Baron JM, et al.: Osteosclerosis in primary hyperparathyroidism. Am J Med 59:104–113, 1975.

Grech P, Martin TJ, et al.: Diagnosis of Metabolic Bone Disease, Chapman and Hall, London, 1985.

Gupta A, Hruska KA: Hyperphosphatemia and hypophosphatemia. In Favus MJ (ed.) Primer on Metabolic Bone Diseases and Disorders of Mineral Metabolism, 1st ed. Am Soc Bone Miner Res, Kelseyville, CA 51:143–147, 1990.

Hahn TJ: Drug-induced disorders of vitamin D and mineral metabolism. Clin Endocrinol Metab 9:107–129, 1980.

Heath H III, Hodgson SF, Kennedy MA: Primary hyperparathyroidism: Incidence, morbidity, and potential economic impact in a community. N Engl J Med 302:189, 1980.

Kleerekoper M, Krane SM (eds.): Clinical Disorders of Bone and Mineral Metabolism: Proceedings of the Lawrence and Dorothy Fallis International Symposium. Mary Ann Liebert, New York, 1989.

Malluche H, Faugere MC: Renal bone disease 1990: An unmet challenge for the nephrologist. Kidney Int 38:193–211, 1990.

Malluche H, Hartmut H, Faugere MC: Atlas of mineralized bone histology. Karger, Basel, New York, 1986.

Mundy GR: The hypercalcemia of malignancy. Kidney Int 31:142–155, 1987

Nuovo MA, Dorfman HD, Sun CC, et al.: Tumor-induced osteomalacia and rickets. Am J Surg Pathol 13:588–599, 1989.

Parfitt AM: Osteomalacia and related disorders. In Krane SM (ed.) Metabolic Bone Disease, 2nd ed. Grune & Stratton, New York (in press).

Rasmussen H: The calcium messenger system. N Engl J Med 314:1094–1101,1164–1170, 1986.

Roth KS, Foreman JW, Segal S: The Fanconi syndrome and mechanisms of tubular transport dysfunction. Kidney Int 20:705–716, 1981.

Sherrard SJ, Andress DL: Aluminum-related osteodystrophy. Adv Intern Med 34:307–324, 1989.

Sherrard DJ, Andress DL: Renal Osteodystrophy. In Schrier RW, Gottschalk CW (eds.) Diseases of the Kidney. Little, Brown and Co., Boston, 1988.

Stern PH: Vitamin D and bone. Kidney Int (Suppl) 29:S17–21, 1990.

Soft Tissue Calcification

Anderson HC: Calcific diseases: A concept. Arch Pathol Lab Med (in press).

Boskey AL, Vigorita VJ, Spencer O, et al.: Chemical, microscopic and ultrastructural characterization of the mineral deposits in tumoral calcinosis. Clin Orthopaed Relat Res (in press).

O'Conner JM: Soft Tissue Ossification. Springer-Verlag, New York, 1983.

Russell RGG, Kanis JA: Ectopic calcification and ossification. In Nordin BFC (ed.) Metabolic Bone and Stone Disease, 2nd ed. Churchill Livingstone, Edinburgh, 1984.

Chapter 8 Accumulation of Abnormal MetabolicProducts and Various Hematologic Disorders

Oxalosis

Benhamou CL, Pierre D, et al.: Primary bone oxalosis: The roles of oxalate deposits and renal osteodystrophy. Bone 8:59–64, 1987.

Julian BA, Faugere MC, Malluche HH: Oxalosis in bone causing a radiographical mimicry of renal osteodystrophy. Am J Kidney Dis 9:436–40, 1987.

Amyloidosis

Chapman RH, Cotter F: The carpal tunnel syndrome and amyloidosis. Clin Orthopaed Relat Res 169:159, 1982.

Rousselin B, Helenon O, Zingraff J, et al.: Pseudotumor of the craniocervical junction during long-term hemodialysis. Arthritis Rheum 33:1567–1573, 1990.

Tagliabue JR, Stull MA, Lack EE, et al.: Case report 610: Amyloid arthropathy of the left ankle. Skel Radiol 19:448–452, 1990.

Gaucher's Disease

Goldblatt J, Sacks S, Beighton P: The orthopedic aspects of Gaucher disease. Clin Orthopaed Relat Res 137:208, 1978.

Springfield DS, Landried M, Mankin HJ: Gaucher hemorrhagic cyst of bone. A case report. J Bone Joint Surg 71A:141–144, 1989.

Xanthomatosis (Chester-Erdheim Disease of Bone)

Lantz B, Lange TA, Heiner J, Herring GF: Erdheim-Chester disease. A report of three cases. J Bone Joint Surg 71A:456–464, 1989.

Eosinophilic Granuloma

Compere EL, Johnson WE, Coventry MB: Vertebra plana (Calve's disease) due to eosinophilic granuloma. J Bone Joint Surg 36A:969, 1954.

Lieberman PH, Jones CR, Filippa DA: Langerhans cell (eosinophilic) granulomatosis. J Invest Dermatol 75:71, 1980.

Systemic Mastocytosis

Cook JV, Chandy J: Systemic mastocytosis affecting the skeletal system. J Bone Joint Surg 71B:536, 1989.

Fallon MD, Whyte MP, Teitelbaum SL: Systemic mastocytosis associated with generalized osteoporosis. Hum Pathol 12:813–820, 1981.

Skeletal Manifestations of Hematological Diseases

Bennett OM, Namnyak SS: Bone and joint manifestations of sickle cell anaemia. J Bone Joint Surg 72B:794–799, 1990.

Gratwick GM, Bullough PG, Bohne WH, et al.: Thalassemic osteoarthropathy. Ann Intern Med 88:494, 1978.

Mundy GR, Bertolini DB: Bone destruction and hypercalcemia in plasma cell myeloma. Oncology 13:291–299, 1986.

Schumacher HR: Articular cartilage: The degenerative arthropathy of hemochromatosis. Arthritis Rheum 25:1460–1468, 1982.

Visani G, Finelli C, Castelli U, et al.: Myelofibrosis with myeloid metaplasia: Clinical and haematological parameters predicting survival in a series of 133 patients. Br J Haematol 75:4–9, 1990.

SECTION IV—ARTHRITIS

Chapter 9 The Pathophysiology of Arthritis

Andriacchi T, Sabiston P, DeHaven K, et al.: Ligament: injury and repair. In Woo SS-Y, Buckwalter JA (eds.) Injury and Repair of the Musculoskeletal Soft Tissues. Am Assoc Orthop Surg 103–128, 1987.

Bullough PG, Goodfellow JW: The pattern of aging of the articular cartilage of the elbow joint. J Bone Joint Surg 49B:175–181, 1967.

Bullough PG, Goodfellow JW: The significance of the fine structure of articular cartilage. J Bone Joint Surg 50B:852–857; 1968.

Bullough PG, Jagannath A: The morphology of the calcification front in articular cartilage. J Bone Joint Surg 65B:72–78, 1983.

Bullough PG, Yawitz PS, Tafra L, et al.: Topographical variations in the morphology and biochemistry of adult canine tibial plateau articular cartilage. J Orthop Res 3:1–16, 1985.

Gatter RA: A Practical Handbook of Joint Fluid Analysis. Lea & Febiger, Philadelphia, 1984.

Hunter W: Of the structure and diseases of articulating cartilages. Phil Trans 267–271, 1743.

Kuettner KE, Schleyerbach R, Hascall VC (eds.): Articular Cartilage Biochemistry. Raven Press, New York, 1986.

MacConaill MA: The movements of bones and joints. J Bone Joint Surg 32:244, 1950.

Mink JH, Deutsch AL: Magnetic resonance imaging of the knee. Clin Orthop 244:29, 1989.

Wormsley T: The articular mechanism of the diarthroses. J Bone Joint Surg 10A:40, 1928.

Chapter 10 The Noninflammatory Arthritides

Bennett GA, Waine H, Bauer KW: Changes in the Knee Joint at Various Ages with Particular Reference to the Nature and Development of Degenerative Joint Disease. The Commonwealth Fund, New York, 1942.

Brandt KD (ed.): Cartilage Changes in Osteoarthritis. Indiana University School of Medicine, Bloomington, 1990.

Bullough PG, DiCarlo EF: Subchondral avascular necrosis: A common cause of arthritis. Ann Rheum Dis 49:412–420, 1990.

Bullough PG, Goodfellow J, O'Connor JJ: The relationship between degenerative changes and load bearing in the human hip. J Bone Joint Surg 55B:746–758, 1973.

Burwell RG: Perthes' disease: Growth and aetiology. Arch Dis Child 63:1408–1412, 1988.

Eichenholtz SN: Charcot Joints. Charles C Thomas, Springfield, IL, 1966.

Glickstein MF, Burk DL Jr, Schiebler ML, et al.: Avascular necrosis versus other diseases of the hip: Sensitivity of MR imaging. Radiology 169:213–215, 1988.

Harris WH: Etiology of osteoarthritis of the hip. Clin Orthop 213:20–33, 1986.

Kellgren JH, Lawrence JS: Radiological assessment of osteoarthrosis. Ann Rheum Dis 16:494, 1957.

Landin LA, Danielsson LG, Wattsgard C: Transient synovitis of the hip. Its incidence, epidemiology and relation to Perthes' disease. J Bone Joint Surg 69B:238–242, 1987.

Macys JR, Bullough PG, Wilson PD Jr: Coxarthrosis: A study of the natural history based on a correlation of clinical, radiographic and pathologic findings. Semin Arthritis Rheum 10:66–80, 1980.

Mitchell DG, Steinberg ME, Dalinka MK, et al.: Magnetic resonance imaging of the ischemic hip. Alterations within the osteonecrotic, viable, and reactive zones. Clin Orthop 244:60–77, 1989.

Peyron JG: Epidemiologic and etiologic approach to osteoarthritis. Semin Arthritis Rheum 8:288, 1979.

Thompson GH, Salter RB: Legg-Calvé-Perthes disease. Current concepts and controversies. Orthop Clin North Am 18:617–635, 1987.

Chapter 11 The Inflammatory Arthritides

Inflammatory Arthritis Associated with Diffuse ConnectiveTissue Disease
Cassidy JT, Martel W: Juvenile rheumatoid arthritis: Clinicoradiologic correlations. Arthritis Rheum 20 (Suppl 2): 207–211, 1977.

Rodnan GP, Schumacher HR (eds.): Primer on the Rheumatic Diseases, 8th ed. Arthritis Foundation, Atlanta, GA, 1983.

Soren A: Histodiagnosis and Clinical Correlation of Rheumatoid and Other Synovitis. Lippincott, Philadelphia, 1978.

Diseases Resulting from Deposition of Metabolic Products in the Joint Tissues
Boss GR, Seegmiller JE: Hyperuricemia and gout. N Engl J Med 300:1459, 1979.

Gatter RA: Use of the compensated polarizing microscope. Clin Rheum Dis 3:91, 1977.

Hough AJ, Banfield WG, Sokoloff L: Cartilage in hemophilic arthropathy: Arch Pathol Lab Med 100:91–96, 1976.

Resnick D, Niwayama G, Goergen T, et al.: Clinical, radiographic and pathologic abnormalities in calcium pyrophosphate dihydrate deposition disease (CPPD): Pseudogout. Radiology 122:1, 1977.

Schumacher HR, Holdsworth DE: Ochronotic arthropathy. I. Clinicopathologic studies. Semin Arthritis Rheum 6:207, 1977.

Sissons HA, Steiner GC, Bonar F, et al.: Tumoral calcium pyrophosphate deposition disease. Skel Radiol 18:79–87, 1989.

Chapter 12 Spinal Arthritis and Degenerative Disc Disease
Bullough PG, Boachie-Adjei O: Atlas of Spinal Diseases. Gower Medical Publishing, New York, 1988.

Resnick D, Niwayama G: Diagnosis of bone and joint disorders (3 vols.) 2nd ed. WB Saunders, Philadelphia, 1988.

Schmorl G, Junghanns H: The Human Spine in Health and Disease. 2nd Am. ed. Grune & Stratton, New York, 1971.

Chapter 13 Tissue Response to Prosthetic Implants
Black J, Sherk H, et al.: Metallosis associated with a titanium alloy femoral component in total hip arthroplasty. J Bone Joint Surg 72A:126–130, 1990.

Brien WW, Salvati EA, Healey JH, et al.: Osteogenic sarcoma arising in the area of a total hip replacement. A case report. J Bone Joint Surg 72A:1097–1099, 1990.

Christiansen K, Holmes K, Zilko PJ: Metal sensitivity causing loosened joint prostheses. Ann Rheum Dis 38:476, 1979.

DiCarlo EF, Bullough PG: The biologic responses to orthopaedic implants and their wear debris. Clin Mater (in press).

Gordon M, Bullough PG: Synovial and osseous inflammation in failed silicone rubber prostheses. J Bone Joint Surg 64A:574, 1982.

Johanson NA, Bullough PG, Wilson PD, et al.: The microscopic anatomy of the bone-cement interface in failed total hip arthroplasties. Clin Orthop 218:123, 1987.

Kim KC, Ritter MA: Hypotension associated with methyl methacrylate in total hip arthroplasties. Clin Orthop 88:154, 1972.

Mears D: Materials and Orthopedic Surgery. Williams & Wilkins, Baltimore, 1979.

Rae T: A study of the effects of particulate metals of orthopaedic interest on murine macrophages in vitro. J Bone Joint Surg 57B:444, 1975.

Salvati EA, Brause BD: Infection of orthopedic prostheses. In Schlossberg D (ed.) Orthopedic Infection, Chap. 10, Springer-Verlag, New York, 1988.

Santavirta S, Konttinen YT, et al.: Aggressive granulomatous lesions associated with hip arthroplasty. J Bone Joint Surg 72A:252–258, 1990.

SECTION V—TUMORS

Chapter 14 Benign Conditions—Bony and Cartilaginous

Fibrous Dysplasia
Harris WH, Dudley H Jr, Barry RJ: The natural history of fibrous dysplasia. J Bone Joint Surg 44A:207, 1962.

Henry A: Monostotic fibrous dysplasia. J Bone Joint Surg 51B:300, 1969.

Logel RJ: Recurrent intramuscular myxomas associated with Albright's syndrome. Case report and review of the literature. J Bone Joint Surg 58A:565–568, 1976.

Yabut SM Jr, Kenan S, Sissons HA, et al.: Malignant transformation of fibrous dysplasia. A case report and review of the literature. Clin Orthop 228:281–289, 1988.

Ossifying Fibroma
Campanacci M, Laus M: Osteofibrous dysplasia of the tibia and fibula. J Bone Joint Surg 63A:367, 1981.

Enchondromatosis
Liu J, Hudkins PG, Swee RG, et al.: Bone sarcomas associated with Ollier's disease. Cancer 59:1376–1385, 1987.

Paterson DC, Morris LL, Binns MA, et al.: Generalized enchondromatosis. A case report. J Bone Joint Surg 71A:133–140, 1989.

Shapiro F: Ollier's disease. J Bone Joint Surg 64A:95, 1982.

Osteochondroma
D'Ambrosia R, Ferguson A: The formation of osteochondroma by epiphyseal cartilage transplantation. Clin Orthop Relat Res 61:103, 1968.

Multiple Osteochondromas
Peterson HA: Multiple hereditary osteochondromata. Clin Orthop 239:222–230, 1989.

Voegeli E, Laissue J, Kaiser A, et al.: Case report 143. Skel Radiol 6:134, 1981.

Dysplasia Epiphysealis Hemimelica
Mendez AA, Keret D, MacEwen GD: Isolated dysplasia epiphysealis hemimelica of the hip joint. J Bone Joint Surg 70A:921–925, 1988.

Trevor D: Tarso-epiphysial aclasis: A congenital error of epiphysial development. J Bone Joint Surg 32B:204–213, 1950.

Bone Island and Sclerosing Dysplasias
Greenspan A, Steiner GC, Knutzon R: Bone island (enostosis): Clinical significance and radiologic and pathologic correlations. Skel Radiol 20:85–90, 1991.

Greenspan A, Steiner GC, Sotelo D, et al.: Mixed sclerosing bone dysplasia coexisting with dysplasia epiphysialis hemimelica (Trevor-Fairbank disease). Skel Radiol 15:452–454, 1986.

Osteoid Osteoma
Freiberger RH, Loitman BS, et al.: Osteoid osteoma. A report on 80 cases. Am J Roentgenol 82:194, 1959.

Greenspan A, Elguezabal A, Bryk D: Multifocal osteoid osteoma, a case report and review of the literature. Am J Roentgenol Radium Ther Nucl Med 121:103, 1974.

Keim HA, Reina EG: Osteoid osteoma as a cause of scoliosis. J Bone Joint Surg 57A:159, 1975.

Worland RL, Ryder CT, Johnston AD: Recurrent osteoid-osteoma: Report of a case. J Bone Joint Surg 37A:277, 1975.

Osteomas of the Cranium and Facial Bones
Bullough PG: Ivory exostosis of the skull. Postgrad Med 41:277–281, 1965.

Rayne J, Bullough PG: A case of Gardner's syndrome. Br J Surg 53:824–826, 1966.

Chapter 15 Benign Tumors—Cystic, Fibrous and Others

Epidermoid Inclusion Cyst
Roth SI: Squamous cysts involving the skull and distal phalanges. J Bone Joint Surg 46A:1442, 1964.
Rozmaryn LM, Sadler AH, Dorfman HD: Intraosseous glomus tumor in the ulna. A case report. Clin Orthop 220:126–129, 1987.
Sugiura I: Intra-osseous glomus tumor. J Bone Joint Surg 58B:245, 1976.

Ganglionic Cyst of Bone
Bauer TW, Dorfman HD: Intraosseous ganglion, a clinicopathologic study of 11 cases. Am J Surg Pathol 6:207–213, 1982.
Kambolis C, Bullough PG, Jaffe HL: Ganglionic cystic defects of bone. J Bone Joint Surg 55A:496, 1973.

Unicameral Bone Cyst
Makley JT, Joyce MJ: Unicameral bone cyst (simple bone cyst). Orthop Clin North Am 20:407–415, 1989.

Aneurysmal Bone Cyst
Frassica FJ, Amadio PC, Wold LE, et al.: Aneurysmal bone cyst: Clinicopathologic features and treatment of ten cases involving the hand. J Hand Surg 13A:676–683, 1988.
Martinez V, Sissons HA: Aneurysmal bone cyst. A review of 123 cases including primary lesions and those secondary to other bone pathology. Cancer 61:2291–2304, 1988.

Giant Cell Reparative Granuloma
Dorfman HD, Steiner GC, Jaffe HL: Vascular tumors of bone. Hum Pathol 2:349–376, 1971.
Ratner V, Dorfman HD: Giant-cell reparative granuloma of the hand and foot bones. Clin Orthop Relat Res 251–258, 1990.
Sanerkin N, et al.: An unusual intraosseous lesion with fibroblastic, osteoclastic, osteoblastic, aneurysmal and fibromyxoid elements. "Solid" variant of aneurysmal bone cyst. Cancer 51:2278, 1983.
Schajowicz F, Aiello CL, Francone MV, et al.: Cystic angiomatosis (hamartous haemolymphangiomatosis) of bone. A clinicopathological study of three cases. J Bone Joint Surg 60B:100–106, 1978.

Hemangioma
Moon NF: Synovial hemangioma of the knee joint. Clin Orthop 90:183–190, 1972.

Nonossifying Fibroma
Bertoni F, et al.: Benign fibrous histiocytoma of bone. J Bone Joint Surg 68A:1225–1230, 1986.
Marks KE, Bauer TW: Fibrous tumors of bone. Orthop Clin North Am 20:377–393, 1989.
Spjut HJ, Fechner RE, Ackerman LV: Benign fibrous histiocytoma. Supplement to Atlas of Tumor Pathology (2nd series). Tumors of Bone and Cartilage, fascicle 5. Armed Forces Institute of Pathology, Washington, DC, 1981.

Periosteal "Desmoid"
Kimmelstiel P, Rapp I: Cortical defect due to periosteal desmoids. Bull Hosp Joint Dis 12:286, 1951.

Lipoma of Bone
Milgram JW: Intraosseous lipomas. A clinicopathologic study of 66 cases. Clin Orthop 231:277–302, 1988.
Milgram JW: Intraosseous lipomas with reactive ossification in the proximal femur. Report of eight cases. Skel Radiol 7:1–13, 1981.

Hoffa's Disease
Hallel T, Lew S, Bansal M: Villous lipomatous proliferation of the synovial membrane (lipoma arborescens). J Bone Joint Surg 70A:264–270, 1988.

Chapter 16 Neoplasms—Benign and Malignant; Bony and Cartilaginous
Unni KK (ed.): Bone Tumors. Churchill Livingstone, New York, 1988.

Osteoblastoma
Marsh BW, Bonfiglio M, Brady LP, et al.: Benign osteoblastoma: Range of manifestations. J Bone Joint Surg 57A:1, 1975.
Spjut HJ, Fechner RE, Ackerman LV: Aggressive osteoblastoma in tumors of bone and cartilage (Suppl). Armed Forces Institute of Pathology, Washington, DC, 1981.

Osteosarcoma
Ayala AG, Raymond AK, Jaffe N: The pathologist's role in the diagnosis and treatment of osteosarcoma in children. Hum Pathol 15:258–266, 1984.
Bane BL, et al.: Extraskeletal osteosarcoma. A clinicopathologic review of 26 cases. Cancer 65:2762–2770, 1990.
Greenspan A, Steiner GC, Norman A, et al.: Osteosarcoma of the soft tissue. Case report #436. Skel Radiol 16:489–492, 1987.
Jundt G, Schulz A, Berghauser KH, Fisher LW, Gehron-Robey P, Termine JD: Immunocytochemical identification of osteogenic bone tumors by osteonectin antibodies. Virchows Arch [Pathol Anat] 414:345–353, 1989.
Klein MJ, Kenan S, Lewis MM: Osteosarcoma, clinical and pathological considerations. Orthop Clin North Am 20:327–345, 1989.
Kurt AM, Unni KK, McLeod RA, et al.: Low-grade intraosseous osteosarcoma. Cancer 65:1418–1428, 1990.
Parham DM, Pratt CB, Parvey LS, et al.: Childhood multifocal osteosarcoma—Clinico-pathologic and radiologic correlates. Cancer 55:2653–2658, 1985.
Picci P, Campanacci M, Bacci G, Capanna R, Ayala A: Medullary involvement in parosteal osteosarcoma. J Bone Joint Surg 69A:131–136, 1987.
Schajowicz F, McGuire MH, Araujo ES, et al.: Osteosarcomas arising on the surfaces of long bones. J Bone Joint Surg 70A:555–565, 1988.
Sim FH, Unni KK, Beabout JW, et al.: Osteosarcoma with small cells simulating Ewing's tumor. J Bone Joint Surg 61A:207–215, 1979.
Tsuneyoshi M, Dorfman HD: Epiphyseal osteosarcoma: distinguishing features from clear cell chondrosarcoma, chondroblastoma and epiphyseal enchondroma. Hum Pathol 18:644–651, 1987.
Unni KK, Dahlin DC, Beabout JW: Periosteal osteogenic sarcoma. Cancer 37:2476–2485, 1976.

Paget's Sarcoma
Smith J, Botet JF, Yeh SDJ: Bone sarcomas in Paget's disease: A study of 85 patients. Radiology 152:583–590, 1984.

Radiation Sarcoma
Steiner GC: Post-radiation sarcoma of bone. Cancer 18:603–612, 1965.

Enchondroma
Takigawa K: Chondroma of the bones of the hand. J Bone Joint Surg 53A:1591, 1971.

Juxtacortical Chondroma
Lewis MM, Kenan S, Yabut SM, et al.: Periosteal chondroma. A report of ten cases and review of the literature. Clin Orthop 256:185–192, 1990.

Soft-tissue Chondroma
Chung EB, Enzinger FM: Benign chondromas of soft parts. Cancer 41:1414, 1978.

Chondroblastoma
Green P, Whittaker RP: Benign chondroblastoma. J Bone Joint Surg 57A:418, 1975.
Schajowicz F, Gallardo H: Epiphysial chondroblastoma of bone. J Bone Joint Surg 52B:205, 1970.

Chondromyxoid Fibroma
Zillmer DA, Dorfman HD: Chondromyxoid fibroma of bone: Thirty-six cases with clinicopathologic correlation. Hum Pathol 20:952–964, 1989.

Fibromyxoma
Marcove RC, Kambolis C, Bullough PG, et al.: Fibromyxoma of bone. Cancer 17:1209, 1961.

Chordoma
Miettinen M: Chordoma: Antibodies to epithelial membrane antigen and carcinoembryonic antigen in differential diagnosis. Arch Pathol Lab Med 108:891–892, 1984.

Ulich TR, Mirra JM: Ecchordosis physaliphora vertebralis. Clin Orthop 163:,282, 1989.

Valderrama E, Kahn LB, et al.: Chondroid chordoma: Electron-microscopic study of two cases. Am J Surg Pathol 7:625–632, 1983.

Volpe R, Mazabraud A: A clinicopathologic review of 25 cases of chordoma (a pleomorphic and metastasizing neoplasm). Am J Surg Pathol 7:161, 1983.

Primary Synovial Chondromatosis
Norman A, Steiner GC: Bone erosion in synovial chondromatosis. Radiology 161:749–752, 1986.

Villacin A, Brigham L, Bullough P: Primary and secondary synovial chondrometaplasia. Histopathologic and clinicopathologic differences. Hum Pathol 10:439, 1979.

Chondrosarcoma
Barnes R, Catto M: Chondrosarcoma of bone. J Bone Joint Surg 48B:729, 1966.

Culver JE, Sweet DE, McCue FC: Chondrosarcoma of the hand arising from a pre-existent benign solitary enchondroma, case report and pathological description. Clin Orthop Relat Res 113:128–131, 1975.

Harwood AR, Krajbich JI, Fornasier VL: Mesenchymal chondrosarcoma: A report of 17 cases. Clin Orthopaed Relat Res 158:144, 1981.

Johnson S, Tetu B, Ayala AG, et al.: Chondrosarcoma with additional mesenchymal component (dedifferentiated chondrosarcoma): A clinicopathologic study of 26 cases. Cancer 58:278–286, 1986.

Mankin HJ, Cantley KP, Lippiello L, et al.: The biology of human chondrosarcoma I. J Bone Joint Surg 62A:160, 1980.

Mankin HJ, Cantley KP, Schiller AL, et al.: The biology of human chondrosarcoma II. J Bone Joint Surg 62A:176, 1980.

McCarthy EF, Dorfman HD: Chondrosarcoma of bone with dedifferentiation: A study of eighteen cases. Hum Pathol 13:36, 1982.

Nakashima Y, Unni KK, Shives TC, Swee RG, Dahlin DC: Mesenchymal chondrosarcoma of bone and soft tissue. Cancer 57:2444–2453, 1986.

Sanerkin NG, Gallagher P: A review of the behaviour of chondrosarcoma of bone. J Bone Joint Surg 61B:395, 1979.

Wu KK, et al.: Extra-osseous chondrosarcoma. J Bone Joint Surg 62A:189–194, 1980.

Unni KK, Dahlin DC, Beabout JW, et al.: Chondrosarcoma: Clear-cell variant. J Bone Joint Surg 58A:676, 1976.

Chapter 17 Neoplasms—Benign and Malignant; Fibrous, Small Cell and Others

Desmoplastic Fibroma
Gebhardt MC, Cambell CJ, Schiller ML, et al.: Desmoplastic fibroma of bone. J Bone Joint Surg 67A:732–747, 1985.

Fibrosarcoma
Huvos AG, Higinbotham NL: Primary fibrosarcoma of bone. Cancer 35:837, 1975.

Malignant Fibrous Histiocytoma
Enzinger FM: Malignant fibrous histiocytoma 20 years after Stout. Am J Surg Pathol 10 (Suppl 1):43–53, 1986.

Spjut HJ, Fechner RE, Ackerman LV: Malignant fibrous histiocytoma. Supplement to Atlas of Tumor Pathology (2nd series). Tumors of Bone and Cartilage, Armed Forces Institute of Pathology, Washington, DC, 1981.

Giant Cell Tumor
Bertoni F, Present D, et al.: Giant-cell tumor of bone with pulmonary metastases. Six case reports and a review of the literature. Clin Orthop 237:275–285, 1988.

Bliss BO, Reid RJ: Large cell sarcomas of the tendon sheath. Malignant giant cell tumor of the tendon sheath. Am J Clin Pathol 49:776, 1968.

Campanacci M, Baldini N, Boriani S, et al.: Giant-cell tumor of bone. J Bone Joint Surg 69A:106–114, 1987.

Jacobs TP, et al.: Giant cell tumor in Paget's disease of bone—familial and geographic clustering. Cancer 44:742–747, 1979.

Sim FH, Dahlin DC, Beabout JW: Multicentric giant cell tumor of bone. J Bone Joint Surg 59A:1052–1060, 1977.

Sung HW, Kuo DP, Shu YB, et al.: Giant cell tumor of bone: Analysis of two hundred and eight cases in Chinese patients. J Bone Joint Surg 64A:755–761, 1982.

Vascular Neoplasms
Dorfman HD, Steiner GC, Jaffe HL: Vascular tumors of bone. Hum Pathol 2:349–376, 1971.

Gutierrez RM, Spjut HS: Skeletal angiomatosis: Report of three cases and review of the literature. Clin Orthop 85:82–97, 1972.

Tang JS, Gold RH, Mirra JM, et al.: Hemangiopericytoma of bone. Cancer 62:848–859, 1988.

Tsuneyoshi M, Dorfman HD, Bauer TW: Epithelioid hemangioendothelioma of bone. A clinicopathologic, ultrastructural and immunohistochemical study. Am J Surg Pathol 10:754–764, 1986.

Weiss SW, Enzinger FM: Spindle cell hemangioendothelioma: A low-grade angiosarcoma resembling a cavernous hemangioma and Kaposi's sarcoma. Am J Surg Pathol 10:521–530, 1986.

Ewing's Sarcoma
Jaffe R, et al.: The neuroectodermal tumor of bone. Am J Surg Pathol 8:885–898, 1984.

Triche T, Cavazzana A: Round cell tumors of bone. In Unni KK (ed.) Bone Tumors. Churchill Livingstone, New York, 1988.

Lymphoma
Epstein BS: Vertebral changes in childhood leukemia. Radiology 68:65, 1957.

Kyle RA: Multiple myeloma: Review of 869 cases. Mayo Clin Proc 50:29, 1975.

Ostrowski ML, et al.: Malignant lymphoma of bone. Cancer 58:2646–2655, 1986.

Sweet D, Mass D, Simon M, et al.: Histiocytic lymphoma (reticulum cell sarcoma) of bone. J Bone Joint Surg 63A:79–84, 1981.

Triche TJ: Diagnosis of small round cell tumors in childhood. Bull Cancer 75:297–310, 1988.

Valderrama JAF, Bullough PG: Solitary myeloma of the spine. J Bone Joint Surg 50B:82, 1968.

Adamantinoma of Long Bones
Campanacci M, Laus M, Giunti A, et al.: Adamantinoma of the long bones. Am J Surg Pathol 5:533, 1981.

Czerniak B, Rojas-Corona RR, Dorfman HD: Morphologic diversity of long bone adamantinoma. The concept of differentiated (regressing) adamantinoma and its relationship to osteofibrous dysplasia. Cancer 64:2319–2334, 1989.

Schajowicz F, Santini-Araujo E: Adamantinoma of the tibia masked by fibrous dysplasia. Report of three cases. Clin Orthop 238:294–301, 1989.

Weiss SW, Dorfman HD: Adamantinoma of long bone. An analysis of nine new cases with emphasis on metastasizing lesions

and fibrous-dysplasia-like changes. Hum Pathol
8:141–153, 1977.

Synovial Sarcoma
Krall RA, Kostianovsky M, Patchefsky AS: Synovial sarcoma. Am
J Surg Pathol 5:137, 1981.
Wright PH, Sim FH, Soule EH, et al.: Synovial sarcoma. J Bone
Joint Surg 64A:112, 1982.

Epithelioid Sarcoma
Prat J, Woodruff J, Marcove R: Epithelioid sarcoma. Cancer
41:1472, 1978.

Pigmented Villonodular Synovitis
Arthaud JB: Pigmented nodular synovitis: A report of 11
lesions in non-articular locations. Am J Clin Pathol
58:511–517, 1972.
Kahn L: Malignant giant cell tumor of the tendon sheath. Arch
Pathol 96:203, 1973.
Wendt RG, et al.: Polyarticular pigmented villonodular synovitis:
Evidence for a genetic contribution. J Rheumatol
13:921–926, 1986.

Metastatic Cancer
Boland PJ, Lane JM, Sundaresan N: Metastatic disease of the
spine. Clin Orthop 169:95, 1982.
Levy RN: Metastatic disease of bone. Clin Orthop Relat Res
169:2, 1982.
Mir R, Phillips SL, et al.: Metastatic neuroblastoma after 52 years
of dormancy. Cancer 60:2510–2514, 1987.

SECTION VI—COMMON BUT UNEXCITING
ORTHOPEDIC CONDITIONS

Chapter 18 Miscellaneous Orthopedic
BoneConditions

Bone Infarction
Bullough PG, Kambolis CP, Marcove RC, et al.: Bone infarctions
not associated with caisson disease. J Bone Joint Surg
47A:477–491, 1965.

Congenital Pseudarthrosis
Campanacci M, Nicoll EA, Pagella P: The differential diagnosis
of congenital pseudarthrosis of the tibia. J Int Orthopaed
(SICOT) 4:283, 1981.

Slipped Capital Femoral Epiphysis
Boyer DW, Mickelson MR, Ponseti IV: Slipped capital femoral
epiphysis. J Bone Joint Surg 63A:85, 1981.

Congenital Dislocation of the Hip
Tachdjian MO (ed.): Congenital Dislocation of the Hip. Churchill
Livingstone, New York, 1982.

Osteochondritis Dissecans
Barrie HJ: Osteochondritis dissecans 1887–1987. A centennial
look at Konig's memorable phrase. J Bone Joint Surg
69B:693–695, 1987.

Hypertrophic Osteoarthropathy
Resnick D, Niwayama S: Enostosis, hyperostosis, and periostitis.

Chapter 96, in Diagnosis of Bone and Joint Disorders, 2nd ed.
WB Saunders, Philadelphia, 1988.

Infantile Cortical Hyperostosis
Thornberg LP: Infantile cortical hyperostosis (Caffrey-Silverman
syndrome). Animal model: Craniomandibular osteopathy in
the canine. Am J Pathol 95:575, 1979.

Myositis Ossificans
Lagier R, Cox JN: Pseudomalignant myositis ossificans. Hum
Pathol 6:653, 1975.
Norman A, Dorfman HD: Juxtacortical circumscribed myositis
ossificans. Evolution and radiographic features. Radiology
96:301, 1970.
Smith R, Russell RGG, Wood CG: Myositis ossificans progressiva. Clinical features of eight patients and their response
to treatment. J Bone J Surg 58B:48–57, 1976.

Subungual Exostosis
Miller-Breslow A, Dorfman HD: Dupuytren's (subungual)
exostosis. Am J Surg Pathol 12:368–378, 1988.

Reactive Periostitis
Spjut HJ, Dorfman HD: Florid reactive periostitis of the tubular
bones of the hands and feet. Am J Surg Pathol
5:423–433, 1981.

Chapter 19 Miscellaneous Orthopedic
Soft-Tissue Conditions

Ganglion
Burk DL Jr, Dalinka MK, Kanal E, et al.: Meniscal and ganglion
cysts of the knee: MR evaluation. Am J Radiol
150:331–336, 1988.
Lantz B, Singer KM: Meniscal cysts. Clin Sports Med
9:707–723, 1990.

Carpal Tunnel Syndrome
Phalen GS: The birth of a syndrome, or carpal tunnel revisited.
J Hand Surg 6:109, 1981.

Morton's Neuroma
Lassmann G: Morton's toe. Clinical, light and electron microscopic investigations in 133 cases. Clin Orthop Relat Res
142:73, 1979.

Compartment Syndrome
Hargens AR, Schmidt DA, Evans KL, et al.: Quantitation of skele-
tal muscle necrosis in a model compartment syndrome.
J Bone Joint Surg 63A:631, 1981.

Fibromatoses
Enzinger FM, Weiss SW: Fibromatoses. In Soft Tissue Tumors.
CV Mosby, St. Louis, MO, 1983.

Cranial Fasciitis
Lauer DH, Enzinger FM: Cranial fasciitis of childhood. Cancer
45:401–406, 1980.

Elastofibroma
Renshaw TS, Simon MA: Elastofibroma. J Bone Joint Surg
55A:409, 1973.

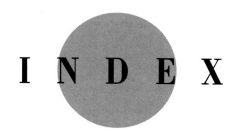

INDEX